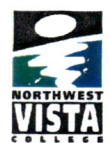

Northwest Vista College
Learning Resource Center
3535 North Ellison Drive
San Antonio, Texas 78251

D1767596

RC
280
.O8

NORTHWEST VISTA COLLEGE

Ovarian cancer.

34009001109330

Ovarian Cancer
Second Edition

Ovarian Cancer
Second Edition

Editors

Stephen C. Rubin, M.D.
Professor and Chief
Division of Gynecologic Oncology
University of Pennsylvania
Philadelphia, Pennsylvania

Gregory P. Sutton, M.D.
Department of Gynecologic Oncology
St. Vincent Hospitals and Health Services
Indianapolis, Indiana

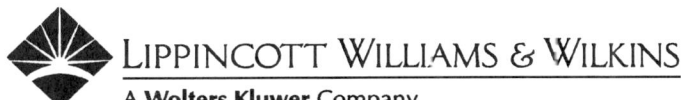

LIPPINCOTT WILLIAMS & WILKINS
A **Wolters Kluwer** Company
Philadelphia • Baltimore • New York • London
Buenos Aires • Hong Kong • Sydney • Tokyo

Acquisitions Editor: Jonathan Pine
Developmental Editors: Lisa Consoli and William Wiebalck
Production Editor: Rakesh Rampertab
Manufacturing Manager: Colin J. Warnock
Cover Designer: Christine Jenny
Compositor: TechBooks
Printer: Maple Press

© 2001 by LIPPINCOTT WILLIAMS & WILKINS
530 Walnut Street
Philadelphia, PA 19106 USA
LWW.com

All rights reserved. This book is protected by copyright. No part of this book may be reproduced in any form or by any means, including photocopying, or utilized by any information storage and retrieval system without written permission from the copyright owner, except for brief quotations embodied in critical articles and reviews. Materials appearing in this book prepared by individuals as part of their official duties as U.S. government employees are not covered by the above-mentioned copyright.

Printed in the USA

Library of Congress Cataloging-in-Publication Data
Ovarian cancer / [edited by] Stephen Rubin, Gregory Sutton.— 2nd ed.
   p. ; cm.
  Includes bibliographical references and index.
  ISBN 0-7817-2408-2
  1. Ovaries—Cancer.   I. Rubin, Stephen C.   II. Sutton, Gregory P.
  [DNLM: 1. Ovarian Neoplasms. WP 322 O963 2001]
  RC280.O8 O883   2001
  616.99′465—dc21   00-067781

Care has been taken to confirm the accuracy of the information presented and to describe generally accepted practices. However, the authors, editors, and publisher are not responsible for errors or omissions or for any consequences from application of the information in this book and make no warranty, expressed or implied, with respect to the currency, completeness, or accuracy of the contents of the publication. Application of this information in a particular situation remains the professional responsibility of the practitioner.

The authors, editors, and publisher have exerted every effort to ensure that drug selection and dosage set forth in this text are in accordance with current recommendations and practice at the time of publication. However, in view of ongoing research, changes in government regulations, and the constant flow of information relating to drug therapy and drug reactions, the reader is urged to check the package insert for each drug for any change in indications and dosage and for added warnings and precautions. This is particularly important when the recommended agent is a new or infrequently employed drug.

Some drugs and medical devices presented in this publication have Food and Drug Administration (FDA) clearance for limited use in restricted research settings. It is the responsibility of the health care provider to ascertain the FDA status of each drug or device planned for use in their clinical practice.

10 9 8 7 6 5 4 3 2 1

To our families

Contents

Contributing Authors ix
Preface to the Second Edition xiii
Preface to the First Edition xiv
Acknowledgments xv

Part I. Basic Science of Ovarian Cancer

1. Molecular Genetics of Hereditary Ovarian Cancer 3
   Jeff Boyd

2. Molecular Alterations in Sporadic Ovarian Cancer 23
   Laura J. Havrilesky and Andrew Berchuck

3. Chemotherapy Resistance in Ovarian Cancer 43
   Stephen J. Williams and Thomas C. Hamilton

4. Advances in Biotherapeutic Approaches to Ovarian Cancer 57
   George Coukos and Carl H. June

Part II. Histopathology of Ovarian Cancer

5. Pathology of Malignant Ovarian Epithelial Tumors and Miscellaneous
   and Rare Ovarian and Paraovarian Neoplasms 99
   James E. Wheeler

6. Pathology of Ovarian Germ Cell Tumors 135
   Helen Michael and Lawrence M. Roth

7. Sex Cord-Stromal and Steroid Cell Tumors 151
   Robert H. Young and Robert E. Scully

Part III. Clinical Aspects of Ovarian Cancer

8. Epidemiology, Etiology, and Screening of Ovarian Cancer 167
   Katherine Y. Look

9. Hereditary Ovarian Cancer: Clinical Syndromes and Management 181
   Jeanne M. Schilder, Dawn V. Holladay, and Holly H. Gallion

10. Primary Surgical Management of Early Epithelial Ovarian Carcinoma 201
    David H. Moore

11. Laparoscopy in the Management of Ovarian Cancer 219
    Tom P. Manolitsas, Parul Gupta, and Jeffrey M. Fowler

12. Primary Surgical Management of Advanced Epithelial Ovarian Cancer 241
    Dennis S. Chi and William J. Hoskins

13.	Primary Chemotherapy for Epithelial Ovarian Cancer *William P. McGuire*	259
14.	Second-Look Laparotomy *Thomas C. Randall and Stephen C. Rubin*	273
15.	Secondary Cytoreductive Operations *Thomas W. Burke and Mitchell Morris*	289
16.	Recent Developments in the Treatment of Recurrent Ovarian Carcinoma *James T. Thigpen and Vincent E. Herrin*	301
17.	Intraperitoneal Chemotherapy *Maurie Markman*	315
18.	Palliative Surgery for Epithelial Ovarian Cancer *Daniel L. Clarke-Pearson, Gustavo C. Rodriguez, and Matthew Boente*	329
19.	Radiotherapy in the Management of Epithelial Ovarian Cancer *Higinia R. Cardenes and Marcus E. Randall*	345
20.	Ovarian Germ Cell Tumors *Jean A. Hurteau and Steven J. Williams*	371
21.	Management of Ovarian Stromal Tumors *Peter E. Schwartz, Fredric V. Price, and Melanie K. Snyder*	383
22.	Ovarian Tumors of Low Malignant Potential *Gregory P. Sutton*	399
23.	Quality of Life Issues in Ovarian Cancer *George J. Olt and Joanna Cain*	419
Subject Index		431

Contributing Authors

Andrew Berchuck, M.D. *Professor, Division of Gynecologic Oncology, Duke University Medical Center, Durham, North Carolina*

Matthew Boente, M.D. *Chief Gynecologic Oncology, Department of Surgical Oncology, Fox Chase Cancer Center, Philadelphia, Pennsylvania*

Jeff Boyd, Ph.D. *Associate Attending Biologist, Departments of Surgery and Human Genetics, Memorial Sloan-Kettering Cancer Center, New York, New York*

Thomas W. Burke, M.D. *Professor, Department of Gynecologic Oncology, The University of Texas M.D. Anderson Cancer Center, Houston, Texas*

Joanna Cain, M.D. *Professor and Chair, Department of Obstetrics and Gynecology, The Milton S. Hershey Medical Center, Pennsylvania State University, Hershey, Pennsylvania*

Higinia R. Cardenes, M.D. *Clinical Assistant Professor, Department of Radiation Oncology, Indiana University School of Medicine, Indianapolis, Indiana*

Dennis S. Chi, M.D. *Gynecology Service, Department of Surgery, Memorial Sloan-Kettering Cancer Center, New York, New York*

Daniel L. Clarke-Pearson, M.D. *James M. Ingram Professor and Director of Gynecologic Oncology, Duke University Medical Center, Durham, North Carolina*

George Coukos, M.D., Ph.D. *Assistant Professor, Division of Gynecologic Oncology, Center for Research on Reproduction & Women's Health, Leonard and Madlyn Abramson Family Cancer Research Institute, Philadelphia, Pennsylvania*

Jeffrey M. Fowler, M.D. *Division of Gynecologic Oncology, Ohio State University, James Cancer Center, Columbus, Ohio*

Holly H. Gallion, M.D. *Professor, Department of Obstetrics and Gynecology, Division of Gynecologic Oncology, University of Kentucky, Lexington, Kentucky*

Parul Gupta, M.D. *Chief Resident, Department of Obstetrics and Gynecology, Ohio State University, Columbus, Ohio*

Laura J. Havrilesky, M.D. *Fellow, Gynecologic Oncology, Department of Obstetrics and Gynecology, Duke University Medical Center, Durham, North Carolina*

Thomas C. Hamilton, Ph.D. *Senior Member, Department of Medical Oncology, Fox Chase Cancer Center, Philadelphia, Pennsylvania*

Vincent E. Herrin, M.D. *Assistant Professor of Medicine, Department of Medicine, Uniformed Services University of the Health Sciences; Staff Physician, Department of Hematology and Oncology, National Naval Medical Center, Bethesda, Maryland*

Dawn V. Holladay, M.S. *Genetic Counselor, Department of Obstetrics and Gynecology, University of Kentucky Medical Center, Lexington, Kentucky*

William J. Hoskins, M.D. *Professor, Department of Obstetrics and Gynecology, Cornell University-Weill Medical College; Chief, Gynecology Service, Memorial Sloan-Kettering Cancer Center, New York, New York*

Jean A. Hurteau, M.D. *Assistant Professor, Section, Gynecologic Oncology, Indiana University School of Medicine; Attending Staff, Department of Obstetrics and Gynecology, Indiana University Medical Center, Indianapolis, Indiana*

Carl H. June, M.D. *Professor of Medicine, Director, Translational Research Leonard and Madlyn Abramson Family Cancer Research Institute, University of Pennsylvania Cancer Center, University of Pennsylvania, Philadelphia, Pennsylvania*

Katherine Y. Look, M.D. *Professor, Department of Obstetrics and Gynecology, Indiana University School of Medicine; Member, Department of Obstetrics and Gynecology, Indiana University Hospital, Indianapolis, Indiana*

Tom P. Manolitsas, M.D. *Department of Obstetrics and Gynecology, Division of Gynecologic Oncology, The Ohio State University College of Medicine, Columbus, Ohio*

Maurie Markman, M.D. *Director, The Cleveland Clinic Taussig Cancer Center, The Cleveland Clinic Foundation, Cleveland, Ohio*

William P. McGuire, M.D. *Professor, Department of Medicine, University of Mississippi, Jackson, Mississippi; Director, Cancer Center, Department of Oncology, Franklin Squar Hospital, Baltimore, Maryland*

Helen Michael, M.D. *Professor, Department of Pathology and Laboratory Medicine, Indiana University School of Medicine; Chief, Department of Pathology and Laboratory Medicine, Wishard Memorial Hospital, Indianapolis, Indiana*

David H. Moore, M.D. *Professor and Chief of Gynecologic Oncology, Department of Obstetrics and Gynecology, Indiana University School of Medicine, Indianapolis, Indiana*

Mitchell Morris, M.D. *Professor of Gynecologic Oncology, Department of Gynecologic Oncology, The University of Texas M. D. Anderson Cancer Center, Houston, Texas*

George J. Olt, M.D. *Associate Professor, Department of Obstetrics and Gynecology, Pennsylvania State College of Medicine, Hershey, Pennsylvania*

Fredric V. Price, M.D. *Attending Physician, Department of Obstetrics and Gynecology, Western Pennsylvania Hospital, Pittsburg, Pennsylvania*

Marcus E. Randall, M.D. *William A. Mitchell Professor and Chair, Department of Radiation Oncology, Indiana University School of Medicine, Indianapolis, Indiana*

Thomas C. Randall, M.D. *Assistant Professor, Department of Obstetrics and Gynecology, University of Pennsylvania; Associate Director, Division of Gynecologic Oncology, Pennsylvania Hospital, Indianapolis, Indiana*

Gustavo C. Rodriguez, M.D. *Associate Professor, Division of Gynecologic Oncology, Duke University Medical Center, Durham, North Carolina*

Lawrence M. Roth, M.D. *Professor, Department of Pathology, Indiana University School of Medicine; Director, Division of Surgical Pathology, Indiana University Hospital, Indianapolis, Indiana*

Stephen C. Rubin, M.D. *Professor and Chief, Division of Gynecologic Oncology, University of Pennsylvania, Philadelphia, Pennsylvania*

Jeanne M. Schilder, M.D. *Clinical Instructor, Department of Obstetrics and Gynecology, University of Kentucky Medical Center, Lexington, Kentucky*

Peter E. Schwartz, M.D. *Professor, Department of Obstetrics and Gynecology, Yale University School of Medicine; Chief, Gynecologic Oncology, Department of Obstetrics and Gynecology, Yale-New Haven Hospital, New Haven, Connecticut*

Robert E. Scully, M.D. *Pathologist, Massachusetts General Hospital, Emeritus Professor of Pathology, Harvard Medical School, New Haven, Connecticut*

Melanie K. Snyder, M.D., S.A.C.S *Department of Obstetrics and Gynecology, Yale University School of Medicine, New Haven, Connecticut*

Gregory P. Sutton, M.D. *Department of Gynecologic Oncology, St. Vincent Hospitals and Health Services, Indianapolis, Indiana*

James T. Thigpen, M.D. *Professor of Medicine, Department of Medicine, University of Mississippi Medical Center, Jackson, Mississippi*

James E. Wheeler, M.D. *Professor of Pathology and Laboratory Medicine, Department of Pathology and Laboratory Medicine, University of Pennsylvania Medical Center, Philadelphia, Pennsylvania*

Stephen J. Williams, Ph.D. *Postdoctoral Associate, Ovarian Cancer Program, Fox Chase Cancer Center, Philadelphia, Pennsylvania*

Robert H. Young, M.D. *Professor, Department of Pathology, Harvard University; Director of Surgical Pathology, Department of Pathology, Massachusetts General Hospital, Boston, Massachusetts*

Preface to the Second Edition

Since the first edition of this book was published, there have been dramatic advances in our understanding of the basic biology of ovarian cancer, and equally important advances in the clinical management of the disease. These exciting new developments in the field, including new chemotherapeutic and surgical approaches, make this an appropriate time to undertake this revision. Now more than ever, ovarian cancer is a disease that requires a true multidisciplinary approach, with the input of specialists in gynecologic oncology, medical oncology, pathology, radiation oncology, obstetrics and gynecology, general surgery, and others. The second edition of this book has once again brought together the nation's leading experts on all aspects of ovarian cancer, to produce a comprehensive yet readable and clinically relevant work on the subject.

The book retains its organization into sections on the basic science, histopathology, and clinical aspects of ovarian cancer. The basic science chapters have been extensively rewritten, and new chapters have been added on the molecular biology of ovarian cancer, including hereditary cancers, and experimental approaches to the disease. The section on histopathology has been updated to reflect new data in this area. The largest section of the book, that on the clinical aspects of ovarian cancer, has been thoroughly revised and updated to reflect the latest available information of the state-of-the-art management of the disease. New information has been added on screening and the management of early stage disease, and the sections on both primary and second-line chemotherapy have been comprehensively rewritten to reflect recent advances and newly developed chemotherapeutic agents. Equally important are the advances in our understanding of the surgical management of ovarian cancer, covered in chapters on primary surgery, secondary surgery, and palliative surgery. New information has been added as well on the management of germ cell and stromal tumors of the ovary, and the role of radiotherapy in the management of the disease. Also covered are new approaches to the management of ovarian cancers of low malignant potential, and quality of life issues.

This progress in the management of ovarian cancer have been so important that, according to recent data from the National Cancer Institute, there has been a significant improvement in the survival of women with this disease over the last decade. Based on the information detailed in this book by our distinguished panel of authors, many of whom have been at the forefront of these advances, we believe this trend will continue. It is our hope that the second edition of this book will serve as a valuable resource for all those who care for patients with ovarian cancer.

Preface to the First Edition

Ovarian cancer is the leading cause of death in women with gynecologic malignancies. Although it accounts for only about 27 percent of new gynecologic cancer cases each year in Western countries, this deadly disease kills more women than all other gynecologic malignancies combined. By this measure, ovarian cancer is surely the most important problem in gynecologic cancer today.

Ovarian cancer is a disease that exemplifies the importance of the multimodal approach to the treatment of cancer, requiring the input of gynecologic oncologists, medical oncologists, radiotherapists, pathologists, basic scientists, nurses, and social workers. In this text we have brought together in a single volume the nation's leading experts on ovarian cancer to produce an authoritative multi-disciplinary reference on the subject. The book begins with a section on the basic science of ovarian cancer, addressing the latest data in the areas of genetics, growth factors and oncogenes, chemotherapy resistance, and immunobiology. This is followed by separate chapters on the histopathology of the three main types of ovarian cancer: epithelial, germ cell, and sex cord-stromal tumors. The third and largest section of the book addresses in detail the clinical aspects of ovarian cancer, opening with chapters on epidemiology and familial ovarian cancer, followed by chapters covering all aspects of the surgical, chemotherapeutic, and radiotherapeutic management of ovarian cancer, including the latest in investigational approaches, and closing with chapters on quality-of-life issues and new surgical approaches.

Our contributors, to whom we are grateful, have adhered to a tight production schedule to allow timely publication of the most current material. We hope that this book will prove to be a valuable reference for all who treat ovarian cancer patients and that it will be of use in our common quest for improving the care of women with this disease.

Acknowledgments

Many people have played important roles in the preparation of the second edition of this book. The editors would like to acknowledge in particular the contributions of J. Stuart Freeman, Jr., William Wiebalck, and Rakesh Rampertab of Lippincott Williams & Wilkins. We also wish to acknowledge the tireless efforts and organizational skills of Carmen Lord, our editorial assistant at the University of Pennsylvania.

PART I

Basic Science of Ovarian Cancer

1
Molecular Genetics of Hereditary Ovarian Cancer

Jeff Boyd

INTRODUCTION

Discoveries over the past 20 years have brought us to a new frontier in cancer research, founded on the identification and understanding of basic cellular processes that become disrupted during cancer development. Historically, many empiric models have received temporary favor in efforts to address the problem of cancer etiology, including those founded on the actions of somatic chromosomal abnormalities, viruses, environmental agents, chemical carcinogens, and congenital predispositions. We now know that all of these models are in fact correct by virtue of their convergence into the genetic paradigm: cancer is the result of an accumulation of mutations in genes that determine the tumor phenotype (1). These mutations give growth and survival advantages to the cells of a tumor, all of which are derived from a single common cell that was transformed through an accumulation of genetic mutations.

Among the most robust of all biologic paradigms is that of the genetic basis of human cancer development. The genetic foundation of carcinogenesis was implied by some of the earliest practitioners of cancer cell biology and cytogenetics. In the mid-nineteenth century, Rudolph Virchow recognized that metastatic cancer cells resemble those of the primary tumor and that all cells of a tumor might arise from a single progenitor cell. Therefore, the neoplastic phenotype is heritable from one tumor cell generation to the next, prompting his aphorism, *onmis cellulae cellula*. In the early 1900s, Theodor Boveri extended this concept to the cytogenetic level, suggesting that gains and losses of specific chromosomes from abnormal segregation might lead to abnormal cell division and other aspects of the cancer phenotype (2). In 1960, Nowell and Hungerford provided strong support for Boveri's hypothesis with the discovery of the Philadelphia chromosome in association with chronic myeloid leukemia (3).

It was not until 1978 that the first vertebrate oncogene was identified, and in the two decades since Bishop and Varmus described the transforming *src* gene of Rous sarcoma virus (4), the genetic paradigm has been defined in sufficient detail to allow an unprecedented optimism regarding the understanding of cancer. The most direct and ultimately the most effective approach to preventing, detecting, diagnosing, and treating cancer is to identify the genes involved in tumorigenesis. Although the number of genes that may be mutated and contribute to the development of the various cancer types is large, perhaps in the hundreds, the problem is not intractable. Indeed, in the relatively short period since the previous edition of this text was published, the genes responsible for hereditary ovarian cancer have been localized, cloned, and characterized; genetic testing and counseling based on this knowledge have been implemented; and the clinical practice of gynecologic oncology has been altered as a result. The purpose of this chapter is to present an brief overview of fundamental aspects of cancer molecular genetics, followed by a detailed presentation of the current state of knowledge on the molecular genetic basis of hereditary ovarian cancer. The clinical implications of this information are discussed in Chapter 9.

PRINCIPLES OF CANCER MOLECULAR GENETICS

All cancers are genetic in origin, in the sense that the driving force of tumor development is genetic mutation. A given tumor may arise through the accumulation of mutations that are exclusively somatic (i.e., acquired) in origin, or through the inheritance of a mutation from one or the other parent through the germline, followed by the acquisition of additional somatic mutations. These two genetic scenarios distinguish what are colloquially referred to as "sporadic" and "hereditary" cancers, respectively (Figure 1.1). Although the neoplastic phenotype is also derived from epigenetic alterations in gene expression, it is the sequential mutation of cancer-related genes, with their subsequent selection and accumulation in a clonal population of cells, that determines whether a tumor develops and the time required for its development and progression. The data to support this multistep, multigenic paradigm of cancer development are extensive (5–8), but perhaps the most compelling evidence is that the age-specific incidence rate for most human epithelial tumors increases at roughly the fourth to eighth power of elapsed time, suggesting that a series of four to eight genetic alterations is rate limiting for cancer development (9).

Genetic alterations in cancer cells have thus far been described in two major families of genes, oncogenes (10) and tumor suppressor genes (11). Proteins encoded by oncogenes may generally be viewed as stimulatory and those encoded by tumor suppressor genes as inhibitory to the neoplastic phenotype; mutational activation of proto-oncogenes to oncogenes and mutational inactivation of tumor suppressor genes must both occur for cancer development to take place.

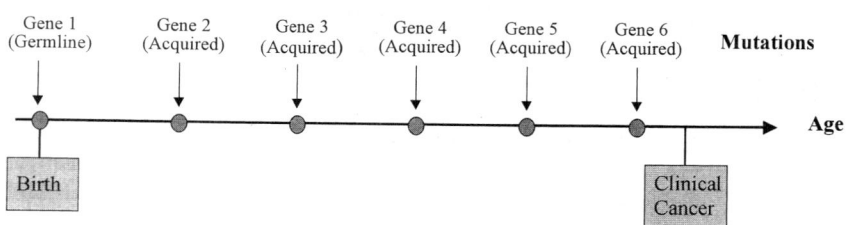

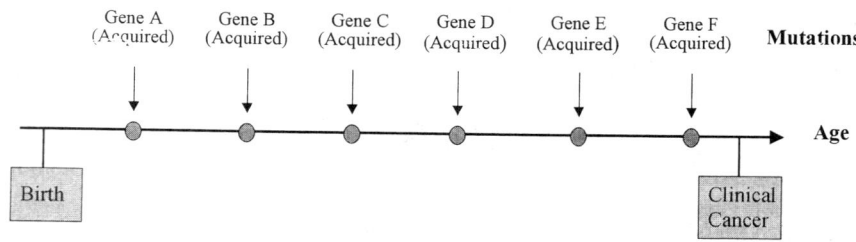

FIG. 1.1. All cancers are genetic. "Hereditary" cancers may be distinguished from "sporadic" cancers according to the mechanism through which the requisite mutations occur. The first rate-limiting genetic alteration is inherited through the germline in hereditary tumorigenesis, and the additional mutations are acquired somatically in the premalignant cell. In sporadic tumorigenesis, all mutations are acquired somatically. The average age at diagnosis for a hereditary cancer is typically younger than for the same cancer occurring sporadically.

Proto-oncogene mutations are almost always somatic; two known exceptions involve the *RET* and the *MET* proto-oncogenes, mutations of which may be inherited through the germline, predisposing to multiple endocrine neoplasia type 2 (12) and papillary renal carcinoma (13), respectively. Tumor suppressor gene mutations may be inherited or acquired somatically. Other than the noted exceptions, all hereditary cancer syndromes for which predisposing genes have been identified are linked to tumor suppressor genes. Genes encoding proteins involved in various DNA repair processes have been proposed to represent a third class of genes involved in cancer development (14). However, these genes share many of the features of tumor suppressor genes and are considered as such in this chapter.

Oncogenes

Oncogenes result from gain-of-function mutations in their normal cellular counterpart proto-oncogenes, the normal function of which is to drive cell proliferation in the appropriate contexts. Activated oncogenes behave in a dominant fashion at the cellular level; that is, cell proliferation or development of the neoplastic phenotype is stimulated after the mutation of only one allele. This class of genes was originally discovered through studies of the mechanism of retroviral tumorigenesis (15), which involves viral transduction of the vertebrate proto-oncogene and reintegration into the host genome under the transcriptional control of viral promoters, so that expression is constitutive and therefore oncogenic. The most common mechanisms for mutational activation of human proto-oncogenes are gene amplification, which typically results in overexpression of an otherwise normal protein product; point mutation, which generally leads to constitutive activation of a mutant form of the protein product; and chromosomal translocation, which usually results in juxtaposition of the oncogene with the promoter region of a constitutively expressed gene, leading to overexpression of the oncogene-encoded protein. The last mechanism is most common in hematopoietic malignancies, whereas the first two are more common in solid cancers. Because oncogenes are not involved in genetic predisposition to ovarian cancer, a more detailed presentation of this topic may be found in Chapter 2.

Tumor Suppressor Genes

The protein products of tumor suppressor genes normally function to inhibit cell proliferation and are inactivated through loss-of-function mutations. Knudson's "two-hit" model established the paradigm for tumor suppressor gene recessivity at the cellular level, wherein both alleles must be inactivated to exert a phenotypic effect on tumorigenesis (16). This two-hit model is frequently misunderstood, especially in the context of hereditary cancers, having become synonymous with the notion that inactivation of both alleles of a single gene is necessary *and* sufficient for tumorigenesis. It is important to recognize that this theory estimates only the number of events that are rate limiting for cancer development (17). As implied by Figure 1.1, all human cancers are likely to require mutations in multiple genes, many of which occur at a relatively high frequency compared with the rate-limiting genetic alterations and therefore do not appear in a kinetic analysis such as that performed by Knudson.

The most common mutations observed in tumor suppressor genes are point mutations (either missense or nonsense), microdeletions or insertions of one or several nucleotides causing frameshifts, large deletions, and, rarely, translocations. A mutation in one allele, whether germline or somatic, is revealed after somatic inactivation of the homologous wild-type allele. In theory, the same spectrum of mutational events could contribute to inactivation of the second allele, but what is typically observed in tumors is homozygosity or hemizygosity for the first mutation, indicating "loss" of the wild-type allele. As originally demonstrated for the retinoblastoma susceptibility gene (18), loss of the second allele may occur through mitotic nondisjunction or recombination mechanisms, or through large deletions (Figure 1.2). This so-called loss of heterozygosity (LOH) has become recognized as the hallmark of tumor suppressor gene inactivation at particular genomic loci.

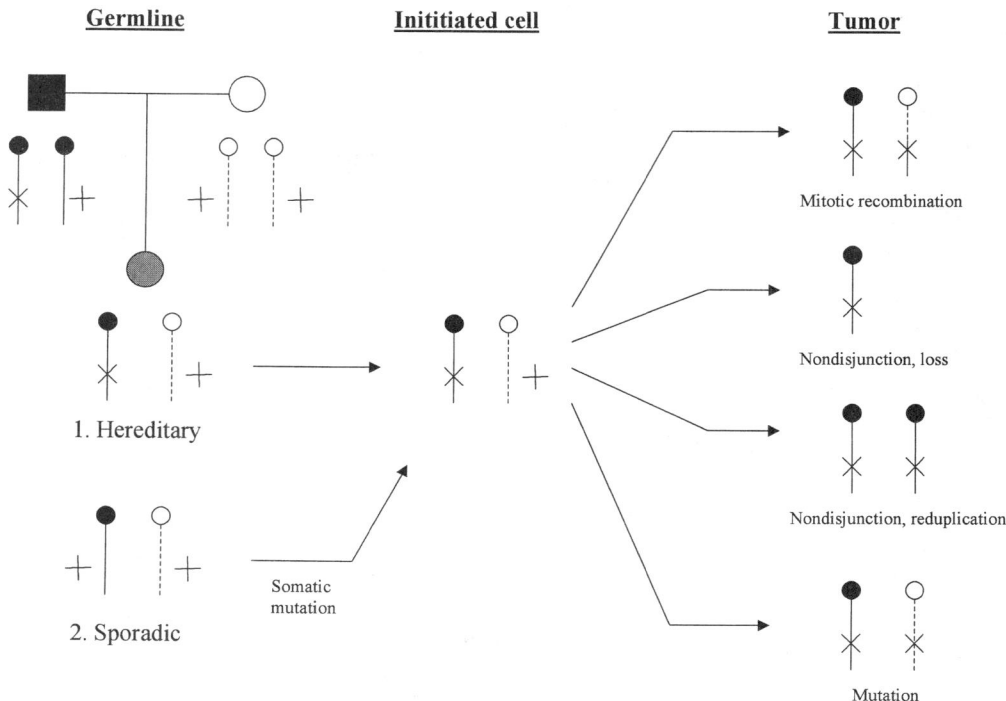

FIG. 1.2. Chromosomal mechanisms for "loss of heterozygosity" affecting a tumor suppressor gene. A cell may be initiated or predisposed to tumorigenic progression by the inheritance of a mutant allele through the germline (in which case the initiated cell is potentially any somatic cell) or by a somatic mutation in one cell (e.g., an ovarian epithelial cell). Inactivation of the remaining wild-type allele may occur through several possible mechanisms, such as mitotic recombination resulting in homozygosity for the mutant allele, chromosomal nondisjunction and loss of the wild-type chromosome (resulting in hemizygosity for the mutant allele), reduplication of the mutant chromosome (resulting in homozygosity for the mutant allele), or an additional somatic mutation affecting the wild-type allele. The result is functionally the same in all cases, in that the wild-type tumor suppressor allele is lost or inactivated and the premalignant cell is homozygous or hemizygous for a mutant tumor suppressor allele.

Several tumor suppressor genes involved in hereditary predisposition to cancer have been shown to function in the recognition and/or repair of various forms of DNA damage. The mutational inactivation of DNA repair genes contributes to tumorigenesis indirectly by promoting one or another type of genetic instability which then leads to the mutation of additional cancer-related genes. This relatively unique mechanism of tumor suppression has led some to suggest that the DNA repair genes should represent a third cancer gene family. In all cases described to date, however, the genetic mechanism appears to be a cellular recessive mechanism involving loss of function, consistent with the tumor suppressor categorization. Perhaps more appropriate is the classification scheme proposed by Kinzler and Vogelstein, in which tumor suppressor genes are subdivided into "gatekeepers" and "caretakers" (14). The former category includes those genes that function directly to inhibit cell proliferation or promote cell death (e.g., *RB, TP53, APC*), while the latter category consists of those genes that function to maintain genomic integrity, such as the mismatch repair (MMR) genes involved in hereditary nonpolyposis colorectal cancer (HNPCC), the nucleotide excision repair genes involved in xeroderma pigmentosum, *ATM,* and possibly the *BRCA1/2* genes. It should be noted that some of these genes do not readily adhere to this distinction; *BRCA1* and *BRCA2,* for example, may function as both.

Molecular Tumorigenesis

A human cancer represents the endpoint of a long and complex process involving multiple changes in genotype and phenotype. Human solid tumors are monoclonal in nature; every cell in a given malignancy may be shown to have arisen from a single progenitor cell. As proposed by Nowell (19), the process through which a cell and its offspring sustain and accumulate multiple mutations, with the stepwise selection of variant sublines, is known as clonal evolution or clonal expansion (Figure 1.3). A long-term goal in the study of the molecular genetics of a particular tumor type is to catalogue the specific genes that are affected by mutations and the relative order in which they are affected and, ultimately, to use this molecular blueprint to improve methods of diagnosis, prognostication, and treatment. This task will undoubtedly prove difficult, however, because a defining characteristic of cancer is genetic instability (20). There are multiple types of such instability, operative at both the chromosomal and molecular levels (21). The ability to differentiate the genetic mutations that are simply byproducts of genetic instability from those that are critical to the neoplastic phenotype or, indeed, responsible for increased genetic instability of one form or another is among the most formidable challenges to be faced in cancer research.

The greatest progress in this context has clearly been achieved for colorectal cancer, and a model has been proposed that applies molecular detail for this particular cancer type to the general paradigm of multistep tumorigenesis and clonal evolution. In addition to the demonstration that most colon cancer cell lines are affected by one

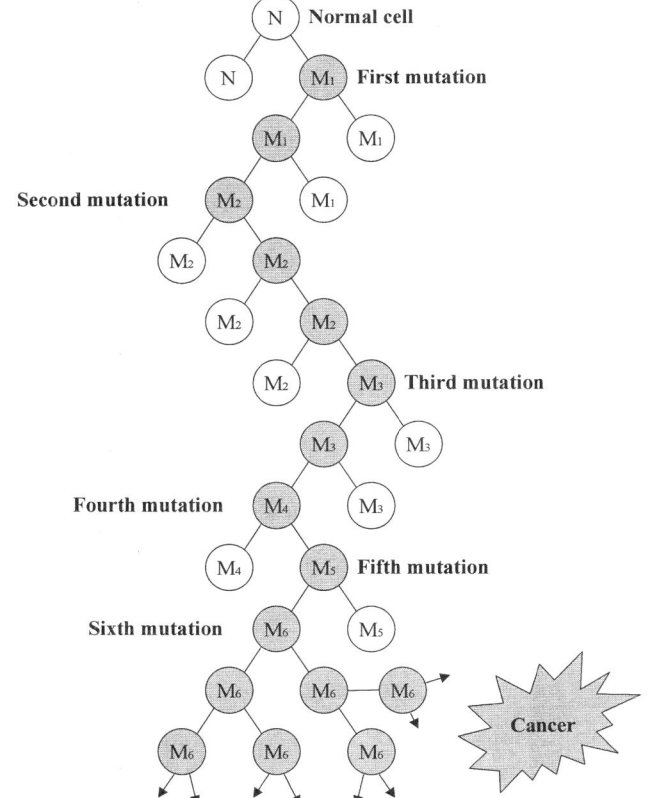

FIG. 1.3. Clonal evolution in neoplasia. A single normal cell is initiated as a result of the first mutation. Additional mutations affecting critical genes, combined with various selective pressures, lead to the development of a cancer consisting of a clonal population of cells that are all derived from the same progenitor cell. Each critical mutation in the developing tumor may be viewed as having provided an important selective advantage leading to subsequent clonal expansion.

of two types of genetic instability (22), specific molecular genetic alterations have been shown to occur at discrete stages of neoplastic progression in the colon—for example, mutation of the *APC* tumor suppressor gene at a very early stage of hyperproliferation, mutation of the *K-RAS* oncogene in the progression of early to intermediate adenoma, and mutation of the *TP53* tumor suppressor gene in the progression of late adenoma to carcinoma (23). Several features of colorectal cancer facilitate this type of characterization, including the well-defined histopathologic progression of normal colonic epithelium to cancer and the accessibility of the various premalignant lesions for molecular analyses, as well as the occurrence of some of these genetic mutations in unusually large fractions of all colorectal tumors. The model is limited in applicability to other cancer types, however, because nonmalignant precursor lesions for many solid tumor types (e.g., ovarian cancer) are not readily detectable, and few molecular genetic changes have been described that occur in major fractions of other cancer types.

HEREDITARY MANIFESTATIONS OF OVARIAN CANCER

A family history of ovarian cancer confers the greatest risk of all known factors, other than age, for development of the disease (24). Consistent with this observation are epidemiology-based estimates that about 10% of all epithelial ovarian carcinoma cases result from hereditary predisposition (25), with the germline inheritance of a mutant gene conferring autosomal dominant susceptibility with variable penetrance. Extraordinary progress has been made in identifying the molecular basis for essentially all of these manifestations of ovarian carcinoma, allowing hereditary ovarian cancer incidence to be estimated directly. These estimates are somewhat higher than those based on genetic epidemiologic studies of familial clustering of ovarian cancer, because molecular analyses of unselected ovarian cancer cases allow for the detection of apparently low-penetrance hereditary cancer cases not associated with family histories of cancer. There are likely to exist other genetic variants that confer ovarian cancer predisposition with low penetrance or in combination with other cancer susceptibility loci, but little is currently known regarding these types of genes. Therefore, it is likely that an even larger fraction of ovarian cancers will eventually be regarded as hereditary in origin, but for the purposes of this discussion the term "hereditary cancer" will refer to that associated with a Mendelian dominant allele acting with relatively high penetrance.

Epidemiologic studies and detailed analyses of familial ovarian cancer pedigrees have consistently confirmed the existence of two distinct manifestations of hereditary ovarian cancer: (a) the breast and ovarian cancer syndrome, in which both cancers are seen in excess and in some cases manifest in the same individual; and (b) ovarian cancers associated with an excess of colorectal and endometrial cancers that define HNPCC syndrome (Figure 1.4). It has been hypothesized that a site-specific form of ovarian cancer may represent a third distinct manifestation of hereditary disease, based on the description of families that contain multiple cases of ovarian cancer and no apparent excess of breast cancer. However, genetic linkage analyses have failed to demonstrate linkage of these families to any locus other than the breast and ovarian cancer susceptibility gene *BRCA1* on chromosome 17q12-21(26), suggesting that these kindreds are likely to represent a variant manifestation of the breast and ovarian cancer syndrome in which early-onset breast cancer is rare or has not yet appeared. Finally, the occurrence of invasive epithelial ovarian cancer in very young women (less than 30 years of age) has been well documented, but a recent study of a large series of these cases suggests that this phenomenon is unlikely to result from genetic predisposition (27).

Breast and Ovarian Cancer Syndrome

The breast and ovarian cancer syndrome accounts for 90% to 95% of all familial ovarian cancer cases (28). The probable genetic relationship of these two malignancies in a hereditary context has been demonstrated in population-based, case-control epidemiologic studies (29–31). Although there is no standardized clinical definition

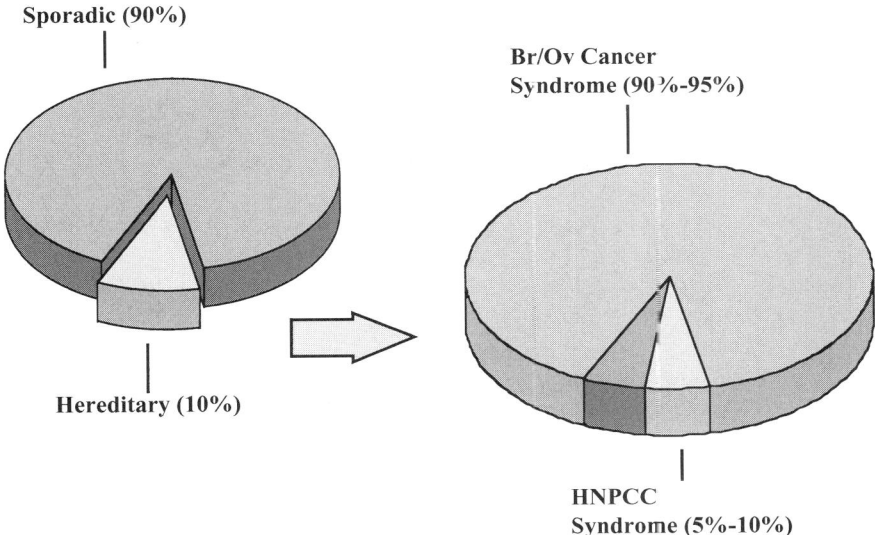

FIG. 1.4. Ovarian cancer attributable to genetic predisposition. Approximately 10% of all epithelial ovarian carcinomas are associated with autosomal dominant genetic predisposition. Of these, the great majority occur within the breast and ovarian cancer syndrome and a small fraction, 5% to 10%, occur within the hereditary nonpolyposis colorectal cancer syndrome.

of this syndrome (as there is for HNPCC), families with a total of five or more breast or ovarian cancers in first- or second-degree relatives have been suggested to qualify as having the breast and ovarian cancer syndrome (32); alternatively, families that contain at least three cases of early-onset (before 60 years of age) breast or ovarian cancer have been similarly classified (33). After the original report of genetic linkage of early-onset breast cancer families to the *BRCA1* locus (34), some breast and ovarian cancer families were shown to demonstrate linkage to *BRCA1* as well (35). This finding has been extended such that it is now clear that most (76% to 92%) breast and ovarian cancer families are linked to *BRCA1* (28,32). The variable estimates of linkage are probably the result of genetic heterogeneity. Lower estimates are obtained if all families, including those with cases of male breast cancer, are considered, whereas higher estimates are obtained if families with cases of male breast cancer or fewer than two cases of ovarian cancer are excluded (28). Most of the breast and ovarian cancer families not linked to *BRCA1* are linked to the *BRCA2* gene on chromosome 13q12-13, especially those with cases of male breast cancer (28,36). A more detailed discussion of these genes is provided later in this chapter.

The penetrance of *BRCA* genes for cancer—that is, the probability of developing cancer after inheriting a mutant *BRCA* allele—is relatively high but incomplete (i.e., less than 100%). Estimates of the lifetime probability of developing ovarian cancer in association with a *BRCA* mutation range from 16% to 63% (36–39), and the penetrance for ovarian cancer appears to be lower in *BRCA2*-linked than in *BRCA1*-linked families (36). An important research priority is to determine what additional factors influence the development of ovarian cancer, breast cancer, or both in *BRCA* heterozygotes. Variable penetrance is widely presumed to reflect the effects of various hormonal, environmental, and/or genetic modifiers, but few such modifying factors have been identified to date. The use of oral contraceptives has been shown to substantially reduce the risk of ovarian cancer in women with *BRCA* mutations (40), and increasing parity has been suggested to increase ovarian cancer risk in *BRCA1* carriers (41). The only genetic modifier of *BRCA* penetrance yet demonstrated is the *HRAS1* locus, rare alleles of which are associated with an increased risk of ovarian cancer in *BRCA1* carriers (42).

Hereditary Nonpolyposis Colorectal Cancer Syndrome

Epithelial ovarian carcinoma is also recognized as a component of the HNPCC syndrome. Also described as the cancer family syndrome or as Lynch syndrome I or II (depending on the absence or presence of extracolonic malignancies, respectively), HNPCC is an autosomal dominant genetic syndrome that accounts for approximately 5% of all colorectal cancers (43). Clinically, the syndrome is characterized by early-onset (average age at diagnosis, 45 years) colorectal cancer with a predominance of proximal or right-sided tumor localization, a high risk of metachronous colorectal cancers, and an increased risk of extracolonic malignancy, especially of the endometrium (44). The so-called Amsterdam criteria have been developed to represent a formal clinical definition of the syndrome (45); the criteria include (a) three or more relatives with colorectal cancer, one of whom is a first-degree relative of the other two; (b) affected family members in at least two generations; (c) at least one case diagnosed before the age of 50 years; and, (d) the exclusion of familial adenomatous polyposis.

In addition to cancers of the colon and endometrium, HNPCC family members are at a substantially increased risk for cancers of other gastrointestinal sites, the upper urologic tract, and the ovary (46). This syndrome is believed to account for essentially all cases of hereditary endometrial carcinoma and 5% to 10% of cases of hereditary ovarian carcinoma. The estimated lifetime risk for endometrial cancer in female HNPCC gene carriers is 40% to 60%, corresponding to a relative risk of 13 to 20, and that of ovarian cancer is 6% to 20%, corresponding to a relative risk of 4 to 8 (46–50). The wide variation in tissue-specific penetrance observed among different HNPCC families is likely to result at least partially from the genetic heterogeneity characterizing this syndrome. The recent cloning and characterization of the genes responsible for HNPCC (discussed later) have provided significant insights into the etiology of HNPCC-associated tumors and the potential for genetic screening for this disorder, although few significant insights into the factors controlling penetrance and tissue specificity of various mutations have yet emerged.

MOLECULAR GENETIC DETERMINANTS OF HEREDITARY OVARIAN CANCER

The molecular bases for both manifestations of hereditary ovarian cancer have been almost completely elucidated (Table 1.1). The structure and function of *BRCA1* and *BRCA2,* responsible for the breast and ovarian cancer syndrome, and of the MMR genes responsible for HNPCC have been determined, and the mechanisms through which inactivation of these genes leads to tumorigenesis have been illuminated in impressive detail. Because most hereditary ovarian cancers are attributable to *BRCA1* or *BRCA2,* these genes are discussed most thoroughly here.

TABLE 1.1. *Molecular genetic determinants of hereditary ovarian cancer*

Syndrome	Gene	Chromosome	Fraction[a](%)
Breast and ovarian cancer	BRCA1	17q21	75–90
	BRCA2	13q12	10–25
	Unknown	?	<5
Hereditary nonpolyposis colorectal cancer	MSH2	2p22-p21	30–35
	MLH1	3p21	30–35
	MSH6	2p16-p15	5
	PMS2	7p22	<5
	PMS1	2q31-q33	<1
	Unknown	?	30

[a] Fraction of specific syndrome attributable to gene indicated.

BRCA1

As discussed earlier, genetic linkage analyses implicated a gene on chromosome 17q12-21, named *BRCA1*, as responsible for most cases of hereditary ovarian cancer occurring in the context of the breast and ovarian cancer syndrome. The discovery of a candidate *BRCA1* gene (51) was confirmed by several subsequent studies describing the segregation of inactivating mutations in this gene with disease phenotype in numerous breast and ovarian cancer families (52–54). Deleterious germline mutations of *BRCA1* confer a relatively high lifetime risk for development of ovarian cancer, consistent with the observation that most unselected cases of ovarian cancer found to be associated with germline *BRCA1* mutations occur in women with remarkable medical or family histories, such as an early age at diagnosis, a previous diagnosis of breast cancer, or relatives with breast or ovarian cancer (55–58). These studies of unselected series of ovarian cancers also indicate that germline mutations in *BRCA1* are associated with approximately 5% of all ovarian cancers.

The *BRCA1* gene consists of 22 coding exons distributed over approximately 100 kb of genomic DNA on chromosome 17q21 (51). The 7.8-kb mRNA transcript is expressed most abundantly in the testis and thymus, and at lower levels in the breast and ovary, and encodes a 1,863-residue protein (51). Mutations of *BRCA1* described to date are located throughout the gene with little evidence of clustering; about 80% of the mutations are loss-of-function nonsense or frameshift alterations (59), consistent with the classification of *BRCA1* as a tumor suppressor gene. Other studies have shown that allelic deletions (as detected by LOH) affecting the 17q21 region in *BRCA1*-linked breast or ovarian cancers invariably involve the wild-type chromosome, as would be expected if *BRCA1* were behaving as a typical tumor suppressor gene (60,61). Two specific founder mutations, 185delAG and 5382insC, are present in approximately 1.0% and 0.1%, respectively, of the Ashkenazi Jewish population (62,63). Relatively high frequencies of other specific *BRCA1* founder mutations have also been described in Dutch, Belgian, Scandinavian, and French Canadian breast and ovarian cancer families (64–67).

The data linking *BRCA1* to most hereditary ovarian cancers are now unequivocal. It was believed that this gene would be found to play a major role in sporadic ovarian carcinomas as well. This speculation centered on the observation that LOH, the genetic hallmark of tumor suppressor gene inactivation, is observed on chromosome 17q in up to 80% of sporadic ovarian carcinomas (68–73). However, analyses of several series of unselected ovarian carcinomas, most of which would be sporadic, suggest that somatic mutations of *BRCA1* are rare (55,56,58,74,75). This finding is supported by fine deletion mapping studies, which implicate one or perhaps two regions distal to *BRCA1* as harboring an additional tumor suppressor gene or genes (76–78). These data suggest that mutational inactivation of *BRCA1* is necessary at a relatively early stage of development in order to contribute to ovarian tumorigenesis. Under this hypothesis, somatic mutation of *BRCA1* in the adult ovarian epithelium seldom provides a significant selective advantage in a developing malignancy and therefore rarely leads to clonal selection and manifestation as a somatic mutation in the ovarian cancer.

BRCA2

Similar approaches were used to localize and clone the *BRCA2* cancer susceptibility gene. Genetic linkage analysis of high-risk breast cancer families that were not linked to *BRCA1* revealed a locus at chromosome 13q12-13 to which some of these families were linked (79). A candidate gene from this region of chromosome 13 was determined to represent *BRCA2* based on the presence of germline inactivating mutations that segregated with disease in linked families (80). Confirmation of this finding was provided by additional studies in which inactivating mutations were identified in breast cancer families, especially those with male breast cancer (81–83). In contrast to *BRCA1*, inherited mutations in *BRCA2* appear to confer a substantially lower risk of ovarian cancer compared with breast cancer, as inferred from tumor incidence rates in linked families (80,81,84) and from penetrance

TABLE 1.2. *Frequencies of BRCA founder mutations in the Ashkenazi Jewish population*

Mutation and reference (ref. no.)	Individuals with mutations/ individuals examined	Percentage
BRCA1 185delAG		
Struewing et al. (1995) (63)	8/858	0.9
Roa et al. (1996) (62)	68/6,216	1.1
BRCA1 5382insC		
Roa et al. (1996) (62)	8/6,232	0.1
BRCA2 6174delT		
Oddoux et al. (1996) (92)	12/1,255	0.9
Roa et al. (1996) (62)	94/6,170	1.5
Total		2.6

analysis studies, which suggest that the lifetime risk of ovarian cancer in *BRCA2* mutation carriers is in the range of 16% to 27% (36,39,85). Furthermore, an analysis of unselected ovarian cancer cases suggests that germline inactivating mutations of *BRCA2* may be found in patients with late-onset disease and no remarkable medical or family history in regard to breast or ovarian cancer (86–88). Taken together, these findings are consistent with the hypothesis that inherited mutations in *BRCA2* contribute to ovarian cancer with a lower penetrance than those in *BRCA1* and that the fraction of all ovarian cancers resulting from hereditary predisposition may be higher than previously suspected based on estimates derived from the study of cancer-prone families segregating highly penetrant alleles.

The *BRCA2* gene consists of 26 coding exons distributed over approximately 70 kb of genomic DNA, encoding a transcript of 11 to 12 kb (81). As with BRCA1, the BRCA2 mRNA is most highly expressed in testis and thymus, with lower levels in breast and ovary (81). In addition to tissue-specific expression profiles, *BRCA1* and *BRCA2* share a number of additional structural and functional similarities. Both are unusually large genes in terms of the number of exons and the size of the encoded message, both have a large exon 11 that contains approximately half of the entire coding region, both contain translation start sites in exon 2, and both are relatively A/T-rich. Mutations of *BRCA2* reported to date, like those for *BRCA1*, are dispersed throughout the gene with little evidence for hotspots or clustering (59). The great majority of mutations are frame shift in nature, with microdeletions being most common; microinsertions, nonsense mutations, and missense mutations occur rarely. LOH at the *BRCA2* locus in tumors from linked individuals invariably involves the wild-type allele, consistent with the classification of *BRCA2* as a tumor suppressor gene (89,90). Some mutations have been observed in multiple unrelated families, suggesting that a subset of *BRCA2* mutations may also occur relatively frequently. A single mutation in *BRCA2*, 6174delT, is found in approximately 1.4% of the Ashkenazi Jewish population (62,91,92); this mutation together with those in *BRCA1* are present in approximately 1 in 40 Ashkenazi Jewish individuals (Table 1.2). As might be expected, a relatively large fraction of all ovarian cancer cases in Ashkenazi Jews may be associated with a germline mutation in *BRCA1* or *BRCA2*; one study suggests that as many as 62% of ovarian cancers in this population are attributable to one of these three founder mutations (88). Relatively high frequencies of other specific *BRCA2* founder mutations have also been described in Scandinavian, Yemenite Jewish, and French Canadian breast and ovarian cancer families (66,67,93,94).

As with *BRCA1*, it was believed that somatic mutations of *BRCA2* might be involved in a significant fraction of sporadic ovarian cancers, based on the high frequency of allelic loss observed on chromosome 13q in these tumors (69,70,95). Analysis of a large sample of unselected ovarian cancers revealed that, although LOH including the *BRCA2* locus is seen in more than half of the tumors, somatic mutations of the gene are rare (86,87), but probably more common than for *BRCA1*. These studies further indicated that approximately 3% to 4% of all ovarian cancers are associated with germline mutations in *BRCA2*.

Function of BRCA Proteins

The precise functions of the BRCA proteins remain to be determined in detail. Published studies to date provide evidence supporting multiple discrete functions, primarily related to transcriptional activation and DNA repair, which is not improbable given the large size of both proteins (Figure 1.5) For BRCA1, multiple specific antibodies detect a 220-kDa protein in the nucleus of cultured cells and normal tissues

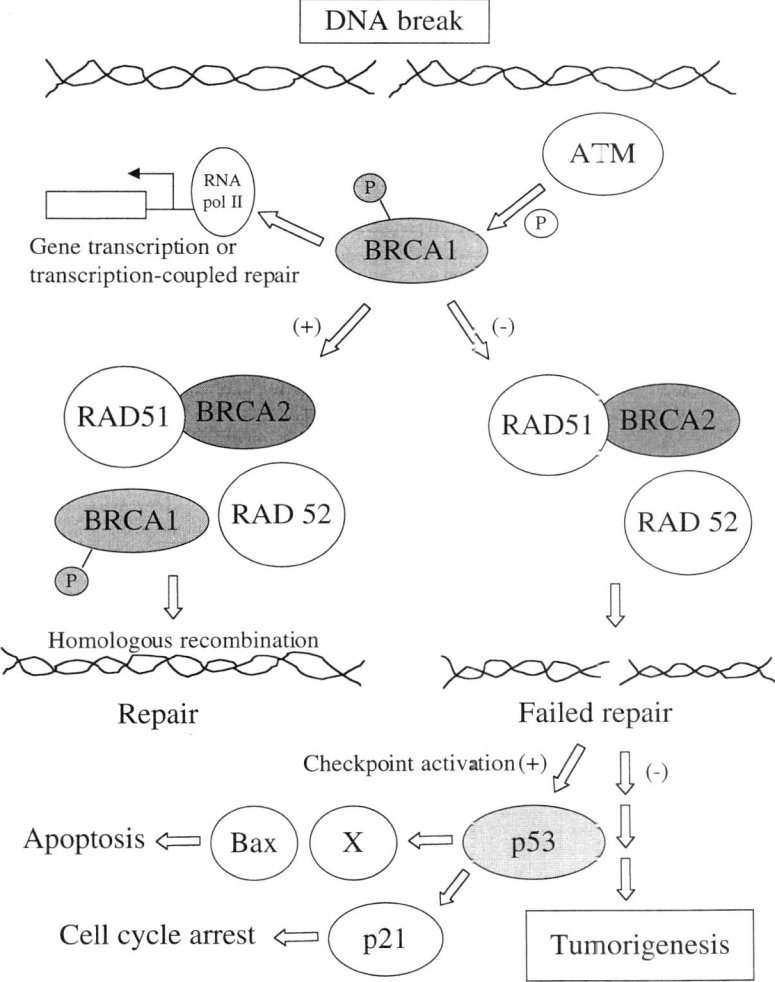

FIG. 1.5. Current model for the function of BRCA proteins. After DNA damage (e.g., a double-strand break), the ATM protein phosphorylates BRCA1. Phosphorylated BRCA1 may regulate gene transcription or transcription-coupled DNA repair. In cooperation with a BRCA2-RAD51 complex and with other RAD52-related proteins, phosphorylated BRCA1 mediates double-strand break repair through homologous recombination. In the absence of BRCA1 (or BRCA2) repair does not occur, leading to activation of the p53-mediated cell cycle checkpoint or checkpoints. The proliferation of cells containing damaged DNA is blocked either through the Bax-mediated induction of apoptosis or through the p21-mediated induction of cell cycle arrest. In the absence of functional p53, cells with DNA damage continue to proliferate, leading to tumorigenesis. Hereditary ovarian cancers associated with *BRCA* have sustained inactivating mutations in *BRCA1* or *BRCA2* and *P53*.

(96–99). Several domains of potential functional significance include an amino-terminal RING-finger domain, a negatively charged region in the carboxyl-terminus, and C-terminal sequences now known as BRCT domains that are partially homologous to yeast RAD9 and a cloned p53-binding protein (51,100). The presence of these motifs is consistent with the ability of BRCA1 to activate gene transcription *in vitro* (101,102). Evidence that BRCA1 is a component of the RNA polymerase II transcription complex (103) and that it interacts physically with RNA helicase (104) and the transcriptional activators p53 (105,106), CtIP (107), and C-MYC (108) further supports its possible function in transcriptional regulation. Therefore, mutational inactivation of *BRCA1* might be expected to affect the expression of other genes that are involved presumably in the regulation of growth or differentiation in breast and ovarian epithelium. The expression pattern of Brca1 during mouse development (109,110) and the cell cycle- (111,112) and hormone-regulated (113,114) expression of BRCA1 suggest a relationship with differentiation and cell proliferation. Finally, functional studies demonstrating the ability of BRCA1 expression to inhibit growth, suppress tumorigenesis, and induce apoptosis support the classification of BRCA1 as a tumor suppressor protein (115–117).

Evidence has also accumulated to suggest a role for BRCA1 in the cellular response to DNA damage. This function was originally inferred from data showing BRCA1 colocalization *in vivo* and physical association *in vitro* with the RAD51 protein, known to function in the repair of double-strand DNA breaks, which implied a role for BRCA1 in the control of recombination and genomic integrity (118). The ability of several distinct DNA-damaging agents to cause changes in the subnuclear localization and phosphorylation state of BRCA1 supports this hypothesis (119–121). Additionally, data derived from the study of embryonic tissues and cells from mice rendered nullizygous for *Brca1* provide strong evidence for the role of Brca1 in the response to DNA damage. An embryonic lethal phenotype is observed in mice with a homozygous null mutation in *Brca1*, suggesting its requirement for embryonic cellular proliferation before gastrulation (122). Partial rescue of this developmental lethality is achieved by simultaneous knockout of either the *p53* or the *p21* gene (123,124); one interpretation of these data is that the accumulation of DNA damage in *Brca1* knockouts leads to the arrest of cell division mediated by p53 and p21, and that their concomitant knockout allows additional cell division to take place before the eventual lethality. Finally, embryonic stem cells from *Brca1* nullizygous mice are defective in transcription-coupled repair of oxidative DNA damage and hypersensitive to ionizing radiation and hydrogen peroxide (125), and mouse embryo fibroblasts with a partial loss-of-function phenotype display chromosomal abnormalities associated with centrosome amplification (126,127). Most recently, the interaction of BRCA1 with other known pathways of DNA repair and apoptosis has been demonstrated. The ATM checkpoint kinase was shown to phosphorylate BRCA1 in response to DNA double-strand breaks (128), and the inducible expression of BRCA1 in human cells was found to result in the p53-independent induction of GADD45 expression and the JNK/SAPK-dependent activation of programmed cell death (129).

The BRCA2 gene product exhibits many functional similarities to BRCA1. BRCA2 is a 460-kDa nuclear phosphoprotein (130–132) that interacts physically with p53 and RAD51 (132). Expression of both genes appears to be coordinately regulated during cell cycle progression (130,133) and in response to estrogen (114) in human cells, and during proliferation and development in embryonic and adult mouse tissues (134–136). Preliminary findings suggest that BRCA2 may also function as a transcription factor, because a small portion of the protein shares homology with the known transcription factor c-Jun and is capable of activating transcription *in vitro* (137).

Substantial evidence also exists for the function of BRCA2 in DNA repair. Studies of the role of Brca2 in mouse development indicate that loss of the protein confers radiation hypersensitivity, consistent with its interaction with the Rad51 protein involved in repair of double-strand DNA breaks (138). Remarkably, BRCA1 and BRCA2 proteins may thus be involved in the same biochemical pathway, mediated by RAD51, regulating genomic integrity (118,138,139). Additional studies with the *Brca2* nullizygous mouse model provide further data implicating Brca2 in the response to DNA damage. The *Brca2* knockout mouse also displays an embryonic lethal phenotype, indicating a critical role for Brca2 in cellular proliferation during embryogenesis (124,138,140). This phenotype is partially rescued in *Brca2/p53* nullizygotes (124), again implying a role for Brca2 in the cellular response to DNA damage. In *Brca2* nullizygotes carrying mutations that allow survival to adulthood, the animals display inefficient DNA repair after X-irradiation and an increased susceptibility to tumors (141,142). Using embryonic fibroblasts from these mice, an increased sensitivity to mutagens and the accumulation of chromosomal abnormalities were also observed (143). Using the human pancreatic carcinoma cell line Capan-1, which is homozygous for the *BRCA2* 6174delT mutation, it was shown that BRCA2 mediates sensitivity to radiation and drugs that induce double-strand DNA breaks (131,144) and, furthermore, that the BRC repeat motif of BRCA2 mediates the physical interaction with RAD51 that is necessary for the normal response to DNA damage (131).

DNA Mismatch Repair Genes

The HNPCC syndrome arises from an inherited defect in any one of at least five known genes, *MSH2* (chromosome 2p), *MLH1* (chromosome 3p), *MSH6* (chromosome 2p), *PMS2* (chromosome 7p), and *PMS1* (chromosome 2q). Although mutations have been described in all five genes, the majority of HNPCC kindreds are linked to either *MSH2* or *MLH1*, and more than 90% of all reported mutations affect one of these two genes (145). Evidence suggests that mutations in the *MSH6* gene may be associated with a significant fraction of "HNPCC-like" kindreds not meeting the full Amsterdam criteria, as well as those with a preponderance of endometrial cancers in female carriers (146–148). As illustrated in Figure 1.6, the proteins encoded by these genes participate in the same pathway of DNA MMR, and loss-of-function mutations are associated with a specific form of genetic instability in the tumors of affected family members (149,150). These MMR genes function as classic tumor suppressors, because the wild-type allele inherited from the unaffected parent is lost or mutated somatically in HNPCC-linked tumors (151–153).

The genetic instability phenotype associated with defective MMR genes is most readily observed through somatic length alterations in simple repeat sequences, such as $(CA)_n$, that are located throughout the genome and known as "microsatellites." Replication errors in these repeat sequences are probably common, and their inefficient repair results in the "microsatellite instability" phenotype. Since the discovery of mutant MMR genes and the corresponding microsatellite instability, a large number of studies have documented microsatellite instability in many sporadic tumor types, including those not associated with the HNPCC syndrome (154,155). Although mutations of the MMR genes have been readily identified in many HNPCC kindreds, somatic MMR gene mutations in sporadic tumors with the microsatellite instability phenotype are not commonly detected (153,156). It appears likely that hypermethylation of the *MLH1* promoter, resulting in downregulation of its expression, is the causative mechanism in most sporadic colorectal, gastric, and endometrial carcinomas with microsatellite instability (156–158).

It is not clear how microsatellite instability *per se* contributes to tumorigenesis in the ovary, endometrium, or other organs affected by the HNPCC syndrome. Microsatellites exist throughout the genome in predominantly noncoding regions of DNA. Simple repeat sequences are known to occur in the coding regions of genes, however, and their somatic mutation may result in loss of function for genes critical to the regulation of proliferation, invasion, or metastasis. Examples include genes encoding the transforming growth factor-β receptor type II (159,160), the regulator of apoptosis BAX (161), the insulin-like growth factor II receptor (162), and caspase-5 (163), all of which contain homopolymeric microsatellite repeats that are mutated in

1. Insertion-deletion loops (in microsatellites)

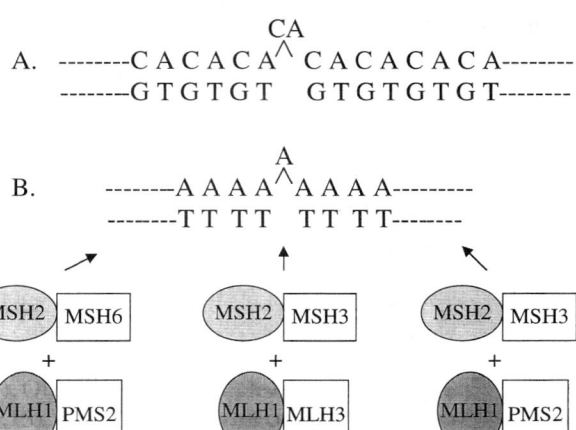

2. Single base mismatches

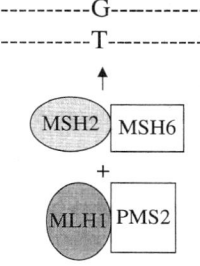

FIG. 1.6. The human mismatch repair system. Two types of DNA replication errors are recognized by the mismatch repair system: insertion-deletion loops in microsatellite repeats and single-base mismatches. The mismatch is recognized by a complex consisting of MSH2 and either MSH3 or MSH6. A second complex consisting of MLH1 and either PMS2 or MLH3 links the MSH2-bases recognition complex to accessory repair proteins. Both MSH2 and MLH1 are required for effective mismatch repair, whereas MSH3, MSH6, PMS2, and MLH3 are redundant.

one or another tumor type with microsatellite instability.

SUMMARY AND CONCLUSION

At least 10% of all cases of epithelial ovarian carcinoma are associated with autosomal dominant genetic predisposition. The large majority of these hereditary cases, approximately 90%, occur in the context of the breast and ovarian cancer syndrome, with 60% attributable to *BRCA1* and 30% to *BRCA2*. Another 5% of hereditary ovarian cancers are associated with the HNPCC syndrome, caused by mutation of one of several DNA MMR genes, and a small fraction may be attributed to one or more as yet undiscovered predisposition genes. The underlying molecular genetic bases for both of these hereditary ovarian cancer syndromes have been elucidated in detail, allowing for the implementation of genetic testing and preventive strategies in routine clinical practice (see Chapter 9). Additionally, elucidation of the function of proteins encoded by ovarian cancer susceptibility genes has substantially affected understanding of the molecular mechanism of ovarian tumorigenesis in the hereditary context. It is likely that this knowledge may be extrapolated to some degree to the process of sporadic ovarian tumorigenesis, ultimately leading to more effective methods for prevention, early detection, and treatment of the more common form of this disease.

REFERENCES

1. Bishop JM. Cancer: the rise of the genetic paradigm. *Genes Devel* 1995;9:1309–1315.
2. Boveri T. *Zur Frage der Entstehung maligner Tumoren.* Jena: Verlag von Gustav Fischer, 1914.

3. Nowell PC, Hungerford DA. A minute chromosome in human chronic granulocytic leukemia. *Science* 1960;132:1497–1499.
4. Spector D, Varmus HE, Bishop JM. Nucleotide sequences related to the transforming gene of avian sarcoma virus are present in DNA of uninfected vertebrates. *Proc Natl Acad Sci USA* 1978;75:4102–4106.
5. Weinberg RA. Oncogenes, antioncogenes, and the molecular basis of multistep carcinogenesis. *Cancer Res* 1989;49:3713–3721.
6. Boyd J, Barrett JC. Genetic and cellular basis of multistep carcinogenesis. *Pharmacol Ther* 1990;46:469–486.
7. Bishop JM. Molecular themes in oncogenesis. *Cell* 1991;64:235–248.
8. Vogelstein B, Kinzler KW. The multistep nature of cancer. *Trends Genet* 1993;9:138–141.
9. Renan MJ. How many mutations are required for tumorigenesis? Implications from human cancer data. *Mol Carcinog* 1993;7:139–146.
10. Hunter T. Cooperation between oncogenes. *Cell* 1991;64:249–270.
11. Weinberg RA. Tumor suppressor genes. *Science* 1991;254:1138–1146.
12. Hofstra RMW, Landsvater RM, Ceccherini I, et al. A mutation in the *RET* proto-oncogene associated with multiple endocrine neoplasia type 2B and sporadic medullary thyroid carcinoma. *Nature* 1994;367:375–378.
13. Schmidt L, Duh F-M, Chen F, et al. Germline and somatic mutations in the tyrosine kinase domain of the MET proto-oncogene in papillary renal carcinomas. *Nature Genet* 1997;16:68–73.
14. Kinzler KW, Vogelstein B. Gatekeepers and caretakers. *Nature* 1997;386:761–763.
15. Bishop JM. Cellular oncogenes and retroviruses. *Annu Rev Biochem* 1983;52:301–354.
16. Knudson AG. Hereditary cancer, oncogenes, and antioncogenes. *Cancer Res* 1985;45:1437–1443.
17. Haber DA, Housman DE. Rate limiting steps: the genetics of pediatric cancers. *Cell* 1991;64:5–8.
18. Cavenee WK, Dryja TP, Phillips RA, et al. Expression of recessive alleles by chromosomal mechanisms in retinoblastoma. *Nature* 1983;305:779–784.
19. Nowell P. The clonal evolution of tumor cell populations. *Science* 1976;194:23–28.
20. Loeb LA. Mutator phenotype may be required for multistage carcinogenesis. *Cancer Res* 1991;51:3075–3079.
21. Lengauer C, Kinzler KW, Vogelstein B. Genetic instabilities in human cancers. *Nature* 1998;396:643–649.
22. Lengauer C, Kinzler KW, Vogelstein B. Genetic instability in colorectal cancers. *Nature* 1997;386:623–627.
23. Fearon ER, Vogelstein B. A genetic model for colorectal tumorigenesis. *Cell* 1990;61:759–767.
24. Parazzini F, Franceschi S, La Vecchia C, Fasoli M. The epidemiology of ovarian cancer. *Gynecol Oncol* 1991;43:9–23.
25. Claus EB, Schildkraut JM, Thompson WD, Risch NJ. The genetic attributable risk of breast and ovarian cancer. *Cancer* 1996;77:2318–2324.
26. Steichen-Gersdorf E, Gallion HH, Ford D, et al. Familial site-specific ovarian cancer is linked to BRCA1 on 17q12-21. *Am J Hum Genet* 1994;55:870–875.
27. Stratton JF, Thompson D, Bobrow L, et al. The genetic epidemiology of early-onset epithelial ovarian cancer: a population-based study. *Am J Hum Genet* 1999;65:1725–1752.
28. Narod S, Ford D, Devilee P, et al. Genetic heterogeneity of breast-ovarian cancer revisited. *Am J Hum Genet* 1995;57:957–958.
29. Go RCP, King MC, Bailey-Wilson J, et al. Genetic epidemiology of breast cancer and associated cancers in high risk families: I. Segregation analysis. *J Natl Cancer Inst* 1983;71:455–461.
30. Lynch HT, Harris RE, Guirgis HA, et al. Familial association of breast/ovarian carcinoma. *Cancer* 1978;41:1543–1548.
31. Schildkraut JM, Risch N, Thompson WD. Evaluating genetic association among ovarian, breast, and endometrial cancer: evidence for a breast/ovarian cancer relationship. *Am J Hum Genet* 1989;45:521–529.
32. Easton DF, Bishop DT, Ford D, Crockford GP. Genetic linkage analysis in familial breast and ovarian cancer: results from 214 families. The Breast Cancer Linkage Consortium. *Am J Hum Genet* 1993;52:678–701.
33. Narod SA, Ford D, Devilee P, et al. An evaluation of genetic heterogeneity in 145 breast-ovarian cancer families. *Am J Hum Genet* 1995;56:254–264.
34. Hall JM, Lee MK, Newman B, et al. Linkage of early-onset familial breast cancer to chromosome 17q21. *Science* 1990;250:1684–1689.
35. Narod SA, Feunteun J, Lynch HT, et al. Familial breast-ovarian cancer locus on chromosome 17q12-q23. *Lancet* 1991;338:82–83.
36. Ford D, Easton DF, Stratton M, et al. Genetic heterogeneity and penetrance analysis of the BRCA1 and BRCA2 genes in breast cancer families. *Am J Hum Genet* 1998;62:676–689.
37. Ford D, Easton DF, Bishop DT, et al. Risks of cancer in BRCA1 mutation carriers. *Lancet* 1994;343:692–695.
38. Easton DF, Ford D, Bishop DT, Breast Cancer Linkage Consortium. Breast and ovarian cancer incidence in BRCA1-mutation carriers. *Am J Hum Genet* 1995;56:265–271.
39. Struewing JP, Hartge P, Wacholder S, et al. The risk of cancer associated with specific mutations of *BRCA1* and *BRCA2* among Ashkenazi Jews. *N Engl J Med* 1997;336:1401–1408.
40. Narod SA, Risch H, Moslehi R, et al. Oral contraceptives and the risk of hereditary ovarian cancer. *N Engl J Med* 1998;339:424–428.
41. Narod SA, Goldgar D, Cannon-Albright L, et al. Risk modifiers in carriers of BRCA1 mutations. *Int J Cancer* 1995;64:394–398.
42. Phelan CM, Rebbeck TR, Weber BL, et al. Ovarian cancer risk in *BRCA1* carriers is modified by the *HRAS1* variable number of tandem repeat (VNTR) locus. *Nat Genet* 1996;12:309–311.
43. Marra G, Boland CR. Hereditary nonpolyposis colorectal cancer: the syndrome, the genes, and historical perspectives. *J Natl Cancer Inst* 1995;87:1114–1125.
44. Lynch HT, Smyrk T. Hereditary nonpolyposis colorectal cancer: an updated review. *Cancer* 1996;78:1149–1167.
45. Vasen HFA, Mecklin J-P, Meera Khan P, Lynch HT. The international collaborative group on hereditary nonpolyposis colorectal cancer (ICG-HNPCC). *Dis Colon Rectum* 1991;34:424–425.
46. Watson P, Lynch HT. Extracolonic cancer in hereditary nonpolyposis colorectal cancer. *Cancer* 1993;71:677–685.

47. Watson P, Vasen HF, Mecklin JP, et al. The risk of endometrial cancer in hereditary nonpolyposis colorectal cancer. *Am J Med* 1994;96:516–520.
48. Aarnio M, Mecklin JP, Aaltonen LA, et al. Life-time risk of different cancers in the hereditary non-polyposis colorectal cancer (HNPCC) syndrome. *Int J Cancer* 1995;64:430–433.
49. Vasen HF, Wijnen JT, Menko FH, et al. Cancer risk in families with hereditary nonpolyposis colorectal cancer diagnosed by mutation analysis. *Gastroenterology* 1996;110:1020–1027.
50. Dunlop MG, Farrington SM, Carothers AD, et al. Cancer risk associated with germline DNA mismatch repair gene mutations. *Hum Mol Genet* 1997;6:105–110.
51. Miki Y, Swensen J, Shattuck-Edens D, et al. A strong candidate for the breast and ovarian cancer susceptibility gene BRCA1. *Science* 1994;266:66–71.
52. Castilla LH, Couch FJ, Erdos MR, et al. Mutations in the *BRCA1* gene in families with early-onset breast and ovarian cancer. *Nature Genet* 1994;8:387–391.
53. Simard J, Tonin P, Durocher F, et al. Common origins of *BRCA1* mutations in Canadian breast and ovarian cancer families. *Nature Genet* 1994;8:392–398.
54. Friedman LS, Ostermyer EA, Szabo CI, et al. Confirmation of *BRCA1* by analysis of germline mutations linked to breast and ovarian cancer in ten families. *Nature Genet* 1994;8:399–404.
55. Takahashi H, Behbakht K, McGovern PE, et al. Mutation analysis of the *BRCA1* gene in ovarian cancers. *Cancer Res* 1995;55:2998–3002.
56. Matsushima M, Kobayashi K, Emi M, et al. Mutation analysis of the *BRCA1* gene in 76 Japanese ovarian cancer patients: four germline mutations, but no evidence of somatic mutation. *Hum Mol Genet* 1995;4:1953–1956.
57. Stratton JF, Gayther SA, Russell P, et al. Contribution of *BRCA1* mutations to ovarian cancer. *N Engl J Med* 1997;336:1125–1130.
58. Berchuck A, Heron KA, Carney ME, et al. Frequency of germline and somatic BRCA1 mutations in ovarian cancer. *Clin Cancer Res* 1998;4:2433–2437.
59. Breast Cancer Information Core, 1999. Available at: http://www.nhgri.nih.gov/Intramural_research/Lab_transfer/Bic.
60. Smith SA, Easton DF, Evans DG, Ponder BA. Allele losses in the region 17q12-21 in familial breast and ovarian cancer involve the wild-type chromosome. *Nat Genet* 1992;2:128–131.
61. Merajver SD, Frank TS, Xu J, et al. Germline *BRCA1* mutations and loss of the wild-type allele in tumors from families with early-onset breast and ovarian cancer. *Clin Cancer Res* 1995;1:539–544.
62. Roa BB, Boyd AA, Volcik K, Richards CS. Ashkenazi Jewish population frequencies for common mutations in *BRCA1* and *BRCA2*. *Nat Genet* 1996;14:185–187.
63. Struewing JP, Abeliovich D, Peretz T, et al. The carrier frequency of the *BRCA1* 185delAG mutation is approximately 1% in Ashkenazi Jewish individuals. *Nat Genet* 1995;11:198–200.
64. Peelen T, van Vliet M, Petrij-Bosch A, et al. A high proportion of novel mutations in BRCA1 with strong founder effects among Dutch and Belgian hereditary breast and ovarian cancer families. *Am J Hum Genet* 1997;60:1041–1049.
65. Petrij-Bosch A, Peelen T, van Vliet M, et al. *BRCA1* genomic deletions are major founder mutations in Dutch breast cancer patients. *Nat Genet* 1997;17:341–345.
66. Huusko P, Paakkonen K, Launonen V, et al. Evidence of founder mutations in Finnish BRCA1 and BRCA2 families. *Am J Hum Genet* 1998;62:1544–1548.
67. Tonin PN, Mes-Masson AM, Futreal PA, et al. Founder *BRCA1* and *BRCA2* mutations in French Canadian breast and ovarian cancer families. *Am J Hum Genet* 1998;63:1341–1351.
68. Sato T, Saito H, Morita R, et al. Allelotype of human ovarian cancer. *Cancer Res* 1991;51:5118–5122.
69. Cliby W, Ritland S, Hartmann L, et al. Human epithelial ovarian cancer allelotype. *Cancer Res* 1993;53:2393–2398.
70. Yang-Feng TL, Han H, Chen KC, et al. Allelic loss in ovarian cancer. *Int J Cancer* 1993;54:546–551.
71. Russell SEH, Hickey GI, Lowry WS, Atkinson RJ. Allele loss from chromosome 17 in ovarian cancer. *Oncogene* 1990;5:1581–1583.
72. Foulkes W, Black D, Solomon E, Trowsdale J. Allele loss on chromosome 4q in sporadic ovarian cancer. *Lancet* 1991;338:444–445.
73. Osborne RJ, Leech V. Polymerase chain reaction allelotyping of human ovarian cancer. *Br J Cancer* 1994;69:429–438.
74. Futreal PA, Liu Q, Shattuck-Eidens D, et al. *BRCA1* mutations in primary breast and ovarian cancers. *Science* 1994;266:120–122.
75. Merajver SD, Pham TM, Caduff RF, et al. Somatic mutations in the *BRCA1* gene in sporadic ovarian tumours. *Nat Genet* 1995;9:439–443.
76. Jacobs IJ, Smith SA, Wiseman RW, et al. A deletion unit on chromosome 17q in epithelial ovarian tumors distal to the familial breast/ovarian cancer locus. *Cancer Res* 1993;53:1218–1221.
77. Godwin AK, Vanderveer L, Schultz DC, et al. A common region of deletion on chromosome 17q in both sporadic and familial epithelial ovarian tumors distal to BRCA1. *Am J Hum Genet* 1994;55:666–677.
78. Saito H, Inazawa J, Saito S, et al. Detailed deletion mapping of chromosome 17q in ovarian and breast cancers: 2-cM region on 17q21.3 often and commonly deleted in tumors. *Cancer Res* 1993;53:3382–3385.
79. Wooster R, Neuhausen SL, Mangion J, et al. Localization of a breast cancer susceptibility gene, *BRCA2*, to chromosome 13q12-13. *Science* 1994;265:2088–2090.
80. Wooster R, Bignell G, Lancaster J, et al. Identification of the breast cancer susceptibility gene BRCA2. *Nature* 1995;378:789–792.
81. Tavtigian SV, Simard J, Rommens J, et al. The complete *BRCA2* gene and mutations in chromosome 13q-linked kindreds. *Nat Genet* 1996;12:333–337.
82. Phelan CM, Lancaster JM, Tonin P, et al. Mutation analysis of the *BRCA2* gene in 49 site-specific breast cancer families. *Nat Genet* 1996;13:120–122.
83. Couch FJ, Farid LM, DeShano ML, et al. *BRCA2* germline mutations in male breast cancer cases and breast cancer families. *Nat Genet* 1996;13:123–125.
84. Thorlacius S, Olafsdottir G, Tryggvadottir L, et al. A single *BRCA2* mutation in male and female breast cancer families from Iceland with varied cancer phenotypes. *Nat Genet* 1996;13:117–119.
85. Easton DF, Steele L, Fields P, et al. Cancer risks in two large breast cancer families linked to BRCA2 on

86. Takahashi H, Chiu H-C, Bandera CA, et al. Mutations of the *BRCA2* gene in ovarian carcinomas. *Cancer Res* 1996;56:2738–2741.
87. Foster KA, Harrington P, Kerr J, et al. Somatic and germline mutations of the *BRCA2* gene in sporadic ovarian cancer. *Cancer Res* 1996;56:3622–3625.
88. Abeliovich D, Kaduri L, Lerer I, et al. The founder mutations 185delAG and 5382insC in BRCA1 and 6174delT in BRCA2 appear in 60% of ovarian cancer and 30% of early-onset breast cancer patients among Ashkenazi women. *Am J Hum Genet* 1997;60:505–514.
89. Collins N, McManus R, Wooster R, et al. Consistent loss of the wild-type allele in breast cancers from a family linked to the *BRCA2* gene on chromosome 13q12-13. *Oncogene* 1995;10:1673–1675.
90. Gudmundsson J, Johannesdottir G, Bergthorsson JT, et al. Different tumor types from BRCA2 mutation carriers show wild-type chromosome deletions on 13q12-q13. *Cancer Res* 1995;55:4830–4832.
91. Neuhausen S, Gilewski T, Norton L, et al. Recurrent *BRCA2* 6174delT mutations in Ashkenazi Jewish women affected by breast cancer. *Nat Genet* 1996;13:126–128.
92. Oddoux C, Struewing JP, Clayton CM, et al. The carrier frequency of the *BRCA2* 6174delT mutation among Ashkenazi Jewish individuals is approximately 1%. *Nat Genet* 1996;14:188–190.
93. Thorlacius S, Sigurdsson S, Bjarnadottir H, et al. Study of a single BRCA2 mutation with high carrier frequency in a small population. *Am J Hum Genet* 1997;60:1079–1084.
94. Lerer I, Wang T, Peretz T, et al. The 8765delAG mutation in BRCA2 is common among Jews of Yemenite extraction. *Am J Hum Genet* 1998;63:272–274.
95. Gallion HH, Powell DE, Morrow JK, et al. Molecular genetic changes in human epithelial ovarian malignancies. *Gynecol Oncol* 1992;47:137–142.
96. Scully R, Ganesan S, Brown M, et al. Location of BRCA1 in human breast and ovarian cancer cells. *Science* 1996;272:123–126.
97. Chen Y, Farmer AA, Chen CF, et al. BRCA1 is a 220-kDa nuclear phosphoprotein that is expressed and phosphorylated in a cell cycle-dependent manner. *Cancer Res* 1996;56:3168–3172.
98. Coene E, Van Oostveldt P, Willems K, et al. BRCA1 is localized in cytoplasmic tube-like invaginations in the nucleus. *Nat Genet* 1997;16:122–124.
99. Wilson CA, Ramos L, Villasenor MR, et al. Localization of human BRCA1 and its loss in high-grade, noninherited breast carcinomas. *Nat Genet* 1999;21:236–240.
100. Koonin EV, Altschul S, Bork P. BRCA1 protein products: functional motifs. *Nat Genet* 1996;13:266–268.
101. Chapman MS, Verma IM. Transcriptional activation by BRCA1. *Nature* 1996;382:678–679.
102. Monteiro ANA, August A, Hanafusa H. Evidence for a transcriptional activation function for BRCA1 C-terminal region. *Proc Natl Acad Sci USA* 1996;93:13595–13599.
103. Scully R, Anderson SF, Chao DM, et al. BRCA1 is a component of the RNA polymerase II holoenzyme. *Proc Natl Acad Sci USA* 1997;94:5605–5610.
104. Anderson S, Schlegel B, Nakajima T, et al. BRCA1 protein is linked to the RNA polymerase II holoenzyme complex via helicase A. *Nat Genet* 1998;19:1–3.
105. Ouchi T, Monteiro ANA, August A, et al. BRCA1 regulates p53-dependent gene expression. *Proc Natl Acad Sci USA* 1998;95:2302–2306.
106. Zhang H, Somasundaram K, Peng Y, et al. BRCA1 physically associates with p53 and stimulates its transcriptional activity. *Oncogene* 1998;16:1713–1721.
107. Yu X, Wu LC, Bowcock AM, et al. The C-terminal (BCRT) domains of BRCA1 interact in vivo with CtIP, a protein implicated in the CtBP pathway of transcriptional repression. *J Biol Chem* 1998;273:25388–25392.
108. Wang Q, Zhang H, Kajino K, Greene MI. BRCA1 binds c-myc and inhibits its transcriptional and transforming activity in cells. *Oncogene* 1998;17:1939–1948.
109. Marquis ST, Rajan JV, Wynshaw-Boris A, et al. The developmental pattern of *BRCA1* expression implies a role in differentiation of breast and other tissues. *Nat Genet* 1995;11:17–26.
110. Lane TF, Deng C, Elson A, et al. Expression of BRCA1 is associated with terminal differentiation of ectodermally and mesodermally-derived tissues in mice. *Genes Devel* 1995;9:2712–2722.
111. Vaughn JP, Davis PL, Jarboe MD, et al. BRCA1 expression is induced before DNA synthesis in both normal and tumor-derived breast cells. *Cell Growth Differ* 1995;7:711–715.
112. Gudas JM, Li T, Nguyen H, et al. Cell cycle regulation of BRCA1 messenger RNA in human breast epithelial cells. *Cell Growth Differ* 1996;7:717–723.
113. Gudas JM, Nguyen H, Li T, Cowan KH. Hormone-dependent regulation of BRCA1 in human breast cancer cells. *Cancer Res* 1995;55:4561–4565.
114. Spillman MA, Bowcock AM. BRCA1 and BRCA2 mRNA levels are coordinately elevated in human breast cancer cells in response to estrogen. *Oncogene* 1995;13:1639–1645.
115. Rao VN, Shao N, Ahmad M, Reddy ES. Antisense RNA to the putative tumor suppressor gene BRCA1 transforms mouse fibroblasts. *Oncogene* 1996;12:523–528.
116. Holt JT, Thompson ME, Szabo C, et al. Growth retardation and tumour inhibition by *BRCA1*. *Nat Genet* 1995;12:298–302.
117. Shao N, Chai YL, Shyam E, et al. Induction of apoptosis by the tumor suppressor protein BRCA1. *Oncogene* 1995;13:1–7.
118. Scully R, Chen J, Plug A, et al. Association of BRCA1 with Rad51 in mitotic and meiotic cells. *Cell* 1997;88:265–275.
119. Scully R, Chen J, Ochs RL, et al. Dynamic changes of BRCA1 subnuclear location and phosphorylation state are initiated by DNA damage. *Cell* 1997;90:425–435.
120. Ruffner H, Verma IM. BRCA1 is a cell cycle-regulated nuclear phosphoprotein. *Proc Natl Acad Sci USA* 1997;94:7138–7143.
121. Thomas JE, Smith M, Tonkinson JL, et al. Induction of phosphorylation of BRCA1 during the cell cycle and after DNA damage. *Cell Growth Differ* 1997;8:801–809.
122. Hakem R, de la Pompa JL, Sirard C, et al. The tumor suppressor gene *Brca1* is required for embryonic cellular proliferation in the mouse. *Cell* 1996;85:1009–1023.

123. Hakem R, de la Pompa JL, Elia A, et al. Partial rescue of Brca1$^{5-6}$ early embryonic lethality by p53 or p21 null mutation. *Nat Genet* 1997;16:298–302.
124. Ludwig T, Chapman DL, Papaioannou VE, Efstratiadis A. Targeted mutations of breast cancer susceptibility gene homologs in mice: lethal phenotypes of Brca1, Brca2, Brca1/Brca2, Brca1/p53, and Brca2/p53 nullizygous embryos. *Genes Devel* 1997;11:1226–1241.
125. Gowen LC, Avrutskaya AV, Latour AM, et al. BRCA1 required for transcription-coupled repair of oxidative DNA damage. *Science* 1998;281:1009–1012.
126. Hsu LC, White RL. BRCA1 is associated with the centrosome during mitosis. *Proc Natl Acad Sci USA* 1998;95:12983–12988.
127. Xu X, Weaver Z, Linke SP, et al. Centrosome amplification and a defective G-M cell cycle checkpoint induce genetic instability in BRCA1 exon 11 isoform-deficient cells. *Mol Cell* 1999;3:389–395.
128. Cortez D, Wang Y, Qin J, Elledge SJ. Requirement of ATM-dependent phosphorylation of Brca1 in the DNA damage response to double-strand breaks. *Science* 1999;286:1162–1166.
129. Harkin DP, Bean JM, Miklos D, et al. Induction of GADD45 and JNK/SAPK-dependent apoptosis following inducible expression of BRCA1. *Cell* 1999;97:575–586.
130. Bertwistle D, Swift S, Marston NJ, et al. Nuclear location and cell cycle regulation of the BRCA2 protein. *Cancer Res* 1997;57:5485–5488.
131. Chen PL, Chen CF, Chen Y, et al. The BRC repeats in BRCA2 are critical for RAD51 binding and resistance to methyl methanesulfonate treatment. *Proc Natl Acad Sci USA* 1998;95:5287–5292.
132. Marmorstein LY, Ouchi T, Aaronson SA. The BRCA2 gene product functionally interacts with p53 and RAD51. *Proc Natl Acad Sci USA* 1998;95:13869–13874.
133. Wang SC, Lin SH, Su LK, Hung MC. Changes in BRCA2 expression during progression of the cell cycle. *Biochem Biophys Res Commun* 1997;234:247–251.
134. Rajan JV, Wang M, Marquis ST, Chodosh LA. Brca2 is coordinately regulated with Brca1 during proliferation and differentiation in mammary epithelial cells. *Proc Natl Acad Sci USA* 1996;93:13078–13083.
135. Connor F, Smith A, Wooster R, et al. Cloning, chromosomal mapping and expression pattern of the mouse Brca2 gene. *Hum Mol Genet* 1997;6:291–300.
136. Rajan JV, Marquis ST, Gardner HP, Chodosh LA. Developmental expression of Brca2 colocalizes with Brca1 and is associated with proliferation and differentiation in multiple tissues. *Dev Biol* 1997;184:385–401.
137. Milner J, Ponder B, Hughes-Davies L, et al. Transcriptional activation functions in BRCA2. *Nature* 1997;386:772–773.
138. Sharan SK, Morimatsu M, Albrecht U, et al. Embryonic lethality and radiation hypersensitivity mediated by Rad51 in mice lacking Brca2. *Nature* 1997;386:804–810.
139. Chen J, Silver DP, Walpita D, et al. Stable interaction between the products of the BRCA1 and BRCA2 tumor suppressor genes in mitotic and meiotic cells. *Mol Cell* 1998;2:317–328.
140. Suzuki A, de la Pompa JL, Hakem R, et al. Brca2 is required for embryonic cellular proliferation in the mouse. *Genes Devel* 1997;11:1242–1252.
141. Connor F, Bertwistle D, Mee PJ, et al. Tumorigenesis and a DNA repair defect in mice with a truncating Brca2 mutation. *Nat Genet* 1997;17:423–430.
142. Friedman LS, Thistlethwaite FC, Patel KJ, et al. Thymic lymphomas in mice with a truncating mutation in Brca2. *Cancer Res* 1998;58:1338–1343.
143. Patel KJ, Yu VPCC, Lee H, et al. Involvement of Brca2 in DNA repair. *Mol Cell* 1998;1:347–357.
144. Abbott DW, Freeman ML, Holt JT. Double-strand break repair deficiency and radiation sensitivity in BRCA2 mutant cancer cells. *J Natl Cancer Inst* 1998;90:978–985.
145. Peltomaki P, Vasen HFA, International Collaborative Group on Hereditary Nonpolyposis Colorectal Cancer. Mutations predisposing to hereditary nonpolyposis colorectal cancer: database and results of a collaborative study. *Gastroenterology* 1997;113:1146–1158.
146. Kolodner RD, Tytell JD, Schmeits JL, et al. Germ-line msh6 mutations in colorectal cancer families. *Cancer Res* 1999;59:5068–5074.
147. Wijnen J, de leeuw W, Vasen H, et al. Familial endometrial cancer in female carriers of MSH6 germline mutations. *Nat Genet* 1999;23:142–144.
148. Wu Y, Berends JW, Mensink RGJ, et al. Association of hereditary nonpolyposis colorectal cancer-related tumors displaying low microsatellite instability with MSH6 germline mutations. *Am J Hum Genet* 1999;65:1291–1298.
149. Fishel R, Kolodner R. Identification of mismatch repair genes and their role in the development of cancer. *Curr Opin Genet Dev* 1995;5:382–395.
150. Kolodner RD. Mismatch repair: mechanisms and relationship to cancer susceptibility. *Trends Biochem Sci* 1995;20:397–401.
151. Leach FS, Nicolaides NC, Papadopoulos N, et al. Mutations of a mutS homolog in hereditary nonpolyposis colorectal cancer. *Cell* 1993;75:1215–1225.
152. Hemminki A, Peltomaki P, Mecklin JP, et al. Loss of the wild-type MLH1 gene is a feature of hereditary nonpolyposis colorectal cancer. *Nat Genet* 1994;8:405–410.
153. Liu B, Nicolaides NC, Markowitz S, et al. Mismatch repair gene defects in sporadic colorectal cancers with microsatellite instability. *Nat Genet* 1995;9:48–55.
154. Loeb LA. Microsatellite instability: marker of a mutator phenotype in cancer. *Cancer Res* 1994;54:5059–5063.
155. Modrich P. Mismatch repair, genetic stability, and cancer. *Science* 1994;266:1959–1960.
156. Gurin CC, Federici MG, Kang L, Boyd J. Causes and consequences of microsatellite instability in endometrial carcinoma. *Cancer Res* 1999;59:462–466.
157. Herman JG, Umar A, Polyak K, et al. Incidence and functional consequences of hMLH1 promoter hypermethylation in colorectal carcinoma. *Proc Natl Acad Sci USA* 1998;95:6870–6875.
158. Leung SY, Yuen ST, Chung LP, et al. hMLH1 promoter methylation and lack of hMLH1 expression in sporadic gastric carcinomas with high-frequency microsatellite instability. *Cancer Res* 1999;59:159–164.
159. Markowitz S, Wang J, Myeroff L, et al. Inactivation of the type II TGF-β receptor in colon cancer cells with microsatellite instability. *Science* 1995;268:1336–1338.
160. Parsons R, Myeroff L, Liu B, et al. Microsatellite instability and mutations of the transforming growth factor

β type II receptor gene in colorectal cancer. *Cancer Res* 1995;55:5548–5550.
161. Rampino N, Yamamoto H, Ionov Y, et al. Somatic frameshift mutations in the *BAX* gene in colon cancers of the microsatellite mutator phenotype. *Science* 1997;275:967–969.
162. Ouyang H, Shiwaku HO, Hagiwara H, et al. The *insulin-like growth factor II receptor* gene is mutated in genetically unstable cancers of the endometrium, stomach, and colorectum. *Cancer Res* 1997;57:1851–1854.
163. Scwartz S, Yamamoto H, Navarro M, et al. Frameshift mutations at mononucleotide repeats in *caspase-5* and other target genes in endometrial and gastrointestinal cancer of the microsatellite mutator phenotype. *Cancer Res* 1999;59:2995–3002.

2

Molecular Alterations in Sporadic Ovarian Cancer

Laura J. Havrilesky and Andrew Berchuck

INTRODUCTION

Malignant transformation of a normal ovarian epithelial cell is caused by genetic alterations that disrupt regulation of proliferation, programmed cell death, and senescence (Table 2.1). About 10% of epithelial ovarian cancers arise in women who have inherited mutations in cancer susceptibility genes such as *BRCA1* or *BRCA2*. The genetic aspects of hereditary ovarian cancers are discussed in Chapter 1. The vast majority of ovarian cancers arise as a result of the accumulation of genetic damage over the course of a lifetime and are referred to as sporadic cancers. Over the past 15 years, several of the alterations involved in the development of sporadic ovarian cancers have been identified, but much remains unknown regarding their molecular pathogenesis. The anticipated identification of all of the genes in the human genome will provide the framework for studies aimed at completing the understanding of this complex disease. This should facilitate the development of new approaches to early diagnosis, treatment, and prevention that will decrease ovarian cancer mortality.

Most ovarian cancers are characterized by a high degree of genetic damage that is manifested at both the chromosomal and molecular levels. Gains and losses of large portions of chromosomes as well as complex translocations initially were described by means of classic karyotype analysis. In one study of 23 ovarian cancers, the average number of chromosomal alterations was 7 (range, 2 to 14) (1). More recently, studies using a technique called comparative genomic hybridization (CGH) have confirmed that most ovarian cancers have gains or losses of large segments of chromosomes. In one study of 44 ovarian cancers, there were 13 areas of chromosomal gain and 5 areas of chromosomal loss that were seen in at least 20% of cases (2). The most common areas of chromosomal loss were 16q and 17pter-q21, and the most frequent areas of chromosomal gain were 3q25-26 and 8q24. In another study that included 20 sporadic ovarian cancers, the average number of alterations in each cancer was 7.5, and gains were more than twice as common as losses (3). In agreement with the previous study (2), losses on 17p and gains on 8q23-24 and 3q26 were confirmed in two other studies to be among the most frequent events in ovarian cancers (3,4).

It has been suggested that differences exist in the pattern of genetic alterations in serous, mucinous, and endometrioid ovarian cancers (5). In one CGH study, gains at 1q were observed frequently in endometrioid and serous tumors. Increased copy number at 10q was seen in endometrioid tumors only, whereas gains at 11q occurred mostly in serous tumors. In mucinous tumors, the most common copy number change was a gain at 17q. The findings of this small study, which included only 24 well or moderately differentiated cancers, cannot be considered definitive, but they add weight to the theory that there are differences in molecular pathogenesis among the various histologic types of ovarian cancers.

Although chromosomal gains are detected more often than losses by CGH, deletion of one allele at many genetic loci has been noted with the use of loss of heterozygosity (LOH) analysis (Figure 2.1). LOH has been demonstrated to occur at a high frequency on many chromosomal

TABLE 2.1. *Cellular processes that inhibit malignant transformation*

Tumor suppressor genes that restrain inappropriate proliferation
DNA repair genes that fix mutations
Apoptosis of genetically damaged cells
Finite replicative capacity of most adult cells due to lack of telomerase leading to senescence

arms, including 5q (6,7) 6q (8–11), 7p (6,12), 8p (13), 11p (14), 11q (15–18), 13q (6,19), 14q (20), 17p (21), 17q (22), 22q (23), and others (6,19,24). It is unclear whether the extent of these genetic alterations reflects the need to inactivate multiple tumor suppressor genes or is the result of generalized genomic instability. With the identification and characterization of thousands of genes through the efforts of the Human Genome Project, it is now possible to assess simultaneously the expression of large arrays of genes. This promises to speed the pace of genetic discoveries in ovarian cancer in the next decade.

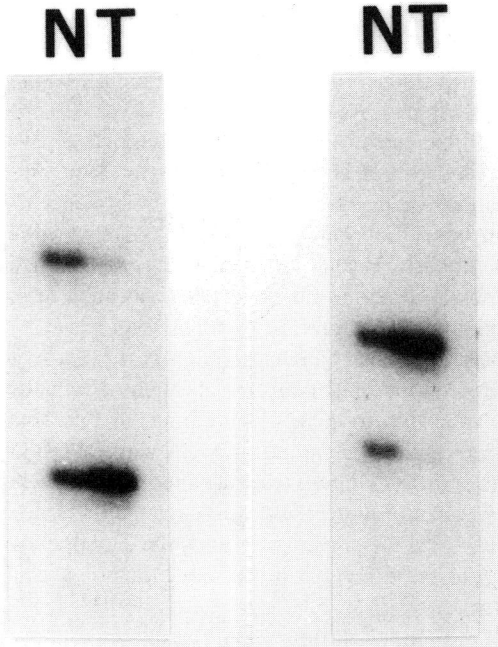

FIG. 2.1. Loss-of-heterozygosity analysis for the p53 gene in ovarian cancer. Tumor-normal pairs in which the upper allele has been lost in the patient on the left and the lower allele has been lost in the patient on the right are shown.

One consistent finding has been that poorly differentiated, advanced-stage cancers have more genetic alterations than early-stage, well-differentiated, or borderline cases (2,19). For example, in one CGH study, the average number of alterations was 5.4 in low-grade ovarian cancers and 11.2 in high-grade cases (2). This finding could be interpreted as reflecting the accumulation of genetic changes with evolution of a cancer. On the other hand, it is equally plausible that advanced-stage, poorly differentiated cancers are intrinsically more virulent, even early in their development, by virtue of their specific mutations or increased genomic instability, or both. If the latter theory is correct, it could have significant implications for early diagnosis of ovarian cancer. Cancers that are inherently more virulent might metastasize fairly rapidly and be less amenable to early detection.

Etiology of Genetic Alterations

In addition to identifying the specific genetic changes involved in ovarian carcinogenesis, an understanding of the etiology of this damage is essential—particularly for the development of effective prevention strategies. Like other sporadic cancers, most epithelial ovarian carcinomas are thought to develop as a result of the accumulation of a series of genetic alterations over a lifetime. The causes of the genetic damage that underlies the development of these cancers are not completely understood (Table 2.2), but epidemiologic and molecular studies have begun to shed some light on the etiology of ovarian cancer. There is evidence to suggest that sporadic ovarian cancer generally is a monoclonal disease that originates in the ovarian surface epithelium or underlying inclusion cysts (25). About 10% of

TABLE 2.2. *Theories regarding the etiology of genetic damage in ovarian cancer*

Spontaneous mutations due to epithelial proliferation after ovulation
Stimulation of epithelial proliferation by steroids and/or gonadotropins
Talc or other carcinogens that migrate up the genital tract
Lack of progestin-induced apoptosis of genetically damaged cells

ovarian cancers arise in women who carry mutations in cancer susceptibility genes (*BRCA1, BRCA2,* DNA repair genes), and there is evidence that some cancers that arise in the peritoneum of these patients may be polyclonal (26). The etiology of acquired genetic damage in the ovarian epithelium remains uncertain, but exogenous carcinogens have not been strongly implicated, except perhaps talc (27).

It has been suggested that ovulation is the main cause of mutations in the ovarian epithelium. Several lines of evidence link ovulation and epithelial ovarian cancer. First, most animals such as rats and mice ovulate reflexively when stimulated appropriately and have a low incidence of epithelial ovarian cancer. In contrast, chickens and women ovulate repetitively and have the highest incidence of epithelial ovarian cancer. Conversely, women with Turner syndrome, who are anovulatory, rarely develop epithelial ovarian cancer. The observation that pregnancy and oral contraceptive pill use, which decrease the number of ovulatory cycles over a lifetime, are protective against ovarian cancer (28) also is consistent with the theory that ovulation is the main driving force underlying the accumulation of genetic damage in the ovarian epithelium.

It is not known with certainty why repetitive ovulation facilitates the development of ovarian cancer; several factors, including stimulation by gonadotropins, may play a role. One appealing theory is that mutations in the epithelium results from errors in DNA synthesis that occur during proliferation required to repair ovulatory defects. There is evidence to suggest that spontaneous mutations are more likely to occur in cells that are proliferating than in those at rest (29). Although the process of DNA synthesis occurs with a high degree of fidelity, it is estimated that spontaneous errors occur in about 1 of every 1,000,000 bases. Several families of DNA repair genes exist, but some types of mutations more readily elude surveillance and repair and become fixed in the genome. In addition, the efficiency of these DNA repair systems may vary among individuals because of inherited differences in the activity of various alleles of DNA repair genes.

A decreased rate of mutations in the ovarian epithelium probably is not solely responsible for the protective effect of pregnancy and oral contraceptive pills against ovarian cancer. This effect is greater in magnitude than would be predicted based on the extent to which ovulation is interrupted. Five years of oral contraceptive use decreases risk by approximately 50% while decreasing lifetime ovulatory cycles by only 10% to 20% (28). However, it has been shown that administration of the progestin levonorgestrel, either alone or in combination with estrogen, stimulates apoptosis of ovarian epithelial cells in macaques (30). This suggests that the progestagenic milieu of pregnancy and use of oral contraceptive pills might protect against ovarian cancer by increasing apoptosis of ovarian epithelial cells, thereby cleansing the ovary of cells that have acquired genetic damage.

MECHANISMS OF MALIGNANT TRANSFORMATION

The mutations that lead to the development of ovarian and other cancers primarily target genes involved in regulating proliferation, programmed cell death (apoptosis), and senescence—processes that determine the number of cells in a population (Table 2.1). Development of a cancer results from disruption of these complex regulatory pathways, with the net effect being an increased number of cells. Mutations that inactivate DNA repair genes also occur in some types of cancers and may accelerate the accumulation of cancer-causing mutations, but this has not yet been demonstrated to be a prominent feature of sporadic ovarian cancers.

In addition to growth of a primary tumor, cancers are characterized by acquisition of a metastatic phenotype. Ovarian cancers have the ability to invade the surrounding stroma due to production of proteases that degrade connective tissue and produce angiogenic factors that stimulate the development of new blood vessels to support their growth and spread. Although these molecular pathways are integral to the process of cancer progression, there is little evidence to date to suggest that evolution of the metastatic phenotype is directly attributable to mutations in genes that encode proteases or other molecules involved in invasion and metastasis.

TABLE 2.3. *Classes of genes involved in growth regulatory pathways and malignant transformation*

Growth Stimulatory (Oncogenes)	
Peptide growth factors	Corresponding receptors
Epidermal growth factor (EGF) and transforming growth factor (TGF-α)	EGF receptor
Heregulin	erbB2 (HER-2/*neu*)
	erbB3, erbB4
Insulin-like growth factors (IGF-I, IGF-II)	IGF-I and II receptors
Platelet-derived growth factor (PDGF)	PDGF receptor
Fibroblast growth factors (FGFs)	FGF receptors
Macrophage-colony stimulating factor (M-CSF)	M-CSF receptor (*fms*)
Cytoplasmic factors	Examples
Nonreceptor tyrosine kinases	*abl, src*, PIK3CA
G proteins	K-*ras*, H-*ras*
Serine-threonine kinases	AKT2
Nuclear factors	Examples
Transcription factors	*myc, jun, fos*
Cell cycle progression factors	cyclins, E2F
Growth Inhibitory (Tumor Suppressor Genes)	
Extranuclear factors	Examples
Cell membrane factors	Transforming growth factors $\beta 1-\beta 3$ and their type I and II receptors
Cell adhesion factors	Cadherins, APC
Phosphatases	*PTEN*
Nuclear factors	Examples
Cell cycle inhibitors	Rb, p53, p16, p27
Unknown function	BRCA1, BRCA2

Proliferation

The rate of proliferation is a major determinant of the number of cells in a population. To prevent excessive proliferation, DNA synthesis and cell division ordinarily are restrained. When proliferation is appropriate, these inhibitory mechanisms are turned off and growth-stimulatory signals are generated. Malignant tumors are characterized by alterations in genes that control proliferation. There is increased activity of genes that stimulate proliferation (oncogenes) and loss of growth-inhibitory (tumor suppressor) genes (Table 2.3). In the past, it was thought that cancer might arise entirely because of more rapid proliferation and/or a higher fraction of cells proliferating. It is now clear that this was an overly simplistic view. Although increased proliferation is a characteristic of many cancers, the fraction of cancer cells actively dividing and the transition time of the cell cycle are not strikingly different from those of some normal cells. Increased proliferation is only one of several factors that contribute to cancerous growth.

The fraction of ovarian cancer cells that are actively proliferating can be measured by various techniques. One approach is to assess the DNA content of cells in a sample. This can be accomplished with flow cytometry using disaggregated nuclei or in frozen sections using image analysis. The fraction of cells with a DNA content consistent with S phase of the cell cycle can be distinguished from those in the G_1 or G_2/M phase to calculate a proliferation index. In one study, about 25% of ovarian cancers had an S-phase fraction of less than 5%, and this result correlated with early stage and favorable survival (31). Proliferation can also be assessed with the use of immunohistochemical techniques to identify cells that express Ki67 or PCNA, antigens that are expressed only in actively proliferating cells. In most such studies, there has been a correlation between higher proliferation indices (greater than 5% to 15%) and more advanced stage, worse grade, and poor survival (32–34).

Apoptosis

Cells are capable of activating a suicide pathway of programmed cell death, referred to as apoptosis. Apoptosis is an active, energy-dependent process that involves cleavage of the DNA by endonucleases and proteins by proteases.

Morphologically, apoptosis is characterized by condensation of chromatin and cellular shrinkage. This is in contrast to the process of necrosis, which is characterized by loss of osmoregulation and cellular fragmentation.

Because the size of a population of cells is normally static due to a balance between the birth rate and the death rate, growth of a neoplasm theoretically could result from either increased proliferation or decreased apoptosis. In addition to restraining the number of cells in a population, apoptosis may serve an important role in preventing malignant transformation by specifically eliminating cells that have undergone mutation. After exposure of cells to mutagenic stimuli, including radiation and carcinogenic drugs, the cell cycle is arrested so that DNA damage may be repaired. If DNA repair is not sufficient, apoptosis occurs so that cells that have undergone significant damage do not survive. This serves as an anticancer surveillance mechanism by which mutated cells are eliminated before they become fully transformed. The p53 tumor suppressor gene is a critical regulator of cell cycle arrest and apoptosis in response to DNA damage, but apoptosis also may be triggered via other pathways under different circumstances.

The molecular events that effect cell death in response to various stimuli have been only partially elucidated thus far, but it appears that a family of genes encoding proteins that reside in the mitochondrial membrane are directly involved (35). The bcl-2 gene, the first of these genes to be identified, was found at a translocation breakpoint in B-cell lymphomas. Expression of bcl-2 acts to inhibit apoptosis (36) and, paradoxically, persistence of bcl-2 expression in ovarian cancers has been associated with favorable prognosis (37,38). The bcl-X_L gene, a structural and functional homolog of bcl-2, also inhibits apoptosis and has been shown to play a role in preventing apoptosis of ovarian cancer cells in response to chemotherapy (39). Conversely, other related genes such as bax and bcl-X_S have pro-apoptotic activity. High bax expression has been reported in 60% of newly diagnosed ovarian cancers and was associated with a favorable response to therapy (40).

It remains unclear exactly how bcl-2 and these other mitochondrial proteins act to regulate apoptosis, but those that increase membrane permeability stimulate apoptosis, whereas those that decrease permeability prevent apoptosis. Activation of a family of cytosolic proteolytic enzymes called caspases also occurs during apoptosis, leading to breakdown of cellular proteins.

Senescence

Normal cells are capable of undergoing division only a finite number of times before becoming senescent. It has been shown that cellular senescence is caused by shortening of repetitive DNA sequences (TTAGGG) called telomeres that cap the ends of each chromosome. Telomeres are thought to be involved in chromosome stabilization and in the prevention of recombination during mitosis. At birth chromosomes have long telomeric sequences that become progressively shorter each time a cell divides. Malignant cells appear to avoid senescence by turning on expression of telomerase activity that acts to lengthen the telomeres (41,42). Telomerase is a ribonucleoprotein complex, and both the protein and RNA subunits have been identified. The RNA component serves as a template for telomere extension, and the protein subunit acts to catalyze the synthesis of new telomeric repeats.

Because telomerase expression in most normal tissues is restricted to development, it has been suggested that telomerase might be a useful diagnostic marker in patients with cancer. Several groups have shown that telomerase activity is detectable in most ovarian cancers (43–45). It has been suggested that persistence of telomerase activity in peritoneal washings after primary therapy for advanced ovarian cancer may predict the presence of microscopic residual disease in some cases despite negative cytologic washings and biopsies (44). Demonstration of the utility of this approach awaits the completion of more definitive studies.

GROWTH-STIMULATORY PATHWAYS—ONCOGENES

Oncogenes encode proteins that are normally involved in stimulating proliferation, but when these gene products are overactive they

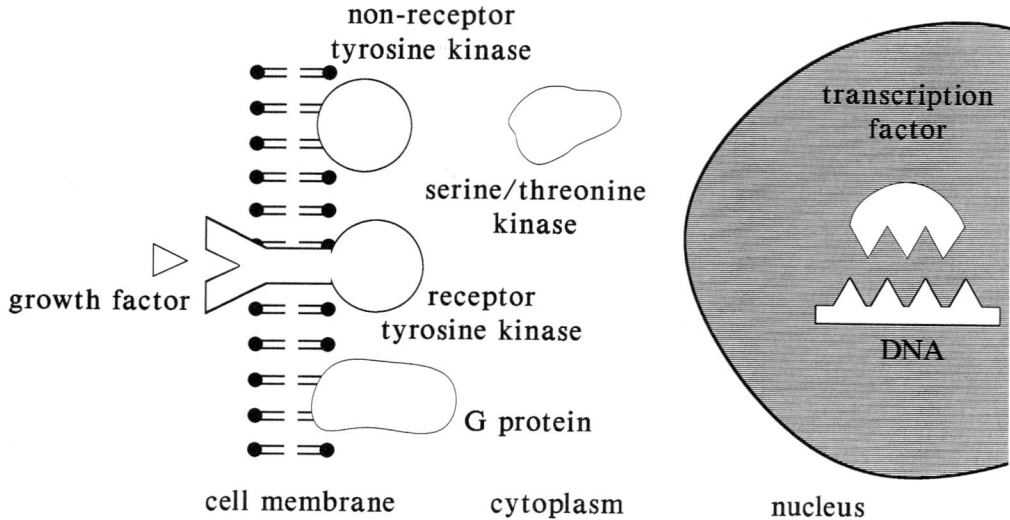

FIG. 2.2. Classes of oncogenes.

contribute to the process of malignant transformation. Oncogenes can be activated via several mechanisms. In some cancers, amplification of oncogenes with resultant overexpression of the corresponding protein has been noted. Some oncogenes may become overactive when affected by point mutations. Finally, oncogenes may be translocated from one chromosomal location to another and then come under the influence of promoter sequences that cause overexpression of the gene. This last mechanism frequently occurs in leukemias and lymphomas but has not been demonstrated in gynecologic cancers or other solid tumors.

In cell culture systems in the laboratory, many genes that are involved in normal growth stimulatory pathways can elicit transformation when altered to overactive forms. On this basis, a large number of genes have been classified as oncogenes (Figure 2.2 and Table 2.4). Studies in human cancers have suggested that the actual spectrum of genes altered in the development of human cancers may be more limited. A number of genes that elicit transformation when activated *in vitro* have not been documented to undergo alterations in human cancers. In this section, the various classes of oncogenes involved in ovarian cancer are discussed.

Peptide Growth Factors

Peptide growth factors in the extracellular space can stimulate a cascade of molecular events that lead to proliferation by binding to cell membrane receptors. Unlike endocrine hormones, which are secreted into the bloodstream to act on distant target organs, peptide growth factors usually act in the local environment where they have been secreted. The concept that autocrine growth stimulation might be a key strategy by which cancer cell proliferation becomes autonomous is intellectually appealing and has received considerable attention. In this model, it is postulated that cancers secrete stimulatory growth factors that then interact with receptors on the same cell. Although increased production of stimulatory growth factors may play a role in enhancing proliferation associated with malignant transformation, these factors also are involved in development, stromal-epithelial communication, tissue regeneration, and wound healing.

It has been shown that ovarian cancers produce and/or are capable of responding to various peptide growth factors. For example, epidermal growth factor (EGF) (46) and transforming growth factor-α (TGF-α) (47) are produced by

TABLE 2.4. *Molecular alterations in sporadic ovarian cancers*

Gene type	Function	Alteration	Approximate frequency (%)
Oncogenes			
Her-2/*neu*	Tyrosine kinase	Overexpression	20
K-*ras*	G protein	Mutation	5
AKT2	Serine/threonine kinase	Amplification	10
PIK3CA	Serine/threonine kinase	Amplification	?40
c-*myc*	Transcription factor	Overexpression	20–30
Tumor suppressor genes			
BRCA1	?DNA repair	Mutation/deletion	5
p53	Transcription factor	Mutation/deletion	60
p16	CDK inhibitor	Homozygous deletion/methylation	?15
p27	CDK inhibitor	Decreased expression	?40

some ovarian cancers that also express the receptor that binds these peptides (EGF receptor) (48,49). Some cancers produce insulin-like growth factor-1 (IGF-1) and IGF-1 binding protein and express type 1 IGF receptor (50). Platelet-derived growth factor (PDGF) also is expressed by many types of epithelial cells, including human ovarian cancer cell lines, but these cells usually are not responsive to PDGF (51–53). In addition, ovarian cancers produce basic fibroblast growth factor (FGF) and its receptor, and basic FGF acts as a mitogen in some ovarian cancers (54). Ovarian cancers produce macrophage colony-stimulating factor (M-CSF) (55), and serum levels of M-CSF are increased in some patients (56). Because the M-CSF receptor (*fms*) is expressed by many ovarian cancers (57), this could comprise an autocrine growth stimulatory pathway in some cancers. In addition, M-CSF could act in a paracrine fashion to stimulate recruitment and activation of macrophages. Because macrophage products such as interleukin-1 (IL-1), IL-6, and tumor necrosis factor-α have been shown to stimulate proliferation of some ovarian cancer cell lines (58–60), the potential for paracrine stimulation of the cancer by macrophages also exists. In addition to expression of peptide growth factors and their receptors, ascites of patients with ovarian cancer contains phospholipid factors that stimulate proliferation of ovarian cancer cells (61,62).

Several groups have demonstrated that normal ovarian epithelial cells produce and are responsive to many of the same peptide growth factors as malignant ovarian epithelial cells (49,63–65). Therefore, despite circumstantial evidence demonstrating the potential for autocrine and paracrine growth regulation of ovarian cancer cells by peptide growth factors, it remains unclear whether alterations in expression of growth factors are critical in the development of ovarian cancer. Peptide growth factors may function as necessary cofactors rather than as the driving force behind malignant transformation.

Growth Factor Receptors Including the Epidermal Growth Factor Receptor Family

Cell membrane receptors that bind peptide growth factors are composed of an extracellular ligand-binding domain, a membrane-spanning region, and a cytoplasmic tyrosine kinase domain. Binding of a growth factor to the extracellular domain results in aggregation and conformational shifts in the receptor and activation of the inner tyrosine kinase (66,67). This kinase phosphorylates tyrosine residues on both the growth factor receptor (autophosphorylation) and targets in the cell interior, leading to activation of secondary signals. For example, phosphorylation of phospholipase C leads to breakdown of cell membrane phospholipids and generation of diacylglycerol and inositol triphosphate, both of which play a role in propagation of the mitogenic signal.

The role of the EGF receptor family of transmembrane receptors and their ligands in growth regulation and transformation has been a prominent focus in cancer research (68). EGF is a peptide growth factor of 53 amino acids that maintains its secondary structure by virtue of disulfide bonds between cysteine residues. At least five other peptide growth factors, including TGF-α, also interact with and activate the EGF receptor. EFG, TGF-α, and other EGF receptor ligands are produced as proforms that are inserted into the cell membrane. The membrane-anchored growth factor can interact with receptors on adjacent cells, a phenomenon known as juxtacrine growth regulation. Alternatively, the active peptide can be cleaved and released into the extracellular space. The free peptide may interact with receptors on the same cell (autocrine) or on nearby cells (paracrine) to stimulate growth.

The EGF receptor is ubiquitously expressed in both epithelial and stromal cells and plays a role in growth stimulation of most cell types. The EGF receptor has been shown to be amplified in some squamous cancers, and the EGF receptor can be targeted therapeutically with monoclonal antibodies (69). EGF receptor is expressed in normal ovarian epithelium, and although the level of expression varies among cancers, it is not a strong predictor of clinical behavior (70).

The EGF receptor family of receptors also often is referred to as the *erb*B family because the first member identified was the v-*erb*B oncogene. The second member of the family (*erb*B2) initially was called *neu* because it was found to be the transforming gene responsible for the generation of neuroblastomas in rats treated with a chemical carcinogen. This **H**uman **E**GF **R**eceptor–like molecule was named both HER-2/*neu* and *erb*B2 by investigators working in the field. The transforming activity of *neu* in the animal model was caused by the presence of a mutation in the transmembrane portion of the molecule that results in constitutive activation of the inner tyrosine kinase domain. Biochemical studies of HER-2/*neu* have shown that activation of this receptor is not driven by ligand binding but rather is dependent on activation of other members of the *erb*B family (*erb*B3, *erb*B4) that heterodimerize with *erb*B2 and activate its tyrosine kinase domain (71).

In contrast to EGF receptor, which normally is expressed in both stromal and epithelial cells, HER-2/*neu* is expressed primarily in epithelial cells. The level of HER-2/*neu* is increased in some human breast, ovarian, and other cancers due to amplification (72,73), and the SKOV3 ovarian cancer cell line and the SKBR3 breast cancer cell line both have amplification of this gene. In human cancers, HER-2/*neu* may also be overexpressed due to alterations in regulation of transcription in the absence of gene amplification. Regardless of the underlying mechanism, it has been shown that overexpression occurs in about 20% of ovarian cancers and 30% of breast cancers and correlates with aggressive features. The level of overexpression in breast cancers generally is higher than in ovarian cancers, however, and some studies have not found overexpression of HER-2/*neu* to adversely affect prognosis in ovarian cancer (74,75). It has been shown that transfection of HER-2/*neu* into normal ovarian epithelial cells can induce a malignant phenotype *in vitro* including the ability of cells to grow in an anchorage-independent fashion and to form tumors in nude mice.

As noted, activation of the *erb*B3 and *erb*B4 transmembrane receptors is requisite for HER-2/*neu* kinase activity. At least four families of ligands, collectively called neuregulins (e.g., heregulin, *neu* differentiating factor), bind to *erb*B3 and *erb*B4 (71). Interestingly, there is considerable promiscuity between *erb*B ligands and receptors. For example, amphiregulin can activate both the EGF receptor (*erb*B1) and *erb*B3. One of the more recently described ligands (epiregulin) can activate heterodimers of any of the *erb*B family members, and these heterodimers are more potent growth stimulators than homodimers of any individual *erb*B receptor. Although their molecular signaling mechanisms have not yet been fully elucidated, the *erb*B family of receptors also has been exploited as therapeutic targets. Monoclonal antibodies that interact with HER-2/*neu* can decrease growth of breast and ovarian cancer cell lines that overexpress this receptor (76,77). In addition, these antibodies may enhance the sensitivity of cancers to cytotoxic chemotherapy by interfering with repair of DNA adducts (78). An anti-HER-2/*neu* antibody that induces breast cancer regression has been approved for clinical use by the

U.S. Food and Drug Administration (79). It is possible that this approach might also benefit some women whose ovarian cancers overexpress HER-2/*neu*.

Other Kinases

Following the interaction of peptide growth factors and their receptors, secondary molecular signals are generated to transmit the mitogenic stimulus towards the nucleus. This function is served by a multitude of complex and overlapping signal transduction pathways that occur in the inner cell membrane and cytoplasm. Many of these signals involve phosphorylation of proteins by enzymes known as kinases (80). Cellular processes other than growth also are regulated by kinases, but one family of kinases appears to have evolved specifically for the purpose of transmitting growth-stimulatory signals. These tyrosine kinases transfer a phosphate group from adenosine triphosphate (ATP) to tyrosine residues of target proteins. Some kinases that phosphorylate proteins on serine and/or threonine residues also are involved in stimulating proliferation. Although several families of intracellular kinases have been identified that can elicit transformation when activated *in vitro,* it remains uncertain whether structural alterations in most of these molecules play a role in the development of human cancers. The activity of kinases is regulated by phosphatases, which act in opposition to the kinases by removing phosphates from the target proteins (81). A number of phosphatases are expressed by ovarian cancers, and some of these oppose the kinase activity of HER-2/*neu* (82).

AKT2 is a gene on chromosome 19q that encodes a serine-threonine protein kinase. AKT2 was shown to be amplified and overexpressed in 2 of 8 ovarian cancer cell lines and in 2 of 15 primary epithelial ovarian cancers (83). This study was confirmed by a larger series of 132 primary ovarian cancers in which 14% had AKT2 amplification or overexpression. AKT2 amplification/overexpression was found have a statistically significant association with higher grade and worse survival (84). Further studies are needed to confirm the functional significance of AKT2 overexpression in ovarian cancers.

The region of chromosome 3p26 that includes the regulatory subunit of phosphatidylinositol 3-kinase (PIK3CA) was shown to be amplified in some ovarian cancer cell lines and in 40% of primary ovarian cancers using CGH (85). The AKT2 gene is one of the downstream targets of PIK3CA. Therefore, theoretically, amplification of either of these two genes could lead to excessive activation of this mitogenic pathway.

G Proteins

G proteins represent another class of molecules involved in transmission of growth-stimulatory signals in toward the nucleus (86,87). They are located on the inner aspect of the cell membrane and have intrinsic guanosine triphosphatase (GTPase) activity that catalyzes the exchange of GTP for guanine diphosphate (GDP). In their active GTP-bound form, G proteins interact with kinases that are involved in relaying the mitogenic signal. Conversely, hydrolysis of GTP to GDP, which is stimulated by GTPase-activating proteins (GAPs), leads to inactivation of G proteins. The *ras* family of G proteins are among the most frequently mutated oncogenes in human cancers (e.g., gastrointestinal and endometrial cancers). Activation of *ras* genes usually involves point mutations in codons 12, 13, or 61 that result in constitutively activated molecules.

Mutations in the *ras* genes do not appear to be a common feature of invasive serous epithelial ovarian cancers (88–90). K-*ras* mutations have been noted more frequently in mucinous ovarian cancers, but these tumors comprise only a small fraction of epithelial ovarian cancers. In contrast, K-*ras* mutations are common in borderline epithelial ovarian tumors, occurring in 20% to 50% of cases (91,92). Thus, studies of the K-*ras* oncogene suggest that the molecular pathology of borderline tumors differs from that of invasive epithelial ovarian cancers.

Nuclear Factors

If proliferation is to occur in response to signals generated in the cytoplasm, these events must lead to activation of nuclear factors responsible for DNA replication and cell division. Expression of several genes that encode nuclear proteins increases dramatically within minutes after treatment of normal cells with peptide growth factors. Once induced, the products of these genes bind to specific DNA regulatory elements and induce transcription of genes involved in DNA synthesis and cell division. When inappropriately overexpressed, however, these transcription factors can act as oncogenes. In regard to the nuclear transcription factors involved in stimulating proliferation, amplification and/or overexpression of members of the *myc* family has most often been implicated in the development of human cancers (93,94). Myc proteins are key regulators of mammalian cell proliferation, and treatment of cells with myc antisense oligonucleotides inhibits proliferation. It has been shown that myc acts as part of a heterodimeric complex with the protein max to initiate transcription of other genes involved in cell cycle progression (93).

Amplification of the c-*myc* oncogene occurs in some epithelial ovarian cancers. In five small studies, c-*myc* was reported to be amplified in 24 (31%) of 77 cases (95–99). In a study in which 51 epithelial ovarian cancers were analyzed, a similar incidence of c-*myc* overexpression was observed (37%) (100). Furthermore, c-*myc* overexpression was more frequently observed in advanced-stage serous adenocarcinomas, suggesting a role for tumor progression.

GROWTH-INHIBITORY PATHWAYS—TUMOR SUPPRESSOR GENES

Tumor suppressor genes encode proteins that are normally involved in inhibiting proliferation, and inactivation of these genes plays a role in the development of most cancers. Knudson's "two-hit" model established the paradigm that both alleles must be inactivated in order to exert a phenotypic effect on tumorigenesis (101). The location and the type of the inactivating mutations in tumor suppressor genes may vary from one cancer to the next. Frequently, mutations in tumor suppressor genes alter the base sequence so that the encoded protein product is truncated because of generation of a premature stop codon. Truncated protein products may result from several types of mutational events including nonsense mutations, in which a single base substitution changes a sequence from a specific amino acid to a stop codon (e.g., AAG to TAG). In addition, microdeletions or insertions of one or several nucleotides that disrupt the reading frame of the DNA (frameshifts) also lead to the generation of stop codons downstream in the gene. In some cases, missense mutations occur that change only a single amino acid in the encoded protein. A mutation in one allele, whether germline or somatic, is revealed after somatic inactivation of the homologous wild-type allele. In theory, the same spectrum of mutational events could contribute to inactivation of the second allele, but what is typically observed in tumors is homozygosity or hemizygosity for the first mutation, indicating "loss" of the wild-type allele. The loss of heterozygosity (LOH) has become recognized as the hallmark of tumor suppressor gene inactivation.

There is also evidence that some tumor suppressor genes may become inactivated as a result of methylation of the promoter region of the gene (102). The promoter is an area proximal to the coding sequence that regulates whether or not the gene is transcribed from DNA into RNA. When the promoter is methylated, it is resistant to activation and the gene is essentially silenced despite remaining structurally intact. Like oncogenes, tumor suppressor gene products are found throughout the cell (Table 2.4). In this section the various classes of tumor suppressor genes involved in sporadic epithelial ovarian cancers are reviewed.

Extranuclear Tumor Suppressor Genes

Although most tumor suppressor gene products are nuclear proteins, some extranuclear tumor suppressors have been identified. Theoretically, any protein that normally is involved in inhibition of proliferation could conceivably act as a tumor suppressor. In this regard, phosphatases that normally oppose the action of the tyrosine kinases by dephosphorylating tyrosine residues are appealing candidates (81). Analysis of deletions on chromosome 10q23 in human cancers led to the discovery of the *PTEN* gene (103). In addition to its phosphatase activity, *PTEN* is homologous to the cytoskeleton proteins tensin and auxin, and it has been postulated that *PTEN* might act to inhibit invasion and metastasis through modulation of the cytoskeleton (104). It has been demonstrated that PIK3CA and AKT2 kinase activity can be specifically opposed by the *PTEN* phosphatase. *PTEN* mutations are rare in serous ovarian cancers, perhaps because amplification of PIK3CA or AKT2 abrogates the need for loss of *PTEN* tumor suppressor function. In contrast, *PTEN* mutations occur in about 20% of endometrioid ovarian cancers (105).

Transforming Growth Factor-β

The TGF-β family of growth factors inhibits proliferation of normal epithelial cells (106). It is thought that TGF-β causes cell cycle arrest in G_1 by triggering pathways that result in inhibition of cyclin-dependent kinases (CDKs). Three closely related forms of TGF-β have been discovered which are encoded by separate genes (TGF-β1, TGF-β2, and TGF-β3). All three forms of TGF-β are 25-kDa homodimers with subunits bound together by disulfide bonds. TGF-β is secreted from cells in an inactive form bound to a portion of its precursor molecule, from which it must be cleaved to release biologically active TGF-β. Active TGF-β interacts with type I and type II cell surface TGF-β receptors and initiates serine/threonine kinase activity (107). Prominent intracellular targets include a class of molecules called Smads that translocate to the nucleus and act as transcriptional regulators (108). Although mutations in the TGF-β receptors and in Smads have been reported in some cancers, this does not appear to be a feature of ovarian cancers.

Normal ovarian epithelial cells produce, activate, and are growth inhibited by TGF-β (109); however, most immortalized ovarian cancer cell lines have lost the ability to either produce, activate, or respond to TGF-β (52,109–113). This suggests that TGF-β might normally act as an autocrine growth-inhibitory factor in normal ovarian epithelium and that loss of this pathway might play a role in the development of some ovarian cancers. Although they are convenient to work with, immortalized cell lines frequently have undergone profound genetic alterations in tissue culture. Examination of primary ovarian cancers obtained directly from patients revealed that in almost all cases cancers were sensitive to the growth-inhibitory effect of TGF-β (114). Therefore, it remains unclear whether alterations in the TGF-β pathway play a role in the development of ovarian cancers.

P53 Tumor Suppressor Gene

Mutation of the p53 tumor suppressor gene is the genetic event most frequently described thus far in human cancers (115–117) (Figure 2.3). The p53 gene encodes a 393-amino-acid protein that appears to play a central role in the regulation

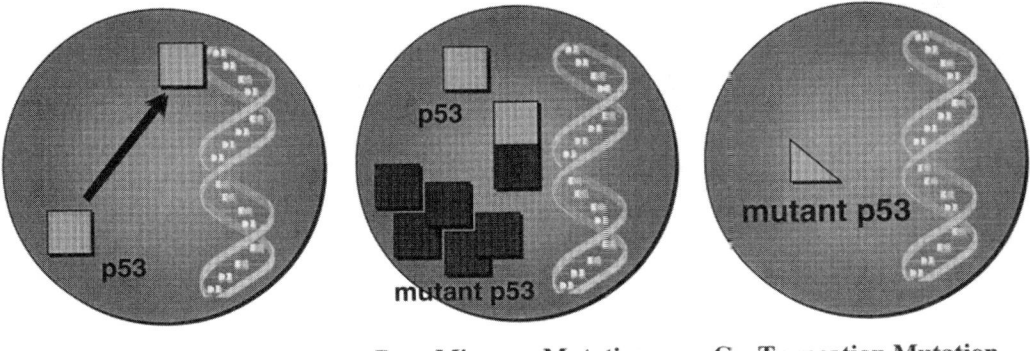

FIG. 2.3. Inactivation of the p53 tumor suppressor gene (**A**) by "dominant negative" missense mutation (**B**) or by truncation mutation (**C**) and deletion.

of both proliferation and apoptosis (118–120). In normal cells, p53 protein resides in the nucleus and exerts its tumor suppressor activity by binding to transcriptional regulatory elements of genes, such as the CDK inhibitor p21, that act to arrest cells in G_1. Beyond simply inhibiting proliferation, normal p53 is thought to play a role in preventing cancer by stimulating apoptosis of cells that have undergone excessive genetic damage (121). In this regard, p53 has been described as the "guardian of the genome," because it delays entry into S phase until the genome has been cleansed of mutations. If DNA repair is inadequate, p53 may initiate apoptosis, thereby eliminating cells with genetic damage.

Many cancers have missense mutations in one copy of the p53 gene that result in substitution of a single amino acid in exons 5 through 8, which encode the DNA binding domains (Figures 2.4 and 2.5). Although these mutant p53 genes encode full-length proteins, they are unable to bind to DNA or regulate transcription of other genes. Mutation of one copy of the p53 gene often is accompanied by deletion of the other copy, leaving the cancer cell with only mutant p53 protein. If the cancer cell does retain one normal copy of the p53 gene, the mutant p53 protein can form a complex with wild-type p53 protein and prevent it from interacting with DNA. Because inactivation of both p53 alleles is not required for loss of p53 function, mutant p53 is said to act in a "dominant negative" fashion. Whereas normal cells have low levels of p53 protein because it is rapidly degraded, missense mutations encode protein products that are resistant to degradation and overaccumulate in the nucleus; this overexpression of mutant p53 protein can be detected immunohistochemically. A smaller fraction of cancers have mutations in the p53 gene that encode truncated protein products (122). Whereas missense mutations in the p53 gene cluster in exons 5 through 8, truncation mutations are more evenly dispersed throughout the gene, presumably because they inactivate the p53 protein regardless of their location (Figure 2.5). In cases of p53 truncation mutations, deletion of the other allele occurs as the second event, as is seen with other tumor suppressor genes (Figure 2.1).

Alteration of the p53 tumor suppressor gene is the most frequently described genetic event in ovarian cancers (122–129). The frequency of overexpression of mutant p53 is significantly higher in advanced stage III/IV disease (40% to 60%) compared with stage I cases (10% to 20%). In addition, p53 inactivation is uncommon in borderline tumors (130). The higher frequency of p53 overexpression in advanced-stage cases may indicate that this is a "late event" in ovarian carcinogenesis. Alternatively, the loss of p53 may confer a more aggressive metastatic phenotype. In advanced-stage ovarian cancer, there is a suggestion that overexpression of p53 may be associated with somewhat worse survival (123,125–129). The literature is not entirely consistent, and most studies have not been large enough or optimally designed to yield reliable prognostic information. Finally, although there is a high concordance between p53 missense mutations and protein overexpression, about 20% of advanced ovarian cancers contain mutations that result in truncated protein products that generally are not overexpressed (122). Overall, about

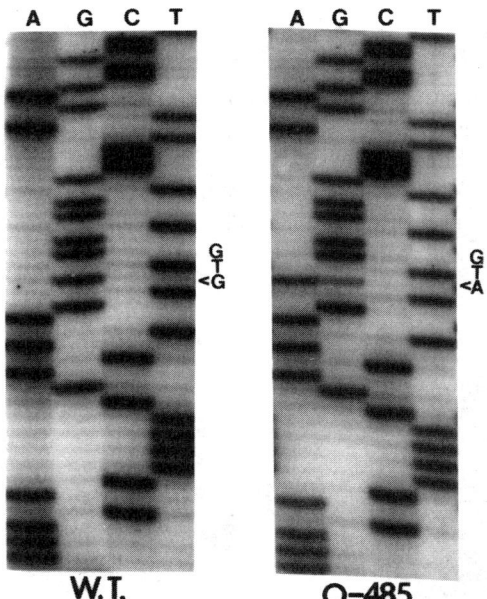

FIG. 2.4. Mutation of codon 216 of the p53 gene in ovarian cancers. Wild-type (WT) sequence GTG; O-485, ovarian cancer with G-to-A mutation changing sequence to GTA. G, guanine; T, thymine; A, adenine.

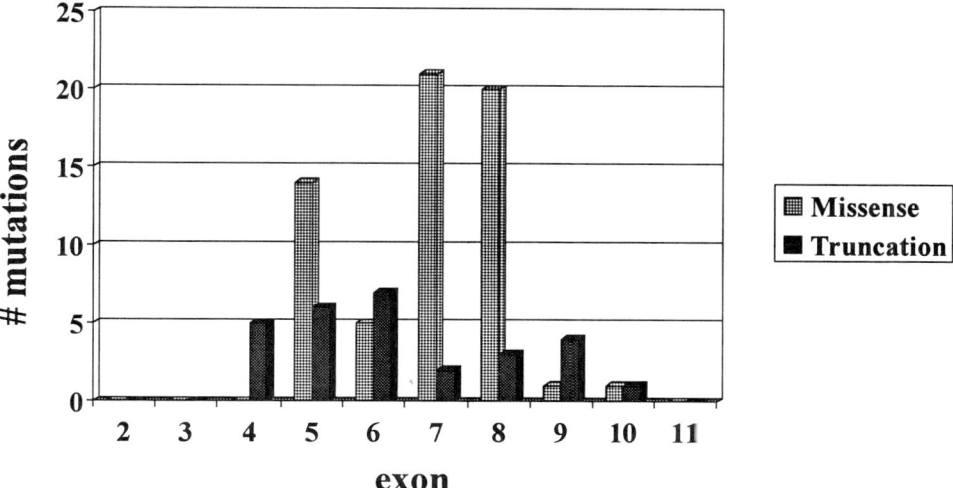

FIG. 2.5. Spectrum of p53 mutations in advanced ovarian cancers ($n = 58$).

70% of advanced ovarian cancers have either missense or truncation mutations in the p53 gene.

The finding that overexpression of mutant p53 tumor suppressor genes is associated with high lifetime ovulatory cycles is consistent with the hypothesis that ovulation-associated proliferation may be the cause of these mutations in the ovarian epithelium (131). In addition, most of the p53 point mutations are transitions rather than transversions (21,132), which also suggests that these mutations occur spontaneously and not because of exogenous carcinogens.

It has been suggested that loss of p53 might confer a chemoresistant phenotype, because p53 plays a role in chemotherapy-induced apoptosis. In this regard, several studies have examined the correlation between chemosensitivity and p53 mutation in ovarian cancers *in vitro* (133–136). Some have suggested a relationship between p53 mutation and loss of chemosensitivity, but in other, equally valid studies such a relationship has not been observed (137). The status of the p53 gene is probably one of a number of factors that determines sensitivity to chemotherapy.

BRCA1

Inherited mutations of the BRCA1 gene on chromosome 17q are the most frequent cause of hereditary ovarian cancers. Before the identification of BRCA1, it had been anticipated that somatic mutations in BRCA1 would be common in ovarian cancers, because more than half of these cancers exhibit LOH on chromosome 17q (22,138,139). Initially, two small studies reported somatic mutations in BRCA1 in about 10% of 54 ovarian cancers (140,141), but somatic mutations were not seen in two larger studies (139,142). In these initial studies, mutational screening was performed with the use of single-stranded conformation analysis.

More recently, a large study in which complete sequencing of the BRCA1 gene was performed in 103 ovarian cancers, somatic mutations were found in at least 7 cases (143). In contrast to women with germline BRCA1 mutations, whose median age at ovarian cancer diagnosis is typically in the mid-forties, the median age of women with somatic mutations was about 60 years. Similar to ovarian cancers with germline BRCA1 mutations, all of the ovarian cancers with somatic BRCA1 mutations were serous. In addition, loss of the wild-type BRCA1 allele invariably accompanied somatic BRCA1 mutations. These data are supportive of the hypothesis that loss of BRCA1 function occurs by way of the classic tumor suppressor paradigm, with mutation of one copy and deletion of the other. The BRCA2

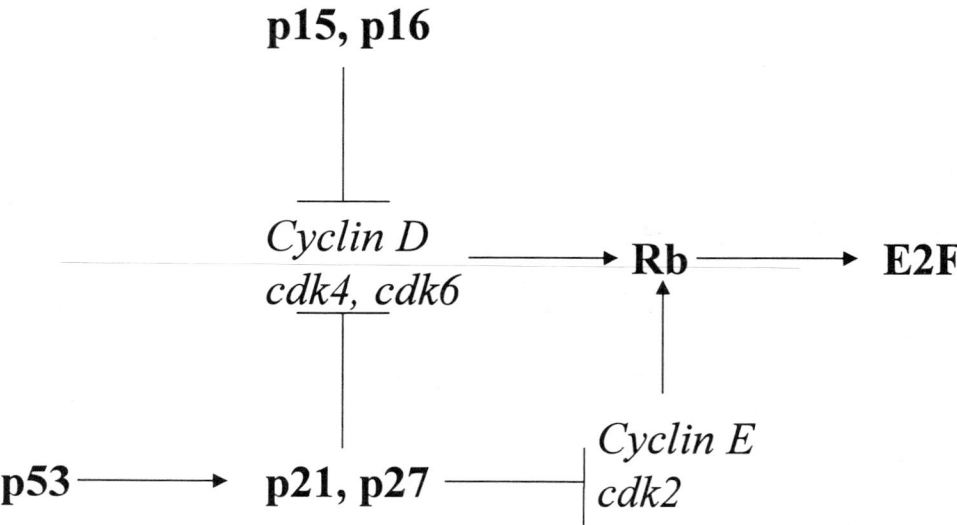

FIG. 2.6. Regulation of G_1 progression by p53, cyclins, cyclin-dependent kinases (CDKs), CDK inhibitors, and Rb.

gene, which is responsible for some hereditary ovarian cancer cases, also has been examined for somatic mutations, but none have been identified (144).

Retinoblastoma Tumor Suppressor Gene

Initiation of the cell cycle with resultant cell division is dependent on progression through the G_1 phase of the cycle into the DNA-synthetic S phase. The retinoblastoma gene (Rb), which was the first tumor suppressor gene discovered, plays a central role in actively regulating this process (145,146). In the early G_1 phase of the cell cycle, Retinoblastoma (Rb) protein binds to the E2F transcription factor and prevents it from activating transcription of other genes involved in cell cycle progression. When Rb is phosphorylated, E2F is released and stimulates entry into the DNA-synthesis phase of the cell cycle (Figure 2.6). Mutations in the Rb gene have been noted primarily in retinoblastomas and sarcomas, but rarely in other types of cancers. LOH at the Rb locus occurs in about 30% of ovarian cancers, but mutations in the gene have not been detected (147), and functional Rb protein is present despite loss of one copy of the gene (148).

Cyclins, Cyclin-Dependent Kinases, and Cyclin-Dependent Kinase Inhibitors

Phosphorylation of Rb serves as a final common pathway with respect to initiation of proliferation, and this process is tightly controlled because of its critical importance (Figure 2.6). Rb is phosphorylated by a family of CDKs (CDK2, CDK4, CDK6) and associated cyclins (cyclin D, cyclin E), which act as regulatory subunits. Conversely, a family of CDK inhibitors (p15, p16, p21, p27) have been described that prevent phosphorylation of Rb by cyclin-CDK complexes. Although many of the intricacies of regulation of G_1 progression remain poorly understood, it is clear that inappropriately high activity of cyclins and CDKs or loss of CDK inhibitors facilitates malignant transformation. Several alterations in these classes of genes have been described in human cancers, including overexpression of cyclin D and loss of p16.

The p16 CDK inhibitor is the most frequently altered of the genes involved in regulating Rb phosphorylation (102). The p16 gene on chromosome 9p21 encodes a protein that inhibits CDK4- or CDK6-cyclin D complexes from phosphorylating Rb. Initially it was noted that both copies of the p16 gene are deleted in a high fraction of immortalized cancer cell lines, including the SKOV3 ovarian cancer cell line (149). The hypothesis that p16 loss plays a significant role in malignant transformation was strengthened by the finding that it is inactivated in some familial melanoma kindreds. Although the p16 gene also is inactivated by mutations or deletion of both alleles in some sporadic cancers, this occurs much less frequently than in immortalized cell lines. More commonly, the p16 gene appears to be silenced through methylation of its promoter, which prevents transcription.

The p16 gene has been studied extensively in ovarian cancers, but the results of various studies are conflicting. Some studies have reported that the p16 gene is homozygously deleted or the promoter is methylated in a fraction of cases (150–152), whereas other studies have not found p16 deletions, mutations, or methylation (153–155). The inconsistency of these various reports most likely reflects the technical difficulty of assaying promoter methylation and homozygous deletions in primary tumor samples. In addition, some groups have reported that some ovarian cancers have very high levels of p16 protein (156), but the underlying mechanism and significance of this observation has not yet been elucidated. Finally, the p14arf protein arises from an alternative reading frame of the p16 gene and has been shown to increase p53 expression by decreasing its degradation (157). Deletions of the p16 locus would also lead to loss of p14arf expression, which could have significant consequences for regulation of G_1 progression.

There is some evidence to suggest that decreased activity of other CDK inhibitors may also play a role in the development of some cancers. In this regard, reduced expression of p27, which is encoded by a gene on chromosome 12p, has been noted in some cancers as a result of increased p27 degradation. About one third of ovarian cancers were noted to have decreased p27 expression, and this correlated with poor outcome (158,159). In addition, overexpression of cyclin D and/or cyclin E has been noted in some cancers. The cyclin D gene on chromosome 11q13 is translocated or amplified in some human cancers. Although the level of cyclin D appears to be high in some ovarian cancers, overexpression has not been shown to be caused by amplification or translocation (159,160). Likewise, cyclin E levels are high in some ovarian cancers, particularly clear cell tumors (161).

Other cyclins, CDKs, and regulatory molecules such as the CHK family are involved in regulating progression from G_2 to M. Alterations in these pathways clearly play a role in the development of some cancers, but the intricacies of the G_2/M transition are less well understood than those of G_1/S. Studies of G_2/M in ovarian cancers to date are preliminary and have not yielded evidence of significant alterations.

Other Genes

Several other known tumor suppressor genes, including *WT1* and *APC*, have been examined but do not appear to be altered frequently in ovarian cancers. Several putative ovarian cancer tumor suppressor genes have been described that are expressed in normal ovarian epithelial cells but not in ovarian cancers. One of these is a ras homolog named *NOEY2* which was described by researchers at the M.D. Anderson Cancer Center (162). The *SPARC* gene, which encodes an extracellular matrix protein that is involved in adhesion (163), and the *DOC2* gene, which is a GRB2 binding protein (164), were described by the group at Brigham and Women's Hospital. Finally, *LOT1*, a transcription factor (165), and the *OVCA1* and *OVCA2* genes on chromosome 17p (166) were described by the group at Fox Chase Cancer Center. The roles of these and other, as yet undiscovered tumor suppressor genes in the development of ovarian cancers remain to be defined by future studies.

REFERENCES

1. Gallion HH, Powell DE, Smith LW, et al. Chromosome abnormalities in human epithelial ovarian malignancies. *Gynecol Oncol* 1990;38:473–477.
2. Iwabuchi H, Sakamoto M, Sakunaga H, et al. Genetic analysis of benign, low-grade, and high-grade ovarian tumors. *Cancer Res* 1995;55:6172–6180.
3. Elledge RM, Allred DC. The p53 tumor suppressor gene in breast cancer. *Breast Cancer Res Treat* 1994;32:39–47.
4. Sonoda G, Palazzo J, du Manoir S, et al. Comparative genomic hybridization detects frequent overrepresen-

tation of chromosomal material from 3q26, 8q24, and 20q13 in human ovarian carcinomas. *Genes Chromosomes Cancer* 1900;20:320–328.
5. Tapper J, Butzow R, Wahlstrom T, et al. Evidence for divergence of DNA copy number changes in serous, mucinous and endometrioid ovarian carcinomas. *Br J Cancer* 1997;75:1782–1787.
6. Cliby W, Ritland S, Dodson M, et al. Human epithelial ovarian cancer allelotype. *Cancer Res* 1993;53:2393–2398.
7. Tavassoli M, Steingrimsdottir H, Pierce E, et al. Loss of heterozygosity on chromosome 5q in ovarian cancer is frequently accompanied by TP53 mutation and identifies a tumour suppressor gene locus at 5q13.1-21. *Br J Cancer* 1996;74:115–119.
8. Saito S, Sirahama S, Matsushima M, et al. Definition of a commonly deleted region in ovarian cancers to a 300-kb segment of chromosome 6q27. *Cancer Res* 1996;56:5586–5589.
9. Tibiletti MG, Bernasconi B, Furlan D, et al. Early involvement of 6q in surface epithelial ovarian tumors. *Cancer Res* 1996;56:4493–4498.
10. Colitti CV, Rodabaugh KJ, Welch WR, et al. A novel 4 cM minimal deletion unit on chromosome 6q25.1-q25.2 associated with high grade invasive epithelial ovarian carcinomas. *Oncogene* 1998;16:555–559.
11. Shridhar V, Staub J, Huntley B, et al. A novel region of deletion on chromosome 6q23.3 spanning less than 500 Kb in high grade invasive epithelial ovarian cancer. *Oncogene* 1999;18:3913–3918.
12. Watson RH, Neville PJ, Roy WJJ, et al. Loss of heterozygosity on chromosomes 7p, 7q, 9p and 11q is an early event in ovarian tumorigenesis. *Oncogene* 1998;17:207–212.
13. Brown MR, Chuaqui R, Vocke CD, et al. Allelic loss on chromosome arm 8p: analysis of sporadic epithelial ovarian tumors. *Gynecol Oncol* 1999;74:98–102.
14. Lu KH, Weitzel JN, Kodali S, et al. A novel 4-cM minimally deleted region on chromosome 11p15.1 associated with high grade nonmucinous epithelial ovarian carcinomas. *Cancer Res* 1997;57:387–390.
15. Gabra H, Langdon SP, Watson JE, et al. Loss of heterozygosity at 11q22 correlates with low progesterone receptor content in epithelial ovarian cancer. *Clin Cancer Res* 1995;1:945–953.
16. Launonen V, Stenback F, Puistola U, et al. Chromosome 11q22.3-q25 LOH in ovarian cancer: association with a more aggressive disease course and involved subregions. *Gynecol Oncol* 1998;71:299–304.
17. Davis M, Hitchcock A, Foulkes WD, Campbell IG. Refinement of two chromosome 11q regions of loss of heterozygosity in ovarian cancer. *Cancer Res* 1996;56:741–744.
18. Gabra H, Watson JE, Taylor KJ, et al. Definition and refinement of a region of loss of heterozygosity at 11q23.3-q24.3 in epithelial ovarian cancer associated with poor prognosis. *Cancer Res* 1996;56:950–954.
19. Dodson MK, Hartmann LC, Cliby WA, et al. Comparison of loss of heterozygosity patterns in invasive low-grade and high-grade epithelial ovarian carcinomas. *Cancer Res* 1993;53:4456–4460.
20. Bandera CA, Takahashi H, Behbakht K, et al. Deletion mapping of two potential chromosome 14 tumor suppressor gene loci in ovarian carcinoma. *Cancer Res* 1997;57:513–515.
21. Kohler MF, Marks JR, Wiseman RW, et al. Spectrum of mutation and frequency of allelic deletion of the p53 gene in ovarian cancer. *J Natl Cancer Inst* 1993;85:1513–1519.
22. Jacobs IJ, Smith SA, Wiseman RW, et al. A deletion unit on chromosome 17q in epithelial ovarian tumors distal to the familial breast/ovarian cancer locus. *Cancer Res* 1993;53:1218–1221.
23. Bryan EJ, Watson RH, Davis M, et al. Localization of an ovarian cancer tumor suppressor gene to a 0.5-cM region between D22S284 and CYP2D, on chromosome 22q. *Cancer Res* 1996;56:719–721.
24. Gallion HH, Powell DE, Morrow JK, et al. Molecular genetic changes in human epithelial ovarian malignancies. *Gynecol Oncol* 1992;47:137–142.
25. Jacobs IJ, Kohler MF, Wiseman RW, et al. Clonal origin of epithelial ovarian carcinoma: analysis by loss of heterozygosity, p53 mutation, and X-chromosome inactivation. *J Natl Cancer Inst* 1992;84:1793–1798.
26. Schorge JO, Muto MG, Welch WR, et al. Molecular evidence for multifocal papillary serous carcinoma of the peritoneum in patients with germline BRCA1 mutations. *J Natl Cancer Inst* 1998;90:841–845.
27. Harlow BL, Cramer DW, Bell DA, Welch WR. Perineal exposure to talc and ovarian cancer risk. *Obstet Gynecol* 1992;80:19–26.
28. Whittemore AS, Harris R, Itnyre J. Characteristics relating to ovarian cancer risk. Collaborative analysis of twelve US case-control studies: IV. The pathogenesis of epithelial ovarian cancer. *Am J Epidemiol* 1992;136:1212–1220.
29. Ames BN, Gold LS. Too many rodent carcinogens: mitogenesis increases mutagenesis. *Science* 1990;249:970–971.
30. Rodriguez GC, Walmer DK, Cline M, et al. Effect of progestin on the ovarian epithelium of macaques: cancer prevention through apoptosis? *J Soc Gynecol Investig* 1998;5:271–276.
31. Reles AE, Gee C, Schellschmidt I, et al. Prognostic significance of DNA content and S-phase fraction in epithelial ovarian carcinomas analyzed by image cytometry. *Gynecol Oncol* 1998;71:3–13.
32. Layfield LJ, Saria EA, Berchuck A, et al. Prognostic value of MIB-1 in advanced ovarian carcinoma as determined using automated immunohistochemistry and quantitative image analysis. *J Surg Oncol* 1997;66:230–236.
33. Hartmann LC, Sebo TJ, Kamel NA, et al. Proliferating cell nuclear antigen in epithelial ovarian cancer: relation to results at second-look laparotomy and survival. *Gynecol Oncol* 1992;47:191–195.
34. Garzetti GG, Ciavattini A, Goteri G, et al. Ki67 antigen immunostaining (MIB 1 monoclonal antibody) in serous ovarian tumors: index of proliferative activity with prognostic significance. *Gynecol Oncol* 1995;56:169–174.
35. Green DR, Reed JC. Mitochondria and apoptosis. *Science* 1998;281:1309–1312.
36. Korsmeyer SJ. BCL-2 gene family and the regulation of programmed cell death. *Cancer Res* 1999;59:1693s–1700s.
37. Herod JJ, Eliopoulos AG, Warwick J, et al. The prognostic significance of Bcl-2 and p53 expression in ovarian carcinoma. *Cancer Res* 1996;56:2178–2184.

38. Henriksen R, Wilander E, Oberg K. Expression and prognostic significance of Bcl-2 in ovarian tumours. *Br J Cancer* 1995;72:1324–1329.
39. Liu JR, Fletcher B, Page C, et al. Bcl-xL is expressed in ovarian carcinoma and modulates chemotherapy-induced apoptosis. *Gynecol Oncol* 1998;70:398–403.
40. Tai YT, Lee S, Niloff E, et al. BAX protein expression and clinical outcome in epithelial ovarian cancer. *J Clin Oncol* 1998;16:2583–2590.
41. Holt SE, Shay JW, Wright WE. Refining the telomere-telomerase hypothesis of aging and cancer. *Nat Biotechnol* 1996;14:836–839.
42. Shay JW. Telomerase in cancer: diagnostic, prognostic, and therapeutic implications. *Sci Am* 1998;4[Suppl 1]:S26–S34.
43. Kyo S, Takakura M, Tanaka M, et al. Quantitative differences in telomerase activity among malignant, premalignant, and benign ovarian lesions. *Clin Cancer Res* 1998;4:399–405.
44. Duggan BD, Wan M, Yu MC, et al. Detection of ovarian cancer cells: comparison of a telomerase assay and cytologic examination. *J Natl Cancer Inst* 1998;90:238–242.
45. Wan M, Li WZ, Duggan BD, et al. Telomerase activity in benign and malignant epithelial ovarian tumors. *J Natl Cancer Inst* 1997;89:437–441.
46. Bauknecht T, Kiechle M, Bauer G, Siebers JW. Characterization of growth factors in human ovarian carcinomas. *Cancer Res* 1986;46:2614–2618.
47. Kommoss F, Wintzer HO, Von Kleist S, et al. In situ distribution of transforming growth factor-α in normal human tissues and in malignant tumours of the ovary. *J Pathol* 1990;162:223–230.
48. Morishige K, Kurachi H, Amemiya K, et al. Evidence for the involvement of transforming growth factor-α and epidermal growth factor receptor autocrine growth mechanism in primary human ovarian cancers in vitro. *Cancer Res* 1991;51:5322–5328.
49. Rodriguez GC, Berchuck A, Whitaker RS, et al. Epidermal growth factor receptor expression in normal ovarian epithelium and ovarian cancer: II. Relationship between receptor expression and response to epidermal growth factor. *Am J Obstet Gynecol* 1991;164:745–750.
50. Yee D, Morales FR, Hamilton TC, Von Hoff DD. Expression of insulin-like growth factor I, its binding proteins, and its receptor in ovarian cancer. *Cancer Res* 1991;51:5107–5112.
51. Sariban E, Sitaras NM, Antoniades HN, et al. Expression of platelet-derived growth factor (PDGF)-related transcripts and synthesis of biologically active PDGF-like proteins by human malignant epithelial cell lines. *J Clin Invest* 1988;82:1157–1164.
52. Berchuck A, Olt GJ, Everitt L, et al. The role of peptide growth factors in epithelial ovarian cancer. *Obstet Gynecol* 1990;75:255–262.
53. Henrikson R, Funa K, Wilander E, et al. Expression and prognostic significance of platelet-derived growth factor and its receptors in epithelial ovarian neoplasms. *Cancer Res* 1993;53:4550–4554.
54. Di Blasio AM, Cremononesi L, Vigano P, et al. Basic fibroblast growth factor and its receptor messenger ribonucleic acids are expressed in human ovarian epithelial neoplasms. *Am J Obstet Gynecol* 1993;169:1517–1523.
55. Ramakrishnan S, Xu FJ, Brandt SJ, et al. Constitutive production of macrophage colony-stimulating factor by human ovarian and breast cancer cell lines. *J Clin Invest* 1989;83:921–926.
56. Kacinski BM, Stanley ER, Carter D, et al. Circulating levels of CSF-1 (M-CSF) a lymphohematopoietic cytokine may be a useful marker of disease status in patients with malignant ovarian neoplasms. *Int J Radiat Oncol Biol Phys* 1989;17:159–164.
57. Kacinski BM, Carter D, Mittal K, et al. Ovarian adenocarcinomas express *fms*-complementary transcripts and *fms* antigen, often with coexpression of CSF-1. *Am J Pathol* 1990;137:1:135–147.
58. Wu S, Rodabaugh K, Martinez-Maza O, et al. Stimulation of ovarian tumor cell proliferation with monocyte products including interleukin-1, interleukin-6 and tumor necrosis factor-α. *Am J Obstet Gynecol* 1992;166:997–1007.
59. Wu S, Boyer CM, Whitaker RS, et al. Tumor necrosis factor-α as an autocrine and paracrine growth factor for ovarian cancer: monokine induction of tumor cell proliferation and tumor necrosis factor-α expression. *Cancer Res* 1993;53:1939–1944.
60. Naylor SM, Stamp GWH, Foulkes WD, et al. Tumor necrosis factor and its receptors in human ovarian cancer. *J Clin Invest* 1993;91:2194–2206.
61. Fang X, Gibson S, Flowers M, et al. Lysophosphatidylcholine stimulates activator protein 1 and the c-Jun N-terminal kinase activity. *J Biol Chem* 1997;272:13683–13689.
62. Mills GB, May C, Hill M, et al. Ascitic fluid from human ovarian cancer patients contains growth factors necessary for intraperitoneal growth of human ovarian adenocarcinoma cells. *J Clin Invest* 1990;86:851–855.
63. Siemans CH, Auersperg N. Serial propagation of human ovarian surface epithelium in culture. *J Cell Physiol* 1991;134:347–356.
64. Lidor YJ, Xu FJ, Martinez-Maza O, et al. Constitutive production of macrophage colony stimulating factor and interleukin-6 by human ovarian surface epithelial cells. *Exp Cell Res* 1993;207:332–339.
65. Ziltener HJ, Maines-Bandiera S, Schrader JW, Auersperg N. Secretion of bioactive interleukin-1, interleukin-6 and colony-stimulating factors by human ovarian surface epithelium. *Biol Reprod* 1993;49:635–641.
66. Pinkas-Kramarski R, Shelly M, Guarino BC, et al. ErbB tyrosine kinases and the two neuregulin families constitute a ligand-receptor network. *Mol Cell Biol* 1998;18:6090–6101.
67. Weiss A, Schlessinger J. Switching signals on or off by receptor dimerization. *Cell* 1998;94:277–280.
68. Gullick WJ. Type I growth factor receptors: current status and future work. *Biochem Soc Symp* 1998;63:193–198.
69. Fan Z, Mendelsohn J. Therapeutic application of anti-growth factor receptor antibodies. *Curr Opin Oncol* 1998;10:67–73.
70. Berchuck A, Rodriguez GC, Kamel A, et al. Epidermal growth factor receptor expression in normal ovarian epithelium and ovarian cancer: I. Correlation of receptor expression with prognostic factors in patients with ovarian cancer. *Am J Obstet Gynecol* 1991;164:669–674.

71. Alroy I, Yarden Y. The ErbB signaling network in embryogenesis and oncogenesis: signal diversification through combinatorial ligand-receptor interactions. *FEBS Lett* 1997;410:83–86.
72. Slamon DJ, Godolphin W, Jones LA, et al. Studies of HER-2/*neu* proto-oncogene in human breast and ovarian cancer. *Science* 1989;244:707–712.
73. Berchuck A, Kamel A, Whitaker R, et al. Overexpression of HER-2/*neu* is associated with poor survival in advanced epithelial ovarian cancer. *Cancer Res* 1990;50:4087–4091.
74. Rubin SC, Finstad CL, Wong GY, et al. Prognostic significance of HER-2/*neu* expression in advanced ovarian cancer. *Am J Obstet Gynecol* 1993;168:162–169.
75. Kacinski BM, Mayer AG, King BL, et al. *Neu* protein overexpression in benign, borderline, and malignant ovarian neoplasms. *Gynecol Oncol* 1992;44:245–253.
76. Rodriguez GC, Boente MP, Berchuck A, et al. The effect of antibodies and immunotoxins reactive with HER-2/*neu* on growth of ovarian and breast cancer cell lines. *Am J Obstet Gynecol* 1993;168:228–232.
77. Pietras RJ, Pegram MD, Finn RS, et al. Remission of human breast cancer xenografts on therapy with humanized monoclonal antibody to HER-2 receptor and DNA-reactive drugs. *Oncogene* 1998;17:2235–2249.
78. Pegram MD, Finn RS, Arzoo K, et al. The effect of HER-2/neu overexpression on chemotherapeutic drug sensitivity in human breast and ovarian cancer cells. *Oncogene* 1997;15:537–547.
79. Pegram MD, Lipton A, Hayes DF, et al. Phase II study of receptor-enhanced chemosensitivity using recombinant humanized anti-p185HER2/neu monoclonal antibody plus cisplatin in patients with HER2/neu-overexpressing metastatic breast cancer refractory to chemotherapy treatment. *J Clin Oncol* 1998;16:2659–2671.
80. Schwartzberg PL. The many faces of Src: multiple functions of a prototypical tyrosine kinase. *Oncogene* 1998;17:1463–1468.
81. Parsons R. Phosphatases and tumorigenesis. *Curr Opin Oncol* 1998;10:88–91.
82. Wiener JR, Kassim SK, Yu Y, et al. Transfection of human ovarian cancer cells with the HER-2/neu receptor tyrosine kinase induces a selective increase in PTP-H1, PTP-1B, PTP-alpha expression. *Gynecol Oncol* 1996;61:233–240.
83. Cheng JQ, Godwin AK, Bellacosa A, et al. AKT2, a putative oncogene encoding a member of a subfamily of protein-serine/threonine kinases, is amplified in human ovarian carcinomas. *Proc Natl Acad Sci USA* 1992;89:9267–9271.
84. Bellacosa A, de Feo D, Godwin AK, et al. Molecular alterations of the AKT2 oncogene in ovarian and breast carcinomas. *Int J Cancer* 1995;64:280–285.
85. Shayesteh L, Lu Y, Kuo WL, et al. PIK3CA is implicated as an oncogene in ovarian cancer. *Nat Genet* 1999;21:99–102.
86. Campbell SL, Khosravi-Far R, Rossman KL, et al. Increasing complexity of Ras signaling. *Oncogene* 1998;17:1395–1413.
87. Gutkind JS. Cell growth control by G protein-coupled receptors: from signal transduction to signal integration. *Oncogene* 1998;17:1331–1342.
88. Enomoto T, Inoue M, Perantoni AO, et al. K-*ras* activation in neoplasms of the human female reproductive tract. *Cancer Res* 1990;50:6139–6145.
89. Feig LA, Bast RC Jr, Knapp RC, Cooper GM. Somatic activation of *ras*K gene in a human ovarian carcinoma. *Science* 1984;223:698–701.
90. Haas M, Isakov J, Howell SB. Evidence against *ras* activation in human ovarian carcinomas. *Mol Biol Med* 1987;4:265–275.
91. Teneriello MG, Ebina M, Linnoila RI, et al. p53 and ki-*ras* gene mutations in epithelial ovarian neoplasms. *Cancer Res* 1993;53:3103–3108.
92. Mok SCH, Bell DA, Knapp RC, et al. Mutation of K-*ras* protooncogene in human ovarian epithelial tumors of borderline malignancy. *Cancer Res* 1993;53:1489–1492.
93. Facchini LM, Penn LZ. The molecular role of Myc in growth and transformation: recent discoveries lead to new insights. *FASEB J* 1998;12:633–651.
94. Bouchard C, Staller P, Eilers M. Control of cell proliferation by Myc. *Trends Cell Biol* 1998;8:202–206.
95. Baker VV, Borst MP, Dixon D, et al. c-*myc* amplification in ovarian cancer. *Gynecol Oncol* 1990;38:340–342.
96. Zhou DJ, Gonzalez-Cadavid N, Ahuja H, et al. A unique pattern of proto-oncogene abnormalities in ovarian adenocarcinomas. *Cancer* 1988;62:1573–1576.
97. Serova DM. Amplification of c-*myc* proto-oncogene in primary tumors, metastases and blood leukocytes of patients with ovarian cancer. *Eksp Onkol* 1987;9:25–27.
98. Sasano H, Garrett C, Wilkinson D, et al. Protoocogene amplification and tumor ploidy in human ovarian neoplasms. *Hum Pathol* 1990;21:4:382–391.
99. Berns EMJJ, Klijn JGM, Henzen-Logmans SC, et al. Receptors for hormones and growth factors (onco)-gene amplification in human ovarian cancer. *Int J Cancer* 1992;52:218–224.
100. Tashiro H, Niyazaki K, Okamura H, et al. c-*myc* overexpression in human primary ovarian tumors: its relevance to tumor progression. *Int J Cancer* 1992;50:828–833.
101. Knudson AG. Hereditary predisposition to cancer. *Ann NY Acad Sci* 1997;833:58–67.
102. Liggett WHJ, Sidransky D. Role of the p16 tumor suppressor gene in cancer. *J Clin Oncol* 1998;16:1197–1206.
103. Steck PA, Pershouse MA, Jasser SA, et al. Identification of a candidate tumour suppressor gene, MMAC1, at chromosome 10q23.3 that is mutated in multiple advanced cancers. *Nat Genet* 1997;15:356–362.
104. Li J, Yen C, Liaw D, et al. PTEN, a putative protein tyrosine phosphatase gene mutated in human brain, breast, and prostate cancer. *Science* 1997;275:1943–1947.
105. Obata K, Morland SJ, Watson RH, et al. Frequent PTEN/MMAC mutations in endometrioid but not serous or mucinous epithelial ovarian tumors. *Cancer Res* 1998;58:2095–2097.
106. Serra R, Moses HL. Tumor suppressor genes in the TGF-beta signaling pathway? *Nat Med* 1996;2:390–391.
107. Shi Y, Wang YF, Jayaraman L, et al. Crystal structure of a Smad MH1 domain bound to DNA: insights on DNA binding in TGF-beta signaling. *Cell* 1998;94:585–594.
108. Kretzschmar M, Massague J. SMADs: mediators and regulators of TGF-beta signaling. *Curr Opin Genet Dev* 1998;8:103–111.

109. Berchuck A, Rodriguez GC, Olt GJ, et al. Regulation of growth of normal ovarian epithelial cells and ovarian cancer cell lines by transforming growth factor-β. *Am J Obstet Gynecol* 1992;166:676–684.
110. Marth C, Lang T, Koza A, et al. Transforming growth factor-beta and ovarian carcinoma cells: regulation of proliferation and surface antigen expression. *Cancer Lett* 1990;51:221–225.
111. Bartlett JMS, Rabiasz GJ, Scott WN, et al. Transforming growth factor-β mRNA expression in growth control of human ovarian carcinoma cells. *Br J Cancer* 1992;65:655–660.
112. Jozan S, Guerrin M, Mazars P, et al. Transforming growth factor-β-1 (TGF-β-1) inhibits growth of a human ovarian cancer cell line (OVCCR-1) and is expressed in human ovarian tumors. *Int J Cancer* 1992;52:766–770.
113. Zhou LI, Leung BS. Growth regulation of ovarian cancer cells by epidermal growth factor and transforming growth factors-α and β-1. *Biochem Biophys Acta* 1992;1080:130–136.
114. Hurteau J, Rodriguez GC, Whitaker RS, et al. Effect of transforming growth factor-β on proliferation of human ovarian cancer cells obtained from ascites. *Cancer* 1994;74:93–99.
115. Berchuck A, Kohler MF, Marks JR, et al. The p53 tumor suppressor gene frequently is altered in gynecologic cancers. *Am J Obstet Gynecol* 1994;170:246–252.
116. Wang XW, Harris CC. p53 tumor-suppressor gene: clues to molecular carcinogenesis. *J Cell Physiol* 1997;173:247–255.
117. Hainaut P, Hernandez T, Robinson A, et al. IARC Database of p53 gene mutations in human tumors and cell lines: updated compilation, revised formats and new visualisation tools. *Nucleic Acids Res* 1998;26:205–213.
118. Lamb P, Crawford L. Characterization of the human p53 gene. *Mol Cell Biol* 1986;6:1379–1385.
119. Braithwaite AW, Sturzbecher HW, Addison C, et al. Mouse p53 inhibits SV40 origin-dependent DNA replication. *Nature* 1987;329:458–460.
120. Rotter V, Abutbul H, Ben Zeev A. P53 transformation-related protein accumulates in the nucleus of transformed fibroblasts in association with the chromatin and is found in the cytoplasm of non-transformed fibroblasts. *EMBO J* 1983;2:1041–1047.
121. Kuerbitz SJ, Plunkett BS, Walsh WV, Kastan MB. Wild-type p53 is a cell cycle checkpoint determinant following irradiation. *Proc Natl Acad Sci USA* 1992;89:7491–7495.
122. Casey G, Lopez ME, Ramos JC, et al. DNA sequence analysis of exons 2 through 11 and immunohistochemical staining are required to detect all known p53 alterations in human malignancies. *Oncogene* 1996;13:1971–1981.
123. Marks JR, Davidoff AM, Kerns B, et al. Overexpression and mutation of p53 in epithelial ovarian cancer. *Cancer Res* 1991;51:2979–2984.
124. Kohler MF, Kerns BJ, Humphrey PA, et al. Mutation and overexpression of p53 in early-stage epithelial ovarian cancer. *Obstet Gynecol* 1993;81:643–650.
125. Hartmann L, Podratz K, Keeney G, et al. Prognostic significance of p53 immunostaining in epithelial ovarian cancer. *J Clin Oncol* 1994;12:64–69.
126. Eltabbakh GH, Belinson JL, Kennedy AW, et al. p53 overexpression is not an independent prognostic factor for patients with primary ovarian epithelial cancer. *Cancer* 1997;80:892–898.
127. Henriksen R, Strang P, Backstrom T, et al. Ki-67 immunostaining and DNA flow cytometry as prognostic factors in epithelial ovarian cancers. *Anticancer Res* 1994;14:603–608.
128. Berns EM, Klijn JG, van PWL, et al. p53 protein accumulation predicts poor response to tamoxifen therapy of patients with recurrent breast cancer. *J Clin Oncol* 1998;16:121–127.
129. van dZAG, Hollema H, Suurmeijer AJ, et al. Value of P-glycoprotein, glutathione S-transferase pi, c-erbB-2, and p53 as prognostic factors in ovarian carcinomas. *J Clin Oncol* 1995;13:70–78.
130. Berchuck A, Kohler MF, Hopkins MP, et al. Overexpression of the p53 tumor suppressor gene is not a feature of benign and early stage borderline epithelial ovarian tumors. *Gynecol Oncol* 1994;52:232–236.
131. Schildkraut JM, Bastos E, Berchuck A. Relationship between lifetime ovulatory cycles and overexpression of mutant p53 in epithelial ovarian cancer. *J Natl Cancer Inst* 1997;89:932–938.
132. Kupryjanczyk J, Thor AD, Beauchamp R, et al. p53 mutations and protein accumulation in human ovarian cancer. *Proc Natl Acad Sci USA* 1993;90:4961–4965.
133. Brown R, Clugston C, Burns P, et al. Increased accumulation of p53 protein in cisplatin-resistant ovarian cell lines. *Int J Cancer* 1993;55:678–684.
134. Eliopoulos AG, Kerr DJ, Herod J, et al. The control of apoptosis and drug resistance in ovarian cancer: influence of p53 and Bcl-2. *Oncogene* 1995;11:1217–1228.
135. Righetti SC, Della TG, Pilotti S, et al. A comparative study of p53 gene mutations, protein accumulation, and response to cisplatin-based chemotherapy in advanced ovarian carcinoma. *Cancer Res* 1996;56:689–693.
136. Perego P, Giarola M, Righetti SC, et al. Association between cisplatin resistance and mutation of p53 gene and reduced bax expression in ovarian carcinoma cell systems. *Cancer Res* 1996;56:556–562.
137. Havrilesky LJ, Elbendary A, Hurteau JA, et al. Chemotherapy-induced apoptosis in epithelial ovarian cancers. *Obstet Gynecol* 1995;85:1007–1010.
138. Schildkraut JM, Collins NK, Dent GA, et al. Loss of heterozygosity on chromosome 17q11-21 in cancers of women who have both breast and ovarian cancer. *Am J Obstet Gynecol* 1995;172:908–913.
139. Takahashi H, Behbakht K, McGovern PE, et al. Mutation analysis of the BRCA1 gene in ovarian cancers. *Cancer Res* 1995;55:2998–3002.
140. Merajver SD, Pham TM, Caduff RF, et al. Somatic mutations in the BRCA1 gene in sporadic ovarian tumours. *Nat Genet* 1995;9:439–443.
141. Hosking L, Trowsdale J, Nicolai H, et al. A somatic BRCA1 mutation in an ovarian tumour. *Nat Genet* 1995;9:343–344.
142. Futreal PA, Liu Q Shattuck-Eidens D, et al. BRCA1 mutations in primary breast and ovarian carcinomas. *Science* 1994;266:120–122.
143. Berchuck A, Heron K, Carney ME, et al. Frequency of germline and somatic BRCA1 mutations in ovarian cancer. *Clin Cancer Res* 1998;4:2433–2437.
144. Lancaster JM, Wooster R, Mangion J, et al. BRCA2 mutations in primary breast and ovarian cancers. *Nat Genet* 1996;13:1–5.

145. Ewen ME. Regulation of the cell cycle by the Rb tumor suppressor family. *Results Probl Cell Differ* 1998;22:149–179.
146. Bartek J, Bartkova J, Lukas J. The retinoblastoma protein pathway in cell cycle control and cancer. *Exp Cell Res* 1997;237:1–6.
147. Sasano H, Comerford J, Silverberg SG, Garrett CT. An analysis of abnormalities of the retinoblastoma gene in human ovarian and endometrial carcinoma. *Cancer* 1990;66:2150–2154.
148. Dodson MK, Cliby WA, Xu HJ, et al. Evidence of functional RB protein in epithelial ovarian carcinomas despite loss of heterozygosity at the RB locus. *Cancer Res* 1994;54:610–613.
149. Kamb A. Cyclin-dependent kinase inhibitors and human cancer. *Curr Top Microbiol Immunol* 1998;227:139–148.
150. Kanuma T, Nishida J, Gima T, et al. Alterations of the p16INK4A gene in human ovarian cancers. *Mol Carcinog* 1997;18:134–141.
151. Niederacher D, Yan HY, An HX, et al. CDKN2A gene inactivation in epithelial sporadic ovarian cancer. *Br J Cancer* 1999;80:1920–1926.
152. Schultz DC, Vanderveer L, Buetow KH, et al. Characterization of chromosome 9 in human ovarian neoplasia identifies frequent genetic imbalance on 9q and rare alterations involving 9p, including CDKN2. *Cancer Res* 1995;55:2150–2157.
153. Schuyer M, van Staveren IL, Klijn JG, et al. Sporadic CDKN2 (MTS1/p16ink4) gene alterations in human ovarian tumours. *Br J Cancer* 1996;74:1069–1073.
154. Shih YC, Kerr J, Liu J, et al. Rare mutations and no hypermethylation at the CDKN2A locus in epithelial ovarian tumours. *Int J Cancer* 1997;70:508–511.
155. Ryan A, Al-Jehani RM, Mulligan KT, Jacobs IJ. No evidence exists for methylation inactivation of the p16 tumor suppressor gene in ovarian carcinogenesis. *Gynecol Oncol* 1998;68:14–17.
156. Shigemasa K, Hu C, West CM, et al. p16 overexpression: a potential early indicator of transformation in ovarian carcinoma. *J Soc Gynecol Investig* 1997;4:95–102.
157. Kamijo T, Weber JD, Zambetti G, et al. Functional and physical interactions of the ARF tumor suppressor with p53 and Mdm2. *Proc Natl Acad Sci USA* 1998;95:8292–8297.
158. Masciullo V, Sgambato A, Pacilio C, et al. Frequent loss of expression of the cyclin-dependent kinase inhibitor p27 in epithelial ovarian cancer. *Cancer Res* 1999;59:3790–3794.
159. Sui L, Tokuda M, Ohno M, et al. The concurrent expression of p27(kip1) and cyclin D1 in epithelial ovarian tumors. *Gynecol Oncol* 1999;73:202–209.
160. Worsley SD, Ponder BA, Davies BR. Overexpression of cyclin D1 in epithelial ovarian cancers. *Gynecol Oncol* 1997;64:189–195.
161. Session DR, Lee GS, Choi J, Wolgemuth DJ. Expression of cyclin E in gynecologic malignancies. *Gynecol Oncol* 1999;72:32–37.
162. Yu Y, Xu F, Peng H, et al. NOEY2 (ARHI), an imprinted putative tumor suppressor gene in ovarian and breast carcinomas. *Proc Natl Acad Sci USA* 1999;96:214–219.
163. Mok SC, Chan WY, Wong KK, et al. SPARC, an extracellular matrix protein with tumor-suppressing activity in human ovarian epithelial cells. *Oncogene* 1996;12:1895–1901.
164. Mok SC, Chan WY, Wong KK, et al. DOC-2, a candidate tumor suppressor gene in human epithelial ovarian cancer. *Oncogene* 1998;16:2381–2387.
165. Abdollahi A, Godwin AK, Miller PD, et al. Identification of a gene containing zinc-finger motifs based on lost expression in malignantly transformed rat ovarian surface epithelial cells. *Cancer Res* 1997;57:2029–2034.
166. Schultz DC, Vanderveer L, Berman DB, et al. Identification of two candidate tumor suppressor genes on chromosome 17p13.3. *Cancer Res* 1996;56:1997–2002.

3

Chemotherapy Resistance in Ovarian Cancer

Stephen J. Williams and Thomas C. Hamilton

INTRODUCTION

Of the gynecologic cancers, ovarian cancer remains the most lethal, with an estimated 24,000 new cases and 14,500 deaths per year in the United States (1). The most common ovarian malignancies arise from the surface epithelium of the organ. Approximately three quarters of patients present with advanced-stage (International Federation of Gynecology and Obstetrics [FIGO] stage III and IV) cancers, which are surgically incurable. Hence, effective chemotherapy is a critical component of treatment.

Although the survival rate is fairly good when early-stage disease is detected, 5-year survival rates for advanced-stage ovarian cancer remain poor, despite recent advances in the treatment of this malignancy. Table 3.1 summarizes the most common chemotherapeutic regimens and their efficacy. Five-year survival rates for these treatments average approximately 30% for advanced-stage ovarian cancer. Aggressive platinum-based combination chemotherapies are the mainstay for the treatment of this cancer, and they produce 40% to 60% response rates. Therefore, some tumors are resistant to therapy *de novo,* and, even in those patients with initially sensitive tumors, cure is not common.

The underlying reason for the poor outcome of these treatments is the development of resistance and/or the expansion of a resistant subpopulation of cells within the tumor. When resistance is seen, it is not just to the primary agent used; cross-resistance to diverse other drugs is seen both clinically and in drug-resistance models of ovarian cancer. Resistance after anticancer drug treatment has been associated with many molecular and cellular mechanisms. Molecular mechanisms that have been elucidated include alterations in the pharmacokinetic and pharmacodynamic properties of the tumor. These alterations are listed in Table 3.2. In general terms, pharmacokinetic changes include alterations of drug metabolism at both organ and cellular levels, alterations in drug accumulation, and the propensity of tumors to metastasize to areas poorly accessible to chemotherapy (sanctuary sites). Pharmacodynamic changes revolve around the development of cellular adaptations such as increased DNA repair and DNA damage tolerance. Both of these areas are discussed in detail in the following sections.

CROSS-RESISTANCE

It is not surprising that cross-resistance exits among drugs that damage DNA, such as the alkylating agents melphalan and cyclophosphamide and the platinum analogs. To understand this cross-resistance, a brief understanding of the pharmacology of these two classes of drugs is needed. These drugs bind nuclear proteins and DNA, resulting in interstrand and intrastrand crosslinks, as well as protein-DNA crosslinks (2,3). Although these compounds are not cell cycle-specific, in contrast to some of the natural products, cells in late G_1 and S phases are most sensitive to alkylators and cisplatin (4). As shown with cisplatin, the level of platination of the DNA seems to correspond to the cytotoxicity of the drug in a panel of ovarian carcinoma cell lines. However, indirect evidence reveals that certain types of crosslinks may be more cytotoxic than others. This indirect evidence is based on the fact that DNA repair of certain crosslinks and mutations is more predominant, with other, more mutagenic lesions remaining in the DNA. It has been shown in ovarian cancer cell lines that repair

TABLE 3.1. *Response rates to various single agents and drug combinations in treatable and cisplatin-refractory advanced ovarian carcinoma*[a]

Agent used	Untreated tumor (% response rate)	Cisplatin-refractory tumor (% response rate)
Cisplatin	25–60	
Paclitaxel	46[b]	23[c], 21–48[b]
Topotecan	14	18[c], 20[b]
Doxorubicin	n.a.	23[c], 10–30[b]
Cisplatin+paclitaxel	73, 80[b]	53[b]
Cisplatin+cyclophosphamide	60[b]	12–20[b]

n.a., data not available.
[a]Representative response rates are reported from clinical studies of stage III/IV advanced ovarian carcinoma.
[b]Gynecologic Oncology Group.
[c]Gore ME. Proceedings from European Cancer Conference, 1999.

of interstrand crosslinks of cisplatin is increased in resistant cell lines, whereas sensitive and resistant cells maintain the same level of intrastrand crosslink repair (5). Also, the *trans* isomer of cisplatin, which has little antitumor activity, is incapable of forming the major cisplatin-induced GG intrastrand crosslink (6). Although it is generally accepted that drugs in the same class will exhibit some cross-resistance, there have been analogs of cisplatin that do not exhibit cross-resistance; these are discussed later.

The use of drugs with different mechanisms of action led in part to the introduction of paclitaxel in combination therapies for cisplatin-resistant ovarian cancer (7,8). Although taxanes are useful for treatment of cisplatin-refractory ovarian cancer (9), resistant cell populations still develop. Broad cross-resistance seems to be the norm in cisplatin-refractory ovarian carcinoma despite the use of agents that differ in their mechanisms of action (10,11) (Figure 3.1). This seems to suggest some broadly acting resistance mechanism in ovarian carcinomas.

TABLE 3.2. *Mechanisms of resistance to chemotherapy*

Host factors
  Altered pharmacokinetics
    Decreased drug absorption
    Decreased drug activation
    Enhanced drug excretion
    Enhanced degradative metabolism
    Altered binding/transport proteins
Host-tumor factors
  Metastasis of cells to "sanctuary sites"
    Central nervous system/meninges
    Retroperitoneum
Cellular factors
  Decreased drug accumulation
    Decreased influx
    Increased efflux
  Cytoplasmic/nuclear inactivation
    Glutathione (GSH)
    Metallothioneins
    Glutathione-S-transferase (GST)
  Proteins (cellular abrogaters)
    Tumor suppressors
    Cell cycle modulators
    Binding proteins
  DNA repair
  Tolerance to DNA damage

Adapted from Perez RP, Hamilton TC, Ozols RF. Chemotherapy resistance in ovarian cancer. In: Rubin SC, Sutton GP, eds. *Ovarian cancer*. New York: McGraw-Hill, 1993, with permission.

RESISTANCE TO NATURAL PRODUCTS

General Principles

Resistance to anticancer drugs originating from natural products (i.e., vinca alkaloids, epipodophyllotoxins, taxanes, and anthracyclines) has been characterized in detail since the observation that cell lines selected for resistance to drugs of the individual classes also developed resistance to structurally unrelated compounds in other classes. Several excellent reviews have been published of this so-called classic multidrug resistance (12,13), and it is not discussed in detail here. Although resistant cell lines displayed many phenotypic differences compared with the parental cells from which they were

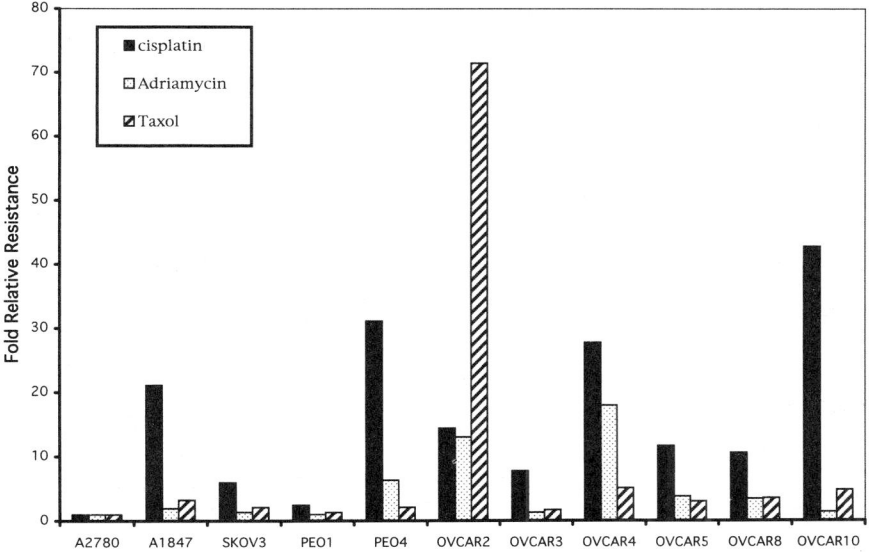

FIG. 3.1. Cross-resistance of human ovarian carcinoma cell lines to cisplatin, Adriamycin, and taxol. Relative resistance was calculated from 50% inhibitory concentration (IC_{50}) values for each cell line relative to the A2780 cell line. (Modified from Johnson S, Laub P, Beesley J, et al. Increased platinum-DNA damage tolerance is associated with cisplatin resistance and cross-resistance to various chemotherapeutic agents in unrelated human ovarian cancer cell lines. *Cancer Res* 1997;57:850–856, with permission.)

derived, reduced drug accumulation was commonly observed. Resistant cell lines were found to overexpress a 170-kDa transmembrane glycoprotein (P170 or P-glycoprotein), which is the product of the *MDR1* gene (14). This glycoprotein, which shares considerable homology with bacterial membrane transport proteins, functions as an energy-dependent drug efflux pump. Transfection of the *MDR1* gene into sensitive cell lines was sufficient to produce the multidrug resistance phenotype. In addition, several well characterized inhibitors of MDR1-mediated drug efflux, including verapamil, cyclosporine, and calmodulin antagonists, have been shown to augment resistance to natural products (15,16) (Table 3.3).

Consistently, investigators have observed reduced drug accumulation in human ovarian carcinoma cell lines selected for natural product resistance *in vitro* (17,18). These cell lines were cross-resistant to other natural products but only minimally cross-resistant with alkylating agents and cisplatin. Resistance was associated with overexpression of the P170 glycoprotein and was partially reversible with verapamil. The classic multidrug resistance phenotype was readily apparent in human ovarian carcinoma cells after selection *in vitro* with natural products. However, the clinical significance of this resistance mechanism remains to be determined.

Given the frequent use of paclitaxel and topotecan in cisplatin-refractory ovarian cancer (7), it seemed possible that P-glycoprotein might begin to play a greater role in ovarian cancer in the future, especially since taxanes are such excellent substrates for P170. As described later, current clinical data do not seem to support this idea. In model systems, paclitaxel resistance has been associated with the MDR phenotype and P-glycoprotein overexpression. For instance, MDR inhibitors KR-30026 and KR-30031 were as effective as verapamil in potentiating paclitaxel-induced cytotoxicity in HCT15 colon cancer cells, yet they had no effect in SKOV3 cells (19). Although cisplatin-resistant cells IGROV-1/Pt0.5 and Pt1 were cross-resistant to alkylating agents, they were as sensitive as their parental lines to paclitaxel, showing no cross-resistance (20). This maintenance of taxol sensitivity was

TABLE 3.3. *Drugs that interfere with p-glycoprotein–mediated drug efflux* in vitro

Calcium channel blockers
  Verapamil and analogs
  Nifedipine and analogs
Calmodulin antagonists
  Trifluoperazine
  Prochlorperazine
  Fluphenazine
  Napthanesulfonamides (W5, W7, W12, W13)
Quinine and derivatives
Steroid hormones
  Tamixofen and analogs
  Progesterone
Cyclosporines
Antibiotics and miscellaneous drugs
  Cephalosporins
    Cefoperazone
    Ceftriaxone
    Cepharanthine
  Erythromycin
  Reserpine
  Dipyridamole
  Amiodarone
Anthracycline and vinca alkaloids

Adapted from Perez RP, Hamilton TC, Ozols RF. Chemotherapy resistance in ovarian cancer. In: Rubin SC, Sutton GP, eds. *Ovarian cancer*. New York: McGraw-Hill, 1993, with permission.

also seen in the cisplatin-resistant A2780/CP8 cell line (21). As expected, P170 expression in clinical specimens is more frequently detected in patients who have been treated with natural products. Bourhis and coworkers (22) found low levels of MDR1 expression in three of ten ovarian cancer patients previously treated with vincristine or Adriamycin (22). Similar findings have been reported by others, but no expression was apparent in any specimen from 35 untreated patients or from 5 patients treated with Cytoxan plus cisplatin (23). Also, no detectable MDR1 expression was found in all but one paclitaxel-resistant ovarian epithelial tumor, whereas paclitaxel-resistant lung tumors showed high levels of MDR1 expression (24). Indeed, a 1999 presentation at the International Gynecologic Cancer Society meeting in Rome (25) reported no relationship to P170 expression and outcome in a large series of ovarian cancer patients. This reveals that the multidrug-resistant phenotype and P-glycoprotein may not play as large a role as anticipated in resistance in ovarian epithelial cancer.

These data are also consistent with clinical observations and *in vitro* data suggesting that resistance to cisplatin and alkylating agents is not associated with MDR1 overexpression. For example, expression of MDR1 was detected in the tumors of 4 of 57 ovarian cancer patients (33 untreated) (26). Moreover, serial specimens obtained from 8 patients showed no change in the level of P-glycoprotein expression during the course of treatment.

Hence, the clinical mechanisms responsible for loss of responsiveness to natural product drugs are unclear. Until recently, natural products were not the major components in the treatment of ovarian cancer. However, with the incorporation of paclitaxel into the first-line therapy for ovarian cancer and the activity of topoisomerase inhibitors in the disease, there will be substantial importance to understanding how responsiveness to these agents is lost.

Resistance to Taxanes

Taxol (paclitaxel) is a member of a new class of chemotherapeutic agents which are of clear utility for the treatment of ovarian cancer (9). Their mechanism of action involves stabilization of the microtubule assembly (27), and they may promote apoptosis by increasing the expression of the pro-apoptotic protein BCL2 (28,29). Taxol is clearly a substrate for the P-glycoprotein, and most tumor cell lines (30) made resistant to taxol have increased P-glycoprotein expression. Inhibitors of the efflux pump reverse this resistance (31). Because the role of P-glycoprotein expression in ovarian cancer seems questionable, many of these models may have limited utility in efforts to understand resistance to taxanes.

The target for taxanes is the β-tubulin of microtubes (32), so alterations in paclitaxel's ability to interact with microtubules might be a mechanism of resistance. Tubulin is made of α and β subunits. Evidence indicates that there are at least six human β-tubulin isoforms, which are expressed in a tissue-specific manner (33,34). In breast and ovarian tumor cell lines, paclitaxel treatment resulted in more polymerized tubules in sensitive but not in resistant cell lines (35). Removal of the β-subunit III isotype resulted in an increase in paclitaxel sensitivity (36), suggesting that alterations in the levels of certain isoforms are responsible for the altered paclitaxel sensitivity. This was confirmed in taxol-resistant A549 human lung cancer cells and in taxol-resistant ovarian tumors. Alterations in the ratios of the various tubulin isoforms correlated with taxol resistance (24). Additionally, altered α- and β-tubulin has been shown in taxol-resistant mutant Chinese hamster ovary cells (37,38).

RESISTANCE TO ALKYLATING AGENTS AND CISPLATIN

Resistance to alkylating agents and resistance to cisplatin are considered together for several reasons. As outlined previously, the cellular target for these agents is DNA and there is a similarity between the types of lesions they produce. The importance of this feature to resistance is seen in the facts that repair-deficient cells are hypersensitive to alkylating agents and cisplatin (39–41) and that repair of platinum-DNA adducts in fibroblasts correlates with cytotoxicity (42). Also, biochemical modulation of DNA repair processes and other resistance mechanisms, common to both drug classes, results in augmentation or reversal of resistance (see later discussion). Finally, selection of human ovarian carcinoma cells for resistance to melphalan or cisplatin results in cross-resistance to other alkylating agents and to irradiation (43).

The complexity of the resistance to platinum and alkylating agents suggests that it occurs by multiple mechanisms. Mechanisms that have been identified include perturbations in drug transport, enhanced detoxification mechanisms (e.g., increased conjugating activities and sulfhydryls), and increased DNA repair and damage tolerance (Figure 3.2). To identify and

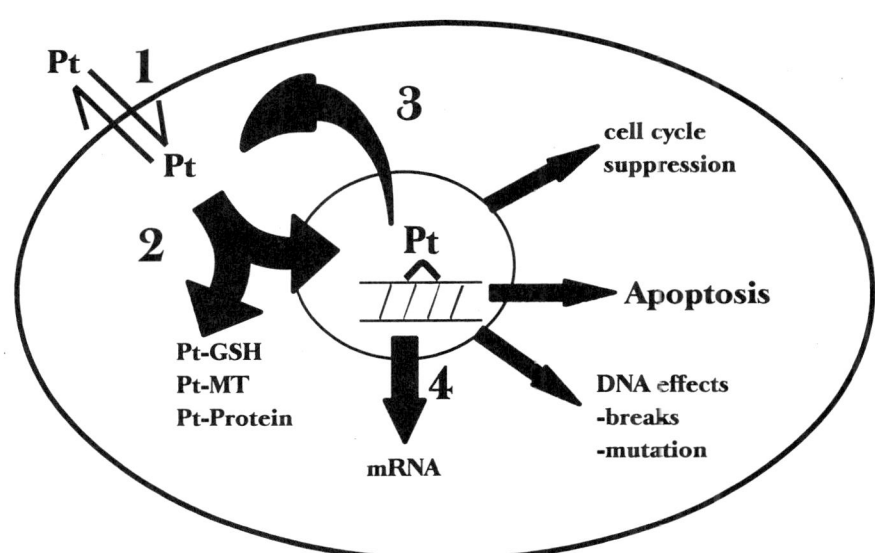

FIG. 3.2. Mechanisms of resistance to cisplatin. Mechanisms of cisplatin (Pt) resistance are shown to the left of the diagram and include (1) decreased influx/increased efflux; (2) inactivation/sequestration by glutathione (GSH), metallothionein (MT), and binding to cellular proteins; (3) increased nucleotide excision repair; and (4) loss of mismatch repair (MMR).

evaluate each of these mechanisms, investigators have used many *in vitro* and *in vivo* model systems of cisplatin-resistant ovarian carcinoma. This review focuses more on the mechanisms of cisplatin-induced resistance, given that mechanisms of resistance to alkylating agents are similar and platinum is the cornerstone of therapy for the disease.

Many advances in the understanding of resistance mechanisms in ovarian cancer have resulted from the development of well-characterized cisplatin-based *in vivo* and *in vitro* model systems. Many nonovarian models have also been developed, which are based on exposing a relatively drug-sensitive cell line to increasing amounts of drug (44–47). This approach may result in individual cell lines with a lower complexity, in regard to resistance mechanisms, than is characteristic of clinical ovarian cancer (48). Most ovarian cancer resistance models also show cross-resistance to alkylating agents such as melphalan (49,50) and have been useful in determining the possible distinct resistance mechanisms for alkylating agents (51,52) and doxorubicin (53).

One resistance system often studied is a panel of human ovarian carcinoma cell lines with quantifiable differences in relative resistance to cisplatin (44). Several resistance mechanisms have been found in this system (54–56). Figure 3.3 shows the sensitivity of these cell lines to cisplatin and the platinum analogs carboplatin and tetraplatin. The platinum resistance of each of these cell lines was determined by clonogenic assay. The parental cell line, A2780, a cisplatin-sensitive cell line, differs in its sensitivity spectrum from its two resistant counterparts, A2780/CP8 and A2780/CP70, which were selected by resistance after incremental, increasing doses of cisplatin up to near-constant exposure to 200 μ mol/L of the drug. Also shown are two unrelated cell lines (OVCAR3 and OVCAR10) obtained from patients with ovarian cancer refractory to cisplatin therapy. PEO1 and PEO4 are additional cell lines obtained from a single ovarian cancer patient before and after the clinical onset of cisplatin resistance. All of these cell lines have been extensively studied (57,58) with respect to their sensitivity and resistance mechanisms (54). As shown in Table 3.4, each resistance mechanism correlated reasonably well with the respective cisplatin sensitivity. The following sections discuss some of these mechanisms in more detail.

DECREASED DRUG ACCUMULATION

Although the clinical relevance of decreased cisplatin and alkylating agent accumulation in resistance is still not known, it is generally accepted that this mechanism contributes to the overall resistance picture. Decreased drug accumulation is common among cisplatin-resistant cell lines (59–62). Mann and colleagues (68) found that decreased accumulation in the human ovarian cancer cell line 2008 was caused by decreased influx. Cisplatin-resistant cell lines that exhibit

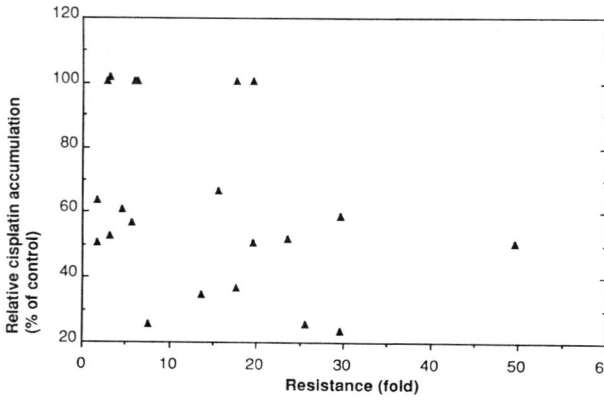

FIG. 3.3. Relative resistance of human ovarian carcinoma cell lines to platinum analogs. Relative resistance was calculated from 50% inhibitory concentration (IC_{50}) values for each cell line relative to the A2780 cell line. (Modified from Perez RP, Hamilton TC, Ozols RF. Chemotherapy resistance in ovarian cancer. In: Rubin SC, Sutton GP, eds. *Ovarian cancer.* New York: McGraw-Hill, 1993, with permission.)

TABLE 3.4. Correlation coefficients relating cisplatin resistance and resistance mechanisms in two human ovarian cancer model systems

Resistance mechanism	In vitro–selected cisplatin-resistance model[a]	Unrelated ovarian tumor cell lines[b]
Glutathione level	0.94	0.13
Cellular platinum accumulation	0.85	−0.11
Platinum-DNA damage formation	0.83	−0.38
Platinum-DNA adduct removal	0.83	0.44
Platinum-DNA damage tolerance	0.99	0.84

[a]A2780/C-series of cell lines derived from the repeated exposure of the A2780 human ovarian cancer cell line to cisplatin.

[b]Panel of human ovarian cancer cell lines derived from untreated or treated patients with platinum-based chemotherapy.

Data from references 44, 47–49, 54–56.

this decrease in drug accumulation also show decreases in accumulation to other drugs. For instance, Shen and colleagues (63) found that cisplatin-methotrexate cross-resistant hepatoma and adenocarcinoma cell lines showed decreased accumulation of cisplatin and methotrexate. A cisplatin-resistant human breast carcinoma cell line, cross-resistant to melphalan, was shown to be deficient in melphalan transport (64). However, the degree to which this mechanism contributes to resistance to cisplatin and alkylating agents and its importance in cross-resistant ovarian cancer is not established (65).

Because the sensitivity to drug is correlated with the number of DNA lesions, decreasing the influx (or increasing the efflux) of drug could naturally lead to reduced potential of DNA damage. Cisplatin enters the cell by either passive diffusion or facilitated transport (66). The uptake is nonsaturable and is not inhibited by platinum analogs (67,68). The carrier-mediated transport is energy dependent, ouabain inhibitable, sodium dependent (69), and potassium dependent (70). This suggests that perturbations of membrane potential may affect cisplatin influx. And although no receptor-mediated channel has been identified for the facilitated diffusion, modulators of adenylate cyclase, forskolin, and 3-isobutyl-1-methylxanthine (IBMX), have been shown to modulate cisplatin influx in human ovarian carcinoma cells (71).

Enhanced drug efflux has been documented in many resistant cell lines. Mann and associates (68) showed a 50% greater efflux of cisplatin in resistant ovarian cancer cells than in their sensitive counterparts. A human squamous carcinoma cell line, resistant to cisplatin, showed decreased binding of cisplatin to intracellular targets (72). Cisplatin-resistant human epidermoid carcinoma KCP-4 cells show increased efflux of cisplatin (73). The cisplatin-resistant human lung adenocarcinoma cell line E-8/0.7 shows an increased efflux phenotype (74).

Mechanisms of cisplatin efflux appear to be passive as well as active. In the resistant E-8/0.7 line and in the C13 resistant human ovarian carcinoma line derived from the OV2008 cell line, it was found that increased efflux is a result of decreased DNA binding as well as higher intracellular pH (74). The decreased intracellular levels of cisplatin were hypothesized to be a result of decreased DNA binding, presumably because of a higher concentration of the neutral cisplatin species, which would efflux passively from the cell in a concentration-dependent equilibrium.

The clinical relevance of active efflux of cisplatin in ovarian cancer is still in question, because most of the data to support this mechanism have been nonovarian in nature. Hybrid studies with cisplatin-resistant KCP-4 cells suggested that the increased efflux of cisplatin was caused by an active efflux pump (75). However, this efflux pump was not P-glycoprotein, given the lack of cross-resistance to known substrates of P-glycoprotein (e.g., vincristine, daunorubicin, doxorubicin). Although cisplatin is not a substrate for the P-glycoprotein, it was found that cisplatin, as a glutathione conjugate, could be a substrate for the so-called GSX pump (encoded by the *MRP* gene) in murine leukemic cells (76). Membrane vesicles from KCP-4 cells showed ATP-dependent uptake of platinum-glutathione conjugates, evidence of an active, anionic efflux system (77).

The discovery of the GSX pump-related MRP2 efflux pump has sparked interest in the contribution of active drug efflux to platinum resistance. This pump, called the canalicular multispecific organic anion transporter (cMOAT), transports organic anions into the bile (78,79). MRP2 and cMOAT belong to the ABC (ATP-binding cassette) family of transport proteins (80). They share 49% homology and substrate specificity with MRP (81). Kool and associates (82) showed that, in cells selected for cisplatin and doxorubicin cross-resistance, cMOAT mRNA expression correlated well with cisplatin resistance but not with the classic MDR phenotype. cMOAT overexpression was independently detected in other cisplatin-resistant human cancer cell lines (81).

Additional evidence supports the role of cMOAT in cisplatin resistance. Transfection of cMOAT antisense into HepG2 cells that stably expressed cMOAT increased the sensitivity toward cisplatin (83). Cells transfected with human cMOAT were not only cisplatin resistant but cross-resistant to vincristine and camptothecin (84). Membrane vesicles prepared from kidney cells and hepatic cells stably expressing rat or human cMOAT can actively transport glutathione conjugates (78,85,86). These data suggest that cMOAT is directly involved in cisplatin resistance and indicate that cMOAT is a membrane efflux protein. In the future it will be important to determine the relevance of this change to ovarian cancer resistance.

DNA DAMAGE TOLERANCE

DNA damage tolerance is a frequent phenotype among cisplatin-resistant cells. This change occurs when similar levels of drug DNA lesions do not produce equivalent cytotoxicity in two or more cell lines (87). This finding suggests that the cell line with more platinum bound to its DNA has greater capacity to repair the damage, has a different spectrum of lesions in its DNA, can replicate and transcribe past these lesions, and/or has an increased threshold for activating programmed cell death pathways. All of these mechanisms appear to be active in ovarian cancer models of cisplatin resistance. In the A2780 model of cisplatin resistance it was calculated that 40 times more total platinum lesions were required to kill 50% of the C200 resistant cell line, compared with its A2780 parental/sensitive counterpart. When interstrand crosslinks within specific DNA sequences were examined, it was found that greater than 17 times more lesions were required to kill C200 than A2780 cells (54). The potential clinical relevance of this study was suggested by similar findings in a series of unrelated ovarian cancer cell lines that varied in their platinum sensitivity (56). In the A2780 system a part of this difference may be explained by differences in adduct types. Additionally, it has been shown that the resistant cells have an increased ability to repair total platinum DNA lesions as well as gene-specific interstrand crosslinks (5,54,55). This latter ability may be especially important, because it has been hypothesized that these lesions may be highly cytotoxic (88).

Studies have also been performed to investigate the molecular basis for this increased ability to repair platinum DNA lesions in the platinum-resistant variants of A2780. Such lesions are generally considered to be repaired by the nucleotide excision repair (NER) system (89,90). The NER pathway consists of a multitude of interacting proteins with three distinct coordinate activities: damage recognition, incision/excision activity, and a helicase activity (91,92). The bulky lesion is recognized by the XPA protein (93), which recruits a TFIIH transcription factor/helicase preincision complex (94). Dual incisions are made $3'$ to the lesion by ERCC5, and then $5'$ by the ERCC1/ERCC4 complex (95,96). The damaged patch is removed, and new DNA is synthesized. This process has been reviewed by Reed (97).

In the A2780 model, examination of the steady-state levels of components of the NER pathway showed upregulation of several NER gene products in the C200 cisplatin-resistant cell lines, most notably ERCC1 (98–100). The functional significance of this finding is suggested by reconstitution studies showing that complementation of cisplatin-sensitive A2780 extracts with ERCC1-XPF protein increases excision activity in an *in vitro* single-lesion assay comparable to levels seen in the cisplatin-resistant C200 cells.

Another important DNA repair pathway is the mismatch repair (MMR) system. This pathway is responsible for scanning newly synthesized DNA and removing mismatches that result from faulty nucleotide incorporation by DNA polymerases (101,102). It has been suggested that this pathway leads to a cycling of futile repair as the MMR system recognizes and repairs the mismatched base opposite the platinum DNA lesion, leaving the lesion intact and enhancing the toxicity of DNA-damaging agents.

The significance of this pathway to platinum sensitivity was suggested by studies in two carcinoma cancer models of MMR deficiency/proficiency. The HCT-116 colon and HEC59 endometrial carcinoma cell lines are MMR-deficient owing to, respectively, the loss of one allele of hMLH1 and both alleles of hMSH2 (103). Adding chromosome 3 restores the hMLH1 allele and MMR proficiency (104). Using these cell lines, Ferry and colleagues found that loss of MMR was associated with a 2.8- to 3.0-fold reduction in cisplatin-induced DNA synthesis in the HCT and HEC cell lines, respectively (105). However NER activity was not impaired by loss of MMR, suggesting an important role of intact MMR for cisplatin sensitivity. This is further suggested by studies using the control HCT+ch2 cells (with chromosome 2 added, hence MMR-deficient), which were 2.1 times more resistant to cisplatin than the HCT+ch3 cells, showing that loss of MMR is involved in low-level resistance to cisplatin (106). The significance of these findings to ovarian cancer was indicated by studies using the MMR-proficient A2780 cell line and its MMR-deficient cisplatin-resistant A2780/CP70 cell line. Comparison of these cell lines revealed that loss of MMR mediates tolerance to cisplatin damage by resulting in the replicative bypass of the lesion (107), as shown in Figure 3.4. However, MMR proficiency contributes to the overall sensitivity to cisplatin by creating more strand breaks and signaling cell cycle arrest.

In summary, it is apparent that cancer cells can develop a variety of ways to cope with platinum-DNA lesions. What is especially interesting is that this so-called DNA damage tolerance phenotype must include activation of an even more pervasive tolerance pathway since, in the models where it has been shown to exist, the platinum-tolerant cells are relatively insensitive to diverse other drugs (108–110).

TOWARD A MOLECULAR BASIS FOR RESISTANCE

Although the aforementioned resistance mechanisms limit the total burden of cellular damage, they compete with damage-initiated intracellular signaling cascades that lead to programmed cell death (apoptosis), conferring sensitivity to the drug. This apoptotic signaling cascade is mediated by a host of proteins, a mutation in any of which would contribute to the ability of the cell to survive damaging insults. Likewise, overexpression of anti-apoptotic proteins in a resistant population could lead to an aberrant apoptotic process. Examples of these include mutations of TP53 (formerly known as p53) and BCL2.

Cisplatin and other DNA-damaging agents induce the expression of wild-type TP53 (111). The upregulation is accompanied by an increase in TP53's ability to transactivate a host of cell cycle regulatory proteins (112), including the cell cycle inhibitor $p21^{Waf1/Cip1}$ (113,114). The role of TP53 mutation in ovarian cancer and in sensitivity or resistance to cisplatin has only recently been investigated. Mutations of TP53 in ovarian cancers and cell lines are common (115,116); they appear late in tumor development (11) and correlate with overall lower survival rates (117,118). Transfection and dominant-negative studies with mutant TP53 in ovarian cancer cells confirm that mutant TP53 results in cisplatin resistance (111,119)).

The *BCL2* oncogene family contains agonists and antagonists of apoptosis (120). The pro- or anti-apoptotic effect is a result of the differential combination of these proteins into homodimers and heterodimers. Overexpression of BCL-X_L or BCL2 has anti-apoptotic effects in a variety of

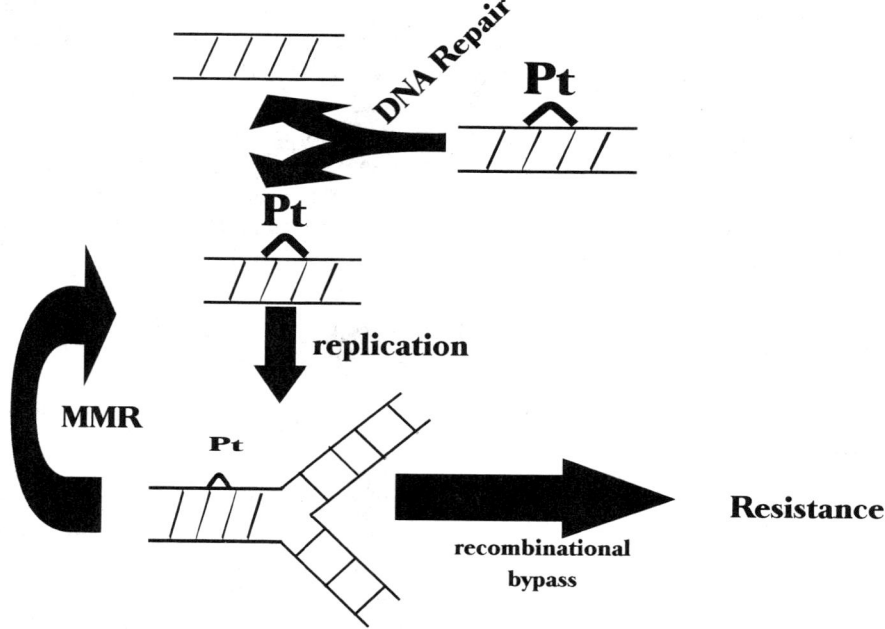

FIG. 3.4. Loss of mismatch repair (MMR) leads to DNA damage tolerance toward cisplatin. The current model explaining the relation between MMR, cisplatin sensitivity, and resistance involves the ability of MMR to maintain the DNA lesion, thereby circumventing replicative bypass of the lesion. In MMR-proficient cells, a cisplatin lesion may be repaired by excision repair or may persist in a futile cycle. However, loss of the MMR activity results in the recombinational bypass of the lesion, conferring resistance to the drug.

cells (121,122). The relationship between overexpression of these proteins and clinical outcome in ovarian cancer is unclear (123), suggesting that a more complex mechanism is involved (124). Although further experimentation is needed to clarify the role of these pathways in resistance, they offer new targets for therapeutic development and new insights into the development of resistance in ovarian cancer.

CONCLUSIONS

It is apparent that resistance to the drugs used to treat ovarian cancer occurs by multiple mechanisms in the models of the disease thus far studied. The importance of altered repair mechanisms (NER and MMR) and modified regulatory proteins (TP53, BCL2, and p21$^{Waf1/Cip1}$) in ovarian cancer drug sensitivity/resistance were discussed here with regard to their individual cellular adaptations to drug. However, it is unclear how these systems may interact, which may explain the complicated picture of the cellular adaptations that occur in resistant ovarian cancer models. For instance, if an MMR-deficient cell, in order to protect itself, overcompensates the lack of repair by increasing expression of cell cycle-suppressive proteins, resistance to cisplatin may be augmented. Conversely, MMR proficiency may promote a cellular environment in which the need for tight all cycle regulation is precluded, increasing the sensitivity to cisplatin.

The cross-resistance to diverse drugs in ovarian cancer was also discussed. Soon after the arrival of paclitaxel in the standard treatment regimen of advanced-stage ovarian cancer, cross-resistance to cisplatin and paclitaxel emerged. On the surface, this may seem surprising, given the differing mechanisms of action of the two drugs. However, one may envision that subpopulations of ovarian tumors could contain adaptive cellular machinery that promotes survival regardless of the type of insult it receives. Alteration of that machinery may lead to increased sensitivity and loss of resistance to the particular drug.

What is lacking is an understanding of which of these mechanisms are relevant in clinical ovarian cancer, and to what degree. It is hoped that the availability of systems such as cDNA expression arrays and proteonomics will allow the gene and protein expression repertoires of clinical ovarian cancer specimens to be comprehensively examined. This information should be suggestive of the resistance pathways involved and of possible targets for drug development. Such information should ultimately result in individualized, improved care for patients with ovarian cancer.

ACKNOWLEDGMENTS

T.C.H. is supported by CA56916, CA84242, CA51228, CA06927, The Evy Lessin Fund, The Adler Foundation, and an appropriation from the Commonwealth of Pennsylvania. S.J.W. is supported by NIH Pharmacology Training Grant T32 CA75266-02.

REFERENCES

1. Wingo PA, Tong T, Bolden S. Cancer statistics, 1995. *CA Cancer J Clin* 1995;45:8.
2. Bellon SF, Coleman JH, Lippard SJ. DNA unwinding produced by site-specific intrastrand cross-links of the antitumor drug cis-diamminedichloroplatinum (II). *Biochemistry* 1991;30:8026–8035.
3. Chu G. Cellular responses to cisplatin. *J Biol Chem* 1994; 269:787–790.
4. Katzung BG. *Basic and clinical pharmacology*, vol 4. San Mateo: Appleton and Lange, 1994.
5. Zhen W, Link C, O'Connor P, et al. Increased gene-specific repair of cisplatin interstrand cross-links in cisplatin-resistant human ovarian cancer cell lines. *Mol Cell Biol* 1992;12:3689–3698.
6. Brabec V, Leng M. DNA interstrand cross-links of trans-diamminedichloroplatinum(II) are preferentially formed between guanine and complementary cytosine. *Proc Natl Acad Sci USA* 1993;90:5345–5349.
7. Ozols RF. Paclitaxel plus carboplatin in the treatment of ovarian cancer. *Semin Oncol* 1999;26(1 Suppl 2):84–89.
8. Pazdur R, Kudelka AP, Kavanagh JJ, Cohen PR. The taxoids: paclitaxel (taxol) and docetaxel (taxotere). *Cancer Treat Rev* 1993;19:351–386.
9. Runowitz C, Wiernik P, Einzig A, et al. Taxol in ovarian cancer. *Cancer* 1993;71:1591–1596.
10. van der Zee AG, Hollema HH, de Bruijn HW, et al. Cell biological markers of drug resistance in ovarian carcinoma. *Gynecol Oncol* 1995;58:165–178.
11. Coukos G, Rubin SC. Chemotherapy resistance in ovarian cancer: new molecular perspectives. *Obstet Gynecol* 1993;91:783–792.
12. van de Vrie W, Marquet RL, Stoter G, et al. In vivo model systems in P-glycoprotein-mediated multidrug resistance. *Crit Rev Clin Lab Sci* 1998;35:1–57.
13. Volm M. Multidrug resistance and its reversal. *Anticancer Res* 1998;18:2905–2917.
14. Nielsen D, Skovsgaard T. P-glycoprotein as multidrug transporter: a critical review of current multidrug resistant cell lines. *Biochim Biophys Acta* 1993;1139:169–183
15. Ford J, Hait W. Pharmacology of drugs that alter multidrug resistance in cancer. *Pharmacol Rev* 1990; 42:155–199.
16. Fisher GA, Lum BL, Hausdouff J, Sikic BO. Pharmacological considerations in the modulation of multidrug resistance. *Eur J Cancer* 1996;32:A6.
17. Bradley G, Naik M, Ling V. P-glycoprotein expression in multidrug-resistant human ovarian carcinoma cells. *Anticancer Res* 1989;49:2790–2796.
18. Rogan A, Hamilton T, Ozols R. Reversal of Adriamycin resistance by verapamil in human ovarian cancer. *Science* 1984;224:994–996.
19. Choi SU, Lee BH, Kim KH, et al. Novel multidrug-resistance modulators, KR-30026 and KR-30031, in cancer cells. *Anticancer Res* 1997;17:4577–4582.
20. Perego P, Romanelli S, Carenini N, et al. Ovarian cancer cisplatin-resistant cell lines: multiple changes including collateral sensitivity to taxol. *Ann Oncol* 1998;9:423–430
21. Zaffaroni N, Silvestrini R, Orlandi L, et al. Villa. Induction of apoptosis by taxol and cisplatin and effect on cell cycle-related proteins in cisplatin-sensitive and -resistant human ovarian cells. *Br J Cancer* 1998;77:1378–1385.
22. Bourhis J, Goldstein LJ, Riou G, et al. Expression of a human multidrug resistance gene in ovarian carcinomas. *Cancer Res* 1989;49:5062–5065.
23. Kavallaris M, Leary J, Barrett J, Friedlander M. MDR1 and multidrug resistance-associated protein (MRP) gene expression in epithelial ovarian tumors. *Cancer Lett* 1996;102:7–15.
24. Kavallaris M, Kuo DYS, Burkhart CA, et al. Taxol-resistant epithelial ovarian tumors are associated with altered expression of specific beta-tubulin isotypes. *J Clin Invest* 1997;100:1282–1293.
25. Aalders JG, Van der Zee AGJ, Arts HJG, et al. Drug resistance associated markers P-glycoprotein, multidrug resistance related proteins 1 and 2, and lung resistance associated protein as prognostic factors in ovarian cancer. *Int J Gynecol Cancer* 1999;9[Suppl 1]:A76.
26. Rubin S. Expression of P-glycoprotein in epithelial ovarian cancer. *Am J Obstet Gynecol* 1990;163:69–73.
27. Schiff PB, Horwitz SB. Taxol stabilizes microtubules in mouse fibroblast cells. *Proc Natl Acad Sci USA* 1980;77:1561–1565.
28. Chadebech P, Brichese L, Baldin V, et al. Phosphorylation and proteasome-dependent degradation of Bcl-2 in mitotic-arrested cells after microtubule damage. *Biochem Biophys Res Commun* 1999;262:823–827.
29. Tang C, Willingham MC, Reed JC, et al. High levels of p26BCL-2 oncoprotein retard taxol-induced apoptosis in human pre-B leukemia cells. *Leukemia* 1994;8:1960–1969.

30. Eck L, Pavich D, Fruehauf JP. MDR-1 expression by human ovarian tumors is associated with taxol resistance. *Proc Am Assoc Cancer Res* 1993;34:232.
31. Isonishi S, Jekunen AP, Hom DK, et al. Modulation of cisplatin sensitivity and growth rate of an ovarian carcinoma cell line by bombesin and tumor necrosis factor-alpha. *J Clin Invest* 1992;90:1436–1442.
32. Rao S, Orr GA, Chaudhary AG, et al. Characterization of the taxol binding site on the microtubule. *J Biol Chem* 1995;270:20235–20238.
33. Sullivan KF, Cleveland DW. Identification of conserved isotype-defining variable region sequences for four vertebrate β-tubulin polypeptide classes. *Proc Natl Acad Sci USA* 1986;83:4327–4331.
34. Sullivan KF. Structure and utilization of tubulin isotypes. *Annu Rev Cell Biol* 1988;4:687–716.
35. Zhan Z, Kang YK, Giannakakou P, et al. Tubulin expression and polymerization in normal tissues, human tumors and paclitaxel (PTX) selected ovarian and breast carcinoma cell lines. *Proc Am Assoc Cancer Res* 1994;35:2326.
36. Lu Q, Luduena RF. Removal of β_{III} isotype enhances taxol induced microtubule assembly. *Cell Struct Funct* 1993;18:173–182.
37. Cabral FR, Brady RC, Schibler MJ. A mechanism of cellular resistance to drugs that interfere with microtubule assembly. *Ann N Y Acad Sci* 1986;466:745–756.
38. Cabral F, Wible L, Brenner S, Brinkley BR. Taxol requiring mutant of Chinese hamster ovary cells with impaired mitotic spindle assembly. *J Cell Biol* 1983;97:30–39.
39. Eastman A. The formation, isolation and characterization of DNA adducts produced by anticancer platinum complexes. *Pharmacol Ther* 1987;34:155–166.
40. Plooy A, Fichtinger-Scepman A, Schutte H, et al. The quantitative detection of various Pt-DNA-adducts in Chinese hamster ovary cells treated with cisplatin: application of immunochemical techniques. *Carcinogenesis* 1985;6:561–566.
41. Blommaert F, van Kijk-Knijnenburg H, Dijt F, et al. Formation of DNA adducts by the anticancer drug carboplatin: different nucleotide sequence preferences in vitro and in cells. *Biochemistry* 1995;34:8474–8480.
42. Sherman S, Lippard S. Structural aspects of platinum anticancer drug interactions with DNA. *Chem Rev* 1987;87:1153–1181.
43. Szymkowski D, Yarema K, Essigmann J, et al. An intrastrand d(GpG) platinum crosslink in duplex M13 DNA is refractory to repair by human cell extracts. *Proc Natl Acad Sci USA* 1992;89:10772–10776.
44. Perez R, Hamilton T, Ozols R. Resistance to alkylating agents and cisplatin: insights from ovarian carcinoma model systems. *Pharmacol Ther* 1990;48:19–27.
45. Perez R, Godwin A, Hamilton T, Ozols R. Ovarian cancer biology. *Semin Oncol* 1991;18:186–204.
46. Perez RP, Hamilton TC, Ozols RF. Chemotherapy resistance in ovarian cancer. In: Rubin SC, Sutton GP, eds. *Ovarian cancer.* New York: McGraw-Hill, 1993.
47. Andrews PA, Murphy MP, Howell SB. Differential potentiation of alkylating and platinating agent cytotoxicity in human ovarian carcinoma cells by glutathione depletion. *Cancer Res* 1985;45:6250–6253.
48. Hamilton T. Ovarian cancer: part I. Biology. *Curr Probl Cancer* 1992;16:1–57.
49. Hamaguchi K, Godwin AK, Yakushiji M, et al. Cross-resistance to diverse drugs is associated with primary cisplatin resistance in ovarian cancer cell lines. *Cancer Res* 1993;53:5225–5232.
50. Mistry P, Kelland L, Abel G, et al. The relationships between glutathione, glutathione-S-transferase and cytotoxicity of platinum drugs and melphalan in eight human ovarian carcinoma cell lines. *Br J Cancer* 1991;64:215–220.
51. Colvin M, Russo JE, Hilton J, et al. Enzymatic mechanisms of resistance to alkylating agents in tumor cells and normal tissue. *Adv Enzyme Regul* 1988;27:211–221.
52. Ozols R, Louie K, Plowman J, et al. Enhanced melphalan cytotoxicity in human ovarian cancer in vitro and in tumor bearing mice by buthionine sulfoximine depletion in glutathione. *Biochem Pharmacol* 1987;36:147–153.
53. Broxterman HJ, Kuiper CM, Schuurhuis GJ, et al. Increase of daunorubicin and vincristine accumulation in multidrug resistant human ovarian carcinoma cells by a monoclonal antibody reacting with P-glycoprotein. *Biochem Pharmacol* 1988;2389–2393.
54. Johnson S, Perez R, Godwin A, et al. Role of platinum-DNA adduct formation and removal in cisplatin resistance in human ovarian cancer cell lines. *Biochem Pharmacol* 1994;47:689–697.
55. Johnson SW, Swiggard PA, Handel LM, et al. Relationship between platinum-DNA adduct formation, removal, and cytotoxicity in cisplatin sensitive and resistant human ovarian cancer cells. *Cancer Res* 1994;54:5911–5916.
56. Johnson S, Laub P, Beesley J, et al. Increased platinum-DNA damage tolerance is associated with cisplatin resistance and cross-resistance to various chemotherapeutic agents in unrelated human ovarian cancer cell lines. *Cancer Res* 1997;57:850–856.
57. Saris C, van de Vaart P, Rietbroek R, Blommaert F. In vitro formation of DNA adducts by cisplatin, lobaplatin and oxaliplatin in calf thymus DNA in solution and in cultured cells. Carcinogenesis 1996;17:2763–2769.
58. Shea T, Flaherty M, Elias A, et al. A phase I clinical and pharmacokinetic study of carboplatin and autologous bone marrow support. *J Clin Oncol* 1989;7:651–661.
59. Andrews PA. Mechanisms of acquired resistance to cisplatin. In: Goldstein LJ, Ozols RF, eds. *Anticancer drug resistance: advances in molecular and clinical research.* Boston: Kluwer, 1994:217–248.
60. Hamilton TH. Mechanisms of resistance to cisplatin and alkylating agents. In: Ozols R, ed. *Drug resistance in cancer therapy.* Boston, Kluwer, 1989:151–169.
61. Andrews PA, Mann SC, Howell SB. cis-Diamminechloroplatinum(II) accumulation in sensitive and resistant human ovarian carcinoma cells. *Cancer Res* 1988;48:68–73.
62. Jekunen AP, Homm DK, Alcaraz JE, et al. Cellular pharmacology of dichloro(ethylenediamine)platinum(II) in cisplatin sensitive and resistant human ovarian carcinoma cells. *Cancer Res* 1994;54:2680–2687.
63. Shen DW, Pastan I, Gottesman M. Cross-resistance to methotrexate and metals in human cisplatin-resistant cell lines results from a pleiotropic defect in accumulation of these compounds associated with reduced plasma membrane binding proteins. *Cancer Res* 1998;58:268–275.

64. Moscow JA, Swanson CA, Cowan KH. Decreased melphalan accumulation in a human breast cancer cell line selected for resistance to melphalan. *Br J Cancer* 1993;68:732–737.
65. Green JA, Vistica DT, Young RC, et al. Potentiation of melphalan cytotoxicity in human ovarian cancer cell lines by glutathione depletion. *Cancer Res* 1984;44:5427–5431.
66. Gately DP, Howell SB. Cellular accumulation of the anticancer agent cisplatin: a review. *Br J Cancer* 1993;67:1171–1175.
67. Gale G, Morris C, Atkins L, Smith A. Binding of an antitumor platinum compound to cells as influenced by physical factors and pharmacologically active agents. *Cancer Res* 1973;33:813–818.
68. Mann S, Andrews P, Howell S. Short-term cis-diamminedichloroplatinum (II) accumulation in sensitive and resistant human ovarian carcinoma cells. *Cancer Chemother Pharmacol* 1990;25:236–240.
69. Andrews P, Mann S, Huynh H, Albright K. Role of the Na+, K(+)-adenosine triphosphatase in the accumulation of cis-diamminedichloroplatinum(II) in human ovarian carcinoma cells. *Cancer Res* 1991;51:3677–3681.
70. Andrews P, Albright K. Role of membrane ion transport in cisplatin accumulation. In: Howell S, ed. *Platinum and other metal coordination compounds in cancer chemotherapy.* New York: Plenum, 1991; 151–159.
71. Mann S, Andrews P, Howell S. Modulation of cis-diamminedichloroplatinum(II) accumulation and sensitivity by forskolin and 3-isobutyl-1-methylxanthine in sensitive and resistant human ovarian carcinoma cells. *Int J Cancer* 1991;46:866–872.
72. Teicher BA, Holden SA, Kelley MJ, et al. Characterization of a human squamous carcinoma cell line resistant to cis-diamminedichloroplatinum(II). *Cancer Res* 1987;47:388–393.
73. Fuji R, Mutoh M, Sumizawa T, et al. Adenosine triphosphate-dependent transport of leukotriene C4 by membrane vesicles prepared from cisplatin-resistant human epidermoid carcinoma tumor cells. *J Natl Cancer Inst* 1994;86:1781–1784.
74. Chau Q, Stewart DJ. Cisplatin efflux, binding and intracellular pH in the HTB56 human lung adenocarcinoma cell line and the E-8/0.7 cisplatin-resistant variant. *Cancer Chemother Pharmacol* 1999;44:193–202.
75. Fujii R, Mutoh M, Niwa K, et al. An active efflux system for cisplatin-resistant human KB cells. *Jpn J Cancer Res* 1994;85: 426–433.
76. Ishikawa T, Ali-Osman F. Glutathione-associated cis-diamminedichloroplatinum (II) metabolism and ATP-dependent efflux from leukemia cells. *J Biol Chem* 1993;268:20116–20125.
77. Ueda K, Suzuki H, Akiyama S, Sugiyama Y. Differences in substrate specificity among glutathione (GS-X) pump family members: comparison between multidrug resistance-associated protein and a novel transporter expressed on a cisplatin-resistant cell line (KCP-4). *Jpn J Cancer Res* 1999;90:439–447.
78. Ishikawa T, Muller M, Klunemann C, et al. ATP-dependent primary active transport of cysteinyl leukotrienes across liver canalicular membrane: role of the ATP-dependent transport system for glutathione S-conjugates. *J Biol Chem* 1990;265:19279–19286.
79. Ouce-Elferink R, Meijer D, Kuipers F, et al. Hepatobiliary secretion of organic compounds: molecular mechanisms of membrane transport. *Biochim Biophys Acta* 1995;1241:215–268.
80. Keppler D, Konig J. Hepatic canalicular membrane 5: expression and localization of the conjugate export pump encoded by the MRP2 (cMRP/cMOAT) gene in liver. *FASEB J* 1997;11:509–516.
81. Taniguchi K, Wada M, Kohno K, et al. A human canalicular multispecific organic anion transporter (cMOAT) gene is overexpressed in cisplatin-resistant human cancer cell lines with decreased drug accumulation. *Cancer Res* 1996;56:4124–4129.
82. Kool M, de Haas M, Scheffer G, et al. Analysis of expression of cMOAT (MRP2), MRP3, MRP4, and MRP5, homologues of the multidrug resistance-associated protein gene (MRP1), in human cancer cell lines. *Cancer Res* 1997;57:3537–3547.
83. Koike K, Kawabe T, Tanaka T, et al. A canalicular multispecific organic anion transporter (cMOAT) antisense cDNA enhances drug sensitivity in human hepatic cancer cells. *Cancer Res* 1997;57:5475–5479.
84. Chen ZS, Kawabe T, Ono M, et al. Effect of multidrug resistance-reversing agents on transporting activity of human canalicular multispecific organic anion transporter. *Mol Pharmacol* 1999;56:1219–1228.
85. Chu XY, Kato Y Sugiyama Y. Multiplicity of biliary excretion mechanisms for irinotecan, CPT-11, and its metabolites in rats. *Cancer Res* 1997;57:1934–1938.
86. Chu XY, Kato Y, Ueda K, et al. Biliary excretion mechanism of CPT-11 and its metabolites in humans: involvement of primary active transporters. *Cancer Res* 1998;58:5137–5143.
87. Eastman A, Schulte N. Enhanced DNA repair as a mechanism of resistance to *cis*-diamminedichloroplatinum(II). *Biochemistry* 1988; 27:4730–4734.
88. Sancar A. Excision repair in mammalian cells. *J Biol Chem* 1995;270:15915–15918.
89. Friedberg EC. *DNA repair,* vol 2. San Francisco: WH Freeman, 1985.
90. Reardon JT, Vaisman A, Chaney SG, Sancar A. Efficient nucleotide excision repair of cisplatin, oxaliplatin, and bis-aceto-ammine-dichloro-cyclohexylamine-platinum(IV) (JM216) platinum intrastrand DNA diadducts. *Cancer Res* 1999;59:3968–3971.
91. Aboussekhra A, Biggerstaff M, Shivji MKK, et al. Mammalian DNA nucleotide excision repair reconstituted with purified protein components. *Cell* 1995;80:859–868.
92. Mu D, Hsu DS, Sancar A. Reaction mechanism of human DNA repair excision nuclease. *J Biol Chem* 1996;271:8285–8294.
93. Koberle B, Masters JR, Hartley JA, Wood RD. Defective repair of cisplatin-induced DNA damage caused by reduced XPA protein in testicular germ cell tumours. *Curr Biol* 1999;9:273–276.
94. Mu D, Park CH, Matsunaga T, et al. Reconstitution of human DNA repair excision nuclease in a highly defined system. *J Biol Chem* 1995;270:2415–2418.
95. Moggs J, Yarema K, Essigmann J, Wood R. Analysis of incision sites produced by human cell extracts and purified proteins during nucleotide excision repair of a 1,3-intrastrand d(GpTpG)-cisplatin adduct. *J Biol Chem* 1996;271:7177–7186.

96. Houtsmuller AB, Rademakers S, Nigg AL, et al. Action of DNA repair endonuclease ERCC1/XPF in living cells. *Science* 1999;284:958–961.
97. Reed E. Platinum-DNA adduct, nucleotide excision repair and platinum based anti-cancer chemotherapy. *Cancer Treat Rev* 1998;24:331–344.
98. Li Q, Gardner K, Zhang L, et al. Cisplatin induction of ERCC-1 mRNA expression in A2780/CP70 ovarian cancer cells. *J Biol Chem* 1998;36:23419–23425.
99. Li Q, Tsang B, Bostick-Bruton F, Reed E. Modulation of excision repair cross complementation group 1 (ERCC1) mRNA expression by pharmacologic agents in human ovarian carcinoma cells. *Biochem Pharmacol* 1999;57:347–353.
100. Ferry KU, Hamilton TC, Johnson SW. Increased nucleotide excision repair in cisplatin-resistant ovarian cancer cells. Role of ERCC1-XPE. *Biochem Pharmacol* 2000;60:1305–1313.
101. Karran P, Bignami M. DNA damage tolerance, mismatch repair and genome instability. *BioEssays* 1994;16:833–839.
102. Sibghat-Ullah, Day RS. DNA-substrate sequence specificity of human G:T mismatch repair activity. *Nucleic Acids Res* 1993;21:1281–1287.
103. Boyer J, Umar A, Risinger J, et al. Microsatellite instability, mismatch repair deficiency, and genetic defects in human cancer cell lines. *Cancer Res* 1995;55:6063–6070.
104. Koi M, Umar A, Chauhan D, et al. Human chromosome 3 corrects mismatch repair deficiency and microsatellite instability and reduces N-Methyl-N'-nitro-N-nitrosoguanidine tolerance in colon tumor cells with homozygous cells with homozygous $hMLH1$ mutation. *Cancer Res* 1994;54:4308–4312.
105. Ferry KV, Fink D, Johnson SW, et al. Decreased cisplatin damage-dependent DNA synthesis in cellular extracts of mismatch repair deficient cells. *Biochem Pharmacol* 1999;57:861–867.
106. Fink D, Nebel S, Aebi S, et al. The role of DNA mismatch repair in platinum drug resistance. *Cancer Res* 1996;56:4881–4886.
107. Moreland NJ, Illand M, Kim YT, et al. Modulation of drug resistance mediated by loss of mismatch repair by the DNA polymerase inhibitor aphidicolin. *Cancer Res* 1999;59:2102–2106.
108. Colella G, Marchini S, D'Incalci M, et al. Mismatch repair deficiency is associated with resistance to DNA minor groove alkylating agents. *Br J Cancer* 1999;80:338–343.
109. Anthoney D, McIlwrath A, Gallagher W, et al. Microsatellite instability, apoptosis, and loss of p53 function in drug-resistant tumor cells. *Cancer Res* 1996;56:1374–1381.
110. Aebi S, Kurdi-Haidar B, Gordon R, et al. Loss of DNA mismatch repair in acquired resistance to cisplatin. *Cancer Res* 1996;56:3087–3090.
111. Lowe SW, Ruley HE, Jacks T, Housman DE. p53-dependent apoptosis modulates the cytotoxicity of anticancer agents. *Cell* 1993;74:957–967.
112. el-Deiry WS. Regulation of p53 downstream genes. *Semin Cancer Biol* 1998;8:345–357.
113. el-Deiry WS, Tokino T, Velculescu VE, et al. WAF1, a potential mediator of p53 tumor suppression. *Cell* 1993;75:817–825.
114. Kim TK. In vitro transcriptional activation of p21 promoter by p53. *Biochem Biophys Res Commun* 1997;234:300–302.
115. McManus DT, Yap EP, Maxwell P, et al. p53 expression, mutation, and allelic deletion in ovarian cancer. *J Pathol* 1994;174:159–168.
116. Yaginuma Y, Westphal H. Abnormal structure and expression of the p53 gene in human ovarian carcinoma cell lines. *Cancer Res* 1992;52:196–199.
117. Kohler MF, Marks JR, Wiseman RW, et al. Spectrum of mutation and frequency of allelic deletion of the p53 gene in ovarian cancer. *J Natl Cancer Inst* 1993;85:1513–1519.
118. Levesque MA, Katsoros D, Yu H, et al. Mutant p53 protein overexpression is associated with poor outcome in patients with well or moderately differentiated ovarian carcinoma. *Cancer* 1995;75:1327–1338.
119. Kuerbitz SJ, Plunkett BS, Walsh WV, Kastan MB. Wild-type p53 is a cell cycle checkpoint determinant following irradiation. *Proc Natl Acad Sci USA* 1992;89:7491–7495.
120. Reed JC, Miyashita T, Takayama S, et al. BCL-2 family proteins: regulators of cell death involved in the pathogenesis of cancer and resistance to therapy. *J Cell Biochem* 1996;60:23–32.
121. Minn A, Rudin C, Boise L, Thompson C. Expression of Bcl-x_L can confer a multidrug resistance phenotype. *Blood* 1995;86:1903–1910.
122. Miyashita T, Reed J. bcl-2 gene transfer increases relative resistance of S49.1 and WEHI7.2 lymphoid cells to cell death and DNA fragmentation induced by glucocorticoids and multiple chemotherapeutic drugs. *Cancer Res* 1992;52:5407–5411.
123. Herod J, Eliopoulos A, Warwick J, et al. The prognostic significance of Bcl-2 and p53 expression in ovarian carcinoma. *Cancer Res* 1996;56:2178–2184.
124. Auersperg N, Edelson MI, Mok SC, et al. The biology of ovarian cancer. *Semin Oncol* 1998;25:281–304.

4

Advances in Biotherapeutic Approaches to Ovarian Cancer

George Coukos and Carl H. June

INTRODUCTION

The recent advances in cell and molecular biology have improved our understanding of the mechanisms underlying tissue differentiation, malignant transformation, and host-tumor interactions. As the pathways of programmed cell death and cell cycle control are being elucidated, several key genes have been identified that play a central role in maintaining the integrity of the genome and regulating the cell cycle. Specific gene alterations have been associated with sporadic or hereditary tumors and cell response to chemotherapy. Tumor cell migration, invasion, metastasis, and angiogenesis are being elucidated at a molecular level. The immune response to tumors has also been extensively studied, and particular defects have been identified in patients with established malignancies. This growing bulk of information has allowed for the design of specific molecular strategies aimed at suppressing tumor growth and controlling tumor progression. Several approaches have emerged as potentially promising, and some are being tested in the management of epithelial ovarian cancer (EOC). These are the focus of the present review.

One strategy targets the tumor cells directly. Gene therapy is based on the introduction of specific genes into target tumor cells in order to cause cytostatic or cytocidal effects. A second approach, also targeting the tumor cells directly, consists of the use of recombinant viruses with oncolytic activity. These manifest tropism toward the tumor and kill the tumor cells by direct infection. A third approach targets the immune system, based on the observation that tumor cells possess specific antigens against which an immune response may be generated. Nevertheless, tumor cells are poorly immunogenic in patients with established malignancies. Immune therapies aim at enhancing immune recognition and immune-mediated tumor destruction.

CANCER GENE THERAPY

Gene therapy is defined as a therapeutic approach that utilizes the introduction of a cloned gene, a gene fragment, or other nucleic material into tumor cells in order to modify the behavior of tumor cells or induce their death. Three fundamental approaches have been undertaken in cancer gene therapy (1). First, the *cytotoxic* (or suicide) gene approach utilizes genes encoding enzymes that transform inactive prodrugs into cytotoxic active drugs. Only transfected cells expressing the specific enzyme become susceptible to killing. Second, the *corrective* gene approach consists of the introduction of specific genes into tumor cells in order to cause cell cycle arrest, induce programmed cell death, or make tumor cells susceptible to conventional therapeutic agents such as chemotherapy drugs or radiation. This approach is based on the observation that particular tumors display alterations in specific genes involved in pathways controlling programmed cell death and/or the cell cycle. Third, the *immunopotentiating* approach introduces specific genes into tumor cells in order to enhance their recognition by the host immune system.

Although gene therapy strategies have been designed based on the identification of specific

TABLE 4.1. *Gene delivery vectors*

Viral
  Adenovirus
  Adeno-associated virus
  Herpes simplex virus
  Vaccinia virus
  Polyoma virus
  Papilloma simian virus
  Oncoretroviral vectors
    Moloney murine leukemia virus
    Harvey murine sarcoma virus
    Avian spleen neurosis virus
  Lentiviruses
    Human immunodeficiency virus
    Simian immunodeficiency virus
    Feline immunodeficiency virus
Nonviral
  Cationic lipids
  Cationic liposomes
  Stealth liposomes
  Naked plasmid DNA
  Gene gun

TABLE 4.2. *General methodology for the construction of a viral vector*

Identification of genes essential for viral replication (packaging genes)
Replacement of packaging genes with transgenes flanked by a packaging sequence ψ (5' end) and a poly-A tail (3' end)
Insertion of an enhancer and/or promoter upstream of transgene (5' end)
Insertion of a reporter gene

gene functions and have yielded promising results in preclinical *in vitro* and animal models, their application in the clinical practice has proved much more difficult. A fundamental problem relates to the vectors used for gene transfer. To date, several vectors have been developed and tested (Table 4.1), but they all have significant limitations related to low efficacy, inability to penetrate deeply into tumor nodules, inactivation by the immune system, and undesired side effects. The National Institutes of Health Recombinant DNA Advisory Committee has approved hundreds of protocols for gene therapy for the treatment of cancer. (Visit the Web site ww.nih.gov/od/oba for details of approved protocols.) The vast majority of these are phase I trials that use viral vectors; some use DNA-protein complexes, DNA particles, ribozymes, or lipid-based vehicles (2). Viruses remain the vectors of choice mainly because of their high efficiency of transfection. After all, viruses already have evolved successful strategies for introducing their genome into eukaryotic cells and using the host cell biochemical machinery.

Wild-type viruses have the ability to infect several cell types, in which they carry out a replicative cycle under permissive circumstances, leading to the death of the host cell. Gene therapy viral vectors have been engineered to become replication-incompetent through deletion of portions of the viral genome that are critical for viral replication. Transgenes are inserted to replace the excised genes, often under the control of a strong exogenous promoter (Table 4.2). A reporter gene is often also inserted to assess the efficacy of gene transduction. The *Escherichia coli* lacZ gene encoding β-galactosidase allows for blue staining of transduced cells after incubation with the substrate X-gal. Other reporter genes include the luciferase gene, the green fluorescent protein, chloramphenicol transferase (CAT), and human placental alkaline phosphatase.

Adenovirus

At present, the most extensive experience is with adenoviral vectors for human gene therapy trials, including cancer gene therapy (2,3). They are stable, they can be produced relatively easily on a large scale (Table 4.3), and they can be manufactured without contamination by replication-competent adenovirus (4). They accommodate inserts of transcripts of up to 7.5 kb. Backbones have been derived from adenovirus 2 (Ad2) and Ad5 serotypes, both of which belong to the wild-type-C adenovirus subgroup. These

TABLE 4.3. *Construction of replication-defective recombinant adenovirus*

Cloning of transgene cDNA into appropriate plasmid (padCMVlink)
Linearization of plasmid
Linearization of adenovirus genomic DNA
Cotransfection of plasmid and adenovirus in permissive 293 cells supplying the missing packaging adenoviral gene (E1, E3, E4)
Intracellular homologous recombination allowing for replacement of the packaging gene by the transgene

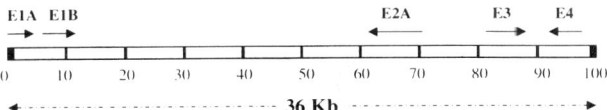

FIG. 4.1. Schematic representation of the adenovirus 5 genome. Conventionally, the adenoviral genome is divided in 100 map units (mu). At either end, there are inverted terminal repeats (ITRs) that act as sites of viral DNA replication. Commonly, the E1A and E1B regions may be replaced with a transgene. Additional DNA can be removed from the E3 or E4 region to make space for larger transgenes and to prevent formation of replication-competent adenovirus within packaging cells.

are nonenveloped DNA viruses which, in the wild form, carry out a lytic infection in a large variety of dividing or quiescent human cells. The vitronectin receptor ($\alpha v\beta 3$ integrin) and a newly identified coxsackie/adenovirus receptor (CAR) mediate the entry of the virus into human cells through clathrin-coated vesicles (5). The viral genome is quickly transported into the nucleus, where the viral chromosome remains extrachromosomal. Transcription is initiated within a few hours after infection, and the viral cycle is completed within 20 to 24 hours in human cells. Adenoviruses do not mediate long-term expression of genes in dividing cells, because the inserted gene is not integrated into the human genome, and therefore the vector is diluted with each successful cell division. In addition, adenovirus is highly immunogenic. Although these are serious limitations for treatment of genetic disorders, these properties may prove to be an advantage for cancer gene therapy (6).

Modification of the viral genome (Figure 4.1) was undertaken in order to produce replication-incompetent strains. The early (E) gene E1 was first targeted, because E genes control viral replication and regulate the expression of late genes. Substitution of E1A and E1B genes by a designated transgene led to the first generation of adenoviral vectors (7). Adenoviral vectors are remarkably efficient. For example, almost 100% of hepatocytes could be transfected after the delivery of 10^{10} particles of an E1-deleted virus in the portal system of an adult mouse. Recombinant adenovirus that is replication defective is produced on appropriate packaging cell lines complementing the missing genes. Because of the high likelihood of recombination events occurring during manufacturing *in vitro*, engineering of strains lacking only one gene was characterized by a prohibitive degree of contamination by replication-competent adenovirus (8). This translated into high toxicity, particularly hepatotoxicity, considering the liver tropism of the replication-competent wild-type virus. A second-generation virus was then produced by adding an additional mutation in the E2A or E3 region (4). This improved the toxicity profile of the vector by dramatically decreasing contamination by replication-competent adenovirus.

Administration of adenovirus is followed by an intense inflammatory and immune response. Activation of human Toll receptor 2 probably mediates the early innate response consisting of the release of inflammatory cytokines such as interferon-γ (IFN-γ), interleukin (IL)-1, and IL-6, as well as the recruitment of an acute inflammatory infiltrate followed by a specific neutralizing antibody and a T-cell response (9). Both the transgene and viral genes expressed by transfected cells are cross-presented on major histocompatibility complex (MHC) class I or II sites, triggering activation of specific $CD8^+$ and $CD4^+$ T cells (10). The generation of an intense inflammatory reaction in proximity to the tumor may not be undesirable, because it may enhance tumor immune recognition. However, immune-mediated vector neutralization may impose marked limitations on the transduction efficacy of the vector. Our group and others have recently demonstrated the presence of neutralizing antibodies in serum and in the peritoneal fluid of patients with EOC that significantly decrease the efficacy of adenoviral vectors *in vitro* (Figure 4.2). The presence of anti-adenoviral antibody titers did not appear to compromise the efficiency of gene transfer in a phase I trial of adenoviral-based gene therapy for pleural

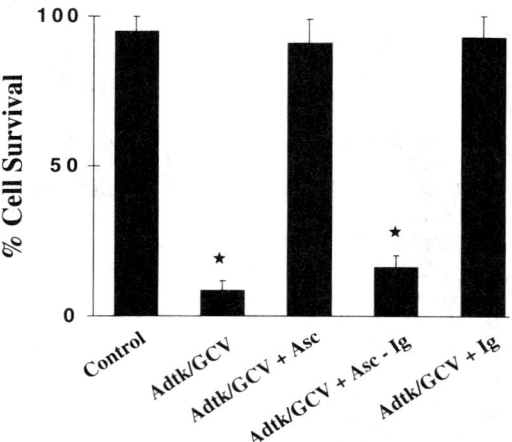

FIG. 4.2. Malignant ascites neutralizes the cytotoxic activity of adenoviral-based gene therapy. Malignant ascites was harvested from patients with advanced ovarian cancer and deprived of its immunoglobulin fraction with the use of a protein-A sepharose column. Ovarian cancer SKOV3 cells were infected with an E1/E3-deleted adenoviral vector carrying the herpes simplex virus thymidine kinase (Adtk) and exposed to 100 μmol/L ganciclovir (GCV). Significant killing was observed 4 days after the addition of GCV (Adtk/GCV). Ascites diluted at 30% completely neutralized the cytotoxic effect of Adtk (Adtk/GCV+Asc), whereas ascites containing a 100-fold lower amount of immunoglobulin lost its neutralizing ability (Adtk/GCV+Asc-Ig). The immunoglobulin fraction of ascites retained entirely the neutralizing ability of ascites (Adtk/GCV+Ig). (Stars indicate statitistical significance, $p < .01$.)

mesothelioma (11). However, there is still considerable concern about the limitations posed by the immune system, particularly when repeated vector administrations are planned. A third-generation adenoviral vector with somewhat decreased immunogenicity has been produced by deletion of the E4 region (in addition to the E1 region) and preservation of the E3 region (4). The protein product of E3 inhibits MHC class I transport to the cell surface, thereby limiting immune recognition of adenovirus-infected cells.

EOC cells are susceptible to infection by adenoviral vectors (12). We recently demonstrated that an E1/E4-deleted adenovirus and an E1/E3-deleted virus had similar efficacy in several EOC cell lines. Adenoviral vectors are currently finding clinical applications (discussed later). Recent investigation has focused on the tissue selectivity of adenoviral infection, and various techniques have been used to enhance tissue targeting of adenoviral vectors. Cross-linking of adenoviral particles to basic fibroblast growth factor (FGF2) was shown to significantly increase the affinity of adenovirus toward an EOC cell line, resulting in a ten-fold enhancement of its efficacy *in vitro* (13).

Adeno-Associated Virus

Adeno-associated virus (AAV) is a 4.7-kb virus that is not autonomous and is not associated with any known disease in humans. In the absence of a helper virus, AAV enters a latent state of infection; coinfection by adenovirus or herpes virus enables AAV to replicate (14). Its genome has at least six transcripts with three internal promoters and two inverted terminal repeats (ITRs). Construction of recombinant AAV vectors can be accomplished by stripping off the gene sequences that encode viral structural proteins and generating a backbone with the two ITRs surrounding the inserted transgene (15). A packaging cell line is necessary for viral replication and production. Several cell types are susceptible to infection by AAV, including nondividing cells (16). Its ability to infect both dividing and nondividing cells may offer a major advantage in eradicating tumors that contain a low S-phase component. EOC cells directly harvested from patients are susceptible to infection by AAV, making AAV a promising vector that awaits further testing in cancer gene therapy and immune gene therapy for EOC (17,18). The major advantages offered by AAV include efficient transfection, high stability, and integration into the host genome. Although 80% of the population is seropositive to AAV, an existing immune response does not appear to interfere with transfection efficiency. Moreover, AAV infection is not accompanied by inflammation or generation of a strong recall immune response (19). The size of the transgene is of importance in AAV-based gene therapy because of the inability of AAV to carry transcripts larger than 4.5 kb.

Herpes Simplex Virus

Herpes simplex virus (HSV) is an enveloped double-stranded DNA virus of approximately 150 kb that is capable of infecting a wide variety of human tissues. HSV enters the cells through at least three identified receptors (20–22). After fusion of the viral envelope with the cell membrane, the virus enters the cell and is transported to the nucleus. Manipulation of the HSV genome (Figure 4.3) has generated a great variety of vectors, including replication-incompetent virus vectors and amplicons (23). Amplicon vectors are derived from plasmids that carry HSV genes, including the HSV origin of DNA replication and the packaging signals, together with bacterial genes (24). Amplicon vectors require the presence of a helper virus or additional HSV-1 genes to carry out transgene expression. Recombinant vectors contain full-length HSV genomes in which various viral genes have been deleted and substituted by transgenes (23). Various strategies have been followed for the generation of replication-incompetent HSV vectors, but some key genes controlling viral replication are invariably disrupted including the ribonucleotide reductase, thymidine kinase, UL5, and ICP34.5 genes (25). In addition, because the HSV genome contains at least 30 nonessential genes (i.e., genes not essential for viral propagation in culture), multiple genes may be deleted without compromising vector production. HSV vectors therefore have the desirable property of being able to deliver transgenes. A unique phenomenon associated with HSV is that of latent infection. During latency, both early genes that encode the regulatory proteins and late genes that encode the proteins required for viral replication are shut off and only latency-associated transcripts are encoded (26).

Ongoing research is aimed at designing HSV vectors that undergo latency in nonneuronal cells. This system may offer unique opportunities for transfection of nondividing cells and the permanent expression of multiple transgenes. As opposed to HSV mutants which are prone to undergo latency, HSV strains that are replication incompetent can still induce cytotoxicity in the host cell by expressing toxic viral proteins such as ICP0, ICP4, ICP22, ICP27, and the UL13 gene products (27). HSV vectors may therefore generate cytotoxicity in infected cells independently of the transgene.

Ovarian cancer cells are susceptible to infection by HSV vectors. We found that approximately 75% of cells are infected at 1 multiplicity of infection (MOI) with an ICP34.5-deleted HSV vector *in vitro*, whereas a comparable infection with replication-incompetent adenovirus required 50 to 500 MOI (28). The sensitivity of EOC to HSV infection was confirmed by Wang and associates, who reported a high efficiency of

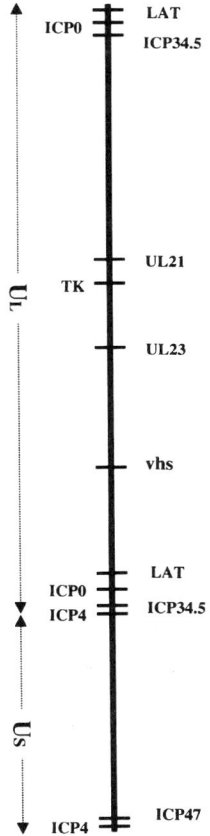

FIG. 4.3. Schematic representation of the herpes simplex virus 1 (HSV-1) genome. Some nonessential genes used in the preparation of replication-incompetent vectors are depicted. Note that ICP34.5 and ICP0 are represented by two copies. The unique long (UL) and unique short (US) segments are connected by inverted terminal repeats.

transduction provided by a replication-defective HSV-1 vector (29). The advantages of HSV vectors include the feasibility of large-scale production, the versatility of the vector system, the ability to carry large or multiple transgenes, and the ability to induce direct toxicity even in the absence of viral replication. The application of HSV vectors may be potentially hindered by preexisting immunity against HSV-1, which is prevalent in the adult population (30). It is possible that HSV-neutralizing antibodies present in the serum or in peritoneal fluid may decrease the efficacy of HSV-mediated gene therapy.

Retroviruses

Retroviruses are diploid positive-strand RNA viruses that replicate in the host through an intermediate step of DNA reverse transcription. The DNA transcribed on the viral RNA template is subsequently integrated into the host genome in a pseudorandom fashion, and the host nuclear machinery is used to produce RNA copies of the virus (31). Oncoretroviruses such as the murine leukemia virus were first used to construct vectors, but lentiviruses such as recombinant human immunodeficiency virus (HIV) strains are also currently undergoing testing. Oncoretroviruses require the target cells to enter S phase, whereas lentiviruses have the distinct advantage of also targeting nondividing cells. Because of viral genomic integration, retroviruses offer the advantage of long-term gene expression (32).

Almost 20 years of experience accumulated with oncoretroviral vectors has proven their feasibility and safety of administration. The major concern with retroviral vectors relates to insertional mutagenesis (31,33). The pseudorandom insertion of genes into the host genome could potentially disrupt a tumor suppressor gene or modify (amplify) a growth-promoting gene, resulting in tumorigenesis, as exemplified by the action of the murine leukemia virus in the mouse. A second potential concern is related to incidental insertion of transgenes into the germline. In the case of a suicide gene this would cause sterility, but in the corrective gene therapy approach it could cause propagation of the transgene into the progeny. Although this result has been described in the mouse, no further animal experiment has substantiated such concern. A third concern is that they may recombine to generate infectious replication-competent retrovirus, with subsequent dissemination to other individuals. The safety of current retroviral vectors has been substantially enhanced to ensure that they remain replication defective. However, as a consequence of these concerns, the U.S. Food and Drug Administration (FDA) currently requires that all patients enrolled in retroviral gene therapy trials undergo lifelong annual testing for the presence of replication-competent retrovirus. A potentially attractive characteristic of retroviruses is related to the lack of immune response after their administration, because retroviral vectors result in the production of one single transgene but no significant viral proteins. In addition, unlike adenovirus, no prior recall immune responses have been encountered in humans. These properties would, in principle, facilitate repeated administration of the virus.

Liposomes

Direct gene delivery of plasmid DNA by relatively inert vehicles may represent a feasible alternative to the use of viral vectors. Liposomes are amphipathic lipids that contain a hydrophobic domain and a hydrophilic domain composed of hydrocarbon chains such as fatty acids. Anionic liposomes do not bind DNA directly and offer limited packaging ability for gene therapy. However, cationic liposomes are positively charged owing to the presence of one or more amine groups and bind DNA with great affinity (34). Cationic lipids are mixed with a fusogenic lipid such as dioleylphospha tidylcholine (DOPE) to form liposomes. Nonspecific ionic interactions often facilitate liposome binding to the cell surface; the complexes cross the cell membrane, possibly through a fluid-phase endocytosis mechanism, but fusion mechanisms may also be involved with some compounds (35). Liposomes currently represent the best vehicle to deliver plasmid DNA into mammalian cells. They are not associated with the toxicity of viral vectors and do not generate as potent an immune response. They are easily produced in large scale. Liposomes also offer the advantage of carrying large transgenes, up to 50 kb, and the cationic types have been shown to deliver transgenes to a large variety of malignant cells *in vitro*. *In vivo*, liposomes have been used intraperitoneally and intravenously and have been proven to be safe. Intratumoral injections have also been described. EOC cells uptake liposomes efficiently (36), and cisplatin sensitizes EOC cells for liposome-mediated gene transfer (37), supporting their use in intraperitoneal or systemic gene therapy for EOC.

A major potential advantage for the use of nonviral vectors relates to the immune response. Although liposomes are reported to be poorly immunogenic, therefore permitting transgene expression with multiple administrations (38), they were shown to trigger a strong direct cytokine response even in the absence of a transgene that induces significant tumor regression (39). One potential problem with cationic liposomes is that they are scavenged by the reticuloendothelial cell system (40). Stealth technologies may need to be implemented to increase tumor selectivity of these agents. However, a major disadvantage of liposome use relates to their poor *in vivo* transduction efficiency, which is very low compared with that of viral vectors. Furthermore, expression of liposome-delivered transgenes is also quite transient. Current research is directed at improving the transfer efficiency of liposomes and improving their tumor selectivity.

CYTOTOXIC (SUICIDE) GENE THERAPY

This therapeutic strategy entails the introduction into tumor cells of a specific gene that encodes an enzyme capable of converting a prodrug into a highly toxic drug. This conversion takes place only within the cells that express the transgene. The most frequently used system is the thymidine kinase of HSV (HSVtk), which allows for the phosphorylation of ganciclovir (GCV) into GCV-monophosphate in cells expressing the transgene (41). GCV-monophosphate is subsequently further phosphorylated twice into GCV-triphosphate by mammalian kinases, to become a very potent inhibitor of DNA and RNA synthesis. Multiple other systems of enzymes/prodrugs have been tested (Table 4.4). The enzyme cytosine deaminase, which converts 5-fluorocytosine (5-FC) into 5-fluorouracil (5-FU) (42), has been approved for human clinical trials. However, this approach is more suitable for tumors that are sensitive to 5-FU, such as colorectal cancer, rather than EOC. A novel "suicide switch" system has been described that exploits the dimeric nature of caspases. Caspases are a family of cysteine proteases that function as the downstream mediators in the signal transduction cascades of programmed cell death or apoptosis. Intra-cellular cross-linking of caspase-1/interleukin-1β-converting enzyme (ICE) or caspase-3/YAMA by a nontoxic lipid-permeable dimeric FK506 analog, which binds to the attached FK506-binding proteins (FKBP), triggers rapid apoptosis (43). This newly developed suicide system may prove extremely versatile and powerful in cancer gene therapy.

The mechanisms of action of suicide gene therapy have been the matter of intense investigation. Incorporation of GCV-triphosphate into DNA inhibits DNA polymerase and ultimately leads to DNA fragmentation followed by apoptosis (44). GCV induces cell death in a cell cycle-dependent manner, because incorporation of the triphosphate metabolite into DNA requires the cell to enter S phase. This provides a mechanism for partial tumor selectivity of the cytotoxic therapy. Cytosine deaminase induces cell death in a cell cycle-independent manner: it converts 5-FC to 5-FU, which is then converted by cellular enzymes into various metabolites, including a monophosphate and a triphosphate form. These cause disruption not only of DNA but also of RNA synthesis. Because of the decreased tumor selectivity of 5-FU and metabolites, a mechanism to increase tumor targeting with cytosine deaminase-based cytotoxic gene therapy might be to link the transgene to a tissue-specific promoter (45). Carcinoembryonic antigen (CEA) is a suitable candidate, particularly in the treatment of gastric and colorectal cancer and potentially for some ovarian cancers.

Suicide gene therapy with HSVtk/GCV was initially expected to affect only transfected tumor cells and was predicted to spare nontransfected tumor. Increased enthusiasm was, however, generated by studies indicating the existence of amplification mechanisms causing unexpected

TABLE 4.4. *Cytotoxic (suicide) genes for cancer gene therapy*

Transgene	Prodrug	Toxic metabolite
Herpes simplex virus thymidine kinase	Ganciclovir (GCV)	GCV-triphosphate
	Acyclovir (ACV)	ACV-triphosphate
	D-arabinofuranosylthymine (araT)	AraT-triphosphate
	(E)-5-[2-Iodovinyl]-2′-deoxyuridine	IVDU-triphosphate
	5-Iodo-5′-Amino-2′-5′-dideoxyuridine	AIU-triphosphate
β-Glucuronidase	Adriamycin-glucuronide	Adriamycin
β-Glucosidase	Amygdalin	Cyanide
β-Lactamase	Adriamycin-cephalosporin	Adriamycin
β-Galactosidase	Cytosine arabinoside (araC)-5′-galactoside	Cytosine arabinoside (araC)
Cytochrome P450 2B1	Cyclophosphamide	4-Hydroxy cyclophosphamide
Thymidine phosphorylase	5′Deoxy-5-fluorouridine	5-Fluorouracil (5-FU)
Alkaline phosphatase	Doxorubicin-phosphate	Doxorubicin
	Mitomycin phosphate	Mitomycin C
	Etoposide-phosphate	Etoposide
Penicillin amidase	Doxorubicin-phenoxyacetamide	Doxorubicin
	Melphalan-phenoxyacetamide	Melphalan
Cytosine deaminase	5-Fluorocytosine (5-FC)	5-Fluorouracil (5-FU)
Xanthine oxidase	Hypoxanthine	Hydrogen peroxide, OH and O_2 radicals
Carboxypeptidase A	Methotrexate-alanine	Methotrexate
Xanthine-guaninephosphoribosyl transferase (XGPRT)	6-Thioxanthine	6-Thioguanosine monophosphate
Varicella zoster virus thymidine kinase	6-Methoxypurine arabinucleoside (araM)	6-Methoxypurine arabinucleoside monophosphate
Purine nucleoside phosphorylase	6-Methylpurine-2′-deoxyribonucleotide	6-Methylpurine
Nitroreductase	5-(Aziridine-1-yl)-2,4-dinirobenzamide (CB 1954)	5-(Aziridin-1-D-4-hydroxyl amino-2-nitrobenzamide

cell death in neighboring, nontransfected cells. These mechanisms have been collectively termed the "bystander effect" of suicide gene therapy (46) (Figure 4.4). Initial studies indicated that it was enough to transfect 5% to 15% of the cells *in vitro* to achieve 100% killing with the HSVtk/GCV system. This observation was later confirmed by *in vivo* experiments and with a variety of vectors. Further studies indicated that other cytotoxic systems, such as the cytosine deaminase/5-FC, cytochrome P450/cyclophosphamide, CPG2/CMDA, XGPRT/6PX, and DOD/MEPDR systems, are associated with similar amplification cascades (47). Several mechanisms may account for this phenomenon. In the HSVtk/GCV system, diffusion of GCV-triphosphate toxic metabolite occurs through gap junctions into neighboring cells (48). This is also true for other systems that generate nonlipid-soluble metabolites, such as DOD/MEP. On the other hand, the cytosine deaminase/5-FC and the P450/cyclophosphamide systems generate lipid-soluble metabolites that propagate freely to nearby cells (49).

Evidence also indicates that additional factors may contribute to the bystander effect. Cytotoxic cytokines released from dying cells may induce apoptosis in neighboring cells (50). Moreover, the Fas/Fas ligand (FasL) system may be involved in apoptosis induced by HSVtk, because Fas, FasL, and two downstream apoptosis mediators such as ICE and caspase-3/YAMA were found to be increased in HSVtk/GCV-treated tumor cells undergoing cell cycle arrest and apoptosis (51). Further, enthusiasm was generated by observations indicating that use of HSVtk could result in the generation of an antitumor immune response (Table 4.5), which could also amplify the effect of cytotoxic gene therapy (52). The use of viral vectors may generate an intense inflammatory response involving tumor cells, which may lead to immune recognition of tumor-specific antigens. This may trigger an antitumor immune response potentiating

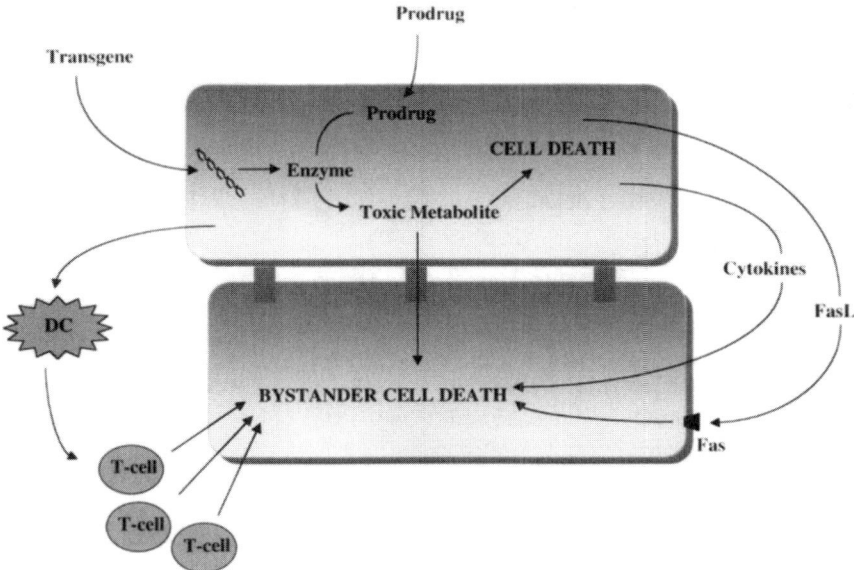

FIG. 4.4. Schematic representation of mechanisms mediating the "bystander" effect of cytotoxic (suicide) gene therapy. Some tumor cells are transduced by a transgene encoding a specific enzyme, becoming sensitive to a specific nontoxic prodrug by virtue of their ability to transform it into a cytotoxic metabolite. Toxic metabolites may diffuse into neighboring cells via gap junctions or membrane diffusion/transport mechanisms, causing cell death in nontransduced cells. Dying infected cells release toxic cytokines and Fas ligand, amplifying the cytotoxic cascade. Furthermore, infected or dying cells may display enhanced presentation of tumor-specific antigens, triggering a tumor-specific cellular immune response. DC, dendritic cell.

the effects of suicide gene therapy (53). Consistent with this notion, HSVtk/GCV cytotoxic therapy proved more efficacious in immunocompetent than in immunodeficient mice (54). The immunogenicity of tumors treated with HSVtk and GCV appears to be related to the modality of cell death. In one report, tumors undergoing apoptosis were not as immunogenic as tumors undergoing necrosis, and the intensity of the immune response generated against tumor cells was correlated with the levels of heat shock protein induced. A specific CD4$^+$ and CD8$^+$ T-cell infiltrate was seen in tumors undergoing necrosis after HSVtk/GCV treatment (55). The cytokine response observed suggested a Th1 lymphocyte response, including IL-2, IL-12, IFN-γ, tumor necrosis factor-α (TNF-α), and granulocyte-macrophage colony-stimulating factor (GM-CSF) (50). Furthermore, costimulatory molecules such as B7 and ICAM were upregulated together with MHC class I molecules in treated cells (55,56).

Preclinical studies demonstrated that ovarian cancer cells are sensitive to the HSVtk/GCV cytotoxic system delivered through adenoviral or retroviral vectors as well as liposomes (57–59). Multiple studies *in vitro* and *in vivo* in the immunodeficient mouse model have documented the ability of the HSVtk/GCV system to induce cytotoxicity, reduce tumor burden, and increase survival (12,60-63). Other suicide systems, such as the prodrug CP1954 combined with the *E. coli*

TABLE 4.5. *Antitumor immune mechanisms involved in suicide gene therapy*

Upregulation of major histocompatibility class I molecules
Expression of tumor-specific antigens
Upregulation of nonspecific enhancers (e.g., B7, ICAM)
Upregulation of heat shock proteins
Upregulation of a specific cytokine promoting TH1 response (IL-1, IL-12, TNF-α, IFN-γ)

nitroreductase gene, have been tested and found to be efficacious in ovarian cancer models (64). We found that EOC cell lines SKOV3, CaOV3, OVCAR3, and A2780 were susceptible to killing by HSVtk/GCV in a dose-dependent manner (65). A single intraperitoneal administration of 1×10^9 particles of an E1/E3-deleted adenoviral vector carrying thymidine kinase under an RSV promoter resulted in significant reduction of tumor burden. This effect was even more dramatic after repeated intraperitoneal administrations (Figure 4.5). Rosenfeld and colleagues (63) also evaluated the efficacy of HSVtk carried by an adenovirus in immunocompetent animals and reported that preimmunization of the animals did not reduce the therapeutic efficacy of HSVtk/GCV. In a mouse model of intraperitoneal ovarian carcinoma, LTKOSN.2VPC cells transduced with a retroviral vector carrying the HSVtk were injected intraperitoneally. This resulted in decreased tumor burden when compared with the parental tumor cells; the therapeutic effect was particularly pronounced in immunocompetent mice.

The use of HSVtk/GCV to enhance the antitumor immune response in ovarian cancer was explored by Freeman and colleagues (66). They engineered the PA-1 human ovarian teratocarcinoma cell line to express HSVtk through retroviral transduction. Intraperitoneal inoculation of these cells in mice, followed by GCV treatment, led to the regression of established intraperitoneal adenocarcinoma. Bystander and/or immune mechanisms probably mediated the tumor response, because established tumors were not directly transduced with HSVtk. It is possible that inflammation in proximity to tumor may contribute to breaking tolerance to the tumor and generation of the immune response. In fact, histologic analysis of tumors revealed that PA-1 cells were adherent on tumor nodules and an intense inflammatory reaction had developed within tumors where PA-1 cells had adhered.

Based on promising preclinical studies, clinical trials using HSVtk/GCV cytotoxic gene therapy have been implemented in patients with advanced or recurrent EOC (67) (Table 4.6). Dose-escalation studies with intraperitoneal administration of an adenoviral vector carrying HSVtk have indicated that this strategy is safe, but no significant tumor responses have yet been reported. Ongoing studies are assessing the therapeutic efficacy of this approach.

Several strategies have been implemented to improve the efficacy of suicide gene therapy. One approach is to improve the efficacy of the promoter. There is convincing evidence *in vitro* that the choice of the promoter has a role in the efficacy of tk transduction and the ultimate outcome of the treatment (68). An approach undertaken by Rancourt and associates entails the cross-linking of adenoviral vectors with specific ligands for cell surface receptors expressed on tumor cells (13). Preliminary evidence indicates

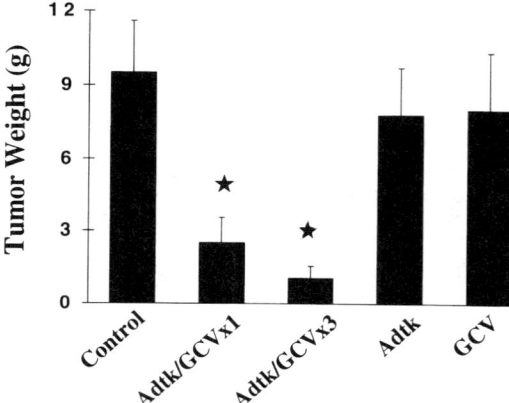

FIG. 4.5. Adenoviral-mediated suicide gene therapy results in tumor control *in vivo*. Human ovarian cancer A2780 tumors were established intraperitoneally (i.p.) in severe combined immunodeficient (SCID) mice. A group of mice were inoculated i.p. with 1×10^9 pfu of E1/E3-deleted adenoviral vector carrying the herpes simplex virus thymide kinase (Adtk) and treated with ganciclovir (GCV) for 10 days (Adtk/GCV×1). Another group of mice were treated with 1×10^9 pfu Adtk and GCV for three consecutive cycles (Adtk/GCV×3). Control animals were not treated, and additional control groups were inoculated with Adtk but did not receive GCV (Adtk) or were treated with GCV without prior inoculation of the vector (GCV). Mice treated with Adtk/GCV one time displayed significantly lower tumor burden than control animals (*left star, p < .01*). Mice treated with Adtk/GCV three times displayed significantly lower tumor burden compared with animals treated once (*right star, p < .05*).

TABLE 4.6. *Gene therapy approaches tested clinically in ovarian cancer*[a]

Gene	Rationale
Herpes simplex virus–thymidine kinase	Cancer cells transduced with thymidine kinase die after administration of ganciclovir. Bystander killing mechanisms mediated by toxic metabolites and cytokines amplify the toxic effect. A T-cell response may be triggered against the tumor.
p53	More than 50% of advanced ovarian cancers display loss of p53. Overexpression of p53 induces apoptosis or cell cycle arrest and sensitizes cancer cells to chemotherapy drugs. Bystander mechanisms of cell killing and inhibition of angiogenesis may also occur.
BRCA1	Overexpression of BRCA1 in sporadic ovarian cancer cells induces tumor growth suppression.
Adenoviral E1A	Approximately 30% of ovarian cancers overexpress the HER-2/neu proto-oncogene. Adenoviral E1A gene product counteracts HER-2 protein and inhibits tumor growth in ovarian cancer cells overexpressing HER-2/neu.
Gene encoding an anti–HER-2/neu single-chain intracellular antibody	Expression of the gene results in decreased expression of surface HER-2 and induces growth suppression in ovarian cancer cells overexpressing HER-2/neu.

[a] For an up-dated reference on current clinical trials, visit the Web sites www.ovarian.org/, www.centerwatch.com/, or cancertrials.nci.nih.gov/.

that cross-linking of adenovirus carrying HSVtk to basic FGF leads to a ten-fold increase in transduction efficacy in ovarian carcinoma cell lines. An attractive vehicle for the intraperitoneal delivery of gene therapy may be represented by microspheres of biodegradable polymer such as l-lactide/glycolide copolymer (PLG) (69). This material has previously been tested and proven safe for the intraperitoneal delivery of chemotherapy drugs. Biodegradable polymer microspheres release suspended drugs at a sustained fashion, depending on the rate of degradation of the polymer and the stability of the drug. The theoretic advantage of this delivery system relates to problems inherent to intraperitoneal drug delivery, which is often hampered by adhesion formation. If the spheres are administered shortly after a surgical procedure, they are able to coat and provide sustained release of a drug to peritoneal (tumor) surfaces to which access later will be precluded because of the formation of peritoneal adhesions. A 1999 report indicates that suspension of adenovirus vector in copolymer microspheres is feasible and does not compromise the stability of the vector (70). We recently provided evidence that GCV may also be suspended in PLG microspheres, resulting in significantly increased efficacy *in vitro* against EOC cells transfected with adenovirus carrying the HSVtk (71). It is possible that application of this technology may result in optimization of the conditions of intraperitoneal gene therapy. Finally, the combination of cytotoxic HSVtk/GCV gene therapy with conventional chemotherapy agents may significantly improve the therapeutic efficacy of chemotherapy drugs through a possible synergistic effect (72).

CORRECTIVE GENE THERAPY

The information accumulated regarding the genetic alterations of cancer has encouraged gene therapy approaches aimed at correcting specific molecular defects in cancer. Corrective gene therapy strategies may be categorized in two main approaches: replacement and neutralization. In tumors with documented loss of a gene function, wild-type genes are delivered to achieve normal levels of expression or overexpression of the wild-type gene within tumor cells, resulting in apoptosis or cell cycle arrest (Table 4.7). Examples include the administration of p16, p21, p53, and BRCA1 genes. In tumors with documented overexpression of oncogenes, ablative gene therapies may be carried out to neutralize oncogene function (73) (Table 4.8).

A large number of solid tumors, including approximately 50% to 75% of specimens from patients with EOC, have been shown to harbor alterations in the p53 tumor suppressor gene,

TABLE 4.7. *Genes used in corrective gene therapy for cancer*

Gene	Action
p53	Induces apoptosis (upregulates Bax, down-regulates Bcl-2). Induces cell cycle arrest (upregulates p21 and Gadd45). Blocks DNA replication and transcription.
p21	Induces cell cycle arrest (inhibits cyclin D kinase, inactivates retinoblastoma [Rb] gene and PCNA).
p16	Induces cell cycle arrest downstream of p21 (inhibits cyclin D).
BRCA1	Induces cell cycle arrest (interacts with p21 and Rb).
Bax	Induces apoptosis downstream of p53 (induces activation of caspases).
ICE	(Interleukin-1β converting enzyme). Large family of proteases that induce apoptosis (cleave a large number of regulatory proteins).
Rb	Induces cell cycle arrest and loss of *in vivo* tumorigenic potential (inhibits E2F transcription factor, c-*myc* and c-*fos*).
Bcl-X_s	Induces apoptosis (binds to and inhibits Bcl-2 or Bcl-X_L).

leading to defective apoptosis and alterations in cell cycle control. Loss of p53 is believed to represent a fairly late event in multistep carcinogenesis leading to ovarian cancer, but it may contribute to chemotherapy resistance and represents an independent prognostic factor for poor outcomes (74). Other molecular alterations of genes partaking in cell cycle control have been identified in ovarian cancer, namely p21 and p16 cyclin inhibitors. Approximately 30% of EOC specimens have been shown to overexpress HER-2/neu protein (75), an epidermal growth factor receptor-related protein that is involved in uninhibited tumor growth and malignant transformation. Several oncogenes, such as H-ras and c-myc, are overexpressed in ovarian cancer (74). The molecular aspects of hereditary ovarian cancer have been partially elucidated with the identification and cloning of the BRCA1 and BRCA2 genes, which appear to be mutated in a proportion of patients with hereditary breast and ovarian cancer syndrome. Although the function of their protein products has not been entirely elucidated, BRCA1 appears to be involved in DNA repair and tumor suppressor pathways.

The observation that BRCA1 blocks cell cycle progression via p21 (76) and causes tumor growth inhibition via the retinoblastoma (Rb) gene (77) led to preclinical gene therapy studies with a splice variant of the wild-type BRCA1 gene (BRCA1sv) delivered via a retroviral vector to EOCs *in vitro* and to animals bearing established ovarian cancer (78). These studies indicated that overexpression of BRCA1 induced arrest of tumor growth. A phase I clinical trial was then carried out at Vanderbilt University Cancer

TABLE 4.8. *Targets of gene suppressive strategies*

Gene	Action
HER-2/neu	Encodes human epidermal growth factor receptor 2 (HER-2), a membrane tyrosine kinase receptor promoting cell replication. HER-2 overexpression is associated with malignant transformation. It is overexpressed in approximately 30% of ovarian cancers.
c-fos	Proto-oncogene encoding a portion of AP-1 transcription factor mediating postreceptor activation of mitogenic pathways normally activated in growth factor-stimulated cells; activates cell proliferation.
c-myc	Proto-oncogene encoding a transcription factor activating mitogenic pathways.
K-ras	Proto-oncogene encoding a guanosine triphosphate-binding protein mediating activation of mitogenic pathways including activation of Raf protein-serine kinase and MAP kinase pathways; is overexpressed in ovarian mucinous adenocarcinomas.
Bcl-2	Major anti-apoptotic factor. Promotes cell survival by counteracting p53-dependent and p53-independent apoptosis. Implicated in chemotherapy resistance.
Bcl-X_L	Promotes cell survival and chemotherapy resistance; counteracts p53-dependent and p53-independent apoptosis.
NF-κB	Transcription factor involved in lymphocyte activation. Overexpressed in many solid tumors. Inhibits apoptosis.
VEGF	Promotes tumor angiogenesis. Inhibits T-cell and dendritic cell maturation and function.

Center, including patients with sporadic, recurrent, or persistent ovarian cancer (79). None of these patients harbored germline mutations in the BRCA1 gene. Patients received one to three intraperitoneal injections of a retroviral vector carrying the BRCA1sv gene at a dose of 10^8 to 10^{10} vector particles. Toxicity was limited: self-limiting clinical peritonitis was observed in 25% of the patients. An antiretroviral antibody response was seen at the higher doses, and gene transfer was documented by Southern blot in approximately 5% to 10% of tumor cells in laparoscopic biopsy material. Of 12 initially reported patients, 4 progressed, 7 displayed stable disease, and 1 demonstrated a partial response.

Gene therapy with tumor suppressor genes and genes involved in control of the cell cycle have also been tested in EOC and other solid malignancies. In vitro and in vivo experiments showed that Bax, a pro-apoptotic gene that is a transcriptional target of p53 (80), and p16, a cyclin D inhibitor involved in regulation of the cell cycle (81), may be appropriate targets for corrective gene therapy. However, most experience to date is with the p53 tumor suppressor gene. Preclinical evidence suggests that p53 corrective gene therapy via adenoviral or retroviral vectors or liposome-plasmid DNA complexes results in an increased amount of apoptosis or cell cycle arrest in EOC cells in vitro; in addition, tumor regression was seen in vivo in intraperitoneal mouse models (82–84). Moreover, EOC cells transfected with the wild-type p53 gene become more sensitive to DNA-damaging agents such as platinum (85), and a synergistic effect between adenovirus-delivered p53 and platinum was described (86). A surprising synergistic effect of p53 overexpression with paclitaxel has also been described in EOC in vitro (87). Bystander mechanisms including the release of toxic metabolites and/or cytokines from apoptotic cells as well as inhibition of tumor angiogenesis have been implicated in p53 gene therapy, because decreased expression of vascular endothelial growth factor (VEGF) (88) and increased Fas/FasL (89) have been observed in cancer cells after exposure to adenovirus-carrying wild-type p53.

The group of Roth and colleagues at the M.D. Anderson Cancer Center at the University of Texas has accumulated significant clinical experience with p53 gene therapy in non-squamous-cell lung cancer (NSCLC). Early studies confirmed the safety of intratumoral bronchoscopic administration of the adenoviral vector. This group recently published results on 52 patients with NSCLC who received Ad. p53 by intratumoral injection with or without cisplatin. The vector was administered bronchoscopically or under computed tomographic guidance monthly for 6 months. The authors documented transgene expression in p53⁻ tumors and observed partial responses or tumor stabilization in 16 of 26 patients who received Ad.p53 alone. The addition of cisplatin increased the progression-free survival rate (90). Adenoviral p53 gene therapy has also been initiated in patients with EOC: 37 heavily pretreated women received intraperitoneal inoculation of p53 at a single dose of 7.5×10^{10} to 7.5×10^{13} particle-forming units (pfu). No significant complications were seen, and reductions in CA125 were observed in more than half of the patients (91).

Neutralization gene therapy strategies target overexpressed oncogenes with ribozymes, triplex-forming or anti-sense oligonucleotides, and intracellular antibodies. Hammerhead ribozymes are catalytic RNA sequences of at least 20 to 30 ribonucleotides that bind to specific mRNA molecules and mediate their enzymatic cleavage (92). AT- and GC-rich stretches of DNA are prone to formation of stable triple helices, which results in their functional inactivation due to disruption of recognition and binding of their cognate transcription factors. Triplex-forming oligonucleotides may be engineered to target specific DNA sequences of oncogenes or growth factors (93). Antisense oligonucleotides are short nucleotide sequences synthesized in a complementary fashion to targeted mRNA sequences, which they bind and inactivate (94). K-ras oncogene mutations have been observed in some mucinous ovarian cancers, whereas c-myc amplification occurs in approximately 30% of ovarian cancers and is especially prevalent in serous adeno-carcinomas (74). The latter oncogene could therefore represent a suitable target for knockout strategies in specific patients.

HER-2/neu (c-erbB-2) is an oncogene that encodes a 185-kDa epidermal growth factor receptor-related protein with tyrosine kinase activity (95) that is overexpressed in about 30% of EOCs (74, 75) and other solid tumors. HER-2/neu overexpression is correlated with malignant transformation and metastasis (96). Therapy with trastuzumab (Herceptin; Genentech, San Francisco, CA), a monoclonal antibody directed against HER-2/neu, has been recently approved by the FDA for breast cancer treatment and is currently being tested experimentally in patients with EOC. An interesting strategy of HER-2/neu oncogene neutralization has been designed by DeShane and colleagues, who engineered a gene encoding a monoclonal single-chain antibody (sFv) against HER-2/neu (97), which remains expressed in an intracytoplasmic location. Measurable levels of intracytoplasmic antibody were obtained after transfection of EOC cells with the gene. This was associated with decreased cell surface expression of HER-2/neu, probably because of entrapment of newly synthesized receptors within the endoplasmic reticulum. Preclinical data in the mouse showed regression of intraperitoneal tumors (98) and led to the initiation of a phase I clinical trial at the University of Alabama (99).

The adenoviral E1A gene product specifically suppresses the HER-2/neu promoter and functions as a tumor suppressor gene in tumors overexpressing HER-2/neu (100). Stable transfection of SKOV3.ip1 cells with the E1A gene led to a dramatic reduction of the malignant phenotype *in vitro* and *in vivo* (101). A replication-incompetent adenoviral vector with an intact E1A gene (Ad.E1A$^+$) lacking E1B and E3 administered intraperitoneally to immunosuppressed mice bearing EOC tumors in intratumoral expression of the E1A protein product, suppressed expression of HER-2/neu, and prolonged survival (102). A phase I clinical trial with adenoviral E1A delivered through liposomes was initiated at the M.D. Anderson Cancer Center in patients with metastatic breast or ovarian cancer with documented overexpression of HER-2/neu. Cationic liposomes carrying E1A were delivered weekly starting at an intraperitoneal dose of 1.8 mg/m^2. The study reached a maximal tolerated dose of 3.6 mg/m^2, and in several patients there was disease stabilization. Downregulation of HER-2/neu was observed in two patients, and E1A gene expression was documented in tumors and in normal organs such as kidney, lungs, and liver (57).

ONCOLYTIC AGENTS

Unlike gene therapy, the direct treatment of tumors with replication-competent viruses is not a novel idea. A number of studies were undertaken in the 1950s and 1960s with direct intratumoral injections of wild-type viruses, with limited success. The viral approaches were abandoned because of the inability to manipulate viruses. With the advent of molecular biology and recombinant technologies, mutant viruses have been generated, renewing the interest in virus-based oncolytic tumor therapies. Many viruses have been used experimentally, including HSV-1, adenovirus, Newcastle disease virus (NDV), influenza virus, vaccinia virus, and vesicular stomatitis virus. Here we update recent advances with direct intratumoral injections of HSV and adenovirus. Later we review recent studies with viral oncolysates prepared by *in vitro* infection of tumors.

Replication-restricted HSV-1 mutants have been generated in several laboratories by alteration of genes controlling viral replication, such as tk (UL23) (103–105) or the ICP6 gene (UL39) that encodes the large subunit of HSV ribonucleotide reductase (106). UL23 and UL39 mutants have shown tumor selectivity for neuronal (104,107) and nonneuronal (108) malignancies. HSV oncolytic agents have also been generated by alterations of both copies of the RL1 gene (109–111). Its product, the ICP34.5 protein, is critical for neurovirulence (112,113) and plays an important role in viral replication (114), viral exit from infected cells (115), and prevention of the premature shutoff of protein synthesis in the infected host cells (116).

Recombinant replication-competent HSV-1 mutants are emerging as potent oncolytic agents. Initially they were designed for the treatment of central nervous system (CNS) tumors (104). Two clinical trials are currently ongoing with intracerebral tumor administration of such ICP34.5$^-$ mutants for the treatment of malignant gliomas

(117,118). HSV-1 recombinant strains are also displaying efficacy and tumor selectivity against various extra-CNS malignancies. An expanding number of tumors are proving sensitive to HSV oncolysis, including mesothelioma (119), malignant melanoma (120), metastatic colon carcinoma (121), head and neck squamous cancer (122), breast cancer (123), and prostate cancer (124). In the animal studies, no spread of the virus could be documented outside the tumors by immunohistochemistry or polymerase chain reaction after intraperitoneal administration of the virus, and no toxicity was seen (28,119). Together, these results suggested that HSV-based oncolytic therapy may provide an attractive approach for the treatment of solid tumors (25).

To test the ability of recombinant HSV-1 to infect EOC cells, we performed immunofluorescence and flow cytometry evaluation of HSV antigen expression by several established ovarian cancer cells 16 hours after exposure to a recombinant HSV-1 strain lacking ICP34.5, a viral gene involved in neurotoxicity. EOCs were found to be quite susceptible to infection by recombinant HSV-1, with approximately 70% of the cells infected at 1 MOI and approximately 99% infected at 1.5 MOI (28). Several strains of HSV-1 lacking ICP34.5 were tested and found to exert a potent oncolytic activity on established EOC cell lines. Importantly, primary cultures were significantly more susceptible to HSV killing than established lines (28,125). Furthermore, HSV-1 lacking ICP34.5 was shown to be equally efficient in chemotherapy-sensitive and chemotherapy-resistant EOC *in vitro* and *in vivo* (126). Additional evidence that recombinant HSV-1 lacking ICP34.5 is efficacious against chemotherapy-sensitive and chemotherapy-resistant EOCs was provided by *in vivo* experiments in two human EOC xenograft models in the severe combined immunodeficient (SCID) mouse (28).

The mechanism of cell death was investigated after infection by a recombinant HSV-1 lacking ICP34.5. Established EOC lines incubated with recombinant HSV1 were evaluated with cell cycle analysis and *in situ* DNA fragmentation analysis. EOC cells were found to undergo a variable degree of apoptosis, depending on the cell line. Apoptosis was detected within 24 to 48 hours after infection and was not dependent on the p53 status of the cells, which may partially account for the fact that chemotherapy resistance does not affect the sensitivity of EOC to HSV oncolysis. We further investigated the tumor specificity of HSV-G207, a doubly-deleted strain of HSV-1 lacking ICP34.5 and ribonucleotide reductase (RR), which regulates viral proliferation. HSV-G207 induced a dose-dependent lysis in EOC cells *in vitro* but spared normal human mesothelial cells (125). An increasing bulk of evidence supports the safety of these agents for *in vivo* oncolytic therapy (Table 4.9).

The oncolytic agent most advanced in clinical testing is an E1B-defective adenovirus termed ONYX-015 (127). The adenoviral E1B gene encodes a 55-kDa protein that inactivates the p53 tumor suppressor gene. Based on evidence suggesting that p53 inhibits adenoviral replication, a recombinant adenovirus lacking E1B was engineered. This virus was anticipated to replicate in p53-deficient tumor cells but not in cells possessing wild-type p53. Great enthusiasm was generated by the observation that intratumoral

TABLE 4.9. *Evidence for safety of oncolytic herpes simplex virus 1 (HSV-1) mutants*

1. SCID mice show no toxicity after i.p. injection of 1×10^6 pfu ICP34.5-deficient HSV-1716 but are readily killed by 1×10^2 pfu wild-type HSV-1.
2. Human skin xenotransplants in SCID mice show no toxicity after inoculation of ICP34.5-deficient HSV-1716, but are rapidly lysed by wild-type HSV-1.
3. After i.p. inoculation in the SCID mouse, ICP34.5-deficient HSV-1716 remains confined within tumor nodules and is not detected by immunohistochemistry or by polymerase chain reaction in any normal murine tissues, whereas wild-type HSV-1 rapidly spreads in extraperitoneal and distant tissues, including the brain.
4. ICP34.5/ICP6-deleted HSV-G207 causes no toxicity after systemic administration in HSV-sensitive nonhuman primates.
5. ICP34.5-deficient HSV-1716 and ICP34.5/ICP-6-deleted HSV-G207 cause no peritonitis in the SCID mouse.
6. ICP34.5/ICP6-deleted HSV-G207 rapidly kills ovarian cancer cells but not normal peritoneal cells.

SCID, severe combined immunodeficiency.

injection of ONYX-015 into human cervical carcinomas grown in nude mice led to complete regression in 60% of the tumors (127). The rationale for these studies was that in cervical tumors p53 is rapidly degraded owing to the presence of the human papilloma virus E6 protein product. Further reports confirmed that intratumoral or intravenous administration of ONYX-015 to nude mice bearing human xenografts from a variety of tumors had antitumoral efficacy and that the virus was not toxic to normal human cells. Moreover, a synergism with platinum-based chemotherapy was seen. However, conflicting results were obtained by different authors, who reported that intact p53 function and p53-dependent apoptosis was required for adenoviral replication (128). Clinical trials with ONYX-015 are ongoing for head and neck cancer and lung cancer. Despite the controversy regarding the mechanism of action and tumor selectivity of ONYX-015, preliminary results from a phase II study of ONYX-015 plus 5-FU/cisplatin chemotherapy in 30 patients with head and neck cancer indicated significantly higher response rates and disease-free intervals in those patients receiving the virus (129). A randomized phase III trial currently under preparation in head and neck cancer will further clarify the efficacy of ONYX-015. Because EOCs often display mutations in the p53 pathway, ONYX-015 may represent a useful tool also for recurrent or persistent EOC.

IMMUNOTHERAPY

Immunologists have categorized immunotherapies as either active or passive. Active immunizations require an intact host immune system and are typically delivered as prophylactic or therapeutic vaccines. In contrast, passive or adoptive immunotherapies consist of the transfer of serum, antibodies, or lymphocytes to the host and do not require an intact host immune system to generate the response. In most experimental animal tumor models, adoptive immunotherapies have been most effective at eradicating large established tumor masses, whereas active immunization strategies are probably best suited for patients with premalignant conditions and for those patients rendered to a minimal residual disease status.

Immune-based strategies have been tested extensively during the past three decades as experimental tumor therapeutics. Antibody therapies, cytokines, and biologic response modifiers, as well as lymphokine-activated killer (LAK) cell, T-lymphocyte, and dendritic cell (DC) adoptive immuno-therapy strategies have been implemented in various tumors (Figure 4.6). Most of the immunotherapy trials have been carried out in small groups of patients and without adequate controls or randomization procedures. Often results were disappointing, since clinical responses were at best partial and transient and immune responses were not always documented or correlated poorly with clinical responses.

Tumors are antigenic—that is, they possess specific antigenic epitopes that can be recognized by the immune system. Specific antitumor antibodies have been isolated from patients with solid malignancies, and antigens recognized by cytotoxic T cells have been identified and cloned. Nevertheless, with rare exceptions, established malignancies are not immunogenic: they fail to generate a specific immune response of sufficient potency to cause tumor rejection (Table 4.10). Evidence accumulated over the past decades indicates that the humoral component of the immune response against tumors plays virtually no protective role. In part, this may be related to escape mechanisms that tumors develop to evade complement-mediated cytotoxicity. This may explain why immune therapies based on antibody-mediated cytotoxicity have failed to produce any significant responses. However, there is now a resurgence of interest in passive serotherapy, the intravenous administration of monoclonal antibodies. The antibodies used are either unmodified monoclonal antibodies, engineered antibody fragments that have better tumor penetration, or antibodies conjugated to radioisotopes or to toxins. Hundreds of antibodies are currently in clinical trials, and the FDA has approved three, including indications for treatment of breast cancer, T-cell leukemia, and B-cell lymphoma.

Cellular immune responses, including T lymphocytes and natural killer (NK) cells play an important role in tumor regression (130). NK cells are effector cells of both innate and acquired

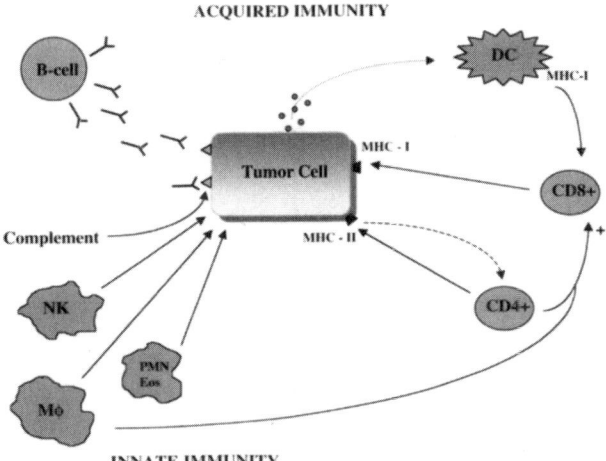

FIG. 4.6. Schematic representation of antitumor immune mechanisms. Innate immunity is composed of complement and major histocompatibility (MHC)-independent cytotoxic cell effectors such as macrophages (Mφ) and natural killer (NK) cells. Polymorphonucleate granulocytes (PMN) and eosinophils (Eos) may also participate in antitumor innate responses. Acquired immunity responses include humoral antibody-mediated response and MHC-dependent cellular responses. Antibodies may facilitate complement-mediated cell killing. Professional antigen-presenting cells such as dendritic cells (DCs) or macrophages phagocytose tumor debris and cross-present tumor-specific antigens on MHC class I sites. These are recognized and induce clonal proliferation of CD8$^+$ T lymphocytes with cytotoxic activity. MHC class II-associated tumor antigens are recognized by CD4$^+$ T-helper lymphocytes. Cytokines produced by T-helper cells and other immune cells enhance CD8$^+$ function.

immunity. They recognize target cells independently of the MHC, and their tumoricidal activity is stimulated by TNF, IFN, IL-2 and IL-12 (131). Cytotoxic T lymphocytes, on the other hand, recognize MHC class I-restricted tumor-specific antigens (i.e., antigens that are associated with class I MHC molecules) (132). Some of the mechanisms of tumor antigen presentation have been elucidated. T cells require antigen presentation by professional cells, such as DCs or macrophages. DCs appear to play a particularly important role in tumor recognition (133). They are recruited in tumor sites and have been shown to phagocytose debris from tumor cells, from which they elaborate antigenic peptides that are ultimately expressed on their cell surface in association with MHC molecules (134). Pioneering work has been carried out in melanoma, where over the past decade several antigens have been characterized (135). Many of these are intracellular antigens, and some are also expressed by normal human tissues (135–137).

Increasing evidence suggests that patients with established malignancies including EOC may display defects in the mechanisms of tumor recognition and tumor rejection (138–140). In EOC, these include defective maturation and function of professional antigen-presenting cells (APCs) such as DCs and defects in T-cell function (141,142). The tumor microenvironment appears to play a paramount role in mediating immune evasion (143). Putative factors released by EOCs, including TGF-β, IL-10, and VEGF (Table 4.11), and cell surface molecules such as Muc-1 may impair expression of MHC molecules, DC maturation, antigen presentation by DCs, and/or activation of T cells (144–146). EOCs express a novel molecule, termed RCAS1, that is a member of the TNF ligand family (147). RCAS1 has been proposed to mediate immunosuppression in EOC by killing tumor-reactive T cells. Tumor-infiltrating T cells from patients with advanced EOC exert only weak cytotoxicity against autologous tumor cells *in vitro* (148). Inactivation of these pathways at multiple sites

TABLE 4.10. *Immune escape mechanisms identified in tumors*

Humoral Immunity
   Loss of antigenic determinants recognized by antitumor antibodies
   Escape from complement-mediated cytotoxicity
   Complement inactivation
Cellular Immunity
   Loss of antigenic determinants recognized by tumor-specific T cells
   Downregulation of major histocompatibility class I molecules (inhibition of TAP)
   Induction of T-cell anergy
      Loss of costimulatory signals (B7)
      Release of counterstimulatory signals (CTLA-4)
   Inhibition of T-cell function (by IL-10 & TGF-β)
   Loss of T-cell receptor (inhibition of NF-κB and loss of TCR$_\zeta$)
   Inhibition of dendritic cell maturation (by VEGF)
   Induction of T-cell apoptosis (by tumor-released Fas ligand)
   Escape from T-cell–induced apoptosis (loss of apoptotic machinery, production of Fas ligand)

may explain why previous attempts at tumor immunotherapy with cell extract vaccination or infusion of poorly selected or poorly activated T cells have failed to produce clinically meaningful results (149,150). Newer therapeutic strategies target these defects, taking advantage of advances in molecular biology and biotechnology. Tumor immunology is evolving into a sophisticated field in which molecular and cellular engineering strategies are employed to correct or bypass these defects.

VACCINE THERAPIES

Tumor vaccines are classified as preventive or therapeutic. An example of an FDA-approved vaccine is the recombinant hepatitis B vaccine, which is being used to prevent hepatocellular carcinoma in some regions of the world. Preventive vaccines for cervical carcinoma are being evaluated for women infected with carcinogenic serotypes of papillomavirus. There are no FDA-approved therapeutic cancer vaccines, but phase II and III trials are in progress for melanoma, breast cancer, and ovarian cancer, leading to optimism that clinically beneficial treatments are on the horizon.

The design and application of tumor vaccines is based on the founding hypothesis that tumor antigens are not strongly immunogenic (151). This hypothesis has been largely confirmed by animal and clinical observations. Pioneering experiments with tumor vaccines used tumor extracts that were processed and administered to patients with the intention of generating a stronger antitumor immune response. Two fundamental approaches have been used (Table 4.12). Initially, tumor cell extracts of varying purity were directly administered to patients in various locations (e.g., intratumoral, intraperitoneal, subcutaneous). As the role of DCs in mediating antigen presentation to T cells has been elucidated and the technology to generate *ex vivo* large numbers of patient-derived DCs from peripheral blood and bone marrow progenitor cells has evolved, DC-based vaccines have been designed in which autologous DCs are primed ("pulsed") with tumor antigens *ex vivo* and then reinfused to patients (152). Three general types of tumor-derived material have been used: whole tumor cell extracts, partial tumor extracts, and individual tumor antigens. Approaches have

TABLE 4.11. *Effects of immunosuppressive tumor-derived cytokines*

	Transforming growth factor-β	Interleukin-10	Vascular endothelial growth factors
Inhibition of T-cell growth or differentiation	Y	Y	Y
Induction of T-cell anergy	Y	N	N
Induction of T-cell cytotoxic activity	Y	Y	N
Inhibition of cytokine production	Y	Y	N
Inhibition of antigen presentation	Y	Y	N
Inhibition of Th1 response	Y	Y	N
Stimulation of Th2 response	Y	Y	N
Inhibition of costimulatory molecules	Y	Y	N
Inhibition of dendritic cell maturation	Y	N	Y

TABLE 4.12. *Strategies for the preparation of tumor vaccines*

I. Whole-cell vaccines
  A. Administration of autologous or allogeneic tumor cells
    1. Tumor cells modified with physical or chemical agents
      a. Ultraviolet radiation
      b. Ionizing radiation
      c. Dinitrophenyl (DNP)
      d. Acetic acid
      e. Keyhole limpet hemocyanin
      f. Incomplete Freund's adjuvant
      g. Semustine
      h. *Vibrio cholerae* neuraminidase
    2. Tumor cells modified with biologic extracts
      a. Bacille Calmette-Guérin
      b. *Corynebacterium parvum*
      c. *Candida* antigens
    3. Tumor cells lysed by genetically modified virus
    4. Tumor cells infected by genetically modified *salmonella typhimurium*
  B. Administration of autologous dendritic cells
    1. Dendritic cells incubated with whole tumor cells modified by the following:
      a. Ultraviolet radiation
      b. Ionizing radiation
      c. Cell fragmentation
    2. Dendritic cells incubated with the following derived from whole tumor cells:
      a. Apoptotic bodies
      b. Total RNA
II. Antigen-based vaccines
  A. Administration of tumor-specific antigen
    1. Recombinant tumor-specific antigen enriched by adjuvants
  B. Administration of autologous dendritic cells
    1. Incubated with recombinant antigen
    2. Transduced with specific antigen cDNA
  C. DNA vaccine
    1. Recombinant virus carrying tumor-specific antigen cDNA

become more sophisticated as antitumor immune mechanisms have been elucidated and specific tumor antigens have been recognized.

Whole-Cell Vaccines

Whole-cell vaccines represent the prototype of antitumor vaccines (153). Specific advantages from the use of whole-cell vaccines include the relative simplicity of preparation and the polyvalent nature of these preparations, which theoretically comprise the broadest repertoire of potential tumor rejection antigens present in one specific tumor. Disadvantages include limitations in recovery of autologous tumor cells, time-consuming and cumbersome isolation, *ex vivo* processing, and cost. For some tumors autologous cells are never easily available. However, ovarian cancer is readily accessible within the peritoneal cavity, often manifests with ascites from which large numbers of cells can be recovered, and has often included surgical debulking in experimental second-line approaches.

Several approaches have been undertaken to increase the immunogenicity of tumor cells. One early approach was to associate cells with bacille Calmette-Guérin (bCG). Such trials have been undertaken in cutaneous melanoma, colorectal cancer, and renal cell carcinoma. Some clinical responses have been obtained (153). Another way to potentiate whole-cell vaccines has been that of associating with a specific hapten, such as dinitrophenyl (DNP), which leads to a marked inflammatory response (154). DNP-modified autologous ovarian tumor cells also were used in a clinical phase I trial at Jefferson Medical Center in stage III patients clinically free of disease after surgery and chemotherapy (155). No acute toxicity was reported, and a measurable cell-mediated immune response to autologous ovarian cancer cells was detected in some patients. Although studies have reported a statistically significant prolongation of survival in patients who developed a response to DNP-modified tumor cells, no clinically meaningful responses were reported in this trial.

Based on the observation that viral extracts are inflammatory and viruses generate potent immune responses, several investigators have attempted to generate whole tumor cell vaccines through the use of viruses. Viral oncolysates, prepared with different viruses, have been used in trials against melanoma, gastric cancer, cervical cancer, ovarian cancer, vulvar cancer, and renal cancer (156,157) (Table 4.13). The theoretical mechanisms by which the use of viruses

TABLE 4.13. *Virus used for oncolysate vaccine preparation*

Herpes simplex virus
Newcastle disease virus
Polyoma virus
Vaccinia virus
Influenza virus
Friend leukemia virus
Vesicular stomatitis virus
Measles virus

TABLE 4.14. *Theoretic mechanisms of tumor immune enhancement by viruses*

Increased tumor antigen presentation directly by tumor cells
Increased apoptosis
Increased uptake of apoptotic bodies by antigen-presenting cells (macrophages, dendritic cells)
Release of stimulatory cytokines and chemokines enhancing dendritic cells
Release of costimulatory molecules
Modification of tumor antigens

enhances the antitumor immune response are multiple: (a) inflammatory cytokines or chemokines released by tumor cells may activate immune cells (158); (b) the association of viral antigens with tumor antigens may increase the uptake of tumor antigens by DCs; (c) recall immune mechanisms against viral antigens may activate helper T cells, which may enhance the expansion of tumor-specific T lymphocytes (159); and (d) heat shock protein-mediated immune enhancement may play a role as a chaperone to increase immunogenicity (160).

The choice of viruses has been an important factor. Original work was limited to nonpathogenic viruses (e.g., NDV, vesicular stomatitis virus) to ensure safety (156,157). Pathogenic viruses carrying out a lytic cycle in human cells, such as influenza A and vaccinia virus, were also studied, but prior inactivation by ultraviolet (UV) radiation was mandated, which significantly reduced the immunogenicity of the oncolysate and led to unsatisfactory clinical results (161) (Table 4.15). The M.D. Anderson group described the use of influenza A virus to produce oncolysate vaccines prepared with established EOC cell lines (162). Allogeneic cells were used because of the inability of influenza A virus to efficiently infect and lyse primary autologous ovarian cancer cells. Extracts were UV-irradiated and subjected to membrane purification procedures. Patients received several courses of intraperitoneal or intrapleural oncolysate administration. In these studies, some patients displayed progression-free intervals lasting several months, and in few a complete pathologic response was documented. Although specific T-cell responses against vaccine antigens were detected (163), the use of allogeneic cells made it difficult to determine the specificity of the antitumor immune response.

Important work with viral oncolysates has been also carried out by the Heidelberg group in Germany with NDV, a poultry pest virus that is nonpathogenic in the human (164). The use of live inactivated NDV with intact tumor cells yielded superior results compared with tumor lysates or membrane preparations (165). Remarkably, maximal therapeutic effect was noted when a low dose of NDV was used to modify tumor cells, leading to the generation of specific cytotoxic T lymphocytes with antitumor but no antiviral activity. The authors postulated that NDV-infected cells were transformed into professional APCs, directly generating an antitumor specific T-cell response. The mechanisms affording this transformation include (a) improved adhesion of lymphocytes to NDV-infected tumor cells (owing to the expression of new cell surface adhesion molecules), which provided costimulatory T-cell activation, and (b) secretion of activating cytokines such as IFN-α, IFN-β, TNF-α, IL-1, and IL-6, as well as chemokines such as RANTES and IP10, which enhanced tumor recognition (Table 4.16). In a phase II trial carried out in Germany, repeated

TABLE 4.15. *Clinical trials performed in ovarian cancer with viral oncolysate*

Virus	Responses
Autologous	
Vaccinia virus[a]	9/29 Partial response
Newcastle disease virus	50% 2-yrs survival with high-quality vaccine
Allogeneic	
Influenza-A	9/40 Partial response

[a] Includes also other solid tumors.

TABLE 4.16. *Mechanisms of action of Newcastle disease virus*

Virus replicates selectively in tumor cells.
Viral infection increases tumor cell adhesiveness to T cells (mediated by hemagglutinin-neuraminidase).
Viral infection induces stimulatory cytokines, chemokines, and other stimulatory molecules.
Virus provides CD4+ cell costimulation.
Virus provides CD8+ cell costimulation.
Virus reverses T-cell anergy.

administration of NDV-modified autologous tumor cells resulted in a 50% survival rate at 2 years in 31 patients with advanced EOC (166). In addition to proving the safety of viral tumor vaccines, these studies provided significant information on the paramount importance of the conditions used for the preparation of virally modified cells, especially the viral titers and UV inactivation.

Viral applications have several advantages in the field of tumor vaccines because of their immunogenic potential, their stability, their versatility, and their ready availability. Advances in molecular biology have allowed for the generation of attenuated viral strains that are unable to replicate or that replicate preferentially in malignant cells. In addition to modifying the tumor tropism for tumor cells, based on tumor-specific promoters driving important viral genes, viruses can be engineered to encode specific genes that enhance tumor immunogenicity (167). Examples include MHC class I or II molecules, immunodominant tumor-rejection antigens, costimulatory molecules, and cytokines. If prevention of viral-induced lysis proves to be critical for the generation of highly immunogenic tumor vaccines, multiattenuated replication-incompetent viruses can be used. The engineering and application of HSV encoding IL-12 and GM-CSF provide extraordinary examples of how viruses can be modified to enhance the immunogenicity of tumors (168,169).

Gene therapy has been used as an alternative tool to alter tumor cells. Freeman and coworkers modified the ovarian teratocarcinoma cell line PA-1 to permanently express HSVtk (66). Preclinical data suggested that HSVtk$^+$ PA-1 cells administered intraperitoneally followed by systemic GCV produced a vaccine effect. In fact, the PA-1 cells adhered on tumor surfaces and their death generated an inflammatory response within tumor nodules after the administration of GCV. Preliminary results of a clinical trial support the safety of intraperitoneal administration of HSVtk$^+$ PA-1 cells. An alternative approach was undertaken by Link and colleagues (170), who engineered a murine ovarian carcinoma line to permanently express HSVtk. Administration of these cells intraperitoneally to patients with EOC followed by GCV systemic administration was proven to be safe, but no clinically beneficial results have been reported.

Antigen-Based Vaccines

Recent developments in molecular biology have allowed for the identification and cloning of specific tumor rejection antigens (135–137). T-cell clones, which recognize *in vivo* or *in vitro* autologous tumor cells, have been matched with tumor DNA libraries expressed on various expression systems, leading to the identification of specific tumor rejection antigens. Pioneering work has been carried out in melanoma (171,172), but other tumors were demonstrated to possess similar antigens. In general, these may be tumor-specific peptides that are absent in all adult normal tissues except germline cells such as MAGE, BAGE, or GAGE. Other tissue rejection antigens were identified as tissue-specific differentiation antigens, which may be recognized as nonself by virtue of their temporally inappropriate expression within a specific tissue. Tumor-specific antigens result also from mutations such as those occurring in tumor suppressor genes and oncogenes, as described in many malignancies. Examples include p53, caspase-8, and bcr-abl. Overexpressed peptides may also represent tumor-specific antigens; an example is HER-2/neu, an oncogene overexpressed in approximately 30% of breast and ovarian cancers. Finally, cytotoxic lymphocytes may recognize epitopes of mucin, a surface glycoprotein containing multiple tandem repeats of 20 amino acids (173). Although this protein is heavily glycosylated in normal cells, the peptide repeats are unmasked by underglycosylation in some tumors, including breast and ovarian carcinomas (174).

The identification of tumor-specific antigens has generated a great deal of enthusiasm, given the prospects of generating peptide-based vaccines (175). This tool provides for the first time the opportunity to monitor the antitumor specific immune response and to make correlations with clinical responses. Multiple trials are ongoing to test the validity of this hypothesis. Purified peptides have been either administered to patients with direct conjugation to carrier proteins such as keyhole limpet hemocyanin (KLH) (176) or used to pulse *ex vivo* autologous DCs, which are then reinfused to patients. It appears that DC-based vaccines may be superior to peptide-based vaccines, particularly if supplemented by cytokines.

Despite the significant advancements in the field of T-cell-defined tumor antigens, their exact potential in clinical applications is far from understood. For example, a clinical trial with MAGE-A1 peptide in 25 patients with melanoma was reported. Five patients with regional metastases and 2 with distant metastases displayed a clinical response; 3 patients had a complete response. However, no clear cytotoxic lymphocyte response was detected in the blood of 4 patients analyzed, including 2 with complete tumor regression. In addition, patients at relapse harbored tumors that were MAGE-A1 positive (177). It is clear that more clinical experimentation needs to be carried out to better define the role of peptide-based tumor vaccines. Moreover, analysis of the molecular pathways underlying antigen presentation by DCs, T-cell signal transduction, and the factors implicated in immune evasion within the tumor microenvironment will be critically important for understanding of the clinical potential of vaccine- and cell-based immunotherapy.

Most of the present knowledge of tumor-specific antigens is derived from preclinical and clinical data in melanoma. Few tumor-specific antigens have been recognized in patients with EOC (178) (Table 4.17). HER-2/neu is one of them; cytotoxic lymphocytes from patients with ovarian cancer have been shown to target peptides from HER-2/neu, which are human leukocyte antigen (HLA)-A2 restricted (179). HER-2/neu provides an excellent paradigm of peptide-based vaccines and illustrates the possible limitations of such an approach. First, its HLA-A2 restriction limits its application to HLA-A2+ individuals, who represent approximately 40% of the adult population. Second, HER-2/neu is expressed by only about 30% of EOCs. Moreover, because of tumor heterogeneity, HER-2/neu is overexpressed in a variable percentage of tumor cells within the same tumor. It is easy to envision failure of HER-2/neu-targeted vaccine therapy resulting from the ability of the tumor to select HER-2/neu− clones, which may evade the immune attack. Third, HER-2/neu does not appear to encode MHC class II-restricted antigens that are sufficient to generate a CD4+ T-helper response, and this is likely to limit the efficacy of the HLA-A2-restricted cytotoxic T-lymphocyte response.

TABLE 4.17. *Tumor-associated antigens identified in ovarian cancer*

Antigen type	Prevalence in ovarian cancer (%)	MHC restriction
Tumor-specific antigens		
MAGE-1	+28	HLA-A1
MAGE-3	+17	HLA-A1/2/B44
MAGE-6	—	HLA-CW16
BAGE	+15	HLA-CW16
GAGE-1,2	+31	HLA-CW6
RAGE-1	—	HLA-B7
Mucins		Non-restricted
Differentiation antigens		
CEA	+30	HLA-A2
Mutated antigens		
p53	+50 or more	HLA-A2
Ras		
MUM-1	Melanoma	HLA-B44
β-catenin		HLA-A24
CASP-8		HLA-B35
Overexpressed antigens		
p53	+(30–40)	HLA-A2
HER-2/neu	+(30)	HLA-A2

HLA, human leukocyte antigen; MHC, major histocompatibility complex.

Other tumor-associated antigens in ovarian cancer include peptides from the amino enhancer of split protein (180), the folate-binding protein (which is overexpressed in more than 90% of ovarian cancers) (181), and mucin carbohydrate-derived antigens such as O-linked mutant glycans TN, T, and sialylated TN (sTN), which are not expressed by normal cells. In a recent clinical trial, a synthetic analog of sTN, ([NANA2-6]-GAL-NAC), was conjugated with KLH, mixed with DOX-B SE adjuvant, and administered to patients with advanced EOC. Vaccine administration was well tolerated and an immune response was documented; a number of patients displayed stable disease for a prolonged period (150). In another trial, 7 patients with advanced-stage ovarian cancer and 33 with advanced-stage

TABLE 4.18. *T-Cell deficiency in ovarian cancer*

Cause		Effect
Tumor microenvironment cytokines (IL-10, TGF-β, VEGF)	$\longrightarrow$	Inhibition of T-cell differentiation Decrease Th1/Th2 ratio
Counterstimulatory signals Loss of costimulatory signals	$\longrightarrow$	T-cell anergy
Fas ligand	$\longrightarrow$	T-cell apoptosis
Cytotoxic chemotherapy	$\longrightarrow$	T-cell death (? Deletion of tumor-specific clones)
Aging	$\longrightarrow$	Decreased T-cell reserve and replicative senescence

breast cancer received high-dose chemotherapy with stem cell rescue followed by vaccine treatment with an sTN-KLH conjugate. Antitumor response was documented in some patients with decreasing CA125 levels, and 17 of the 27 evaluable patients demonstrated sTN-specific T-cell proliferation (182). Investigators found that the chance of death was more than two times greater among patients in the control group than among those who received the sTN-KLH vaccine. The chance of relapse was approximately 1.7 times greater for patients in the control group compared with those vaccinated. This sTN-KLH therapeutic vaccine is currently being evaluated in a phase III clinical trial that will involve 900 evaluable patients with metastatic breast cancer.

DNA vaccines entail the administration of DNA encoding for tumor-associated peptide sequences (183). This may be a more efficient way of engineering vaccines, because DNA is stable and easy to manufacture. DNA vaccines may be incorporated into microgold particles or plasmids and inserted into target cells via gene guns or liposomes, respectively. In addition, DNA encoding tumor-rejection antigens can be inserted into recombinant viruses under the control of a strong promoter (184). DNA vaccines may directly target DCs (185,186). In this case, the DCs express the tumor-rejection antigens, bypassing the process of uptake and processing of tumor antigens. This approach may significantly enhance antigen presentation. Modified DCs can then be reinfused into patients. Moreover, DNA vaccines may target cancer cells, which may be induced to overexpress immunodominant tumor-rejection antigens, costimulatory molecules, or cytokines (187,188).

Adoptive T-cell Immunotherapy

The idea of using autologous or allogeneic T lymphocytes to attack established tumors is not new, since intravenous and intracavitary injections of lymphocytes have been given to patients by various investigators over the past 40 years. The fundamental hypothesis is that although T cells generally cannot generate a strong response spontaneously against autologous tumors *in vivo* (Table 4.18), their manipulation *ex vivo* might result in enhancement of their antitumor activity. Initial approaches with adoptive immunotherapy used autologous or allogeneic (donor) lymphocytes. In some early studies, tumor-infiltrating lymphocytes were successfully isolated from the peritoneal cavities of 50% of patients with EOC and then expanded with low-dose recombinant IL-2 (189). The T-cell lines harvested displayed features of $CD8^+$ and $CD4^+$ T lymphocytes and were anticipated to display antitumor activity because they had previously been recruited to the tumor site.

To increase the tumor specificity of autologous T lymphocytes, Canevari and coworkers (190) used a bispecific monoclonal antibody, OC/TR, directed against the folate binding receptor, a tumor-associated antigen expressed on EOC, and against the CD3 molecule on T cells. The patients were treated with injections of T cells, the bispecific monoclonal antibody, and low-dose recombinant IL-2. Their hypothesis was that the use of such a bispecific antibody would enhance the physical interaction between tumor and adoptively transferred T cells. Although this approach increased the recruitment of autologous lymphocytes within the tumor, it did not provide specific pathways for T-cell costimulation. A 27% rate of antitumor response was observed in this study, including three patients (10%) with a complete clinical response. A local antitumor immune response within the peritoneal cavity, but no systemic antitumor immune response after intraperitoneal administration, was reported in a follow-up study (191). Recent observations indicate that tumor-infiltrating lymphocytes may be inactivated within the tumor microenvironment by tumor-derived factors. Analysis of tumor-infiltrating and peripheral blood lymphocytes from patients with EOC indicated that tumor-infiltrating lymphocytes display suppressed function (141). This may explain the relatively weak responses obtained with *in vitro* expanded autologous T cells isolated from ovarian tumors. A further potential problem with this approach is the immunogenicity of the bispecific murine monoclonal antibody, which provokes a vigorous immune response against the antibody conjugate, preventing repeated use of the reagent.

Activation of cytotoxic antigen-specific T lymphocytes requires the presentation of antigens on MHC molecules. Tumor antigens may be presented directly by the tumor cells to T cells, or they may be cross-presented. Cross-presentation refers to the uptake and processing of tumor cells or tumor antigens by professional APCs such as DCs. Cross-presentation is generally a better way to prime T-cell immune responses, whereas direct presentation at the site of the tumor is required for tumor elimination by T cells. In addition, T-lymphocyte activation also requires stimulation by a costimulatory pathway, which may involve the T-cell CD28 receptor (192,193), although other costimulatory pathways also exist (194). CD28 stimulation may be afforded by antigen-presenting cells expressing B7.1 and B7.2 molecules, which are specific CD28 ligands expressed on the cell surface. In the absence of costimulatory signals accompanying binding of T-cell receptor (TCR) to a specific antigen, T cells not only fail to become activated but may enter a permanent state of anergy, in which they become tolerant to that antigen or undergo apoptosis (195). Tumors expressing MHC class I molecules may present antigens directly. Because this can occur in the absence of costimulatory signals, it could result in T-cell tolerance towards tumor-specific antigens. EOCs express low levels of MHC class I molecules (178), and this may induce a state of immune nonresponsiveness, termed immune ignorance. Tolerance may also be induced by downregulatory costimulatory signals, such as those provided by the CTLA-4 receptor (196).

Multiple studies have indicated that tumors escape immune recognition in part through failure to provide the appropriate costimulatory signals that are required to activate the cellular immune system. Occupation of the CD28 receptor facilitates tumor recognition because it reduces the number of TCR molecules that have to be occupied by tumor antigen and increases the affinity of binding between TCR and tumor antigens (197). Incubation of naïve T cells and peripheral monocytes with CD28 ligands induces activation of $CD4^+$ T-helper cells, cytotoxic $CD8^+$ T cells, and NK cells. Of note, once cytotoxic lymphocytes have been activated with CD28 ligands, they become CD28 independent for their effector phase and efficiently kill MHC class I-bearing tumor cells in the absence of further costimulatory signals (198). Animal evidence indicates that restoration of T-cell function and reversion of tolerance may be achieved with the addition of CD28 ligands and may lead to eradication of established tumors. Costimulation, therefore, provides a potential tool for the generation of functionally active autologous lymphocytes in adoptive T-cell immunotherapy strategies.

Several tumor immunotherapy strategies have been designed to enhance T-cell costimulation (194) (Table 4.19). Autologous lymphocytes have been expanded and costimulated *ex vivo* and then reinfused into patients or stimulated *in vivo* by systemic administration of CD28 ligands. Alternatively, vaccine approaches have been undertaken that manipulate the tumor to increase

TABLE 4.19. *Therapeutic strategies for induction of T-Cell costimulation*

Ex vivo expansion and activation of autologous T-cells; *ex vivo* generation of tumor antigen-specific T-cells
Systemic augmentation of T-cell function with cytokines
Genetic manipulation of tumors to produce costimulatory signals
Vaccination with tumor antigens and costimulatory ligands

its ability to produce costimulating ligands. The first trials testing this approach are now underway using B7-transfected tumors as a vaccine. *Ex vivo* costimulation of T cells may be accomplished by incubation of cells with CD28 and CD3 ligands such as anti-CD28 or B7 and anti-CD3 monoclonal antibodies linked to polymer beads (199). The preparation of cells *ex vivo* offers distinct advantages. First, by controlling the costimulating conditions *in vitro,* T cells are removed from suppressive influences within the tumor microenvironment. Moreover, if autologous T cells are harvested before the administration of chemotherapy, tumor-specific T cells may be salvaged from the deleterious effects of chemotherapy (see later discussion). Furthermore, CD3/CD28 costimulation results in clonal proliferation not only of $CD8^+$ T cells but also of $CD4^+$ T cells (199). This approach is believed to lead to preferential enhancement of T-cell effector responses and activation of antitumor memory mechanisms, which are most suitable for tumor growth control. *In vivo* administration of ligands to CD3 and CD28 used in experimental models of prostate and colon carcinoma resulted in tumor regression (200). In that study, the ligands comprised monoclonal antibody fragments that were combined with monoclonal antitumor antibodies to form bispecific molecules in order to enhance costimulation.

Three phase I trials of T-cell adoptive immunotherapy using T-cell costimulation in EOC are currently under way. A trial conducted at the National Cancer Institute entails *ex vivo* expansion of autologous T cells followed by anti-CD3 activation and retroviral transduction with a folate receptor-binding ligand, an antigen that is expressed in 90% of ovarian cancers. A trial is being conducted at the University of Milan, Italy, with autologous T cells coated with bispecific anti-CD3/CD28 antibodies (194). Finally, a trial of costimulated allogeneic T-cell infusions given after nonmyeloablative stem cell transplantation is currently underway at the University of Pennsylvania (for an updated reference on current clinical trials, visit the following Web sites: www.ovarian.org/, www.centerwatch.com/, cancertrials.nci.nih.gov/).

An attractive approach to adoptive immunotherapy is that of combining costimulation procedures with methodologies yielding clonal *ex vivo* expansion of tumor-specific T cells (201). One possible approach is that of using APCs such as DCs primed with whole tumor or with tumor-rejection monovalent antigens (202). Tumor-specific T cells may be generated with this approach and may be subjected to CD3/CD28 costimulation, yielding large numbers of tumor-specific activated T cells (203,204). The DCs provide the appropriate pathways for recruitment of not only $CD8^+$ clones but also $CD4^+$ T-helper clones. Furthermore, the use of CD3/CD28 costimulation may further enhance the expansion of $CD8^+$ and $CD4^+$ antitumor T-cell clones. The presence of $CD4^+$ T-helper antitumor clones may offer a significant advantage, because it mediates the specific antigen memory mechanisms that may provide long-term antitumor protection. Another approach is that of rendering tumor cells able to provide CD28-mediated costimulation by transducing them with B7 molecules. Ectopic expression of B7.1 melanoma cells resulted in improved primary T-cell activation, compared with nontransduced tumor cells, and, most importantly, allowed for the generation of large numbers of long-term proliferating MHC class I-restricted tumor-specific T cells (205).

The utilization of T-cell-based adoptive immunotherapy still has obvious limitations. First, a large portion of infused T cells are "trapped" in the lungs (206,207). There are indications that trapping and sequestration of the T cells is minimized if the duration of *ex vivo* T-cell culture is minimized. A second obstacle relates to immunogenicity of the adoptively transferred T cells. Some culture systems contain fetal bovine serum or other components that may trigger the immune system to recognize the adoptively transferred T cells as foreign, resulting in their subsequent elimination. Other manipulations, such as the transduction of foreign genes into T cells, can also render the cells immunogenic and decrease their survival after infusion. A third obstacle relates to the survival of T lymphocytes and their ability to undergo prolonged clonal expansion, both of which are limited (208). Infusion of autologous tumor-infiltrating T lymphocytes transfected with neomycin gene to melanoma patients demonstrated that cells persist *in vivo* for up to 2 months. T cells also display a finite ability to undergo clonal expansion, which reaches about 30 to 40 population doublings. After that, T cells senesce and enter a replicative arrest. The notion of generating T lymphocytes that persist for longer periods and have the ability to undergo indefinite clonal expansion is an attractive one. Intense work is being carried out on the role of telomerases in affecting the lifespan of somatic cells including T lymphocytes (209). Potentially, gene therapy approaches targeting telomerase could generate T lymphocytes with significantly enhanced clonal ability (210). An alternative approach could be to use cytokines known to activate T cells (e.g., IL-2) and expand their clonal abilities. Because systemic administration of cytokines can be fairly toxic, gene therapy approaches may be undertaken to activate postreceptor transduction pathways dependent on IL-2. This approach, however, mandates the presence of "fail safe" mechanisms capable of preventing uncontrolled T-cell expansion. Retroviral transduction of T cells with HSVtk provides a suitable suicide gene tool for this purpose.

Several defects have been identified in immune cells of patients harboring malignancies. Signal transduction abnormalities have been described in T cells of patients with established malignancies and have been validated by animal models (140,211). Peripheral blood lymphocytes from some patients with solid malignancies display decreased expression of the ζ chain of the TCR/CD3 and of p56^{lck}, a cytoplasmic protein tyrosine kinase of the src family associated with the cytoplasmic domain of the TCR/CD3 complex. The latter participates in postreceptor mechanisms after occupation of the TCR. Moreover, suppressed p56^{lck} expression was observed in tumor-infiltrating lymphocytes compared with peripheral lymphocytes from patients with malignancies (212). There is some controversy in this area, because normal levels of the various components of the TCR/CD3 complex and associated protein tyrosine kinases were detected in other studies, but tumor-infiltrating lymphocytes of some patients displayed decreased tyrosine phosphorylation compared with peripheral blood lymphocytes after activation (213). Defects at the transcriptional level involving factors of the NF-κB/REL family have also been described in patients with established tumors (214). Alterations in the NF-κB system may lead to inefficient production of IL-2. Importantly, these lymphocytes can be rescued and activated *ex vivo*, indicating that damage is not irreversible (211).

The factors that cause suppression of lymphocyte function in patients with tumors have not been fully characterized, but several mechanisms have been hypothesized. These include the lack of costimulatory signals leading to tolerance; the secretion of soluble inhibitory factors such as TGF-β and IL-10 by tumors; and the release of factors activating CTLA-4. In particular, TGF-β is a potent immunosuppressive factor that inhibits T-lymphocyte activation, downregulates cell surface receptors mediating T-cell proliferation, and blocks the production of stimulatory cytokines such as IL-12 (215). TGF-β may also induce a switch in T-helper response, favoring the development of Th2-type cells and inhibiting Th1-type responses (216). Because Th1-type cytokines promote cell-mediated immunity and delayed hypersensitivity responses, TGF-β exerts a potent inhibition of antitumor immune response and favors tumor survival (217).

An additional mechanism of tumor-reduced T-cell dysfunction involves the Fas/FasL system (218). The Fas receptor (APO-1/CD95) and its ligand (CD95L) are transmembrane proteins belonging to the TNF family. Binding of FasL to Fas triggers apoptosis through downregulation of Bcl-X_L and upregulation of caspase-8, which associates with the intracellular domain of Fas (219). Clonally expanded effector T cells, such as tumor-infiltrating lymphocytes, are particularly sensitive to Fas-induced apoptosis (220). Moreover, lack of costimulatory signal production by tumors may enhance T-cell sensitivity to Fas-mediated programmed cell death. The expression of FasL by solid tumors has been correlated with the incidence of apoptotic depletion of tumor-infiltrating lymphocytes (221). Tissues producing FasL become immunologically privileged sites, as infiltrating lymphocytes undergo Fas-mediated apoptosis. Fas-mediated immune evasion may play an important role in ovarian cancer: FasL expression has been demonstrated in ovarian cancers (222), and ovarian cancer cells expressing FasL are able to induce lymphocyte apoptosis through activation of caspases (223).

An additional important factor affecting the success of autologous T-cell adoptive therapies relates to the T-cell toxicity from chemotherapy (224). Cytotoxic chemotherapy exerts a profoundly depleting effect on peripheral T cells, including $CD4^+$ and $CD8^+$ lymphocytes. $CD4^+$ cells reconstitute very slowly after intensive chemotherapy, especially in older patients, because of depleted thymic reserve (225). $CD8^+$ cells recover more quickly after chemotherapy, and their kinetics are unrelated to age. However, recovering $CD8^+$ T cells are mainly $CD45RO^+$ and $CD28^-57^+$ cells, which are probably senescent lymphocytes with very low replication reserve (226). In addition, cytotoxic chemotherapy appears to specifically affect lymphocytes that undergo clonal expansion, such as tumor-specific lymphocytes. Evidence obtained in melanoma patients indicates that chemotherapy induces a specific depletion of antitumor lymphocytes directed against tumor-associated antigens (227). If this finding is confirmed, it is likely that the combination of T-cell defects induced by the tumor and those imposed by cytotoxic chemotherapy would lead to a state of profound suppression of tumor-specific immunity.

For these reasons, specific approaches need to be undertaken to restore and, in fact, enhance the activity of APCs, autologous T cells, and NK cells against the tumor. How can this be accomplished in the presence of chemotherapy treatments? One solution is that of harvesting autologous T cells before the induction of chemotherapy through apheresis. T cells can be stored until completion of chemotherapy treatment and then subjected to expansion through costimulation protocols and/or clonal expansion by exposure to tumor-primed DCs. Oncostatin M is a recently identified member of the IL-6 family that is capable of inducing repletion of peripheral $CD4^+$ and $CD8^+$ T cells in the mouse (228). IL-7 has similar effects. Purification of such factors might tremendously benefit the ability to carry out adoptive T-cell therapies. However, a human counterpart of oncostatin M has not yet been identified, and, in contrast to the mouse, the thymus is the only known site of T-cell production in the human. Age induces a severe decrease in the ability of the thymus to produce new T cells, but evidence indicates that thymic reserve is not completely depleted. Moreover, cytokines such as IL-7, epidermal growth factor (EGF) (229), and insulin-like growth factor-1 (IGF-1) could enhance the residual thymic function, offering possible therapeutic tools.

CYTOKINES

There is abundant evidence that cytokines play an important role in tumor immune biology in at least two different ways. First, cytokines affect the function of immune cells, including APCs and various classes of T lymphocytes. Among them, IL-2, IL-12, IL-18, TNF-α, IFN-γ, and GM-CSF exert an activating function, whereas IL-6, IL-10, TGF-β, and VEGF suppress DC and/or T-cell function (230). Second, abundant evidence indicates that cytokines directly influence tumor cell proliferation and survival. Numerous studies have shown that IL-1, IL-2, IL-4, and TGF-β may exert a direct effect on tumor cell growth, depending on the type of cytokines produced by the tumor itself or the cytokine receptors tumor cells express, the surrounding extracellular matrix, and the intrinsic immunogenicity of tumors. A clear example is provided by IL-1, which demonstrates cytocidal effects on certain tumor cells but favors metastatic spread in others (231,232).

There is evidence that cytokines may influence the immunogenicity of tumors. For instance, IFN-γ can increase the expression of MHC class I and enhance tumor immune recognition and immune-mediated destruction in different cell types (233). The pattern of cytokines present within the tumor environment can strongly influence the type of inflammatory/immune cell infiltrate activated by the tumor. Cytokines, together with chemokines, control leukocyte migration and profoundly influence the type of memory mechanisms mediated by T-helper cells (217,230). A Th1-type response mediates the delayed hypersensitivity response that is probably instrumental in tumor rejection, whereas a Th2-type response mediates allergic reactions and may be ineffective against tumors.

This wealth of information has stimulated the initiation of clinical trials with systemic administration of interleukins, including interferons, TNF-α, IL-1, IL-2, and IL-12 (234,235). Objective clinical responses and occasionally complete tumor responses have been seen in patients with melanoma, renal cell carcinoma, colon carcinoma, or ovarian cancer. Based on preclinical evidence suggesting that IL-2 promotes the activation of LAK cells, a subset of NK cells, and cytotoxic T cells and enhances the cytotoxic effect of autologous T cells against EOC cells, a phase I/II study of intraperitoneal administration of IL-2 was conducted in patients with recurrent or progressive EOC. Infusion over 24 hours was better tolerated than a 7-day infusion. An overall response rate of 25% was seen among 35 evaluable patients, including six surgically confirmed complete responses (236). IL-12 was tested in patients with renal carcinoma in a phase II clinical trial conducted by Genetics Institute. Marked toxicity was seen in that trial, with fatal multisystem failure in two patients. It appears that dose and scheduling may have been important parameters in determining toxicity, because toxicity has been mild in other studies (237). A study (protocol 170-B) is currently in progress with the Gynecologic Oncology Group (GOG) to evaluate systemic (intravenous) administration of IL-12 in recurrent or refractory ovarian cancer. Recombinant IL-12 is being administered for 5 days at 16-day interval cycles. IFN-α has been administered to patients with ovarian cancer via intravenous or repeated intraperitoneal infusions. Although intravenous IFN-α yielded poor results (238), better responses were observed with intraperitoneal administration (239). In a recent GOG trial, intraperitoneal IFN-α_{2b} was well tolerated and resulted in measurable responses in a favorable group of patients with minimal residual disease and documented sensitivity to platinum (28% overall response, including 16% surgically documented complete responses), but it was ineffective in patients with platinum-resistant disease (240). Similar results were reported in a recent European study. Because of its ability to upregulate expression of MHC class I molecules, IFN-γ may be a cytokine of potential interest in immune therapy for cancer. A small phase II study carried out in patients with recurrent ovarian cancer resulted in a clinical response in approximately 25% of patients (241).

Overall, clinical results obtained with systemic (intravenous or intraperitoneal) administration of cytokines in patients with ovarian cancer and other malignancies have been disappointing, and in some cases significant toxicity was observed. The advent of gene therapy has generated a renewed interest in cytokine therapy because it has made possible the intratumoral expression of high doses of cytokines. A growing bulk of preclinical evidence suggests that *in situ* cancer vaccination is feasible and, in many cases, effective. Very intense preclinical and clinical investigations are ongoing on the role of cytokines in tumor immune therapy. Preclinical experimentation has been undertaken with several cytokines, including IL-1 through IL-12, IP-10, IFN-α, IFN-β, IFN-γ, TNF-α, TGF-β, M-CSF, G-CSF, and GM-CSF (234).

The rationale for using gene therapy approaches to modify tumor cells was based on the observation that intratumoral injections of cytokines induced protective systemic immune responses with less toxicity than was observed with systemic cytokine administration. Seminal studies with *in situ* vaccination were carried out with IL-2 in colon cancer, in which it was demonstrated that IL-2 transfection rendered tumor cells independent of T-helper cooperation and maximized the immunogenicity of tumor cells, inducing protective systemic immunity in animal models (242). Further classic studies were performed by Dranoff and colleagues (243), who compared the effects of several cytokines on the immunologically inactive melanoma cell line B16 by transfecting cells with a replication-defective retroviral vector. Among 20 different cytokines, GM-CSF emerged as the most powerful in enhancing tumor immunogenicity and triggering protective systemic responses. In key experiments, the authors demonstrated an intense inflammatory infiltrate at the vaccination site comprising mononuclear cells, neutrophils, eosinophils, macrophages, and lymphocytes, while the regional lymph nodes displayed an engorgement of paracortical T-cell areas, suggesting the intervention of professional APCs and the activation of CD4$^+$ and CD8$^+$ T lymphocytes. *In vitro* studies indicated that GM-CSF induces DC precursors to mature and acquire characteristics of professional APCs, further confirming the potential utility of GM-CSF in cancer vaccination. Importantly, preclinical experiments indicated that GM-CSF tumor vaccination can induce an immune response against tumors that are refractory to conventional chemotherapy and/or hormonal therapy as well as tumor types previously thought to be refractory to immunotherapy (244). Multiple trials have been approved by the National Institutes of Health Recombinant DNA Advisory Committee entailing cytokine gene transfer for the treatment of cancers, with the predominant cytokines being IL-2 and GM-CSF.

The optimal way to induce cytokine secretion in the microenvironment of the tumor has been a matter of investigation (245). One possible approach is transfection of autologous cancer cells with a cytokine gene through the use of high-efficiency vectors such as adenoviruses. This results in high local levels of released cytokine, leading to a strong local inflammatory response specific to the particular cytokine. Enhanced tumor recognition may therefore ensue. An alternative approach entails mixture of the tumor cells with cytokine-containing biodegradable polymer microspheres. Toda and coworkers (169) undertook an interesting approach using a replication-competent oncolytic HSV that was engineered to produce GM-CSF. The direct administration of the virus into tumors resulted in GM-CSF expression within the tumor microenvironment and significantly augmented the efficacy of the oncolytic agent as a result of the generation of tumor-specific immune response. This effect persisted after the tumor was eradicated as a protective delayed hypersensitivity response.

A novel approach was undertaken by investigators at Johns Hopkins University, who engineered an MHC-negative lymphoma cell line to secrete high doses of GM-CSF (246). Thanks to the absence of MHC molecules, this line was able to function as a universal carrier cell line, to aid in the induction of immunity to the patient's autologous tumor without inducing a dominant allogeneic anti-MHC response against the GM-CSF-secreting cell line. These investigators undertook preclinical studies in which the GM-CSF carrier leukemia cell line was irradiated and administered together with irradiated autologous tumor cells to tumor-harboring animals, resulting in sustained tumor regressions. Preliminary reports indicated that clinical application of this GM-CSF$^+$ leukemia cell line also results in sustained clinical responses in humans. Immune responses and clinical responses were documented in renal cell cancers treated with irradiated autologous cells with genetic modification to secrete GM-CSF in a dose-escalating double-blind study. As in animal models, an inflammatory infiltrate was seen in intradermal sites of injection comprising macrophages, DCs, neutrophils, eosinophils, and T cells. Vaccinated patients displayed delayed-type hypersensitivity against autologous irradiated tumor cells.

ANTIBODIES

Solid tumors, including EOCs, trigger a humoral immune response. Specific antitumor antibodies have been identified in patients with EOC. However, tumors evade antibody-mediated cytotoxicity through multiple mechanisms, including evasion from complement-mediated cell lysis. Potentially improved antibody-based immunotherapies have been developed that use immunoconjugates composed of antibody molecules or fragments of antibody molecules directed against a tumor-specific antigen which are linked to cell toxins, radioactive particles, or cytokine molecules. Murine monoclonal antibodies were initially used, but their bioavailability was limited by immune-mediated neutralization. Recombinant technology allowed for the engineering of humanized antibodies, in which the Fc domain had a chimeric structure containing human sequences (247). Although this resulted in an increased half-life, immune responses against the therapeutic protein remained problematic. A second generation of antibodies was then produced by engineering of low-molecular-weight single-chain antibody variable domains (sFv) (248). These are much less immunogenic and display rapid localization within tumor sites, but their tumor retention is low.

Monoclonal antibodies have been raised against tumor antigens and tested clinically. A murine monoclonal antibody against the extracellular domain of HER-2 receptor exerted significant antiproliferative effects on breast cancer cells overexpressing HER-2/neu (249). Preclinical evidence in mouse models confirmed the efficacy of this strategy (250). Later a humanized anti-HER-2 antibody was engineered by inserting the binding region or complementarity-determining region of murine monoclonal antibody 4D5 into a consensus human immunoglobulin-1 framework (251). Further preclinical studies with this antibody indicated that it displayed increased affinity for the HER-2 receptor, it exhibited similar cytostatic effects to the murine 4D5 antibody, and it mediated antibody-dependent cell-mediated (252) and complement-mediated (253) cytotoxicity. Trastuzumab (Herceptin), a recombinant humanized anti-HER-2 monoclonal antibody, was tested in a phase II study in 46 patients with metastatic breast cancer whose tumors overexpressed HER-2. The treatment was well tolerated, but an overall response rate of only 11.6% was seen, including 1 complete response out of 43 evaluable patients (2.3%). Similar results were reported by the GOG in protocol 160, a phase II study in which 27 evaluable patients exhibited no complete responses and a partial response rate of just 7.4% (GOG Statistical Report, January 2000). Based on the heterogeneity of protein overexpression among tumor cells within the same patient (254), perhaps it is not surprising that monotherapy based on an anti-HER-2 strategy was not effective.

Bispecific antibodies directing immune cells (T cells) against tumor cells have been engineered by linking a TCR-binding fragment to a moiety directed against a specific tumor antigen. Canevari and colleagues (190) reported an overall 27% response rate after intraperitoneal administration of autologous *ex vivo* expanded T cells retargeted with the bispecific monoclonal antibody OC/TR and low-dose IL-2 in advanced EOC. As discussed earlier, such a methodology does not afford costimulatory signals, possibly accounting for the modest clinical results.

Other cytotoxic agents have been linked to monoclonal antibodies, including plant and bacterial toxins, recombinant cytokines, cytotoxic drugs, and gene therapy vectors. Immunotoxins such as truncated *Pseudomonas* exotoxin A (PE), truncated diphtheria toxin, and ricin, a plant holotoxin isolated from castor beans, have been tested in preclinical and clinical studies in patients with solid malignancies including ovarian cancer (255). The use of antibody-based immune therapies poses specific problems related to the stability of the immunoconjugates and their characteristics of binding to the targeted tumor cells, which translates to their affinity (efficacy) and their specificity (safety). Because these are foreign proteins, an immune reaction always ensues against the immunoconjugates. For example, a PE-carrying murine monoclonal antibody (OVB3-PE) directed against EOC was administered intraperitoneally in 23 patients with advanced refractory EOC (256). All patients developed antibodies against PE within 2 weeks, and no tumor response was seen.

Another issue with the use of antibody-based therapies relates to their specificity of binding. Because these therapies are usually directed against only one tumor antigen, they are restricted to patients with tumors that are rich in that specific protein. Tumor heterogeneity is of concern, in that the targeted antigen may not be expressed by a large portion of tumor cells (254). However, bystander mechanisms provided by radiation or by cytotoxic molecules may partially compensate for this limitation. Again, the propensity of tumors for mutation may result in selection of antigen-negative clones that may ultimately escape monovalent antibody-based therapy.

In addition, the specificity of the antibody is critical for safety issues, because cross-reactivity with normal tissues may result in significant toxicity. The paradigm of onconeuronal antigens clearly illustrates this point (257). Some patients with solid malignancies, including breast and ovarian cancers, develop during the course of their disease paraneoplastic disorders affecting the CNS. A well-characterized disorder is paraneoplastic cerebellar degeneration, in which specific antitumor antibodies and antitumor CD8$^+$ cytotoxic lymphocytes recognize onconeuronal antigens expressed by Purkinje cells, resulting in Purkinje cell destruction. Although antibodies against Purkinje cells have been identified in up to 3% of patients with EOC (258), T cells recognizing the cdr2 antigen are the main effectors of immune toxicity (259). Nevertheless, these disorders illustrate the fact that ovarian tumors and normal human tissues may share immunodominant antigens. In the phase I trial of intraperitoneal OVB3-PE administration, dose-limiting toxicity at doses of 5 and 10 µg/kg was manifested with severe encephalopathy in 3 of 23 patients, resulting in one death (256). In another phase I study of recombinant ricin administration, two patients developed progressive central neurologic toxicity, resulting in one death. Hemorrhagic necrotic vasculitis was seen within the basal ganglia (149).

Radioimmunoconjugates offer the distinct advantage of eliciting a wide bystander effect. Even if only a small percentage of tumor cells express a specific antigen, binding of the radioantibody provides radiation-induced damage to a radius that depends on the energy of the radioisotope. The choice of radioisotope has therefore been a matter of intense investigation (260). Theoretically, β-particle emitters are ideal for radiotherapy because their lethal doses are exhausted within a small radius of penetration. Radioactive iodine 131 and ytrium 90 have been the two isotopes most studied. Although ^{131}I has been widely available and is readily chelated with antibodies, its clinical application is limited by its physical properties (261). A lethal dose of radiation applied to tumor is approximately 500 to 2,000 cGy, depending on the tumor type. Such doses have proved efficacious against hematologic malignancies, but ovarian cancer may be more radioresistant. Dosimetry calculations indicate that ^{131}I delivers this dose up to a depth of less than 0.1 cm. Tissue distribution of monoclonal antibodies may be extremely variable due to patchy antigen presentation and tumor vascularization. It is therefore anticipated that a lethal dose of radiation would not be delivered to the entire tumor, even if the radioconjugate were delivered intravenously. ^{90}Y appears to be more suitable, because it delivers lethal radiation to a tissue depth of approximately 1 cm (262). It is anticipated that the bystander effect delivered by ^{90}Y would be much greater than that of ^{131}I, possibly resulting in better tumor control.

Several studies have been carried out with ^{131}I or ^{90}Y radioantibodies. Most of these studies were designed to administer radioactive antibody to patients via the intraperitoneal route. As predicted, the most critical factor affecting clinical response was the volume of intraperitoneal disease throughout all studies. Minimal responses were seen in patients with nodules larger than 2 cm, whereas patients with smaller-volume disease displayed clinical responses at an average rate of approximately 25%. Importantly, patients with minimal residual or microscopic disease displayed a response rate of approximately 35% to 40% (263). In one study, 15 patients with negative second-look laparoscopy for stage IIb-IV EOC underwent treatment with ^{90}Y HMFG1; 14 of them were alive at after 3 years. A small British study of 25 patients suggested a benefit from the administration of single-dose adjuvant intraperitoneal radioimmunotherapy after complete remission with platinum-based chemotherapy and tumor debulking (264). Obviously, the intraperitoneal route of administration precludes therapeutic benefits in patients with extraabdominal disease or retroperitoneal lymph node involvement. As an alternative, intravenous administration of radioimmunoconjugates might prove more advantageous. A significantly higher tumor uptake of radioantibodies was documented in one study, even in patients with minimal-volume disease (265). Further studies are needed to fully assess the efficacy of this approach.

CONCLUSION

The Human Genome Project is currently completed with the identification of some 30,000–40,000 protein encoding genes. The wealth of information derived from this project will provoke explosive advancements in cancer molecular therapy, including gene, immune, and biologic therapies. These future studies will lead to more exact understanding of the applicability of these approaches to the treatment of solid malignancies, including ovarian cancer. For the time being, the existing evidence indicates that both cancer gene therapy and immune therapy are probably best applied in patients with minimal volume of disease. It is likely that multimodality approaches with cytoreductive surgery, chemotherapy, radiation therapy, gene therapy, and immune therapy in various combinations will be advantageous compared with single-modality treatments. Gene therapy technology may be best suited to elicit cancer vaccination until better and safer vectors are available. It is likely that the implementation of tumor vaccines together with strategies aimed at improving effector cell function and treatments aimed at rendering tumor cells more susceptible to immune-mediated killing may all be necessary for controlling tumor growth. Although it is fair to say that the fields of cancer gene therapy and cancer immunotherapy are at the very early stages, significant progress is anticipated over the forthcoming few decades. Multicenter, prospective, double-blinded studies need to be designed to test these hypotheses.

REFERENCES

1. Dranoff G. Cancer gene therapy: connecting basic research with clinical inquiry. *J Clin Oncol* 1998;16:2548–2556.
2. Wivel NA, Wilson JM. Methods of gene delivery. *Hematol Oncol Clin North Am* 1998;12:483–501.
3. Yeh P, Perricaudet M. Advances in adenoviral vectors: from genetic engineering to their biology. *FASEB J* 1997;11:615–623.
4. Gao GP, Yang Y, Wilson JM. Biology of adenovirus vectors with E1 and E4 deletions for liver-directed gene therapy. *J Virol* 1996;70:8934–8943.
5. McDonald D, Stockwin L, Matzow T, et al. Coxsackie and adenovirus receptor (CAR)-dependent and major histocompatibility complex (MHC) class I-independent uptake of recombinant adenoviruses into human tumour cells. *Gene Ther* 1999;6:1512–1519.
6. Brenner M. Gene transfer by adenovectors. *Blood* 1999;94:3965–3967.
7. Bett AJ, Haddara W, Prevec L, Graham FL. An efficient and flexible system for construction of adenovirus vectors with insertions or deletions in early regions 1 and 3. *Proc Natl Acad Sci USA* 1994;91:8802–8806.
8. Hehir KM, Armentano D, Cardoza LM, et al. Molecular characterization of replication-competent variants of adenovirus vectors and genome modifications to prevent their occurrence. *J Virol* 1996;70:8459–8467.
9. Dai Y, Schwarz EM, Gu D, et al. Cellular and humoral immune responses to adenoviral vectors containing factor IX gene: tolerization of factor IX and vector antigens allows for long-term expression. *Proc Natl Acad Sci USA* 1995;92:1401–1405.
10. Yang Y, Xiang Z, Ertl HC, Wilson JM. Upregulation of class I major histocompatibility complex antigens by interferon gamma is necessary for T-cell-mediated elimination of recombinant adenovirus-infected hepatocytes in vivo. *Proc Natl Acad Sci USA* 1995;92:7257–7261.
11. Molnar-Kimber KL, Sterman DH, Chang M, et al. Impact of preexisting and induced humoral and cellular immune responses in an adenovirus-based gene therapy phase I clinical trial for localized mesothelioma. *Hum Gene Ther* 1998;9:2121–2133.
12. Behbakht K, Benjamin I, Chiu HC, et al. Adenovirus-mediated gene therapy of ovarian cancer in a mouse model. *Am J Obstet Gynecol* 1996;175:1260–1265.
13. Rancourt C, Rogers BE, Sosnowski BA, et al. Basic fibroblast growth factor enhancement of adenovirus-mediated delivery of the herpes simplex virus thymidine kinase gene results in augmented therapeutic benefit in a murine model of ovarian cancer. *Clin Cancer Res* 1998;4:2455–2461.
14. Richardson WD, Westphal H. A cascade of adenovirus early functions is required for expression of adeno-associated virus. *Cell* 1981;27:133–141.
15. Hermonat PL, Labow MA, Wright R, et al. Genetics of adeno-associated virus: isolation and preliminary characterization of adeno-associated virus type 2 mutants. *J Virol* 1984;51:329–339.
16. Lebkowski JS, McNally MM, Okarma TB, Lerch LB. Adeno-associated virus: a vector system for efficient introduction and integration of DNA into a variety of mammalian cell types. *Mol Cell Biol* 1988;8:3988–3996.
17. Hoerer M, Bogedain C, Scheer U, et al. The use of recombinant adeno-associated viral vectors for the transduction of epithelial tumor cells. *Int J Immunopharmacol* 1997;19:473–479.
18. Maass G, Bogedain C, Scheer U, et al. Recombinant adeno-associated virus for the generation of autologous, gene-modified tumor vaccines: evidence for a high transduction efficiency into primary epithelial cancer cells. *Hum Gene Ther* 1998;9:1049–1059.
19. Fisher KJ, Jooss K, Alston J, et al. Recombinant adeno-associated virus for muscle directed gene therapy. *Nat Med* 1997;3:306–312.
20. Montgomery RI, Warner MS, Lum BJ, Spear PG. Herpes simplex virus-1 entry into cells mediated by a novel member of the TNF/NGF receptor family. *Cell* 1996;87:427–436.
21. Geraghty RJ, Krummenacher C, Cohen GH, et al. Entry of alphaherpesviruses mediated by poliovirus receptor-related protein 1 and poliovirus receptor. *Science* 1998;280:1618–1620.
22. Whitbeck JC, Peng C, Lou H, et al. Glycoprotein D of herpes simplex virus (HSV) binds directly to HVEM, a member of the tumor necrosis factor receptor superfamily and a mediator of HSV entry. *J Virol* 1997;71:6083–6093.
23. Glorioso J, Bender MA, Fink D, DeLuca N. Herpes simplex virus vectors. *Mol Cell Biol Hum Dis Ser* 1995;5:33–63.

24. Fraefel C, Song S, Lim F, et al. Helper virus-free transfer of herpes simplex virus type 1 plasmid vectors into neural cells. *J Virol* 1996;70:7190–7197.
25. Coukos G, Rubin SC, Molnar-Kimber KL. Application of recombinant herpes simplex virus-1 (HSV-1) for the treatment of malignancies outside the central nervous system. *Gene Ther Mol Biol* 1999;3:78–89.
26. Spivack JG, Fraser NW. Expression of herpes simplex virus type 1 (HSV-1) latency-associated transcripts and transcripts affected by the deletion in avirulent mutant HFEM: evidence for a new class of HSV-1 genes. *J Virol* 1988;62:3281–3287.
27. Johnson PA, Miyanohara A, Levine F, et al. Cytotoxicity of a replication-defective mutant of herpes simplex virus type 1. *J Virol* 1992;66:2952–2965.
28. Coukos G, Makrigiannakis A, Kang EH, et al. Use of carrier cells to deliver a replication-selective herpes simplex virus-1 mutant for the intraperitoneal therapy of epithelial ovarian cancer. *Clin Cancer Res* 1999;5:1523–1537.
29. Wang M, Rancourt C, Navarro JG, et al. High-efficacy thymidine kinase gene transfer to ovarian cancer cell lines mediated by herpes simplex virus type 1 vector. *Gynecol Oncol* 1998;71:278–287.
30. Gange RW, de Bats A, Park JR, et al. Cellular immunity and circulating antibody to herpes simplex virus in subjects with recurrent herpes simplex lesions and controls as measured by the mixed leukocyte migration inhibition test and complement fixation. *Br J Dermatol* 1975;93:539–544.
31. Boris-Lawrie K, Temin HM. The retroviral vector: replication cycle and safety considerations for retrovirus-mediated gene therapy. *Ann N Y Acad Sci* 1994;716:59–70.
32. Gordon EM, Anderson WF. Gene therapy using retroviral vectors. *Curr Opin Biotechnol* 1994;5:611–616.
33. Powell SK, Kaloss M, Burimski I, et al. In vitro analysis of transformation potential associated with retroviral vector insertions. *Hum Gene Ther* 1999;10:2123–2132.
34. Felgner PL, Holm M, Chan H. Cationic liposome mediated transfection. *Proc West Pharmacol Soc* 1989;32:115–121.
35. Stamatatos L, Leventis R, Zuckermann MJ, Silvius JR. Interactions of cationic lipid vesicles with negatively charged phospholipid vesicles and biological membranes. *Biochemistry* 1988;27:3917–3925.
36. Xing X, Zhang S, Chang JY, et al. Safety study and characterization of E1A-liposome complex gene-delivery protocol in an ovarian cancer model. *Gene Ther* 1998;5:1538–1544.
37. Son K, Huang L. Exposure of human ovarian carcinoma to cisplatin transiently sensitizes the tumor cells for liposome-mediated gene transfer. *Proc Natl Acad Sci USA* 1994;91:12669–12672.
38. Liu Y, Liggitt D, Zhong W, et al. Cationic liposome-mediated intravenous gene delivery. *J Biol Chem* 1995;270:24864–24870.
39. Whitmore M, Li S, Huang L. LPD lipopolyplex initiates a potent cytokine response and inhibits tumor growth. *Gene Ther* 1999;6:1867–1875.
40. Qi XR, Maitani Y, Nagai T. Rates of systemic degradation and reticuloendothelial system uptake of calcein in the dipalmitoylphosphatidylcholine liposomes with soybean-derived sterols in mice. *Pharm Res* 1995;12:49–52.
41. Moolten FL. Tumor chemosensitivity conferred by inserted herpes thymidine kinase genes: paradigm for a prospective cancer control strategy. *Cancer Res* 1986;46:5276–5281.
42. Nishiyama T, Kawamura Y, Kawamoto K, et al. Antineoplastic effects in rats of 5-fluorocytosine in combination with cytosine deaminase capsules. *Cancer Res* 1985;45:1753–1751.
43. MacCorkle RA, Freeman KW, Spencer DM. Synthetic activation of caspases: artificial death switches. *Proc Natl Acad Sci USA* 1998;95:3655–3660.
44. Wallace H, Clarke AR, Harrison DJ, et al. Ganciclovir-induced ablation non-proliferating thyrocytes expressing herpesvirus thymidine kinase occurs by p53-independent apoptosis. *Oncogene* 1996;13:55–61.
45. Lan KH, Kanai F, Shiratori Y, et al. Tumor-specific gene expression in carcinoembryonic antigen-producing gastric cancer cells using adenovirus vectors. *Gastroenterology* 1996;111:1241–1251.
46. Freeman SM, Aboud CN, Whartenby KA, et al. The "bystander effect": tumor regression when a fraction of the tumor mass is genetically modified. *Cancer Res* 1993;53:5274–5283.
47. Connors TA. The choice of prodrugs for gene directed enzyme prodrug therapy of cancer. *Gene Ther* 1995;2:702–709.
48. Mesnil M, Piccoli C, Tiraby G, et al. Bystander killing of cancer cells by herpes simplex virus thymidine kinase gene is mediated by connexins. *Proc Natl Acad Sci USA* 1996;93:1831–1835.
49. Huber BE, Austin EA, Richards CA, et al. Metabolism of 5-fluorocytosine to 5-fluorouracil in human colorectal tumor cells transduced with the cytosine deaminase gene: significant antitumor effects when only a small percentage of tumor cells express cytosine deaminase. *Proc Natl Acad Sci USA* 1994;91:8302–8306.
50. Ramesh R, Marrogi AJ, Munshi A, et al. In vivo analysis of the 'bystander effect': a cytokine cascade. *Exp Hematol* 1996;24:829–838.
51. Wei SJ, Chao Y, Shih YL, et al. Involvement of Fas (CD95/APO-1) and Fas ligand in apoptosis induced by ganciclovir treatment of tumor cells transduced with herpes simplex virus thymidine kinase. *Gene Ther* 1999;6:420–431.
52. Gagandeep S, Brew R, Green B, et al. Prodrug-activated gene therapy: involvement of an immunological component in the "bystander effect." *Cancer Gene Ther* 1996;3:83–88.
53. Freeman SM, Ramesh R, Marrogi AJ. Immune system in suicide-gene therapy. *Lancet* 1997;349:2–3.
54. Vile RG, Nelson JA, Castleden S, et al. Systemic gene therapy of murine melanoma using tissue specific expression of the HSVtk gene involves an immune component. *Cancer Res* 1994;54:6228–6234.
55. Yamamoto S, Suzuki S, Hoshino A, et al. Herpes simplex virus thymidine kinase/ganciclovir-mediated killing of tumor cell induces tumor-specific cytotoxic T cells in mice. *Cancer Gene Ther* 1997;4:91–96.
56. Ramesh R, Munshi A, Abboud CN, et al. Expression of costimulatory molecules: B7 and ICAM up-regulation after treatment with a suicide gene. *Cancer Gene Ther* 1996;3:373–384.
57. Tong XW, Kieback DG, Ramesh R, Freeman SM. Molecular aspects of ovarian cancer: is gene therapy the

solution? *Hematol Oncol Clin North Am* 1999;13:109–133,viii.
58. Barnes MN, Deshane JS, Rosenfeld M, et al. Gene therapy and ovarian cancer: a review. *Obstet Gynecol* 1997;89:145–155.
59. Robertson MW 3rd, Barnes MN, Rancourt C, et al. Gene therapy for ovarian carcinoma. *Semin Oncol* 1998;25:397–406.
60. Tong XW, Block A, Chen SH, et al. In vivo gene therapy of ovarian cancer by adenovirus-mediated thymidine kinase gene transduction and ganciclovir administration. *Gynecol Oncol* 1996;61:175–179.
61. Tong XW, Agoulnik I, Blankenburg K, et al. Human epithelial ovarian cancer xenotransplants into nude mice can be cured by adenovirus-mediated thymidine kinase gene therapy. *Anticancer Res* 1997;17:811–813.
62. Al-Hendy A, Auersperg N. Applying the herpes simplex virus thymidine kinase/ganciclovir approach to ovarian cancer: an effective in vitro drug-sensitization system. *Gynecol Obstet Invest* 1997;43:268–275.
63. Rosenfeld ME, Wang M, Siegal GP, et al. Adenoviral-mediated delivery of herpes simplex virus thymidine kinase results in tumor reduction and prolonged survival in a SCID mouse model of human ovarian carcinoma. *J Mol Med* 1996;74:455–462.
64. McNeish IA, Green NK, Gilligan MG, et al. Virus directed enzyme prodrug therapy for ovarian and pancreatic cancer using retrovirally delivered E. coli nitroreductase and CB1954. *Gene Ther* 1998;5:1061–1069.
65. Benjamin I, Coukos G, Albelda SM, et al. Gene therapy of ovarian cancer utilizing an E1/E4-deleted type 5 adenoviral vector (H5.001RSVTK). *Society of Gynecologic Oncologists 29th Annual Meeting,* Orlando, FL, February 7–11, 1998.
66. Freeman SM, McCune C, Robinson W, et al. The treatment of ovarian cancer with a gene modified cancer vaccine: a phase I study. *Hum Gene Ther* 1995;6:927–939.
67. Alvarez RD, Curiel DT. A phase I study of recombinant adenovirus vector-mediated intraperitoneal delivery of herpes simplex virus thymidine kinase (HSV-TK) gene and intravenous ganciclovir for previously treated ovarian and extraovarian cancer patients. *Hum Gene Ther* 1997;8:597–613.
68. Elshami AA, Cook JW, Amin KM, et al. The effect of promoter strength in adenoviral vectors containing herpes simplex virus thymidine kinase on cancer gene therapy in vitro and in vivo. *Cancer Gene Ther* 1997;4:213–221.
69. Coombes AG, Heckman JD. Gel casting of resorbable polymers: 1. Processing and applications. *Biomaterials* 1992;13:217–224.
70. Matthews C, Jenkins G, Hilfinger J, Davidson B. Poly-L-lysine improves gene transfer with adenovirus formulated in PLGA microspheres. *Gene Ther* 1999;6:1558–1564.
71. Shalaby WSW, Lannuti M, Coukos G, et al. Ganciclovir delivery systems for gene therapy of ovarian cancer. *Society of Gynecologic Oncologists 31st Annual Meeting,* San Diego, CA, February 6–9, 2000.
72. Wildner O, Blaese RM, Morris JC. Synergy between the herpes simplex virus tk/ganciclovir prodrug suicide system and the topoisomerase I inhibitor topotecan. *Hum Gene Ther* 1999;10:2679–2687.
73. Stass SA, Mixson J. Oncogenes and tumor suppressor genes: therapeutic implications. *Clin Cancer Res* 1997;3:2687–2695.
74. Berchuck A, Carney M. Human ovarian cancer of the surface epithelium. *Biochem Pharmacol* 1997;54:541–544.
75. Meden H, Kuhn W. Overexpression of the oncogene c-erbB-2 (HER2/neu) in ovarian cancer: a new prognostic factor. *Eur J Obstet Gynecol Reprod Biol* 1997;71:173–179.
76. Somasundaram K, Zhang H, Zeng YX, et al. Arrest of the cell cycle by the tumour-suppressor BRCA1 requires the CDK-inhibitor p21WAF1/CiP1. *Nature* 1997;389:187–190.
77. Aprelikova ON, Fang BS, Meissner EG, et al. BRCA1-associated growth arrest is RB-dependent. *Proc Natl Acad Sci USA* 1999;96: 11866–11871.
78. Holt JT, Thompson ME, Szabo C, et al. Growth retardation and tumour inhibition by BRCA1. *Nat Genet* 1996;12:298–302.
79. Tait DL, Obermiller PS, Redlin-Frazier S, et al. A phase I trial of retroviral BRCA1sv gene therapy in ovarian cancer. *Clin Cancer Res* 1997;3:1959–1968.
80. Tai YT, Strobel T, Kufe D, Cannistra SA. In vivo cytotoxicity of ovarian cancer cells through tumor-selective expression of the BAX gene. *Cancer Res* 1999;59:2121–2126.
81. Wolf JK, Kim TE, Fightmaster D, et al. Growth suppression of human ovarian cancer cell lines by the introduction of a p16 gene via a recombinant adenovirus. *Gynecol Oncol* 1999;73:27–34.
82. Song K, Cowan KH, Sinha BK. In vivo studies of adenovirus-mediated p53 gene therapy for cis-platinum-resistant human ovarian tumor xenografts. *Oncol Res* 1999;11:153–159.
83. Kim J, Hwang ES, Kim JS, et al. Intraperitoneal gene therapy with adenoviral-mediated p53 tumor suppressor gene for ovarian cancer model in nude mouse. *Cancer Gene Ther* 1999;6:172–178.
84. Mujoo K, Maneval DC, Anderson SC, Gutterman JU. Adenoviral-mediated p53 tumor suppressor gene therapy of human ovarian carcinoma. *Oncogene* 1996;12:1617–1623.
85. Song K, Li Z, Seth P, Cowan KH, Sinha BK. Sensitization of cis-platinum by a recombinant adenovirus vector expressing wild-type p53 gene in human ovarian carcinomas. *Oncol Res* 1997;9:603–609.
86. Gurnani M, Lipari P, Dell J, et al. Adenovirus-mediated p53 gene therapy has greater efficacy when combined with chemotherapy against human head and neck, ovarian, prostate, and breast cancer. *Cancer Chemother Pharmacol* 1999;44:143–151.
87. Nielsen LL, Lipari P, Dell J, et al. Adenovirus-mediated p53 gene therapy and paclitaxel have synergistic efficacy in models of human head and neck, ovarian, prostate, and breast cancer. *Clin Cancer Res* 1998;4: 835–846.
88. Bouvet M, Ellis LM, Nishizaki M, et al. Adenovirus-mediated wild-type p53 gene transfer down-regulates vascular endothelial growth factor expression and inhibits angiogenesis in human colon cancer. *Cancer Res* 1998;58:2288–2292.
89. Owen-Schaub LB, Zhang W, Cusack JC, et al. Wild-type human p53 and a temperature-sensitive mutant

induce Fas/APO-1 expression. *Mol Cell Biol* 1995; 15:3032–3040.
90. Roth JA, Molldrem J, Smythe WR. The current status of cancer gene therapy trials. In: *Principles and Practice of Oncology Updates.* 1999;13:1–15.
91. Buler RE, Pegram M, Runnebaum I. A phase I study of gene therapy with recombinant intraperitoneal p53 in recurrent ovarian carcinoma. *Cancer Gene Ther* 1998;5:S25.
92. Scanlon KJ, Kashani-Sabet M. Ribozymes as therapeutic agents: are we getting closer? *J Natl Cancer Inst* 1998;90:558–559.
93. Helene C, Giovannangeli C, Guieysse-Peugeot AL, Praseuth D. Sequence-specific control of gene expression by antigene and clamp oligonucleotides. *Ciba Found Symp* 1997;209:94–102.
94. Mercola D, Cohen JS. Antisense approaches to cancer gene therapy. *Cancer Gene Ther* 1995;2:47–59.
95. Semba K, Kamata N, Toyoshima K, Yamamoto T. A v-erbB-related protooncogene, c-erbB-2, is distinct from the c-erbB-1/ epidermal growth factor-receptor gene and is amplified in a human salivary gland adenocarcinoma. *Proc Natl Acad Sci USA* 1995;82:6497–501.
96. Guy CT, Cardiff RD, Muller WJ. Activated neu induces rapid tumor progression. *J Biol Chem* 1996;271:7673–7678.
97. Deshane J, Loechel F, Conry RM, et al. Intracellular single-chain antibody directed against erbB2 downregulates cell surface erbB2 and exhibits a selective antiproliferative effect in erbB2 overexpressing cancer cell lines. *Gene Ther* 1994;1:332–337.
98. Deshane J, Siegal GP, Wang M, et al. Transductional efficacy and safety of an intraperitoneally delivered adenovirus encoding an anti-erbB-2 intracellular single-chain antibody for ovarian cancer gene therapy. *Gynecol Oncol* 1997;64:378–385.
99. Alvarez RD, Curiel DT. A phase I study of recombinant adenovirus vector-mediated delivery of an anti-erbB-2 single-chain (sFv) antibody gene for previously treated ovarian and extraovarian cancer patients. *Hum Gene Ther* 1997;8:229–242.
100. Yu DH, Scorsone K, Hung MC. Adenovirus type 5 E1A gene products act as transformation suppressors of the neu oncogene. *Mol Cell Biol* 1991;11:1745–750.
101. Hung MC, Matin A, Zhang Y, et al. HER-2/neu-targeting gene therapy: a review. *Gene* 1995;159:65–71.
102. Zhang Y, Yu D, Xia W, Hung MC. HER-2/neu-targeting cancer therapy via adenovirus-mediated E1A delivery in an animal model. *Oncogene* 1995;10:1947–1954.
103. Martuza RL. Conditionally replicating herpes vectors for cancer therapy. *J Clin Invest* 2000;105:841–846.
104. Martuza R, Malick A, Markert J, et al. Experimental therapy of human glioma by means of a genetically engineered virus mutant. *Science* 1991;252:854–856.
105. Sanders P, Wilkie N, Davison A. Thymidine kinase deletion mutants of herpes simplex virus type 1. *J Gen Virol* 1982;63:277–295.
106. Idowu A, Fraser-Smith E, Poffenberger K, Herman R. Deletion of the herpes simplex virus type 1 ribonucleotide reductase gene alters virulence and latency in vivo. *Antiviral Res* 1992;17:145–156.
107. Boviatsis E, Scharf J, Chase M, et al. Antitumor activity and reporter gene transfer into rat brain neoplasms inoculated with herpes simplex virus vectors defective in thymidine kinase or ribonucleotide reductase. *Gene Ther* 1994;1:323–331.
108. Carroll N, Chiocca E, Takahashi K, Tanabe K. Enhancement of gene therapy specificity for diffuse colon carcinoma liver metastases with recombinant herpes simplex virus. *Ann Surg* 1996;224:323–329.
109. Mineta T, Rabkin S, Yazaki T, et al. Attenuated multi-mutated herpes simplex virus-1 for the treatment of malignant gliomas. *Nat Med* 1995;1:938–943.
110. Kesari S, Randazzo B, Valyi-Nagy T, et al. Therapy of experimental human brain tumors using a neuroattenuated herpes simplex virus mutant. *Lab Invest* 1995;73:636–648.
111. Chambers R, Gillespie GY, Soroceanu L, et al. Comparison of genetically engineered herpes simplex viruses for the treatment of brain tumors in a SCID mouse model of human malignant glioma. *Proc Natl Acad Sci USA* 1995;92:1411–1415.
112. Chou J, Kern E, Whitley R, Roizman B. Mapping of herpes simplex virus-1 neurovirulence to g_1 34.5, a gene nonessential for growth in culture. *Science* 1990;250:1262–1265.
113. MacLean M, Ul-Fareed M, Roberson L, et al. Herpes simplex virus type 1 deletion variant 1714 and 1716 pinpoint neurovirulence-related sequences in Glasgow strain 17+ between immediate early gene 1 and the "a" sequence. *J Gen Virol* 1991;72:63–639.
114. Bolovan CA, Sawtell NM, Thompson RL. ICP34.5 mutants of herpes simplex virus type 1 strain 17syn+ are attenuated for neurovirulence in mice and for replication in confluent primary mouse embryo cell cultures. *J Virol* 1994;68:48–55.
115. Brown S, MacLean A, Aitken J, Harland J. ICP34.5 influences herpes simplex virus type I maturation and egress from infected cells in vitro. *J Gen Virol* 1994;75:3767–3686.
116. He B, Gross M, Roizman B. The gamma(1)34.5 protein of herpes simplex virus 1 complexes with protein phosphatase 1 alpha to dephosphorylate the alpha subunit of the eukaryotic translation initiation factor 2 and preclude the shutoff of protein synthesis by double-stranded RNA-activated protein kinase. *Proc Natl Acad Sci USA* 1997;94:843–848.
117. Brown S, Rampling R, Cruikshank G, et al. A phase 1 dose escalation trial of intratumoral injection with ICP34.5-ve HSV1 into recurrent malignant glioma. In: Twenty-third International Herpesvirus Workshop, York, UK, 1998:A386.
118. Markert J, Medlock M, Martuza R, et al. Initial report of phase I trial of genetically engineered HSV-1 in patients with malignant glioma. In: Twenty-third International Herpesvirus Workshop, York, UK, 1998:A384.
119. Kucharczuk JC, Randazzo B, Elshami AA, et al. Use of a replication-restricted, recombinant herpes virus to treat localized human malignancy. *Cancer Res* 1997;57:466–471.
120. Randazzo B, Bhat M, Kesari S, et al. Treatment of experimental subcutaneous human melanoma with a replication-restricted herpes simplex virus mutant. *J Invest Dermatol* 1997;108:933–937.
121. Kooby DA, Carew JF, Halterman MW, et al. Oncolytic viral therapy for human colorectal cancer and liver metastases using a multi-mutated herpes simplex virus type-1 (G207). *FASEB J* 1999;13:1325–1334.

122. Carew JF, Kooby DA, Halterman MW, et al. Selective infection and cytolysis of human head and neck squamous cell carcinoma with sparing of normal mucosa by a cytotoxic herpes simplex virus type 1 (G207). *Hum Gene Ther* 1999;10:1599–606.
123. Toda M, Rabkin SD, Martuza RL. Treatment of human breast cancer in a brain metastatic model by G207, a replication competent multimutated herpes simplex virus 1. *Hum Gene Ther* 1998;9:2173–2185.
124. Advani SJ, Chung SM, Yan SY, et al. Replication-competent, nonneuroinvasive genetically engineered herpes virus is highly effective in the treatment of therapy-resistant experimental human tumors. *Cancer Res* 1999;59:2055–2058.
125. Coukos G, Makrigiannakis A, Montas S, et al. Multi-attenuated herpes simplex virus-1 mutant G207 exerts cytotoxicity against epithelial ovarian cancer but not normal mesothelium, and is suitable for intraperitoneal oncolytic therapy. *Cancer Gene Ther* 2000;7:275–283.
126. Coukos G, Makrigiannakis A, Kang E, et al. Herpes simplex virus-1 lacking ICP34.5 induces p53-independent death and exerts a potent oncolytic effect against chemotherapy-resistant ovarian cancer in vitro and in vivo. In: Society of Gynecologic Oncologists 31st Annual Meeting, San Diego, CA, February 6–9, 2000.
127. Heise C, Sampson-Johannes A, Williams A, et al. ONYX-015, an E1B gene-attenuated adenovirus, causes tumor-specific cytolysis and antitumoral efficacy that can be augmented by standard chemotherapeutic agents [see comments]. *Nat Med* 1997;3:639–645.
128. Hall AR, Dix BR, O'Carroll SJ, Braithwaite AW. p53-dependent cell death/apoptosis is required for a productive adenovirus infection. *Nat Med* 1998;4:1068–1072.
129. Kirn D, Hermiston T, McCormick F. ONYX-015: clinical data are encouraging. *Nat Med* 1998;4:1341–1342.
130. Markiewicz MA, Gajewski TF. The immune system as anti-tumor sentinel: molecular requirements for an anti-tumor immune response. *Crit Rev Oncog* 1999;10:247–260.
131. Warren HS, Smyth MJ. NK cells and apoptosis. *Immunol Cell Biol* 1999;77:64–75.
132. Wang RF. Tumor antigens discovery: perspectives for cancer therapy. *Mol Med* 1997;3:716–731.
133. Lynch DH. Induction of dendritic cells (DC) by Flt3 Ligand (FL) promotes the generation of tumor-specific immune responses in vivo. *Crit Rev Immunol* 1998;18:99–107.
134. Albert ML, Sauter B, Bhardwaj N. Dendritic cells acquire antigen from apoptotic cells and induce class I-restricted CTLs. *Nature* 1998;392:86–89.
135. Kawakami Y, Rosenberg SA. Human tumor antigens recognized by T-cells. *Immunol Res* 1997;16:313–339.
136. Van den Eynde BJ, van der Bruggen P. T cell defined tumor antigens. *Curr Opin Immunol* 1997;9:684–693.
137. Boon T, Coulie PG, Van den Eynde B. Tumor antigens recognized by T cells. *Immunol Today* 1997;18:267–268.
138. Bukowski RM, Rayman P, Uzzo R, et al. Signal transduction abnormalities in T lymphocytes from patients with advanced renal carcinoma: clinical relevance and effects of cytokine therapy. *Clin Cancer Res* 1998;4:2337–2347.
139. Kurts C, Heath WR, Carbone FR, et al. Cross-presentation of self antigens to CD8+ T cells: the balance between tolerance and autoimmunity. *Novartis Found Symp* 1998;215:172–181.
140. Finke J, Ferrone S, Frey A, et al. Where have all the T cells gone? Mechanisms of immune evasion by tumors. *Immunol Today* 1999;20:158–160.
141. Schondorf T, Engel H, Lindemann C, et al. Cellular characteristics of peripheral blood lymphocytes and tumour-infiltrating lymphocytes in patients with gynaecological tumours. *Cancer Immunol Immunother* 1997;44:88–96.
142. Melichar B, Savary C, Kudelka AP, et al. Lineage-negative human leukocyte antigen-DR+ cells with the phenotype of undifferentiated dendritic cells in patients with carcinoma of the abdomen and pelvis. *Clin Cancer Res* 1998;4:799–809.
143. Ganss R, Limmer A, Sacher T, et al. Autoaggression and tumor rejection: it takes more than self-specific T-cell activation. *Immunol Rev* 1999;169:263–272.
144. Seliger B, Maeurer MJ, Ferrone S. TAP off–tumors on. *Immunol Today* 1997;18:292–299.
145. Petersson M, Charo J, Salazar-Onfray F, et al. Constitutive IL-10 production accounts for the high NK sensitivity, low MHC class I expression, and poor transporter associated with antigen processing (TAP)-1/2 function in the prototype NK target YAC-1. *J Immunol* 1998;161:2099–2105.
146. Ishida T, Oyama T, Carbone DP, Gabrilovich DI. Defective function of Langerhans cells in tumor-bearing animals is the result of defective maturation from hemopoietic progenitors. *J Immunol* 1998;161:4842–4851.
147. Nakashima M, Sonoda K, Watanabe T. Inhibition of cell growth and induction of apoptotic cell death by the human tumor-associated antigen RCAS1. *Nat Med* 1999;5:938–942.
148. Schondorf T, Engel H, Kurbacher CM, et al. Immunologic features of tumor-infiltrating lymphocytes and peripheral blood lymphocytes in ovarian cancer patients. *J Soc Gynecol Investig* 1998;5:102–107.
149. Bookman MA. Biological therapy of ovarian cancer: current directions. *Semin Oncol* 1998;25:381–396.
150. Vanderkwaak TJ, Alvarez RD. Immune directed therapy for ovarian carcinoma. *Curr Opin Obstet Gynecol* 1999;11:29–34.
151. Pardoll DM. Cancer vaccines. *Nat Med* 1998;4:525–531.
152. Tarte K, Klein B. Dendritic cell-based vaccine: a promising approach for cancer immunotherapy. *Leukemia* 1999;13:653–663.
153. Mastrangelo MJ, Maguire HC, Lattime EC, Berd D. Whole cell vaccines. In: De Vita VT, Hellman S, Rosenberg SA, eds. *Biological therapy of cancer*, 2nd ed. Philadelphia: JB Lippincott, 1996:648–658.
154. Berd D, Maguire HC Jr, Schuchter LM, et al. Autologous hapten-modified melanoma vaccine as postsurgical adjuvant treatment after resection of nodal metastases. *J Clin Oncol* 1997;15:2359–2370.
155. Berd D, Kairys J, Dunton C, et al. Autologous, hapten-modified vaccine as a treatment for human cancers. *Semin Oncol* 1998;25:646–653.
156. Sinkovics JG. Viral oncolysates as human tumor vaccines. *Int Rev Immunol* 1991;7:259–287.
157. Sivanandham M, Wallack MK. Viral oncolysates. In: De Vita VT, Hellman S, Rosenberg SA, eds. *Biological*

therapy of cancer. Philadelphia: JB Lippincott, 1996: 659–667.
158. Howard OM, Oppenheim JJ, Wang JM. Chemokines as molecular targets for therapeutic intervention. *J Clin Immunol* 1999;19:280–292.
159. Boone CW, Paranjpe M, Orme T, Gillette R. Virus-augmented tumor transplantation antigens: evidence for a helper antigen mechanism. *Int J Cancer* 1974;13:543–551.
160. Melcher A, Todryk S, Hardwick N, et al. Tumor immunogenicity is determined by the mechanism of cell death via induction of heat shock protein expression. *Nat Med* 1998;4:581–587.
161. Livingston PO, Albino AP, Chung TJ, et al. Serological response of melanoma patients to vaccines prepared from VSV lysates of autologous and allogeneic cultured melanoma cells. *Cancer* 1985;55:713–720.
162. Ioannides CG, Den Otter W. Concepts in immunotherapy of cancer: introduction. *In Vivo* 1991;5:551–552.
163. Ioannides CG, Platsoucas CD, Freedman RS. Immunological effects of tumor vaccines: II. T cell responses directed against cellular antigens in the viral oncolysates. *In Vivo* 1990;4: 17–24.
164. Schirrmacher V, Ahlert T, Probstle T, et al. Immunization with virus-modified tumor cells. *Semin Oncol* 1998;25:677–696.
165. Schirrmacher V. Tumor vaccine design: concepts, mechanisms, and efficacy testing. *Int Arch Allergy Immunol* 1995;108:340–344.
166. Mobus V, Horn S, Stock M, Schirrmacher V. Tumor cell vaccination for gynecological tumors. *Hybridoma* 1993;12:543–547.
167. Restifo NP. The new vaccines: building viruses that elicit antitumor immunity. *Curr Opin Immunol* 1996;8:658–663.
168. Krisky DM, Marconi PC, Oligino TJ, et al. Development of herpes simplex virus replication-defective multigene vectors for combination gene therapy applications. *Gene Ther* 1998;5:1517–1530.
169. Toda M, Martuza R, Kojima H, Rabkin S. In situ cancer vaccination: an IL-12 defective vector/replication-competent herpes simplex virus combination induces local and systemic antitumor activity. *J Immunol* 1998; 160:4457–4464.
170. Link CJ Jr, Moorman D, Seregina T, et al. A phase I trial of in vivo gene therapy with the herpes simplex thymidine kinase/ganciclovir system for the treatment of refractory or recurrent ovarian cancer. *Hum Gene Ther* 1996;7:1161–1179.
171. Rosenberg SA. The immunotherapy of solid cancers based on cloning the genes encoding tumor-rejection antigens. *Annu Rev Med* 1996;47:481–491.
172. Diederichs K, Boone T, Karplus PA. Novel fold and putative receptor binding site of granulocyte-macrophage colony-stimulating factor. *Science* 1991;254:1779–1782.
173. Taylor-Papadimitriou J, Finn OJ. Biology, biochemistry and immunology of carcinoma-associated mucins. *Immunol Today* 1997;18:105–107.
174. Granowska M, Mather SJ, Jobling T, et al. Radiolabelled stripped mucin, SM3, monoclonal antibody for immunoscintigraphy of ovarian tumours. *Int J Biol Markers* 1990;5:89–96.
175. Wang RF, Rosenberg SA. Human tumor antigens for cancer vaccine development. *Immunol Rev* 1999;170: 85–100.
176. Harris JR, Markl J. Keyhole limpet hemocyanin (KLH): a biomedical review. *Micron* 1999;30:597–623.
177. Nestle FO, Alijagic S, Gilliet M, et al. Vaccination of melanoma patients with peptide- or tumor lysate-pulsed dendritic cells. *Nat Med* 1998;4:328–332.
178. Kuiper M, Peakman M, Farzaneh F. Ovarian tumour antigens as potential targets for immune gene therapy. *Gene Ther* 1995;2:7–15.
179. Peoples GE, Goedegebuure PS, Smith R, et al. Breast and ovarian cancer-specific cytotoxic T lymphocytes recognize the same HER2/neu-derived peptide. *Proc Natl Acad Sci USA* 1995;92:432–436.
180. Babcock B, Anderson BW, Papayannopoulos I, et al. Ovarian and breast cytotoxic T lymphocytes can recognize peptides from the amino enhancer of split protein of the Notch complex. *Mol Immunol* 1998;35:1121–1133.
181. Peoples GE, Anderson BW, Fisk B, et al. Ovarian cancer-associated lymphocyte recognition of folate binding protein peptides. *Ann Surg Oncol* 1998;5:743–750.
182. Sandmaier BM, Oparin DV, Holmberg LA, et al. Evidence of a cellular immune response against sialyl-Tn in breast and ovarian cancer patients after high-dose chemotherapy, stem cell rescue, and immunization with Theratope STn-KLH cancer vaccine. *J Immunother* 1999;22:54–66.
183. Liu MA, Fu TM, Donnelly JJ, et al. DNA vaccines: mechanisms for generation of immune responses. *Adv Exp Med Biol* 1998;452:187–191.
184. Todryk S, McLean C, Ali S, et al. Disabled infectious single-cycle herpes simplex virus as an oncolytic vector for immunotherapy of colorectal cancer. *Hum Gene Ther* 1999;10:2757–2768.
185. Diao J, Smythe JA, Smyth C, et al. Human PBMC-derived dendritic cells transduced with an adenovirus vector induce cytotoxic T-lymphocyte responses against a vector-encoded antigen in vitro. *Gene Ther* 1999;6:845–853.
186. Ishida T, Chada S, Stipanov M, et al. Dendritic cells transduced with wild-type p53 gene elicit potent anti-tumour immune responses. *Clin Exp Immunol* 1999;117:244–251.
187. Nawrocki S, Mackiewicz A. Genetically modified tumour vaccines—where we are today. *Cancer Treat Rev* 1999;25: 29–46.
188. Neglia F, Orengo AM, Cilli M, et al. DNA vaccination against the ovarian carcinoma-associated antigen folate receptor alpha (FRalpha) induces cytotoxic T lymphocyte and antibody responses in mice. *Cancer Gene Ther* 1999;6:349–357
189. Freedman RS, Platsoucas CD. Immunotherapy for peritoneal ovarian carcinoma metastasis using ex vivo expanded tumor infiltrating lymphocytes. *Cancer Treat Res* 1996;82:115–146.
190. Canevari S, Stoter G, Arienti F, et al. Regression of advanced ovarian carcinoma by intraperitoneal treatment with autologous T lymphocytes retargeted by a bispecific monoclonal antibody. *J Natl Cancer Inst* 1995;87:1463–1469.
191. Lamers CH, Bolhuis RL, Warnaar SO, et al. Local but no systemic immunomodulation by intraperitoneal

treatment of advanced ovarian cancer with autologous T lymphocytes re-targeted by a bi-specific monoclonal antibody. *Int J Cancer* 1997;73:211–219.
192. Yang G, Mizuno MT, Hellstrom KE, Chen L. B7-negative versus B7-positive P815 tumor: differential requirements for priming of an antitumor immune response in lymph nodes. *J Immunol* 1997;158:851–858.
193. Greenfield EA, Nguyen KA, Kuchroo VK. CD28/B7 costimulation: a review. *Crit Rev Immunol* 1998;18:389–418.
194. Liebowitz DN, Lee KP, June CH. Costimulatory approaches to adoptive immunotherapy. *Curr Opin Oncol* 1998;10:533–541.
195. Becker JC, Brabletz T, Czerny C, et al. Tumor escape mechanisms from immunosurveillance: induction of unresponsiveness in a specific MHC-restricted CD4+ human T cell clone by the autologous MHC class II+ melanoma. *Int Immunol* 1993;5:1501–1508.
196. Walunas TL, Lenschow DJ, Bakker CY, et al. CTLA-4 can function as a negative regulator of T cell activation. *Immunity* 1994;1:405–413.
197. Bachmann MF, McKall-Faienza K, Schmits R, et al. Distinct roles for LFA-1 and CD28 during activation of naive T cells: adhesion versus costimulation. *Immunity* 1997;7:549–557.
198. Harding FA, Allison JP. CD28-B7 interactions allow the induction of CD8+ cytotoxic T lymphocytes in the absence of exogenous help. *J Exp Med* 1993;177:1791–1796.
199. Levine BL, Ueda Y, Craighead N, et al. CD28 ligands CD80 (B7-1) and CD86 (B7-2) induce long-term autocrine growth of CD4+ T cells and induce similar patterns of cytokine secretion in vitro. *Int Immunol* 1995;7:891–904.
200. Holliger P, Manzke O, Span M, et al. Carcinoembryonic antigen (CEA)-specific T-cell activation in colon carcinoma induced by anti-CD3 x anti-CEA bispecific diabodies and B7 x anti-CEA bispecific fusion proteins. *Cancer Res* 1999;59:2909–2916.
201. Yee C, Riddell SR, Greenberg PD. Prospects for adoptive T cell therapy. *Curr Opin Immunol* 1997;9:702–708.
202. Tsai V, Southwood S, Sidney J, et al. Identification of subdominant CTL epitopes of the GP100 melanoma-associated tumor antigen by primary in vitro immunization with peptide-pulsed dendritic cells. *J Immunol* 1997;158:1796–1802.
203. Hombach A, Tillmann T, Jensen M, et al. Specific activation of resting T cells against tumour cells by bispecific antibodies and CD28-mediated costimulation is accompanied by Th1 differentiation and recruitment of MHC-independent cytotoxicity. *Clin Exp Immunol* 1997;108:352–357.
204. Chen YM, Yang WK, Whang-Peng J, et al. Restoration of the immunocompetence by IL-2 activation and TCR-CD3 engagement of the in vivo anergized tumor-specific CTL from lung cancer patients. *J Immunother* 1997;20:354–364.
205. Mackensen A, Wittnebel S, Veelken H, et al. Induction and large-scale expansion of CD8+ tumor specific cytotoxic T lymphocytes from peripheral blood lymphocytes by in vitro stimulation with CD80-transfected autologous melanoma cells. *Eur Cytokine Netw* 1999;10:329–336.
206. Zhu H, Melder RJ, Baxter LT, Jain RK. Physiologically based kinetic model of effector cell biodistribution in mammals: implications for adoptive immunotherapy. *Cancer Res* 1996;56:3771–3781.
207. Ho M, Armstrong J, McMahon D, et al. A phase 1 study of adoptive transfer of autologous CD8+ T lymphocytes in patients with acquired immunodeficiency syndrome (AIDS)-related complex or AIDS. *Blood* 1993;81:2093–2101.
208. Effros RB, Pawelec G. Replicative senescence of T cells: does the Hayflick limit lead to immune exhaustion? *Immunol Today* 1997;18:450–454.
209. Bodnar AG, Kim NW, Effros RB, Chiu CP. Mechanism of telomerase induction during T cell activation. *Exp Cell Res* 1996;228:58–64.
210. Weinrich SL, Pruzan R, Ma L, et al. Reconstitution of human telomerase with the template RNA component hTR and the catalytic protein subunit hTRT. *Nat Genet* 1997;17:498–502.
211. Zier K, Gansbacher B, Salvadori S. Preventing abnormalities in signal transduction of T cells in cancer: the promise of cytokine gene therapy. *Immunol Today* 1996;17:39–45.
212. Nakagomi H, Petersson M, Magnusson I, et al. Decreased expression of the signal-transducing zeta chains in tumor-infiltrating T-cells and NK cells of patients with colorectal carcinoma. *Cancer Res* 1993;53:5610–5612.
213. Farace F, Angevin E, Vanderplancke J, et al. The decreased expression of CD3 zeta chains in cancer patients is not reversed by IL-2 administration. *Int J Cancer* 1994;59:752–755.
214. Uzzo RG, Clark PE, Rayman P, et al. Alterations in NFkappaB activation in T lymphocytes of patients with renal cell carcinoma. *J Natl Cancer Inst* 1999;91:718–721.
215. de Visser KE, Kast WM. Effects of TGF-beta on the immune system: implications for cancer immunotherapy. *Leukemia* 1999;13:1188–1199.
216. Bellone G, Turletti A, Artusio E, et al. Tumor-associated transforming growth factor-beta and interleukin-10 contribute to a systemic Th2 immune phenotype in pancreatic carcinoma patients. *Am J Pathol* 1999;155:537–547.
217. Sallusto F, Lanzavecchia A, Mackay CR. Chemokines and chemokine receptors in T-cell priming and Th1/Th2-mediated responses. *Immunol Today* 1998;19:568–574.
218. O'Connell J, Bennett MW, O'Sullivan GC, et al. The Fas counterattack: cancer as a site of immune privilege. *Immunol Today* 1999;20:46–52.
219. Muzio M, Chinnaiyan AM, Kischkel FC, et al. FLICE, a novel FADD-homologous ICE/CED-3-like protease, is recruited to the CD95 (Fas/APO-1) death—inducing signaling complex. *Cell* 1996;85:817–827.
220. Uzzo RG, Rayman P, Kolenko V, et al. Mechanisms of apoptosis in T cells from patients with renal cell carcinoma. *Clin Cancer Res* 1999;5:1219–1229.
221. Bennett MW, O'Connell J, O'Sullivan GC, et al. The Fas counterattack in vivo: apoptotic depletion of tumor-infiltrating lymphocytes associated with Fas ligand expression by human esophageal carcinoma. *J Immunol* 1998;160:5669–5675.

222. Baldwin RL, Tran H, Karlan BY. Primary ovarian cancer cultures are resistant to Fas-mediated apoptosis. *Gynecol Oncol* 1999;74:265–271.
223. Rabinowich H, Reichert TE, Kashii Y, et al. Lymphocyte apoptosis induced by Fas ligand-expressing ovarian carcinoma cells: implications for altered expression of T cell receptor in tumor-associated lymphocytes. *J Clin Invest* 1998;101:2579–2588.
224. Greenberg PD, Riddell SR. Deficient cellular immunity—finding and fixing the defects. *Science* 1999;285:546–551.
225. Pawelec G, Adibzadeh M, Solana R, Beckman I. The T cell in the ageing individual. *Mech Ageing Dev* 1997;93:35–45.
226. Mackall CL, Fleisher TA, Brown MR, et al. Distinctions between CD8+ and CD4+ T-cell regenerative pathways result in prolonged T-cell subset imbalance after intensive chemotherapy. *Blood* 1997;89:3700–3707.
227. Lee PP, Yee C, Savage PA, et al. Characterization of circulating T cells specific for tumor-associated antigens in melanoma patients. *Nat Med* 1999;5:677–685.
228. Clegg CH, Haugen HS, Rulffes JT, et al. Oncostatin M transforms lymphoid tissue function in transgenic mice by stimulating lymph node T-cell development and thymus autoantibody production. *Exp Hematol* 1999;27:712–725.
229. Freitas CS, Dalmau SR, Kovary K, Savino W. Epidermal growth factor modulates fetal thymocyte growth and differentiation. *Dev Immunol* 1998;5:169–182.
230. Musiani P, Modesti A, Giovarelli M, et al. Cytokines, tumour-cell death and immunogenicity: a question of choice. *Immunol Today* 1997;18:32–36.
231. Bani MR, Garofalo A, Scanziani E, Giavazzi R. Effect of interleukin-1-beta on metastasis formation in different tumor systems. *J Natl Cancer Inst* 1991;83:119–123.
232. Douvdevani A, Huleihel M, Zoller M, et al. Reduced tumorigenicity of fibrosarcomas which constitutively generate IL-1 alpha either spontaneously or following IL-1 alpha gene transfer. *Int J Cancer* 1992;51:822–830.
233. Fruh K, Yang Y. Antigen presentation by MHC class I and its regulation by interferon gamma. *Curr Opin Immunol* 1999;11:76–81.
234. Simons JW, Mikhak B. Ex-vivo gene therapy using cytokine-transduced tumor vaccines: molecular and clinical pharmacology. *Semin Oncol* 1998;25:661–676.
235. Oppenheim JJ, Murphy WJ, Chertox O, et al. Prospects for cytokine and chemokine biotherapy. *Clin Cancer Res* 1997;3:2682–2686.
236. Edwards RP, Gooding W, Lembersky BC, et al. Comparison of toxicity and survival following intraperitoneal recombinant interleukin-2 for persistent ovarian cancer after platinum: twenty-four hour versus 7-day infusion. *J Clin Oncol* 1997;15:3399–3407.
237. Lamont AG, Adorini L. IL-12: a key cytokine in immune regulation. *Immunol Today* 1996;17:214–217.
238. Abdulhay G, DiSaia PJ, Blessing JA, Creasman WT. Human lymphoblastoid interferon in the treatment of advanced epithelial ovarian malignancies: a Gynecologic Oncology Group Study. *Am J Obstet Gynecol* 1985;152:418–423.
239. Berek JS, Hacker NF, Lichtenstein A, et al. Intraperitoneal recombinant alpha-interferon for "salvage" immunotherapy in stage III epithelial ovarian cancer: a Gynecologic Oncology Group Study. *Cancer Res* 1985;45:4447–4453.
240. Berek JS, Markman M, Stonebraker B, et al. Intraperitoneal interferon-alpha in residual ovarian carcinoma: a phase II Gynecologic Oncology Group Study. *Gynecol Oncol* 1999;75:10–14.
241. D'Acquisto R, Markman M, Hakes T, et al. A phase I trial of intraperitoneal recombinant gamma-interferon in advanced ovarian carcinoma. *J Clin Oncol* 1988;6:689–695.
242. Fearon ER, Pardoll DM, Itaya T, et al. Interleukin-2 production by tumor cells bypasses T helper function in the generation of an antitumor response. *Cell* 1990;60:397–403.
243. Dranoff G, Jaffee E. Lazenby A, et al. Vaccination with irradiated tumor cells engineered to secrete murine granulocyte-macrophage colony-stimulating factor stimulates potent, specific, and long-lasting antitumor immunity. *Proc Natl Acad Sci USA* 1993;90:3539–3543.
244. Sanda MG, Ayyagari SR, Jaffee EM, et al. Demonstration of a rational strategy for human prostate cancer gene therapy. *J Urol* 1994;151:622–628.
245. Pardoll DM. Paracrine cytokine adjuvants in cancer immunotherapy. *Annu Rev Immunol* 1995;13:399–415.
246. Borrello I, Sotomayor EM, Cooke S, Levitsky HI. A universal granulocyte-macrophage colony-stimulating factor-producing bystander cell line for use in the formulation of autologous tumor cell-based vaccines. *Hum Gene Ther* 1999;10:1983–1991.
247. Winter G, Harris WJ. Humanized antibodies. *Immunol Today* 1993;14:243–246.
248. Huston JS, Levinson D, Mudgett-Hunter M, et al. Protein engineering of antibody binding sites: recovery of specific activity in an anti-digoxin single-chain Fv analogue produced in *Escherichia coli*. *Proc Natl Acad Sci USA* 1988;85:5879–5883.
249. Hudziak RM, Lewis GD, Winget M, et al. p185HER2 monoclonal antibody has antiproliferative effects in vitro and sensitizes human breast tumor cells to tumor necrosis factor. *Mol Cell Biol* 1989;9:1165–1172.
250. Shepard HM, Lewis GD, Sarup JC, et al. Monoclonal antibody therapy of human cancer: taking the HER2 protooncogene to the clinic. *J Clin Immunol* 1991;11:117–127
251. Carter P, Presta L, Gorman CM, et al. Humanization of an anti-p185HER2 antibody for human cancer therapy. *Proc Natl Acad Sci USA* 1992;89:4285–4289.
252. Lewis GD, Figari I, Fendly B, et al. Differential responses of human tumor cell lines to anti-p185HER2 monoclonal antibodies. *Cancer Immunol Immunother* 1993;37:255–263
253. Jurianz K, Maslak S, Garcia-Schuler H, et al. Neutralization of complement regulatory proteins augments lysis of breast carcinoma cells targeted with rhumAb anti-HER2. *Immunopharmacology* 1999;42:209–218.
254. Rubin SC, Finstad CL, Hoskins WJ, et al. Analysis of antigen expression at multiple tumor sites in epithelial ovarian cancer. *Am J Obstet Gynecol* 1991;164:558–563.

255. Kreitman RJ. Immunotoxins in cancer therapy. *Curr Opin Immunol* 1999;11:570–578.
256. Pai LH, Bookman MA, Ozols RF, et al. Clinical evaluation of intraperitoneal *Pseudomonas* exotoxin immunoconjugate OVB3-PE in patients with ovarian cancer. *J Clin Oncol* 1991;9:2095–2103.
257. Dropcho EJ. Autoimmune central nervous system paraneoplastic disorders: mechanisms, diagnosis, and therapeutic options. *Ann Neurol* 1995;37[Suppl 1]:S102–S113.
258. Drlicek M, Bianchi G, Bogliun G, et al. Antibodies of the anti-Yo and anti-Ri type in the absence of paraneoplastic neurological syndromes: a long-term survey of ovarian cancer patients. *J Neurol* 1997;244:85–89.
259. Okano HJ, Park WY, Corradi JP, Darnell RB. The cytoplasmic Purkinje onconeural antigen cdr2 downregulates c-Myc function: implications for neuronal and tumor cell survival. *Genes Dev* 1999;13:2087–2097.
260. Kairemo KJ. Radioimmunotherapy of solid cancers: a review. *Acta Oncol* 1996;35:343–355.
261. Crippa F. Radioimmunotherapy of ovarian cancer. *Int J Biol Markers* 1993;8:187–191.
262. Roeske JC, Chen GT, Atcher RW, et al. Modeling of dose to tumor and normal tissue from intraperitoneal radioimmunotherapy with alpha and beta emitters. *Int J Radiat Oncol Biol Phys* 1990;19:1539–1548.
263. Maraveyas A, Epenetos AA. Targeted immunotherapy: an update with special emphasis on ovarian cancer. *Acta Oncol* 1993;32:741–746.
264. Nicholson S, Gooden CS, Hird V, et al. Radioimmunotherapy after chemotherapy compared to chemotherapy alone in the treatment of advanced ovarian cancer: a matched analysis. *Oncol Rep* 1998;5:223–226.
265. Ward BG, Mather SJ, Hawkins LR, et al. Localization of radio-iodine conjugated to the monoclonal antibody HMFG2 in human ovarian carcinoma: assessment of intravenous and intra-peritoneal routes of administration. *Cancer Res* 1987;47:4719–4723.

PART II
Histopathology of Ovarian Cancer

5

Pathology of Malignant Ovarian Epithelial Tumors and Miscellaneous and Rare Ovarian and Paraovarian Neoplasms

James E. Wheeler

The classification of ovarian epithelial tumors currently in use is based on that written and illustrated in the World Health Organization (WHO) publication of 1999 (1) and considered in depth in the *Atlas of Tumor Pathology* published by the Armed Forces Institute of Pathology in 1998 (2). It has been adopted by the International Federation of Gynecology and Obstetrics (FIGO), the International Society of Gynecologic Pathologists, and the Society of Gynecologic Oncologists (Table 5.1). This histogenetically based system is founded on the similarity of the epithelial cells of the tumors to the variety of columnar epithelia of müllerian derivation normally found in areas of the female genital tract. For example, the histologic appearance of endometrioid carcinoma of the ovary recapitulates, albeit abnormally, the glands of the endometrium, and serous carcinoma in its best differentiated areas resembles epithelium of the fallopian tube.

A number of other neoplasms involving the ovary, especially small cell carcinoma and metastatic tumors, are also briefly covered in this chapter. Also discussed are neoplasms that are closely related to ovarian tumors and either occur immediately adjacent to the ovary or may be confused for an ovarian primary (Table 5.2).

GENERAL DIAGNOSTIC PROBLEMS

Not all tumors are uniform or can readily be placed into a histogenetic classification category, and mixed-pattern carcinomas with varying epithelial cellular elements may occur. In addition, the proportion of tumors placed into a given category varies depending on the pathologist's judgment, so that one pathologist's poorly differentiated serous carcinoma may be another's undifferentiated carcinoma. A review of the accuracy of the histologic diagnosis of ovarian cancer, as judged by a panel of gynecologic pathologists, reported overall agreement on 97% of cases classified as epithelial. Nine of 12 cases misdiagnosed as primary epithelial tumors were metastatic carcinoma. Subtyping agreement varied from 100% (clear cell carcinoma) to 73% (endometrioid carcinoma) (3). The panelists found that 15% of tumors classified as malignant were of low malignant potential (LMP) and 8% of those called LMP were invasive. Other observers, using a panel of four pathologists, found complete agreement on histologic type in only 30% to 35% of tumors and agreement on grade in only 20% to 30% (4). Examination of a single slide without clinical information, gross findings, or special stains yields widely varying diagnoses even among highly respected gynecologic pathologists (5). Although these and other studies (6) may call the usefulness of the classification scheme into question, they also serve to emphasize the need for adequate tumor sampling and gathering of all possible ancillary information before a final diagnosis is rendered in any ovarian epithelial tumor. Although the stage of the tumor is currently the best prognostic indicator, morphometric analysis, especially a combination of mitotic index, volume percentage epithelium, and nuclear size, may be more useful than typing and grading of ovarian carcinomas (7). Recurrences of carcinoma after radiation or

TABLE 5.1. Simplified histologic classification of ovarian epithelial tumors

Serous tumors
Mucinous tumors
Endometrioid (including epithelial-stromal) tumors
Clear cell tumors
Transitional cell (Brenner) tumors
Mixed epithelial tumors
Undifferentiated and unclassified carcinoma

chemotherapy may show dedifferentiation in as many as 25% to 30% of the cases (8).

Histologic grading of epithelial tumors has been attempted for years; none of the systems proposed (FIGO, modified Broders [9], combined histologic and cytologic features [10,11]) has independent predictive value in a multifactorial evaluation, or else has not attracted sufficient adherents to test fully its reproducibility and effect on survival. This fact has not prevented the introduction of new grading proposals, however (12).

GENERAL CLINICAL-PATHOLOGIC APPROACH

The clinician needs to be aware of interactions with the surgical pathologist even before the tumor has been removed from the pelvis. Ovarian vein blood may be removed to test for a variety of hormones or tumor markers. Because the presence of capsular invasion may lead to adjuvant therapy, it behooves the gynecologic surgeon to note and mark adhesions between the tumor and surrounding structures for specific study by the pathologist (Figure 5.1). The surface area of an ovarian tumor 15 cm in diameter is greater than 700 cm^2, and even the most dedicated pathologist may not identify the most pertinent areas to study without the help of the surgeon. A simple stitch or two in these areas together with a

TABLE 5.2. Miscellaneous and rare ovarian and paraovarian neoplasms

Small cell carcinoma, hypercalcemic type
Sarcoma
Tumors metastatic to the ovary
Lymphoma and leukemia
Paraovarian epithelial tumors
Peritoneal papillary carcinoma

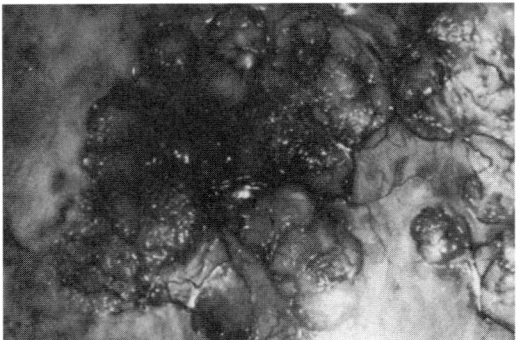

FIG. 5.1. Serosal nodules in an ovarian tumor. The nature of tumor involving the serosal surface cannot always be determined by gross examination. These worrisome nodules represented serosal involvement by a benign cystadenofibroma.

notation on the consultation request being sent to the laboratory are sufficient. With rare exceptions, the tumor should be sent to the laboratory fresh for immediate examination. Even if it is obvious from metastatic deposits that the tumor is malignant, fresh tissue is needed for electron microscopy in the occasional cases with a confusing histologic appearance. In addition, fresh tissue is optimal for study of estrogen, progesterone, and androgen receptors; for the performance of flow cytometric analysis; and to freeze for a variety of research purposes. Diploid tumors and those with a low percentage of cells in the synthetic S phase of the cell cycle, for example, behave in a far more benign fashion, stage for stage, than do tumors that are aneuploid or have a high S-phase fraction (13–15). Tumors containing progesterone receptors tend to behave better than those that do not (16,17). The color and consistency have not been altered by fixative, and a photograph of the gross or sectioned specimen is far more vivid in the original unaltered color. The capsular surface may be inked, unless it is smooth and glistening, so that tumor extension to the surface may be unequivocally demonstrated.

Because of possible variations of histologic appearance within a tumor, sections are made at intervals of 1 cm or less so that a variety of areas may be sampled, including those with different color or consistency and those that are solid or cystic. The gross examination and care with which representative sections are taken is far more important than the exact number of sections. One study of mucinous and serous carcinomas demonstrated that in 11 of 51 cases, fewer than 50% of the histologic sections were diagnostic of cancer, and that in an occasional case up to 75% of the sections showed histology of a benign tumor (18). Hence, the suggestion that one section be taken for every 1 to 2 cm diameter of a tumor may be a lower limit of acceptability, and, especially in tumors of apparent LMP, extra sections may be required to rule out low-grade carcinoma. Sections through the ovarian cortex are useful, not only for finding evidence of capsule invasion, but also for finding possible areas of preexisting benign or LMP neoplasms, endometriosis, and stromal luteinization.

When dealing with a papillary epithelial neoplasm, it is commonly impossible to determine from gross examination whether the lesion is malignant or of LMP (Figure 5.2), and a single frozen section (or two or three) may not be representative. In one study, 23% of tumors, most especially large mucinous tumors, were upgraded from LMP on frozen section to malignant on permanent section (19). In young patients, particularly those who wish to preserve fertility, it is the practice of our gynecologic oncologists, when there exists any conceivable possibility of a less than malignant diagnosis, to wait until the entire tumor can be thoroughly sectioned and sampled and the final diagnosis rendered before proceeding with any procedure that would permanently impair future fertility.

ETIOLOGY AND HISTOGENESIS

The vast majority of epithelial ovarian tumors are thought to arise from the surface cells lining the outside of the ovary. Although these are clearly continuous with the population of mesothelial cells lining of the rest of the pelvis and abdomen, they differ somewhat when studied microscopically and ultrastructurally. The cells lining the peritoneum tend to be flat, and those on the surface of the ovary cuboidal. Peritoneal mesothelium cells and ovarian surface cells have similar surface microvilli, but cytoplasmic tonofilaments, especially in the perinuclear area, are far more prevalent in the former (28% versus 1%). Mucin droplets are occasionally present in peritoneal cells but appear to be lacking in ovarian surface cells (20). Small epithelial cysts found close to the ovarian surface, so-called surface inclusion cysts, which are believed to result from invagination of the surface epithelium, are found in the majority of females from birth onward. Although the epithelium lining them tends to be flat or nonspecifically cuboidal before menarche, afterward most undergo metaplasia so that the epithelium resembles that of the endosalpingeal cells of the fallopian tube (21). Because an unbroken continuum of increasingly enlarging cysts may be found, from the most minute surface inclusion cyst to the most enormous 40- or 50-kg cyst, and because a variety of degrees of cellular metaplasia, atypia, and anaplasia may be seen within a cyst, it seems logical that the vast majority of epithelial tumors should arise from this mechanism even if the neoplastic stimulus is unknown. The cell proliferation marker MIB-1 is present in about half of the inclusion cysts (22). On occasion the surface cells of the ovary may proliferate with or without underlying stromal response and form a surface papillary structure or papilloma composed of or covered by epithelium which may vary from bland to malignant. Attempts to find premalignant changes in ovaries prophylactically removed because of BRCA1 or

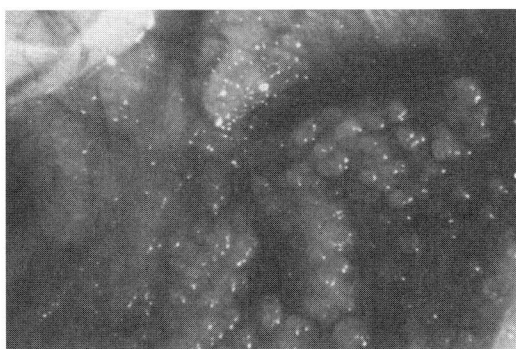

FIG. 5.2. Papillary projections into the cyst cavity of a serous tumor. A tumor of low malignant potential (borderline tumor) cannot safely be distinguished from carcinoma on the basis of examination either of the gross specimen or of a single frozen section.

BRCA2 germline mutations have been almost uniformly unsuccessful (23,24), except in one instance (25). The etiology of the cellular changes eventuating in ovarian epithelial tumors is generally accepted to be of molecular origin, and specific defects, such as the loss of genetic heterozygosity of the BRCA1 and BRCA2 genes (26), are under intense study (Chapter 1). It does appear that differences in underlying gene defects will be shown to relate to the differences in phenotypic histologic appearance (27).

METASTATIC BEHAVIOR

The pathobiology of epithelial ovarian malignancy includes the mass effect of the primary lesion, invasion into adjacent pelvic organs, rare paraneoplastic and endocrine syndromes, and the metastatic behavior of the tumor cells. Knowledge of this behavior is critical to proper preoperative workup, effective staging at laparotomy, and clinical follow-up for recurrent disease. The importance of the spread of tumor cells into ascitic fluid has been recognized by delineation of a unique stage (Ic). Ascites itself may come from some increased transudation from the surface of the ovary or tumor implants, but it is more likely to arise secondary to blockage of normal peritoneal lymph flow by tumorous obstruction of transdiaphragmatic lymphatics (28). Early subclinical involvement of pelvic and aortic lymph nodes (29) and diaphragm (30) is sufficiently frequent that careful examination of these sites has become mandatory at laparotomy. Systematic lymphadenectomy discloses that almost 25% of apparently stage I and 50% of stage II tumors have already spread to pelvic or periaortic lymph nodes or both (29). Distant nodal metastasis, as shown at scalene node biopsy, is present in more than 20% of patients with stage III or IV disease (31). Even LMP tumors may be upstaged from stage I to stage III after pelvic and aortic node sampling (32). Leake and colleagues (33) reported that 4 of 19 otherwise stage I patients with LMP tumors had positive nodes.

The mean interval between clinical diagnosis and death varies according to the metastatic site observed at diagnosis; it is as short as 1 month with central nervous system involvement, 2 months with pericardial effusion, 4 months with bone metastases, 5 months with parenchymal liver involvement, 6 months with pleural effusion, 8 months with parenchymal lung metastases, and 12 months with metastatic subcutaneous nodules (34). Umbilical metastases (Sister Joseph's nodule) are an uncommon complication of ovarian carcinoma and are often caused by another visceral primary (e.g., pancreas, colon) (35).

The most common mechanisms of death for patients are respiratory failure (43%) and infection (12%) (36). At autopsy peritoneal and serosal involvement of abdominal organs is present in about 80% of cases (36,37), and of the pleura in about 30% to 40%. These may or may not be complicated by ascites or pleural effusion. The small and large bowel wall (50% to 55%), liver parenchyma (45%), lung (35% to 40%), fallopian tube and uterus (about 25% each), adrenal gland and spleen (15% to 20% each) are the most common sites of metastatic involvement at autopsy. Serosal involvement of the bowel leads to clinical bowel obstruction in about 30% of affected patients by the time of death, whereas invasion of the bowel wall causes obstruction in 70% of affected patients (37). Bone involvement is claimed to be only about 10%, but since sampling at autopsy is often quite limited this is a minimum figure. Symptomatic central nervous system metastases during life are rare (about 2%) (38) and at autopsy are still uncommon (3% to 6%) (36,37). Thoracic involvement by tumor is found in more than 40% of patients studied radiographically (39), and such involvement lowers the 5-year survival rate to 5%, compared with 50% in the absence of involvement.

Sarcomas, because of their propensity for hematogenous dissemination, may metastasize to distant sites, especially lung, without the initial spread to peritoneum and lymph nodes that is characteristic of epithelial tumors (36)—hence the importance of careful clinical and radiologic evaluation of the lungs and the lack of proven usefulness of lymph node dissection.

ENDOCRINE EFFECTS

Endocrine function is thought of mainly in association with ovarian sex cord-stromal or germ

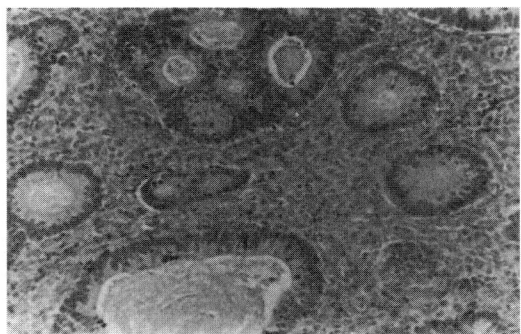

FIG. 5.3. Endometrioid carcinoma with stromal luteinization. The stroma between the invading glands of tumor has become luteinized, with round to oval bland nuclei and plentiful eosinophilic cytoplasm. Hormone production cannot be assessed on the basis of the histologic appearance. Ovarian venous or peripheral blood sampling at the time of oophorectomy may be helpful in this regard.

cell tumors, but it may also result from epithelial tumors. Many of these tumors are mucinous cystadenomas or cystadenocarcinomas, but other epithelial subtypes may also stimulate, in an unknown manner, the ovarian stroma. Stromal cells adjacent to the tumor become enlarged with pink cytoplasm, and the nuclei become round (Figure 5.3). The type of hormone being produced by the luteinized cells cannot readily be determined histologically. Both increased estrogens with associated endometrial hyperplasia and cornification of the genital tract squamous epithelium and increased androgens with virilization have been reported (40). Adenocarcinoma metastatic to the ovary may also cause stromal luteinization and increased estrogen with inappropriate vaginal bleeding (41). Gastrin-secreting cells in benign, borderline, or malignant mucinous tumors can cause clinically apparent Zollinger-Ellison syndrome. Hypercalcemia in small cell carcinoma and, rarely, other epithelial tumors (especially clear cell carcinoma) may result from production of parathyroid hormone-related peptide. This peptide is able to bind to and activate parathyroid hormone receptors. Elevated serum 1,25-dihydroxyvitamin D may contribute to the hypercalcemia. Cushing syndrome, hypoglycemia, and renin secretion associated with epithelial tumors are each represented by single case reports (42). It is clear that sampling of ovarian vein blood at operation in any ovarian tumor patient with unusual clinical manifestations may provide the best means for further investigation.

PARANEOPLASTIC SYNDROMES ASSOCIATED WITH OVARIAN EPITHELIAL TUMORS

A comprehensive review of clinical syndromes associated with gynecologic tumors (42) described several dozen conditions, for most of which the pathophysiology is still uncertain. The enormous diversity of manifestations involving the skin, connective tissue, nervous system, and hematopoietic system serves to emphasize the necessity for the clinician to be alert to signs and symptoms that appear quite removed from the pelvis.

Paraneoplastic syndromes involving skin include acanthosis nigricans, acute neutrophilic dermatosis (Sweet syndrome), multiple sebaceous tumors (Torre-Muir syndrome), multiple seborrheic keratoses (sign of Leser-Trélat), and eruptive keratoacanthomas. The most frequent connective tissue paraneoplastic conditions associated with ovarian carcinoma are dermatomyositis and fasciitis with or without associated arthritis. We have seen fasciitis associated with both benign and malignant epithelial ovarian tumors and have been impressed with the disappearance of the palmar lesions within 1 to 2 weeks after removal of the ovarian tumor.

Acute cerebellar degeneration is the chief paraneoplastic condition involving the central nervous system, and it may predate discovery of the ovarian tumor by weeks or months. It has been traced to circulating anti-Purkinje cell antibodies. Rare patients with carcinoma lose vision as a result of diffuse proliferation of uveal melanocytes. Hematologic effects of ovarian carcinoma include disseminated intravascular coagulation, nonbacterial thrombotic (marantic) endocarditis, and microangiopathic hemolytic anemia. Disseminated intravascular coagulation may be caused by tissue factor on the surface of tumor cells that triggers both intrinsic and extrinsic coagulation pathways. Pyrexia is a rare presenting complaint of patients with carcinoma (42).

TABLE 5.3. *Serous tumors*

Benign
  Serous cystadenoma
Low malignant potential (LMP) or borderline serous tumor
  Serous cystadenoma of LMP
  Serous cystadenofibroma or adenofibroma of LMP
  Serous surface papilloma of LMP
  Serous tumor of LMP with microinvasion
Malignant
  Serous cystadenocarcinoma
  Serous surface papillary carcinoma
  Malignant serous adenofibroma or cystadenofibroma

SEROUS NEOPLASMS

Ovarian serous neoplasms, especially in the benign and LMP categories, are clearly formed of epithelial cells resembling those of the fallopian tube. Higher grade-lesions, especially carcinomas, are characterized by a loss of ciliated cells but retain the ability to form delicate papillary growths of atypical epithelial cells often accompanied by formation of psammoma bodies. Serous neoplasms comprise at least 25% of all epithelial ovarian malignancies; however, because many tumors diagnosed as "papillary" carcinoma or carcinoma not otherwise specified may well be serous, the final proportion of all ovarian carcinomas that are serous is likely to be 40% to 50%. A working classification is as shown in Table 5.3.

Serous Cystadenoma

Histogenetically, the benign serous cystadenoma forms a continuum with the exceedingly common ovarian surface inclusion cyst; a cyst reaching 1 cm in diameter arbitrarily becomes a serous cystadenoma. Genetic changes, including loss of heterozygosity on chromosomes 2 q21 and 17 p13 (43), have been found in serous cystadenomas, but the underlying neoplastic stimulus is still unknown. A unilocular cystadenoma may be examined easily at the gross bench to determine whether any suspicious papillae project into the cyst lumen. A multiloculated cyst needs to be thoroughly sectioned to permit an adequate gross examination. A frozen section is not required in the face of a smooth cyst lining.

Serous Tumors of Low Malignant Potential (Borderline Tumors)

About 15% (44–46) of ovarian tumors (those which Taylor in 1929 called "semimalignant tumors of the ovary" [47]) fall into a group whose degree of histologic malignancy and biologic behavior is intermediate between those that are entirely benign and those that are fully malignant. Because the clinical behavior of these neoplasms is relatively benign, it is exceedingly important that they be correctly evaluated pathologically to arrive at appropriate therapy.

About half of all borderline or LMP tumors are serous (46). Patients present in much the same way as do patients who have malignant tumors: with abdominal swelling or pain, or simply with the incidental finding of a pelvic mass on routine examination. The median age of patients is about 38 or 40 years (48,49), but there is a wide range from the late teens to the ninth decade of life (46,50). Bilateralness, synchronous or metachronous, is exceedingly common, about 40% (46,49), and ipsilateral or contralateral ovarian tissue retained after cystectomy for an LMP tumor may later give rise to another LMP lesion in some 8% to 15% of patients (51,52). If a resection cystectomy has a positive margin, recurrence is highly likely (51).

Almost 80% of patients with LMP tumors have stage I disease when first seen; the rest have extraovarian tumor present, typically on peritoneal surfaces in the pelvis or in both pelvis and abdomen. Centers who see referred patients may well find that 30% of patients with LMP tumors are in stage III (49). As noted earlier, subtle metastatic deposits of tumor may be found in a surprisingly large number of cases if iliac and paraaortic lymph nodes are carefully studied. Benign glandular inclusions are normally found in pelvic or paraaortic lymph nodes in about 15% of adult women (53), and these sometimes are distinguished from metastatic LMP tumor only with great difficulty (54). The thoroughness of the staging procedure has a profound influence in these cases on the proportion of tumors placed in a higher stage. At one institution, for example, the proportion of cases categorized as stage III increased from 6% before 1977 to almost 30% thereafter (55). The latest evidence indicates that staging for LMP tumors remains inadequate in the vast majority of cases (56).

Whether the extraovarian tissue represents metastatic implants or part of a field change related to serous borderline tumors of the peritoneum (57,58) cannot be settled without more clonality studies. At least some LMP serous tumors show evidence for multifocality (59). However, evidence that exophytic tumor growth on the outside of ovaries is highly associated (62%) with extraovarian tumor, whereas only 4% of patients without exophytic tumor have extraovarian tumor, strongly supports the idea of metastatic implantation (50), as do clonality studies (60). Extraabdominal and extrapelvic involvement by serous LMP tumors is rare (61).

On gross examination, the mean tumor size is about 10 cm but may vary from 2 to 25 cm (62) (Figure 5.4). The predominant tumor is a cystic one, lined by numerous papillary projections that fill a varying proportion of the cyst cavity (Figure 5.2). Occasionally only a small area with a slightly raised surface is apparent under optimal illumination; on other occasions large numbers of papillary structures occupy almost the entire cyst or cysts present. The fluid in the cyst may be thin and yellow or have a surprisingly thick mucoid consistency. Because LMP tumors, by definition, lack stromal invasion, any evidence of adhesion between the ovary and surrounding structures must be looked upon as possible evidence for capsular involvement and be carefully marked by the surgeon so that it may be thoroughly studied microscopically.

The less common gross appearance of the serous LMP tumor results from marked stromal proliferation in apparent response to an unknown epithelial stimulus. The tumor forms either a largely solid mass, a serous adenofibroma of LMP, or, more commonly, a mass that is partially solid and partially cystic, a serous cystadenofibroma of LMP (63) (Figure 5.5).

Microscopically, the typical serous LMP tumor shows numerous delicate, complex papillae lined by two or more layers of epithelial cells, usually with at least mild to moderate nuclear atypia (64). They may form little tufts with what appears to be "drop-off" of small papillary cell groups into the lumen (Figure 5.6). Focal areas of bland stromal necrosis or hyalinization are occasionally seen with attenuation or disappearance of the overlying epithelial cells. Because of frequent outpouchings of the cyst lining and a biased cut through epithelium of irregular cysts, invasion must often be diagnosed only after careful evaluation. The diagnosis of definitive invasion depends on the finding of clusters of cells or single cells entering the stroma with a corresponding

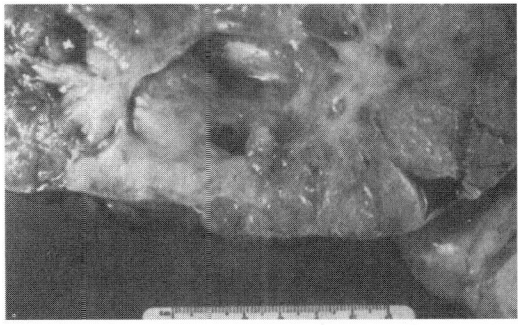

FIG. 5.5. Serous cystadenofibroma with focal tumor of low malignant potential (LMP). The solid areas of tumor are largely composed of benign fibrous stroma, but minute cysts may be seen which, together with the gross cysts, suggest the correct diagnosis of cystadenofibroma. Careful sectioning and histologic study revealed areas of an LMP tumor.

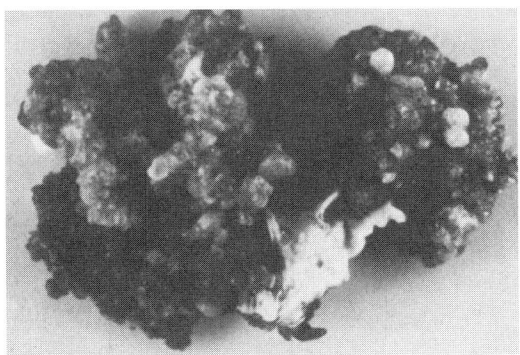

FIG. 5.4. Serous tumor of low malignant potential (borderline tumor) involving the outside of this teenager's ovary. (Courtesy of Dr. Katrina Conard.)

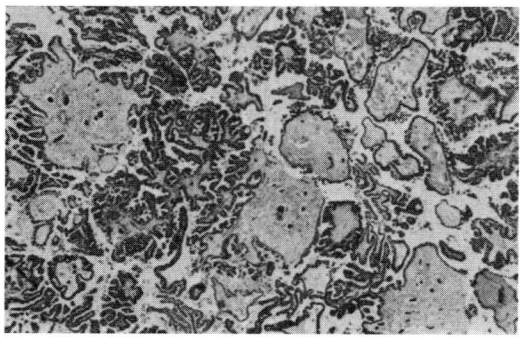 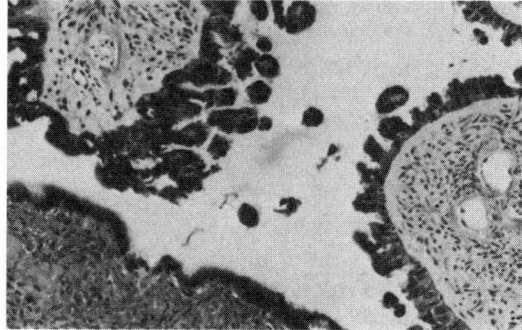

FIG. 5.6. Serous tumor of low malignant potential (borderline tumor). **A:** At low magnification the papillary nature of the tumor is clearly evident. **B:** Adjacent papillae demonstrate the variability of tumor cell growth: the epithelium covering a portion of papilla seen at lower left appears benign, while that on the papilla at the right, shows tufting, and at upper left, the epithelial cells are piled up in papillary groups without apparent stromal support.

desmoplastic reaction, or the piling up and formation of sheets of cells with marked cytologic atypia with loss of any underlying papillary structure. Attempts to quantitate nuclear morphology by image analysis reveal that LMP serous tumors have a nuclear area and an optical density intermediate between those of adenomas and carcinomas (65).

Surface Papillomas of Low Malignant Potential

Warty surface excrescences most often are benign, with a fibrous stroma lined by a single bland cell layer of epithelium. However, an occasional surface papilloma may be covered by several layers of proliferating tufted epithelium with mild to moderate epithelial atypia which may give rise to peritoneal or omental implants in a manner analogous to the usual serous LMP tumor. Over a period of years, such tumors may also lead to complications and death (2).

Low Malignant Potential Serous Tumors with Microinvasion

A small subset of serous LMP tumors may show a few, often eosinophilic, epithelial cells penetrating into stroma immediately underlying an otherwise histologically typical LMP tumor (66,67). Although the significance of this finding may be doubted (64), such tumors may be termed serous LMP tumors with microinvasion. Tumors cells penetrating the basement membrane stain strongly for type IV collagenase, an enzyme useful in initiating metastatic behavior (68,69). In at least one case, similar pink cells were found in a lymph node biopsy (67). Patients with this form of microinvasive LMP serous tumors are clinically similar to other patients with LMP tumors, although the proportion of carefully studied cases with evidence of implants may be increased (70). They are between 22 and 60 years of age with a tumor size from 3 to 20 cm (67), and two thirds of the patients have stage I disease. Because the clinical outcome seems to be virtually identical to that of LMP tumors without microinvasion, these are classified here as a variant of LMP tumors (71). Any area of invasion greater than 3 mm of these microscopically minute and cytologically fairly bland foci would currently be classified as carcinoma.

Peritoneal Implants of Low Malignant Potential Serous Tumors

A variety of epithelial lesions may be seen on the peritoneal surface of patients with LMP serous tumors. Many of them are minute cysts lined by tubal (endosalpingeal)-type epithelium generally lacking papillations in which there is no evidence of desmoplastic reaction in the underlying tissue.

These are the lesions of endosalpingiosis, found in as many as 40% of patients with LMP tumors (72) but also commonly seen, at least in the omentum, in patients who lack ovarian tumor and in whom the only significant lesion may be an underlying chronic salpingitis (73). The presence or absence of these müllerian-like inclusions has no effect on long-term survival (74). However, other peritoneal epithelial structures are papillary and appear histologically identical to the primary ovarian tumor (75). Some of these papillary growths rest on the peritoneal surface, whereas others grow invasively into the underlying stroma with a surrounding desmoplastic reaction. Although it was proposed by Russell in 1984 that the presence of invasive implants might adversely affect the patient's prognosis, some studies (76,77) have been unable to demonstrate any clear effect of the nature of the implants on the prognosis. One other study (78) found that surface implants with or without a superficial desmoplastic reaction did not worsen patient survival, whereas those with implants invading deep into underlying tissue with a desmoplastic reaction in general did poorly. A critical review has confirmed the importance of invasive compared with noninvasive implants (66% versus 95% survival at 7 years) (79). It should be noted that the criteria for "invasive" implants are open for modification, and there is some evidence that histologic features such as micropapillary architecture, intraglandular cribriform growth, and periglandular clefts may become as important as predictors of a poor clinical outcome (80). Pathologic evaluation of implants is frequently difficult; gentle removal of an implant in continuity with a portion of underlying tissue provides an optimal specimen for diagnosis.

The long-term survival rate for patients with stage I serous LMP tumors approaches 100%, and virtually all deaths occur in those with stage III lesions. Recurrent abdominal disease may develop in those with stage III lesions, whether treated or untreated, and deaths from treatment complications of chemotherapy or radiation in some series exceed those from the tumor alone. Attempts to predict prognosis by DNA cytometry have yielded conflicting evidence, suggesting that aneuploidy may not be useful in predicting recurrence or ultimate prognosis (81–83). Analysis of nucleolar organizer regions is not helpful in predicting the clinical behavior (84).

Serous Carcinoma

Patients with serous ovarian carcinoma present clinically in much the same way as patients with any other of the epithelial carcinomas, with pain in 50%, abdominal swelling in 45%, and uterine bleeding, loss of appetite, and nausea and vomiting in a smaller percentage. Almost 50% have a mass discovered on routine physical examination (85). Although most are between the ages of 40 and 70 years, about 7% are younger than this, and some 25% to 30% are nulliparous. About 35% of patients have stage I or II disease, and the remainder have stage III or IV. A disproportionate number of women with stage I tumors (almost 40%) have the best-differentiated tumor (grade 1), double the proportion in the group taken as a whole (85).

Grossly the tumors may not be distinguishable from their LMP counterparts unless the capsule is involved by obvious tumor with adhesion formation, but on section areas of hemorrhage or necrosis are suggestive of possible malignancy (Figure 5.7). Microscopically, with the possible exception of increased nuclear atypia and cell pleomorphism, the most obvious difference between carcinomas and LMP tumors is that of stromal invasion, where groups of cells or single cells invade the stroma and usually initiate a desmoplastic reaction. Vascular space involvement may occur but is uncommonly prominent. Psammoma bodies, which are formed intracellularly, often in neoplastic epithelial cells, by precipitation of calcium-phosphate apatite crystals (86), are found in more than 20% of LMP serous tumors and in more than 30% of serous carcinomas (87). Patients who have tumors with psammoma bodies have above-average survival, possibly because of the diploid DNA content and low S-phase fraction of these tumors (15). Sarcoma-like nodules are rarely seen in the wall of a serous tumor and may be a poor prognostic finding (88).

Serous carcinomas may be graded on the basis of histologic pattern, with grade 1 (well-differentiated) tumors being composed entirely

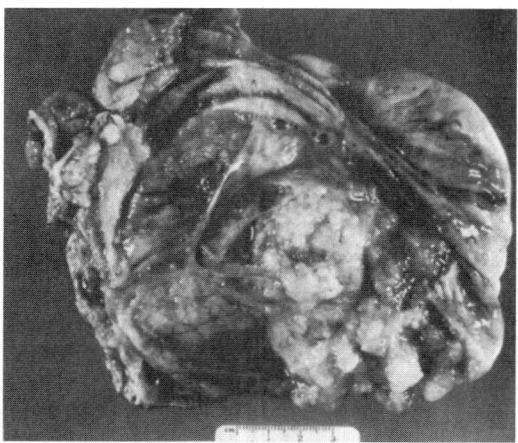

FIG. 5.7. Serous cystadenocarcinoma. One of the bilaterally involved ovaries has been opened to reveal cystic as well as papillary areas. Although the serosal surface seen on the right side of the specimen appears smooth, the entire serosa is best examined *in situ*. In that way adhesions, or any other evidence of possible serosal involvement by tumor, can be marked for special histologic sampling.

of papillae and glands, stage III tumors composed almost entirely of sheets of malignant cells, and grade 2 tumors composed of a mixture of the two patterns. Using these criteria, about 20% of tumors are grade 1, 30% grade 2, and 50% grade 3. Median survival times for patients with grades 1, 2, and 3 tumors are 4.6, 2.3, and 1.5 years, respectively (85). More complex grading systems may be devised, such as that proposed by Bichel and Jakobsen (89), in which not only the histologic grade is considered but also nuclear polymorphism, nucleolar characteristics, nuclear/cytoplasmic ratio, mitoses, invasive margin, capsular penetration, and vascular invasion. Applying these criteria to patients with advanced-stage (III and IV) disease, they were able to distinguish two groups with significantly different prognoses (about 15% versus 45% survival at 5 years); in contrast, the histologic grade or growth pattern did not divide the patients into prognostically significantly groups (89).

Staging divides patients into a group with relatively good prognosis (stages I and II), with a median survival rate of 6.4% after 4 years, and a group with poor prognosis (stages III and IV, with median survival times of 1.6 and 1.0 years, respectively). Stage Ic patients survive no better than these in stage III. Clinical features affecting survival are an asymptomatic versus a symptomatic mass (mean survival time, 2.4 versus 1.5 years, respectively) and age less than versus more than 50 years (3.6 versus 1.8 years, respectively) (85).

Surface Papillary Carcinoma

Serous carcinoma, said to arise directly from the ovarian surface and characterized by early spread to other pelvic and peritoneal surfaces (90), may be difficult to distinguish from peritoneal papillary serous carcinoma (discussed later).

Psammocarcinoma

A few serous tumors of the ovary and peritoneum have been reported (91) in which most epithelial cells of a low-grade papillary carcinoma were massively replaced through the formation of psammoma bodies. Patients (mean age, 57 years; range, 36 to 76 years) present with stage III disease, but despite a high stage and invasion of intraperitoneal viscera, more than 80% of those with follow-up observations extending for longer than 3 years are without evidence of disease. This type of serous tumor, psammocarcinoma, should be distinguished from the multifocal calcification of peritoneal surfaces that may occur after therapy for ovarian cancer (92).

MUCINOUS NEOPLASMS

Mucinous ovarian tumors are traditionally divided into adenomas, tumors of LMP (also known as borderline tumors), and carcinomas (Table 5.4). These superficially simple categories somewhat obscure a number of problem areas. First, the histologic appearance is often not uniform throughout a mucinous tumor, so sampling in excess of that undertaken with other epithelial tumors is required (18). Second, the LMP tumors are of two histologic varieties, whose clinical behavior appears to be significantly different. Third, the definition of exactly what features separate LMP tumors from well differentiated

TABLE 5.4. *Mucinous tumors*

Benign
   Mucinous cystadenoma
Low malignant potential (LMP) or borderline mucinous tumor
   LMP mucinous tumor, endocervical type
   LMP mucinous tumor, intestinal (goblet cell) type
Malignant
   Mucinous adenocarcinoma
   Malignant mucinous adenofibroma or cystadenofibroma

carcinoma has not been unequivocally settled. An additional problem area, the relation of pseudomyxoma peritonei and pseudomyxoma ovarii to mucinous tumors of ovary and appendix, is under active investigation.

Of the 20% of all ovarian tumors that are mucinous, about 85% are benign, 6% are of LMP, and 9% are histologically malignant (1). The histogenetic origin has not been totally settled, although the findings of typical mucinous areas in endometrioid and serous tumors as well as rare mucinous metaplasia in ovarian surface inclusion cysts provide strong evidence for origin from ovarian surface epithelium differentiating along the lines of müllerian epithelium. The frequent association of Brenner tumors, with their foci of mucinous metaplasia, and mucinous cystadenomas suggests that at least some mucinous tumors might arise by this route, whereas the presence of goblet cells, argentaffin cells, and occasionally Paneth cells in some mucinous tumors is consistent with the theory that the tumor originates as an area of a germ cell tumor overexpressing intestinal epithelium. Careful comparative studies, including electron microscopy and lectin histochemistry, support the idea that most, if not all, mucinous tumors are of müllerian (mesodermal) origin (93,94).

The initial evaluation of a mucinous tumor by the pathologist includes all of the standard measurements, but in addition demands more thorough sampling than for a serous tumor of similar size. The reason is that in many mucinous carcinomas one may find one or more areas that, taken by themselves, would be considered diagnostic for either a mucinous cystadenoma or a mucinous LMP tumor. Similarly, many LMP mucinous tumors contain extensive areas diagnostic only of mucinous cystadenoma (18). Sampling of one section per centimeter of tumor diameter is appropriate initially if the diagnosis of malignancy is in any doubt; if malignancy is well established, only sampling of areas of grossly different appearance is indicated.

Mucinous Tumors of Low Malignant Potential (Borderline Tumors)

Patients with mucinous tumors of LMP are reported to have a mean age of 35 years (95) to 54 years (96), and a range of 9 to 70 years (95). About half present with increasing abdominal girth or a palpable abdominal mass, but others have symptoms of pain or fullness (30%) and about 25% are asymptomatic. Bilaterality is reported in 0 to 8% (95,96).

Microscopically, mucinous tumors of LMP are classified as such by most pathologists according to the histologic criteria proposed by Hart and Norris in 1973 (95). Noninvasive mucinous tumors with stratification of two or three atypical epithelial cell layers are considered to be of LMP; tumors, even if not invasive, that have more than three atypical cell layers are classified as malignant, as are all tumors with stromal invasion (Figure 5.8). Using these criteria, long-term follow-up studies show a mortality rate of 4% for patients with LMP tumors and 33% for those with carcinoma (95). If the criteria separating

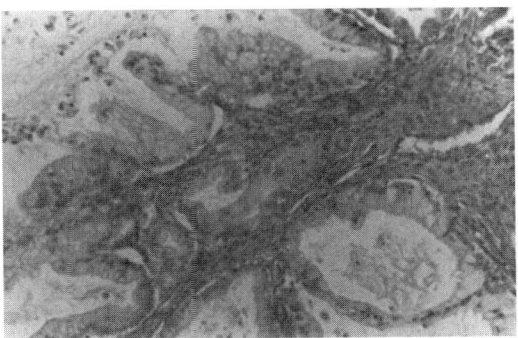

FIG. 5.8. Mucinous tumor of low malignant potential. There is focal loss of nuclear polarity of the mucinous epithelium, seen at center top and left. There is insufficient nuclear piling up and atypia to warrant a diagnosis of low-grade mucinous carcinoma.

carcinoma from LMP tumors were changed to include the degree of nuclear atypia and the presence or absence of pseudomyxoma ovarii and the stratification criterion were reexamined, the proportion of tumors placed in each category would change (97). Many tumors previously designated LMP may be placed in the benign group, and a few tumors previously designated carcinoma may be downgraded to LMP. Unfortunately, all of the criteria needed for the exact classification of mucinous tumors other than those that are clearly benign or malignant are open to at least some question. Attempts to subdivide LMP tumors into several grades (46,98) or to quantitate them morphometrically (99,100) have not been widely adopted.

Nuclear atypia is normally part and parcel of LMP tumors (95,101). Kempson and his coworkers (97,102) placed increased diagnostic importance on nuclear atypia, defining it as nuclei of three times normal size with prominent nucleoli and coarsely clumped chromatin. They placed less importance on increased layers of cell stratification in the absence of this atypia. Of more than 300 patients with complex mucinous tumors without stromal invasion and only minimal to moderate cytologic atypia, only those with mucin dissecting the ovarian stroma (pseudomyxoma ovarii) or with pseudomyxoma peritonei had recurrence. Although it is claimed that carcinomas with stromal invasion behave in a more aggressive manner than those without, after adjustment for stage the significance of invasion, if any, becomes unclear (96,103).

In an important paper, Rutgers and Scully (104) separated the mucinous LMP tumors into two histologic groups with important clinical differences: the müllerian (endocervical-like) group and the intestinal (goblet-cell) group. Those with epithelium resembling endocervix, 15% of their mucinous LMP cases, were clinically benign despite the presence in a few cases of peritoneal implants or lymph node metastases. The patients tended to be younger (34 versus 52 years) than patients in the intestinal cell group, and 80% of the tumors were unilocular or paucilocular, compared with only 28% in the intestinal group. There was also a high degree of bilaterality (40%), and 30% of the endocervical-like tumors were associated with endometriosis. None of these patients had pseudomyxoma peritonei (mucinous ascites). Histologically there was a papillary architectural appearance similar to that of serous LMP tumors, with a characteristic severe acute inflammation of the stroma out of proportion to any necrosis that might be present. The mucinous columnar cells lining the papillae were similar to those of the endocervix.

The intestinal type of mucinous LMP tumor also forms some papillae, but by definition these are lined by mucin-containing goblet cells. This variant is infrequently bilateral (6%) or associated with endometriosis. Histologically, in addition to the goblet cells, they may contain Grimelius-positive enterochromaffin-like cells and Paneth cells but lack the prominent papillae and acute inflammation of the endocervical type of LMP. These intestinal-type tumors have a significant association with pseudomyxoma peritonei (17%), and the prognosis is guarded owing to a 14% mortality rate (104).

Simultaneous or metachronous mucinous tumors of the ovary and cervix have been reported, some of which are diagnosed in patients with the Peutz-Jeghers syndrome (105). Although in some patients the ovarian lesion is most likely metastatic from the cervix, in others the cervical tumor, quite commonly a minimal deviation adenocarcinoma (adenoma malignum), and the ovarian tumor appear to arise independently.

Mural Nodules

A few mucinous tumors, of both endocervical and intestinal type, have been noted with peculiar nodules in the cyst wall. These mural nodules may be sarcoma-like or frankly anaplastic. Grossly the sarcoma-like nodules are circumscribed, usually soft, yellow to dark brown, and hemorrhagic. They range from less than 1 cm to 5 cm in diameter (106). Microscopically, most contain osteoclast-like giant cells in the background with atypical spindle-shaped cells and pleomorphic mononucleated cells (pleomorphic and epulis-like pattern), but in other cases either lack the giant cells (pleomorphic and spindle cells pattern) or appear largely histiocytic (giant cell-histiocytic pattern) (106). Although the lack of immunohistochemical studies or thorough electron microscopy makes it difficult to

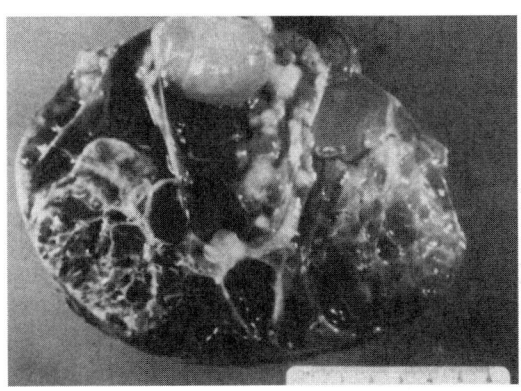 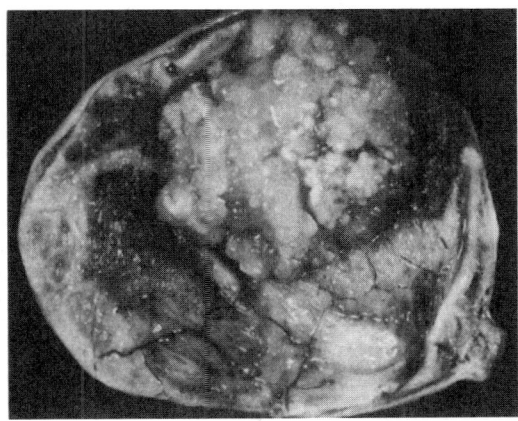

FIG. 5.9. A: Mucinous adenocarcinoma. The multiloculated cut surface demonstrates residual mucin in cysts on the right side. Additional parallel cuts may reveal a solid area of tumor, which would probably be the best area to sample for a frozen section because of the possibility that it might represent an area of frank malignancy. **B:** Mucinous adenocarcinoma. This specimen was composed of a cyst with a smooth serosal surface. When opened, as shown here, the cyst contained a papillary mass of tumor with a mixture of solid and small cystic areas.

rule out a peculiar cellular reaction to invading epithelial cells, the benign follow-up pattern suggests that the process may not be one of malignant degeneration but rather a peculiar reaction secondary to hemorrhage or extravasated mucin.

In rare cases, mucinous tumors have yellowish or red mural nodules that contain frankly anaplastic carcinoma (107–109) or sarcoma (110) which often proves its malignancy by metastasizing and causing death of the patient.

Mucinous Carcinoma

Patients with mucinous carcinoma present with the usual symptoms of ovarian cancer. They have a mean age of about 48 to 54 years (range, late teens to more than 80 years) (96,103). At operation there is only about 10% bilaterality of tumors localized to stages I and II. About 50% to 70% of tumors are in stage I, but most of the rest are in stage III. Reported 5-year survival rates range from about 85% to 95% in stage I, to 25% in stage II, to less than 15% in stages III and IV (103). Lesions of low histologic grade tend to show better 2- and 5-year survival rates at each stage (111). Patients who have carcinoma with stromal invasion have been claimed to have a worse prognosis than those whose tumor is diagnosed on the basis of excessive cellular stratification (103), but after adjustment for stage the difference largely disappears.

On gross examination the tumors range in size from about 8 to 23 cm (103), and they may be huge (2). On section they are formed of one or multiple cystic structures with some papillations projecting from the walls (Figure 5.9). Focal necrosis is relatively common. The cyst fluid often has a mucinous, slippery feel. Histologically, about half of the carcinomas have stromal invasion, with small groups of cells or single cells penetrating into the stroma of the cyst walls or capsule with a desmoplastic reaction. In the other half, the diagnosis is based on the finding of more than three layers of highly atypical cells lining the cyst wall. Papillations tend to be a little blunter and not so fine and delicate as those seen in serous tumors. It is difficult to correlate nuclear grade and mitoses with survival (103).

Pseudomyxoma Ovarii and Peritonei

About 3% or 4% of mucinous ovarian tumors are noted to have irregular strands or pools of mucin (with or without accompanying epithelial cells) dissecting into ovarian stroma, so-called pseudomyxoma ovarii (112,113) (Figure 5.10), and accumulation of mucinous material in the

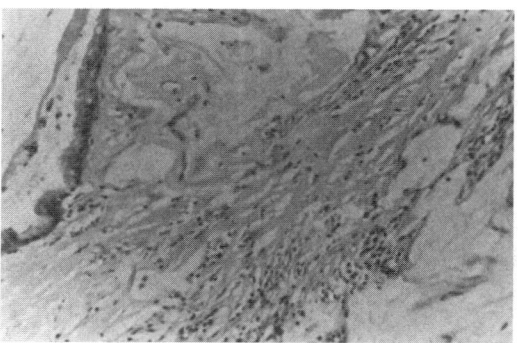

FIG. 5.10. Mucinous tumor with pseudomyxoma ovarii. The epithelium of the mucinous tumor at left appears benign but elsewhere showed changes of a tumor of low malignant potential. Mucin has dissected into the stroma beneath the epithelium and is also apparent at lower right.

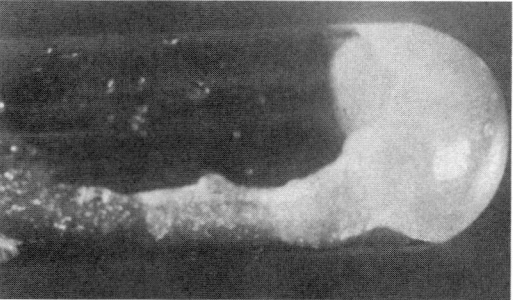

FIG. 5.11. Pseudomyxoma peritonei. The mucin of pseudomyxoma peritonei clings tenaciously to the test tube wall. It may be virtually acellular or contain small clusters of cells from a low-grade mucinous tumor, most likely of appendiceal origin.

peritoneal cavity, known as pseudomyxoma peritonei (mucinous ascites). Although it has been commonly assumed that the mucin arises from the ovarian tumor via dissection and peritoneal spillage, it was noted that some cases were associated with appendiceal lesions, especially appendiceal mucinous cystadenomas. Careful studies of the appendix in the patients with pseudomyxoma peritonei (both men and women) (114,115) disclosed that the appendix almost invariably contains a histologically benign mucinous cystadenoma, and a few contain borderline mucinous tumors or frank mucinous carcinoma. Ovarian tumors associated with pseudomyxoma peritonei tend to be on the right side, and virtually all have pseudomyxoma ovarii and the same histologic appearance as the appendiceal tumor (115). The appendix has some gross abnormality in 90% of cases, usually dilatation at the tip of less than 2.5 cm in diameter, but occasionally it appears grossly normal (115). The lack of appendiceal examination in many cases (116) makes it difficult to exclude pseudomyxoma peritonei as at least occasionally secondary to a mucinous ovarian primary. Molecular studies (117,118) generally support appendiceal origin, but some cases appear to have a dual origin.

The peritoneal mucin, which is often thick and sticky (Figure 5.11), may contain single or small clusters of cells but on occasion appears to be acellular. The condition recurs in more than half the patients and is difficult to manage (119); the mortality rate, usually from recurrent intestinal obstruction, is between 15% and 30%. Analysis of the mucin (120) indicates that it is made up of glycoproteins, largely fucomucins and sialomucins.

ENDOMETRIOID TUMORS

Although the existence of an ovarian carcinoma histologically resembling endometrial carcinoma was noted by Sampson in 1925 (121), it was only in August of 1961 that the Cancer Committee of the FIGO meeting at the Radiumhemmet in Stockholm recommended the establishment of a separate group of "endometrioid" tumors to accommodate this increasingly recognized histologic category of ovarian neoplasm (122). The current classification of endometrioid neoplasms (Table 5.5) also includes mixed epithelial-stromal and stromal neoplasms.

The histogenesis of endometrial carcinoma is unknown, although ovarian endometriosis has been noted, usually in about 10% of cases (123–126), and occasionally transitions are noted between benign epithelium of endometriosis and malignant epithelium of an endometrioid tumor. The admixture of endometrioid carcinoma with epithelium of other müllerian cell types in many cases suggests an origin in common with other primary carcinomas of the ovary.

TABLE 5.5. *Endometrioid and epithelial-stromal tumors*

Benign
  Endometrioid cystadenoma
  Proliferative endometrioid adenofibroma
Low malignant potential (LMP) or borderline tumor
  Endometrioid cystadenoma of LMP
  Endometrioid adenofibroma and cystadenofibroma of LMP
  Endometrioid tumor of LMP with microinvasion
Malignant
  Endometrioid adenocarcinoma
  Endometrioid adenocarcinoma with squamous metaplasia
    Low grade (adenocanthoma)
    High grade (adenosquamous carcinoma)
  Malignant endometrioid adenofibroma or cystadenofibroma
Epithelial-Stromal
  Adenosarcoma
  Malignant mixed mesodermal tumor (MMMT)
Stromal
  Stromal sarcoma, low and high grade

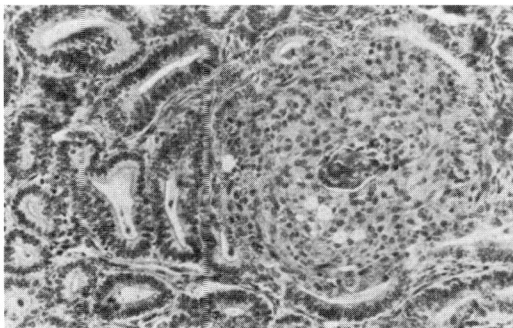

FIG. 5.12. Proliferative endometrioid adenofibroma. Set in a background of benign fibrous stroma are packed endometrioid glands with cytologically bland nuclei (*left*). Foci of squamoid or squamous metaplasia are common in these lesions *right* and should not be confused with the solid tumor growth pattern of a high-grade malignancy.

Although endometriosis of the ovary cannot be considered a tumor, other than in its propensity to form a mass, occasionally the epithelial lining of an endometriotic cyst is composed of cells so atypical as to raise the possibility of an evolving neoplasm. In the absence of stromal invasion or the formation of sheets of clearly malignant cells, follow-up of such cases has indicated a benign course (127).

Proliferative Endometrioid Tumors

A small number of tumors have been reported in which endometrial-like glands proliferate in a largely dense fibromatous background (128–131). Patients are in their mid-thirties to mid-seventies and have an asymptomatic mass discovered on routine examination. The tumors range up to 20 cm in diameter and are composed of endometrioid glands with minor stratification and varying degrees of cell atypia, usually mild to moderate but occasionally more severe (128), and possibly some minor degree of cyst formation. Frequently the endometrioid glands demonstrate some focal areas of squamous metaplasia, and the epithelial glands sit in a bland fibromatous stroma without evidence of infiltration or a desmoplastic reaction (Figure 5.12). Follow-up of proliferative endometrioid adenofibromas is completely benign.

Endometrioid Tumors of Low Malignant Potential (Borderline Tumors)

Endometrioid tumors with increased epithelial proliferation, forming a cribriform pattern of packed glands (128) or occupying foci of more than 5 mm in greatest dimension (131) without stromal invasion, have been termed endometrioid tumors of LMP (borderline) (132). Snyder and others (133) recognize both a papillary and an adenofibromatous growth pattern. The papillary pattern shows an arborizing epithelial growth, often with delicate fibrous stromal support. The adenofibromatous pattern consists of atypical glandular elements set into a bland fibromatous background. Squamous and focal mucinous differentiation is present in up to 50% of both histologic types (133). Mitotic activity varies between rare and brisk, and cytologic atypia is at least moderate to severe. Small areas of serous or clear cell differentiation may be present. Although the follow-up for all these tumors thus far has been quite benign (the only patient with an implant was doing well more than 8 years later), the presence of microscopic areas of invasion in 7% to 10% of these cases is evidence for potentially malignant clinical behavior (128,131). Even those patients whose tumors have more than 5 mm of stromal invasion (currently considered as well-differentiated carcinoma) do very well on follow-up (133).

Endometrioid Carcinoma

Endometrioid carcinoma comprises about 20% of all ovarian malignancies (range, 16% to 24%) (122,125,126,134,135). Clinically most of the women are menopausal, with an average age of about 55 years, but there is a broad age range, from about 28 to 86 years (125,134,135). Presenting symptoms are similar to those of women with other epithelial carcinomas. Grossly the tumors may be as small as 2 cm or as large as 37 cm, but they are most often 12 to 25 cm in diameter (122,126) with a mean weight of about 500 g (134). The majority are cystic, but they may be solid. On section they are soft or rubbery and tan or red with areas of necrosis and cyst formation containing mucoid or brown-tinged fluid (122). With careful staging, about 32% will be designated stage I, 18% stage II, and the remaining 50% stage III or IV (124,125,134,135).

The histologic appearance of endometrial carcinoma is similar to that of the typical uterine endometrial carcinoma. It is composed of ovoid glands with varying amounts of stroma and may demonstrate small or large amounts of epithelial cell necrosis (Figure 5.13). The glands are formed of one or more layers of cuboidal to columnar cells with hyperchromatic nuclei with frequent loss of basal polarization. Papillae are present in about one half of the cases (134), but they are blunt, in contrast to the more finely branching papillae of serous carcinoma (122). Psammoma bodies are noted in 5% to 10% of cases (134). Squamoid or squamous differentiation occurs in some 25% to 50% of cases (126,134) and is most often squamoid without keratin formation. Ovarian endometrioid adenocarcinoma with bland or benign-appearing squamoid or squamous differentiation may also be termed *adenoacanthoma,* whereas endometrioid carcinoma with malignant-appearing squamous elements is termed *adenosquamous carcinoma.* The 5-year survival rate is reported to be about 90% for patients with adenoacanthoma and 20% for those with adenosquamous ovarian carcinoma (136), but some, if not all, of the difference may be explained on the basis of the generally poor differentiation in the glandular portions of the adenosquamous carcinomas together with the higher stage at which adenosquamous carcinomas are found.

Although most cases of endometrioid carcinoma are histologically "pure," as many as 35% contain areas of other histologic epithelial cancer types, most often clear cell carcinoma but occasionally mucinous, papillary serous, or anaplastic carcinoma (125,134,137). No definitive difference in behavior is reported for this admixture except for some indication that patients with high-stage (III and IV) endometrioid carcinoma with a serous or undifferentiated component, even if that component is small, do poorly (8% survival at 5 years, versus 90% if pure) (138).

The clinician should be aware that there are histologic variants of endometrioid carcinoma which may cause diagnostic problems for the pathologist. In one type, which resembles a sex cord-stromal tumor (139) and is also termed the sertoliform variant (140,141), tubules of carcinoma cells invade stroma. These tumors grossly tend to be yellow to gray and solid or focally cystic. Microscopically there are almost always focal areas of typical endometrioid carcinoma, as well as areas of invading solid or hollow tubules mimicking the abortive tubules of a Sertoli cell tumor. Endometrioid carcinomas

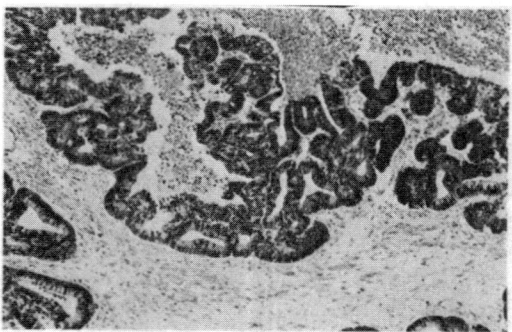

FIG. 5.13. Endometrioid carcinoma. The histologic appearance of this section, with a "garland" of malignant endometrioid glands and "dirty" necrosis at the top, is characteristic of metastatic colon carcinoma. In the absence of a known extraovarian primary, this may be considered a primary endometrioid carcinoma.

demonstrate mucicarmine positivity at the epithelial cell apices, and electron microscopy demonstrates focal formation of lumens with microvilli (140). Clinical masculinization occurs only rarely (141). This histologic pattern may also be confused with some form of Krukenberg tumor or carcinoid. Immunohistochemical staining of this endometrioid variant shows uniform positivity for epithelial membrane antigen, in contrast to almost all Sertoli cell tumors (142). Patients with stage I disease do well (141).

A spindle cell variant of endometrioid carcinoma exists where, by definition, spindle cells comprise more than 90% of the tumor (143). Without extensive sampling, this variant might be confused with a sarcoma or sex cord-stromal tumor. Small areas of inconspicuous gland formation with intraluminal mucin may suggest the correct diagnosis, in which case immunohistochemical staining for keratin and epithelial membrane antigen demonstrates that the spindle cells have epithelial characteristics.

Because of possible confusion caused by these variants, mucicarmine and immunohistochemical stains may be necessary for a definitive diagnosis of endometrioid carcinoma.

More than 10% (and possibly as many as 25%) of cases of primary ovarian endometrioid carcinoma are associated with carcinoma of the endometrium (124,134,135,144,145). Careful study makes it clear that virtually all cases in which the tumors are well differentiated behave as if they represented separate primary lesions rather than ovarian metastases from the uterus, and the 5-year survival rate is excellent. Multinodular disease in the ovary is a hallmark of metastasis from the endometrium, however, and patients with bilateral ovarian involvement, vascular invasion, ovaries less than 5 cm in size, or deep myometrial invasion should be assessed for probable primary uterine tumor metastatic to the ovary (146). The stimulus for synchronous uterine and ovarian carcinomas is unknown, but the finding of endometrial hyperplasia in more than half of the cases (146) suggests hormonal influences.

The differential diagnosis of endometrioid carcinoma includes, more so than any other primary ovarian carcinoma, adenocarcinoma metastatic to the ovary. As noted in the section on metastatic carcinoma, this is most often colonic carcinoma, although other, largely gastrointestinal, primary sites may also give rise to ovarian metastases, histologically simulating endometrioid carcinoma (147,148).

EPITHELIAL-STROMAL TUMORS

Adenosarcoma

Adenosarcoma, a tumor formed of cytologically benign epithelial glands in a cytologically malignant sarcomatous stroma, rarely presents as an ovarian primary (149,150). The glands are generally endometrial-like, and the sarcomatous component resembles endometrial-stromal sarcoma. Only the sarcomatous component has been found in metastases. Variants with atypical cellular stroma rather than frank sarcomatous stroma have a good prognosis (150).

Malignant Mesodermal Mixed Tumors

Malignant mesodermal mixed tumors (MMMT) by definition contain epithelial and mesenchymal elements, both of which are histologically malignant (Figure 5.14). They are classified as endometrioid lesions because the glands often appear endometrial-like and the stroma may resemble that of the endometrium. On rare occasions MMMTs arise from ovarian endometriosis (151). Contiguous ovarian endometriosis is

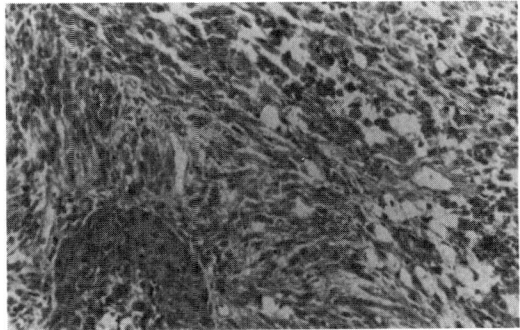

FIG. 5.14. Malignant mixed mesodermal tumor. A clearly defined area of carcinoma (*lower left*) lies in a background of cytologically bizarre, mitotically active spindle cell sarcoma.

found in about 10% of cases (152,153), but a clear transition is not seen. A history of pelvic irradiation is typically lacking (154), in contrast to the high incidence preceding development of uterine MMMTs. Cell line studies support the origin of sarcomatous elements from carcinoma cells (155). The sarcomatous component of MMMTs may be composed solely of homologous elements (so-called carcinosarcomas) (156), but it often contains heterologous elements (e.g., cartilage, bone, striated muscle) not normally found in the ovary. The homologous sarcomatous elements seen are nonspecific spindle cells or stromal cells.

Patients are virtually all perimenopausal or postmenopausal, often of low parity, and usually have advanced disease (stage III or IV) when first seen. The involved ovary is enlarged from about 6 to 21 cm in diameter (mean, 13 cm) (152). On section the tumor is fleshy and gray-white with small to large areas of cystic degeneration; hemorrhage and necrosis usually are present. The carcinomatous areas may be squamous or glandular, and if glandular they may be mucinous, clear cell, serous, or endometrioid (152,153). The sarcomatous areas, if heterologous, are most often cartilaginous and stain positively for the S100 protein. Rhabdomyomatous areas stain for desmin and myosin. Both mesenchymal and epithelial areas often contain eosinophilic hyaline globules from one 1 to 50 μm in diameter that stain positively with periodic acid-Schiff (PAS) stain and have been shown to contain protein reacting as α_1-antitrypsin (157). Although patients with MMMT with heterologous elements may fare slightly worse than those with only homologous mesenchymal components, the usual survival time in both variants is measured in months, with only 10% to 20% of patients surviving to 5 years.

The differential diagnosis includes poorly differentiated carcinoma with areas of spindle cell metaplasia and immature teratoma with epithelial and cartilaginous elements. The latter is readily ruled out by the much younger age of patients with immature teratomas and the presence of a wide variety of immature epithelial and mesenchymal elements in a teratoma without the frankly carcinomatous components of an MMMT. A poorly differentiated carcinoma often shows a gradual transition between the more recognizable epithelial elements and the spindle cell metaplasia. The cells of spindle cell metaplasia contain focal keratin positivity on immunohistochemical stains, and differentiation to heterologous elements such as cartilage is not present. There may be importance in separating the poorly differentiated carcinomas from the MMMTs because, at least in the endometrium, the prognosis for poorly differentiated carcinomas is much better than that of MMMTs (56% versus 11% survival at 5 years) (158).

Stromal Tumors

Endometrioid stromal sarcoma rarely may originate in the ovary, possibly from ovarian endometriosis (159). Histologically it is composed of small spindle cells resembling endometrial stroma with varying numbers of mitoses. Patients whose tumors have fewer than five mitoses per 10 high-powered fields (hpf) do rather well; however, two of the three patients reported with more than 10 mitoses per 10 hpf died within 5 years after diagnosis (160).

CLEAR CELL TUMORS

Clear cell carcinoma of the ovary, although described more than 100 years ago (161) and comprising only a small fraction of ovarian epithelial carcinomas, has provoked disproportionate attention owing to the initial confusion as to its histogenetic origin. Schiller (162) originally proposed origin of a group of clear cell tumors in remnants of the embryologic mesonephros, hence the early term "mesonephroma." Some 15 years later, Teilum (163) noted that Schiller's cases were not homogeneous and that some patients had a germ cell tumor we now recognize as endodermal sinus tumor (EST), whereas others had a tumor that was morphologically somewhat similar but was basically an epithelial neoplasm with prominent clear cytoplasm. The final blow to mesonephric origin came with a 1967 paper of Scully and Barlow (164), which showed that there were very close relationships between clear

TABLE 5.6. *Clear cell tumors*

Benign
  Clear cell cystadenoma
Low malignant potential (LMP) or borderline tumor
  Clear cell tumor of LMP
  Clear cell adenofibroma or cystadenofibroma
    of LMP
Malignant
  Clear cell adenocarcinoma
  Malignant clear cell adenofibroma
    or cystadenofibroma

cell carcinoma and other tumors of müllerian origin, especially endometrioid carcinoma. *Clear cell carcinoma* is the currently accepted name under the WHO classification, but some observers believe that the association with endometrioid carcinoma is so close that clear cell carcinoma might well be considered as simply a variant of endometrioid carcinoma (165). The classification of clear cell tumors is shown in Table 5.6.

Clear Cell Tumors of Low Malignant Potential (Borderline Tumors)

It is difficult to define a cystic clear cell tumor of LMP, but a number of adenofibromatous or cystadenofibromatous lesions contain glands lined by clear cells with only mild to moderate cellular atypia in a fibromatous background without evidence of invasion or any other desmoplastic stromal reaction (129,166,167). These neoplasms appear to represent LMP clear cell tumors, and focally one may occasionally find in one of them a transition to frank clear cell carcinoma. The prognosis appears to be excellent.

Clear Cell Carcinoma

Clear cell carcinomas constitute only about 6% of epithelial ovarian carcinomas (44), with a reported range of about 1% (168) to 17% (169). The mean age of the patients reported is about 53 years, with a range of 28 to 78 years (165, 170).

The signs and symptoms are similar to those found in women with other varieties of epithelial tumors, a symptomatic or asymptomatic mass or ascites being the most common findings. At operation about 60% of women have a stage I lesion (171) (range, 28% to 75% [172,173]), but about 15% to 20% have a stage III or IV tumor. Bilateralism varies between about 12% and 39% (169,174). The tumors are usually about 5 to 20 cm in diameter, but do reach 30 cm (168), and they may be cystic, semisolid, or solid on section. On section, they are usually described as white, yellow, or gray with focal areas of hemorrhage or mucoid material (174). A variety of histologic patterns may be present: solid, papillary-tubular, or glandular with or without hobnail cells (Figure 5.15).

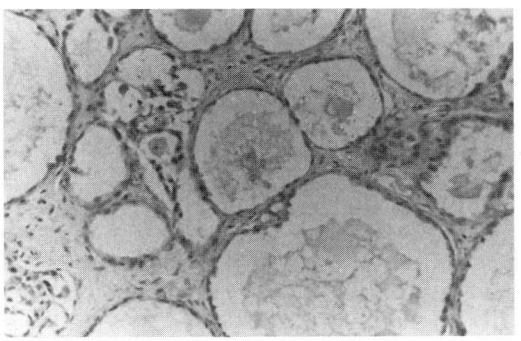 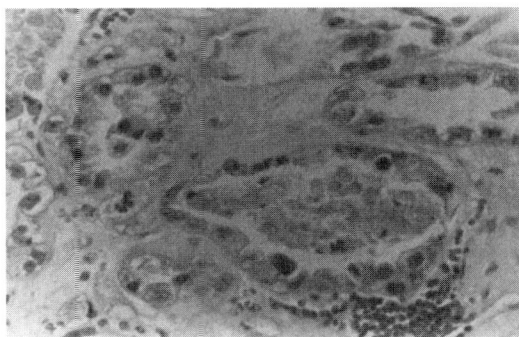

A   B

FIG. 5.15. Clear cell carcinoma. **A:** This pattern of small cystic glands lined by deceptively bland nuclei may mislead the pathologist into making a benign diagnosis. Thorough sampling will inevitably reveal malignant areas such as seen in **(B)**. **B:** These glands are lined by cytologically malignant clear cells. In some cells nuclei are found on the luminal side ("hobnail cells") rather than in the more usual basal location.

The clear cell cytoplasm results mainly from plentiful cytoplasmic glycogen, which may be stained with the PAS stain. Diastase treatment of the slide before PAS staining removes glycogen and PAS positivity. Glycogen granules may also be seen on material prepared for electron microscopy (175). In a few cases there is extensive eosinophilic staining of the tumor cell cytoplasm (oxyphilic clear cell carcinoma) (176,177).

An adenofibromatous component may be present as part of an otherwise typical clear cell carcinoma, and one may find, at least in a consultation service, that some 20% of adenofibromatous tumors are of the clear cell variety. Those with features of marked cellular atypia with stromal invasion, or a stromal desmoplastic, edematous, or myxomatous reaction characteristic of malignancy, qualify as clear cell carcinomas in adenofibroma. Those with lesser nuclear atypia and lack of invasive components are diagnosed as borderline or LMP clear cell tumors in adenofibroma. The association of clear cell carcinoma with endometriosis is more striking than that of endometrioid carcinoma. About 35% of carefully examined cases have ovarian endometriosis (range, 22% [178] to 67% [137]). Clear cell carcinoma may be found in direct continuity with the lining of an endometriotic cyst with or without an intervening lining of atypical epithelial cells (164,165). Clear cell carcinoma may also arise in extraovarian endometriosis (179).

The degree of nuclear atypia and the histologic pattern of clear cell carcinomas have been examined closely for any bearing on the long-term prognosis (164,173,180), and no clinical significance has emerged other than a suggestion that a tubulocystic pattern may indicate a better outcome (170). DNA analysis using flow cytometric techniques (181) of different areas within individual tumors demonstrates that the majority contain both diploid and aneuploid areas. This is in contrast to reports of other ovarian carcinomas (182–184), which found ploidy variability in only about 10% of the 75 tumors examined. Histologic examination is apparently not capable of determining which areas are aneuploid and which are diploid, and aneuploidy *per se* does not appear to confer a clinically worse behavior. Mucin stain shows intraluminal positivity without cytoplasmic staining.

Prognosis in clear cell carcinoma, as with the other epithelial cell types, is most directly related to the stage at the time of laparotomy (137,171). Women with stage IA tumors will virtually all be without evidence of disease at 5 years (180), whereas patients with more advanced lesions may experience a recurrence. Jenison and associates (171), in a summary of 16 series including almost 400 patients with stage I clear cell carcinoma, found an estimated 5-year survival rate of only about 60%. This figure is overly pessimistic, because the thoroughness and extent of the staging procedures carried out in many of the series 20 or 30 years ago were almost certainly deficient by modern standards. Therefore, the understaging of many patients gives a falsely low survival rate for true stage I tumors.

The differential diagnosis of clear cell carcinoma includes metastatic clear cell carcinoma from other gynecologic sites, especially from endometrial clear cell carcinoma, and from nongynecologic sites, especially metastases from renal carcinoma (185). The first of these diagnoses is usually readily apparent on dilation and curettage; the second may cause problems owing to the possible remoteness of the removal of the renal primary (up to 11 years earlier) or the failure of the pathologist or clinician to consider the possibility of a renal primary. Young and Hart (185) note that histologic clues pointing to metastasis from a renal primary include a gross specimen containing a bright yellow tumor (Figure 5.16) with histologic patterns including a prominent sinusoidal vascular growth pattern, an absence of hobnail cells, and a lack of mixture of different histologic patterns typical of clear cell carcinoma. The renal metastases tend to have tubules containing eosinophilic fluid or extravasated red blood cells. They also lack the eosinophilic globules of basement membrane-like material often seen in primary ovarian clear cell carcinomas (185). The eosinophilic or oxyphilic clear cell carcinoma variant is apt to be misdiagnosed as some form of steroid (lipid cell) tumor (176). The steroid tumors as a group, however, not only have frequent endocrine manifestations but also have a more homogeneous appearance on section, and microscopically they usually show less nuclear atypia, less necrosis, and absence of the cyst formation characteristic of most clear cell

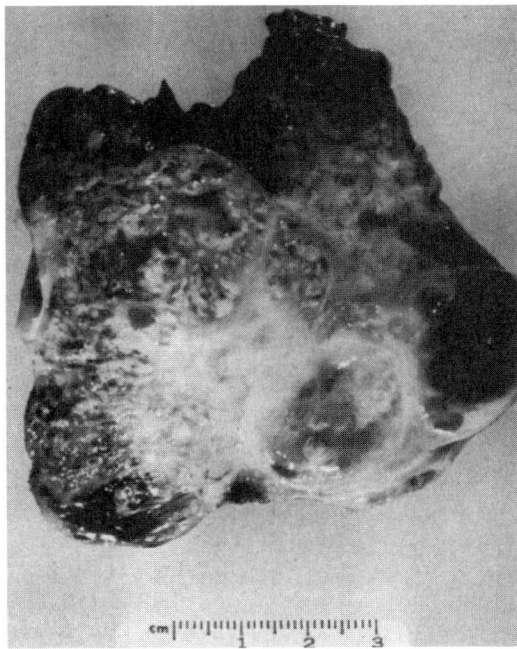

FIG. 5.16. Metastatic renal carcinoma in ovary. The paler areas just left of center were bright yellow and highly suggestive of a stromal tumor. When frozen section revealed an adenocarcinoma with many clear cells rather than a granulosa cell tumor, the surgeon recalled a prior operation for renal cell carcinoma.

carcinomas. The hepatoid variety of EST also enters into the differential diagnosis but may be excluded by its strong immunohistochemical positivity for α-fetoprotein (AFP).

An ovarian tumor found in a woman in her late twenties or early thirties that at first glance appears to be a clear cell carcinoma should also be carefully examined to rule out EST. The EST contains one or more of the patterns described in the chapter on germ cell tumors (see Chapter 6). In addition to elevated serum AFP (186) in the patient, the tumor may be immunohistochemically stained for AFP.

About 10% of clear cell carcinomas have admixed endometrioid carcinoma (125,137), and serous or mucinous areas also may be seen.

If the patient has an elevated preoperative serum concentration of CA 125, the clinician will follow its decline and institute treatment on elevation of this marker with recurrence. A more specific marker for clear cell carcinoma may be the serum cancer-associated galactosyltransferase. It not only is elevated in 75% of ovarian cancer patients but apparently greatly elevated (more than 2,000 mU/ml) specifically in those ovarian cancer patients who have tumors with a clear cell histology (187).

Recurrence of clear cell carcinoma, as with other ovarian and epithelial tumors, is most likely to consist of diffuse spread over abdominal and peritoneal surfaces but lymph node metastases, parenchymal involvement of liver and lung, and bone metastases appear to be more likely with clear cell carcinomas than with serous carcinomas (171).

MALIGNANT BRENNER TUMORS, TRANSITIONAL CELL, AND SQUAMOUS CARCINOMA OF THE OVARY

Although Brenner tumors represent only about 2% of ovarian neoplasms and more than 99% are benign, a small proportion demonstrate atypical proliferative changes and a few are frankly malignant. An overview of the pathology of these lesions demands consideration of the closely related and only recently recognized ovarian transitional cell carcinoma (Table 5.7) (188).

The past 30 years have seen a number of reports relating the epithelium of Brenner tumors to transitional cell epithelium. Ultrastructurally, histochemically, and immunohistochemically, the epithelia are virtually identical, although the grooves seen in nuclei of Brenner tumor epithelium ("coffee bean" nuclei) are not a feature of transitional cells (189). Whether the tumors originate directly from the ovarian surface (190) or from undifferentiated epithelium lining ovarian surface inclusion cysts (191–193),

TABLE 5.7. *Brenner, transitional cell, and squamous tumors*

Benign
  Brenner tumor
Proliferative
  Proliferative brenner tumor
Low malignant potential (borderline)
  Brenner tumor of LMP
Malignant
  Malignant Brenner tumor
  Transitional cell carcinoma, non-Brenner type
  Squamous carcinoma

there appears to be an initial metaplasia into urothelial-like Brenner cells. These cells ramify in tongues of epithelium that penetrate the ovary and stimulate stromal cell proliferation. Ciliated cell or squamous metaplasia is occasionally seen within these transitional cell areas, but most commonly secondary mucinous cell metaplasia occurs and may produce minute mucous cell-lined cysts, similar to cystitis cystica and glandularis (192,193), or even grossly obvious mucinous cystadenomas.

The uncommon Brenner tumors that are not histologically and clinically malignant yet show proliferative activity with or without marked cytologic atypia have been divided into three groups by Roth and coworkers (194). The *metaplastic* Brenner tumor shows marked cyst formation with prominent, often complex, mucinous cell metaplasia and occasional ciliated cell metaplasia. There is no nuclear atypia (Figure 5.17). The *proliferative* Brenner tumor contains cystic spaces with papillary fronds lined by transitional cells with or without mucinous metaplasia which are virtually identical to noninvasive low-grade papillary transitional cell carcinoma. The Brenner tumor of *low malignant potential* is similar to the proliferating Brenner tumor except for areas of high-grade nuclear atypia, similar to a high-grade transitional cell carcinoma *in situ* or a squamous carcinoma *in situ*. All three of these proliferative variants of the Brenner tumor are clinically benign (194), so the brief description given here will serve mainly to alert clinicians to their existence and to possible problems faced by the pathologist who may never have encountered one (195).

The malignant Brenner tumor (196–199) by definition contains an identifiable residual area of benign or proliferating Brenner tumor in addition to a histologically malignant component of infiltrating epithelial carcinoma, which histologically tends to be transitional cell, squamous cell, or undifferentiated. An adenocarcinoma component may also be present (198). Roth and Czernobilsky (198) divided malignant Brenner tumors into well-differentiated and poorly differentiated ones based on the amount of nuclear atypia. The well-differentiated ones have only grade 1 or 2 nuclear atypia, while the poorly differentiated ones have grade 3 (high-grade) epithelial atypia; their biologic behavior seems to parallel the degree of differentiation. Patients with well-differentiated malignant Brenner tumors, with a mean age of 64 years (range, 42 to 76 years) tend to be diagnosed with stage I disease and to remain free of recurrent disease postoperatively. Patients with poorly differentiated lesions, who also have a mean age of 64 years (range, 59 to 68 years) have a 40% mortality at 5 years despite the fact that 80% are originally diagnosed as stage 1A (198). The series reported by Miles and Norris (197), which did not subdivide malignant Brenner tumors by degree of differentiation, demonstrated a 43% mortality rate from the tumor after 3 years of follow-up. As is true with a few benign Brenner tumors, at least one malignant Brenner tumor has been linked with estrogen production and atypical endometrial hyperplasia (199). Flow cytometry may help identify which Brenner tumors are diploid and will behave in a benign fashion, and which are aneuploid and will metastasize (200).

Transitional Cell Carcinoma

Ovarian carcinomas composed of infiltrating transitional cells are occasionally seen in which no Brenner tumor component is identified. These are termed transitional cell carcinomas. Clinically they behave somewhat differently from malignant Brenner tumors. Despite having a histologic appearance identical to the malignant

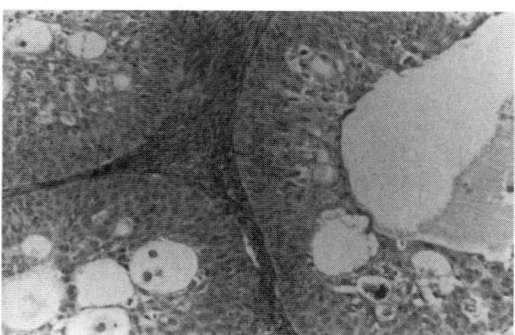

FIG. 5.17. Metaplastic Brenner tumor. The proliferative epithelial cells occupy the majority of the sectioned tumor, and only a little fibrous tissue intervenes. Note the prominent cyst formation. Mucinous cell metaplasia is minimal in this particular microscopic field.

transitional cell component of malignant Brenner tumors, they much more often are diagnosed at a more advanced stage (69% in stage II–IV) and have a worse prognosis (only 43% of patients with stage I transitional cell carcinoma are without evidence of disease at 5 years) (196). Although few pure transitional cell carcinomas exist, more commonly transitional cells make up a component of a serous, endometrioid, or undifferentiated carcinoma. In one large series, 9% of carcinomas contained a transitional cell component (201). Those tumors with a predominant transitional cell component (i.e., more than 50%) do significantly better after chemotherapy than those without (202). Those whose metastases are composed mostly of cells differentiating as transitional cells also have a much better survival.

Primary Squamous Carcinoma

Squamous carcinoma in the ovary almost always represents metastatic disease or arises from a preexisting teratoma. A few cases may also arise in the lining of an endometriotic cyst (203). However, rare cases of apparently primary squamous carcinoma have been reported (204). There is no good evidence of origin in a teratoma in these cases, nor is there an underlying benign squamous (epidermoid) or endometriotic cyst of the ovary (205,206). Those patients with what appears to be a primary squamous carcinoma present with a cystic pelvic mass (7 to 24 cm diameter) that is lined by cytologically malignant squamous epithelium with or without invasion of underlying stroma. If the tumor invades the underlying stroma, it may also metastasize and cause death of the patient. Three of the four patients reported had prior therapy for cervical carcinoma *in situ*, but the relationship, if any, to the ovarian tumor is unknown (204). Because of its rarity, one must sample the tumor carefully to rule out an underlying lesion and clinically rule out a metastasis from another site.

MIXED EPITHELIAL TUMORS OF LOW MALIGNANT POTENTIAL (BORDERLINE TUMORS)

In any reported large series of cases of LMP tumors, a few (3% to 10%) (46) are likely to have a mixed histologic appearance, but how their appearance relates to their biologic behavior is not separately analyzed. In one series of 36 patients with mixed epithelial LMP tumors (207), the mean age was 35 years, and patients presented clinically with symptoms of abdominal pain in 10 and an asymptomatic mass in 9. Almost 80% of the tumors were unilateral, and all were in stage I. More than 50% had associated pelvic or ovarian endometriosis. The gross tumor size ranged from 2 to 16 cm (mean, 8.5 cm), and a granularity or excrescences were noted on the surface of 20% of them. On section, one or more cystic spaces were present with papillary excrescences and often thick mucoid cyst contents. Microscopically, no single cell type formed more than 60% of the lining of the fine delicate or blunt rounded papillae. The lining cells were endocervical-like mucinous cells, ciliated serous cells, and endometrial and squamous cells, and only a few goblet cells were seen. Although a contralateral ovarian tumor or pelvic recurrence developed in 9% of the patients, all were living and well after initial treatment or reexcision (207).

Mixed Epithelial Carcinoma

The presence of a few glands of a different histologic type is so common in an otherwise pure ovarian carcinoma that it is often ignored in the final diagnosis. If more than 10% of a tumor contains another histologic type of epithelium, it should be indicated in the diagnosis, even though the prognostic significance may be doubtful. Certainly the approximate percent of admixture of a second or third cell type present in the carcinoma should be indicated in any study in which histology is correlated with clinical or prognostic factors. For example, one study on clear cell and endometrioid carcinomas termed "mixed" those tumors in which both histologic patterns were present and the lesser element comprised at least 20% of the tumor (137).

UNDIFFERENTIATED CARCINOMA

Carcinomas without clearcut differentiation may constitute as many as 5% to 30% of all epithelial malignancies (208). This proportion depends on the extent of sampling, because additional sections of any tumor may uncover an area of clear diagnostic histology. The skill and experience of the pathologist and the desire to "put a name" on the malignancy may also influence the proportion finally diagnosed as undifferentiated. As noted by Scully (1), the underlying nature of most of these tumors is probably either serous or endometrioid. A study on histologic subtypes and staining for carcinoembryonic antigen (CEA) found that 25% of undifferentiated carcinomas and 19% of serous carcinomas stained positively, in contrast to the endometrioid, clear cell, and mucinous cell types, of which 68% to 80% stained positively (209).

Clinically, patients with undifferentiated carcinoma usually present with symptoms of advanced ovarian carcinoma and at operation more than 90% are found to be in stage III or IV. Tumors tend to be largely solid on section, with areas of necrosis and hemorrhage. Microscopically, as the tumor category implies, there are no uniform histologic criteria, but tumor cells tend to grow in sheets, trabeculae, and clusters. Cytologically marked pleomorphism and tumor giant cells may be present, or the cells may be relatively small and uniform. This latter type of undifferentiated carcinoma must be distinguished from a granulosa cell tumor. The undifferentiated carcinoma is cytokeratin positive and vimentin negative on immunohistochemical staining and lacks the nuclear grooves of granulosa cell tumors. Prognosis in undifferentiated carcinoma is poor; about 12% of patients survive to 10 years (44).

Unclassified Tumors

Tumors composed of cell types, especially intermediate between endometrioid and serous carcinoma, may be placed in this group, but there is a general tendency to lump such tumors with serous carcinomas (2).

Small Cell Carcinoma

In 1982, Dickersin, Kline, and Scully (210) described 11 cases of a small cell ovarian carcinoma with hypercalcemia in young women that had a highly malignant clinical course. The histogenesis of the tumor is controversial, and the cell is of unknown origin (211). No elements of the common epithelial, germ cell, or sex cord-stromal tumors are normally found in association with the neoplastic cells of small cell carcinoma, and Ulbright and associates (212) stressed that there are significant differences between this tumor and the common small cell carcinoma of the lung, where endocrine features are the rule. A few older women (mean age, 59 years) have been described with a small cell ovarian carcinoma of the pulmonary type, most of which had an associated epithelial component with endometrioid or squamous differentiation without hypercalcemia (213). More than 150 cases have been described (214), and the clinicopathologic features are becoming better defined. Patients are young, ranging from 2 to 46 years of age (2), with a mean of 24 years. They present either with typical symptoms of ovarian carcinoma or with signs of hypercalcemia, which is present in two thirds of cases. Ascites or intraabdominal spread may be present at laparotomy.

Grossly the tumors are unilateral and usually larger than 10 cm in diameter. Most are solid and are yellow or grayish-white on section, with small areas of necrosis, hemorrhage, or mucoid degeneration. A few have been described that contained a single large cyst (210,215). Microscopically, there is a diffuse growth of small cells, with slightly ovoid, closely packed, moderately hyperchromatic nuclei with molding. Occasionally nuclei become spindly, giving a slightly sarcomatoid appearance. Cytoplasm is scanty and palely eosinophilic, and cell membranes may be indistinct. Reticulin surrounds groups of cells (210), and there is focal deposition of collagen, which may separate strands of tumor cells. Electronmicroscopic study confirms the epithelial nature of the neoplasm, with definite intracellular junctions and the uniform finding of dilated rough endoplasmic reticulum (210,215). Immunohistochemical stains are often positive for cytokeratin (12 of 15 cases) and epithelial membrane antigen (5/15). Chromogranin A (4/15) and neuron-specific enolase (10/15) may be positive, but convincing neurosecretory granules are not seen ultrastructurally. Hypercalcemia abates after cytoreductive surgery but may return with tumor regrowth. The mechanism of hypercalcemia is probably secondary to production of parathyroid hormone-related protein (216).

The differential diagnosis includes juvenile granulosa cell tumor and undifferentiated carcinoma, as well as intraabdominal desmoplastic small round cell tumor and other rare entities. The first lacks the hypercalcemia of most small cell carcinomas and is vimentin positive and cytokeratin negative. It also has a moderate amount of smooth endoplasmic reticulum on electronmicroscopic analysis (217) and is often estrogenic, unlike typical small cell carcinoma. Undifferentiated carcinoma of the ovary affects older, often postmenopausal, women and most tumors contain areas of papillary serous carcinoma or other identifiable epithelial elements. Hypercalcemia is lacking, and the tumors are almost all bilateral and of high stage when first seen. Intraabdominal desmoplastic small round cell tumor has a prominent nesting pattern with desmoplastic stroma and is cytokeratin, epithelial membrane antigen, desmin, and vimentin positive on immunohistochemical staining; it is seen in the first decade of life in almost one quarter of the cases (218). Metastatic alveolar rhabdomyosarcoma and primitive neuroectodermal tumor are other small cell tumors that enter the differential diagnosis (219,220). A large cell variant of small cell carcinoma, also associated with hypercalcemia, may also be confused with other primary and metastatic ovarian carcinomas (2). Because of potential difficulties with the diagnosis of small round cell tumors, tissue should be saved for possible electronmicroscopy at the time of frozen section, and immunohistochemical stains may be needed. DNA analysis may be useful, because small cell carcinomas tested thus far all appear to be diploid (221), unlike many other tumors with which they might be confused.

Prognosis in small cell carcinoma is only about 12% survival despite radical surgery, radiation, and chemotherapy (210).

Sarcoma

Pure primary sarcomas originating in the ovary are rare, and only a few cases of fibrosarcoma (222), leiomyosarcoma (223), angiosarcoma (224), and other histologic types of sarcoma have been reported (225). The histology is similar to that of the sarcoma originating elsewhere in the body, and the prognosis is usually poor.

Tumors Metastatic to the Ovary

About 7% to 10% (226,227) of ovarian masses are secondary to metastases from some other organ. In many cases, the ovarian metastasis precedes discovery of the primary tumor (228), and the clinician must be aware that the pathologist, even after gross and microscopic study, may mistake a metastatic tumor (especially metastatic colon cancer) for an ovarian primary. Patients with metastases to the ovary range in age from the second to the ninth decade (229) and present with a pelvic mass, pain, or other symptoms consistent with primary ovarian carcinoma (230,231).

With the decreased incidence of gastric carcinoma, metastatic colon carcinoma is now the most common of the metastatic carcinomas to appear as an ovarian primary (229,230,232) that may seem histologically endometrioid, or even clear cell. Up to 3% of women with colonic carcinoma present clinically in that fashion (232). Immunohistochemical staining for cytokeratins 7 and 20 (233) in the endometrioid-appearing tumors or gastric mucin MUC5AC in the mucinous-appearing tumors (234) may help to determine the primary site, but nothing replaces clinical evaluation of the gastrointestinal tract at the time of laparoscopy. Gastric carcinoma is second in frequency (226,229). Carcinoma of the breast, although far more common, is almost always discovered before metastatic ovarian disease becomes apparent (235). The histology of the primary breast cancer, whether ductal or lobular, is reflected in the histology of the ovarian metastases (236). Case reports of numerous other primary sites are available in the literature (237), including ovarian metastases discovered both before and after discovery of the primary.

Gross examination of the sectioned ovary may reveal a solid mass, a diffuse or nodular tumor, or one or more cysts with or without necrosis (227). Bilateral involvement is common (60% to 75%) but not inevitable (227,229). Multiple distinct tumor nodules seen grossly or microscopically, or extensive blood vessel and lymphatic

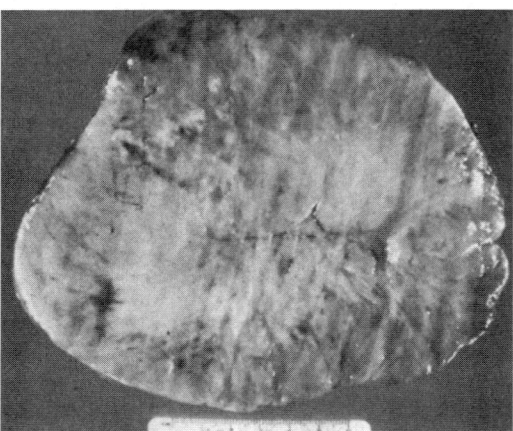

FIG. 5.18. Metastatic gastric carcinoma. Section of enlarged ovary containing metastatic gastric carcinoma. A similarly enlarged contralateral ovary and a slippery, mucoid feel to the cut surface are gross features suggestive of the correct diagnosis.

involvement seen microscopically, are features favoring metastasis over a primary tumor. When representative sections of the primary tumor are available for review, there is usually no problem in diagnosing metastatic disease. However, in the absence of a known primary, the diagnosis may be difficult.

Firm, bilaterally enlarged ovaries are characteristic of metastatic gastric carcinoma (Figure 5.18) and some cases of colonic carcinoma. The ovaries are usually solid on section, and the cut surface may have a mucoid, slippery feel. Microscopically there are infiltrating, mucin-containing signet ring cells with a reactive cellular stromal response. The reactive stromal spindle cells may obscure scanty signet ring cells and lead to an erroneous diagnosis of fibrothecoma both on frozen section (238) and, rarely, on permanent sections (239). Although this form of metastatic tumor was named after Krukenberg (240), it was described grossly by Paget many years earlier (241).

The histologically more common form of metastatic colon cancer shows gland formation instead of signet ring cells and is frequently initially misdiagnosed as primary endometrioid carcinoma. Misdiagnosis of metastatic tumor as primary mucinous or serous carcinoma also occurs (147,227). Most often the metastatic cells form a "pseudoendometrioid" pattern with a prominent "garland" or cribriform pattern of gland formation and striking "dirty" necrosis (147,148) (Figure 5.13). The focal squamous differentiation characteristic of many endometrioid ovarian primaries is lacking. Immunostaining for CEA may be very helpful in the endometrioid-like colonic metastases, because there is strong positivity in both gland lumens and glandular cell cytoplasm. Primary endometrioid carcinomas have only focal positivity (148). When compared with primary mucinous tumors of the ovary, metastatic colon cancer is more often prominently necrotic, with many fewer cases showing a predominance of mucinous cells or evidence of transition from benign-appearing to malignant-appearing epithelium (227). However, CEA staining is not helpful in these cases because both primary and metastatic mucinous tumors are strongly positive (148). Immunohistochemical studies for cytokeratins 7 and 20 are helpful in differentiating colonic metastases from primary ovarian carcinoma, because cytokeratin 7 is negative or only focally positive in metastatic lesions, and cytokeratin 20 is strongly positive. The reverse is true if the tumor is primary (233). Preoperative clinical evaluation of the colon may be exceedingly helpful to clinician, pathologist, and patient alike.

Survival after discovery of metastatic disease in the ovary is usually less than 1 year (231), but some patients, especially those with metastatic colon cancer, may be free of disease at 5 years (226). Uncommonly, metastatic tumor stimulates luteinization of surrounding ovarian stroma, causing clinical production of androgen (239), progesterone (242), or estrogen (41).

In a few patients, metastatic sarcoma in the ovary precedes discovery of the primary by a few months (243). Melanoma will have spread to the ovaries of many patients late in the course of disease, but ovarian metastases may also be the first sign of disease (244). Diagnosis may be difficult if knowledge of a primary melanoma is lacking, because of the multiplicity of histologic patterns that may be seen. These include spindle cell, small cell, pleomorphic, and granulosa cell-like tumor cells and growth patterns that may be nesting or follicle-like (245).

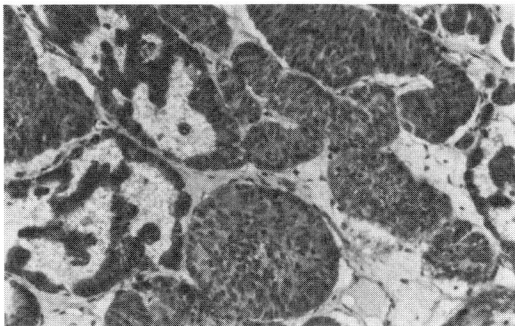

FIG. 5.19. Carcinoid tumor metastatic to the ovary. The precise nature of this malignant epithelial tumor could not be determined at the time of frozen section. An incidentally removed appendix contained the clinically unappreciated primary. Note that edema, characteristic of ovaries containing metastatic tumor, has separated the cells of the trabecula at left, causing a pseudoglandular appearance.

A comprehensive review of diagnostic aspects of metastatic tumors in the ovary (237) noted the problems caused by the variety of cell types and patterns that may be seen. This includes tumors that form small acini, trabecular and insular patterns, cords and columns, and follicle-like spaces, as well as tumors composed of spindle cells, cells with abundant eosinophilic cytoplasm, small cells, clear cells, transitional cells, and mucinous cells (Figure 5.19).

Lymphoma and Leukemia

Rarely, lymphoma or extramedullary leukemia manifests initially as an ovarian tumor primary. Because of the rarity in this location (about 1 in 500 new lymphoma cases) (246), pathologists may overlook the correct diagnosis and think of an anaplastic or metastatic carcinoma (especially breast carcinoma), granulosa cell tumor, or dysgerminoma (247,248).

Patients vary from 3 months to 74 years in age, with about 40% in one series being younger than 20 years of age (248). An abdominal mass or pain is the usual presenting complaint; ascites affects only 5%. About 36% to 50% of the lesions are in stage I, with bilateral involvement in more than half. Tubal, omental, and peritoneal involvement are typical of more advanced disease (248).

Grossly the tumors measure from 2 to 20 cm in diameter, with a mean of 8 to 10 cm, and are lobulated and rubbery (246). On section, they are pinkish- to grayish-white with occasional areas of cystic degeneration. The microscopic appearance is of sheets of noncohesive cells with or without nodularity, with the exact morphology dependent on the lymphoma or leukemia subclassification. If the diagnosis is suspected at the time of frozen section, touch preparations may be made and fresh material may be saved for flow immunologic studies. Cases of diffuse large cell immunoblastic lymphoma comprise about half the patients, and small noncleaved cell lymphomas (Burkitt and non-Burkitt) another 25% (248). Prognosis is poor but stage dependent, with 30% survival at 5 years for patients with stage I lesions and uncommon survival for higher-stage lesions.

Paraovarian Epithelial Tumors

Several topics touched on in this chapter on epithelial ovarian tumors are, strictly speaking, not ovarian, yet are sufficiently related they that seem important for complete understanding of the potential of pelvic tissue to undergo malignant changes similar to those found in the ovary itself. This is additionally important because at operation it is occasionally not entirely clear whether the primary site of origin of the tumor is ovarian or paraovarian. Müllerian-type malignancy may occur in other sites, such as the retroperitoneum (249,250) or on the bowel serosa (251), but these are not considered here. Faced with a large, distorting mass, the operating gynecologist may occasionally have such difficulty pinpointing the origin of a tumor that he or she is tempted simply to remove it and give it to the pathologist with a hope that somehow in the laboratory the true origin will become clear. However, it is frequently the case that the pathologist is also unable to determine the exact site of origin, especially in the case of advanced disease that has overgrown the adnexal area.

A variety of benign cysts, most of which are of paramesonephric or mesonephric origin, are noted in the broad ligament and are often incidental findings (252,253). Cystic epithelial tumors, almost all papillary serous and histologically of LMP, have been reported in the broad ligament (254,255). These patients present with a pelvic mass with or without pain or ascites, and perhaps 10% are pregnant. The age range is from 13 to 76 years, with a mean of about 32 years (255) to 43 years (254). At operation, the cyst is covered by the leaves of the broad ligament, with the fallopian tube often stretched over it. The size ranges from 1 to 28 cm in greatest dimension, and it is rare to have any tumor extending through the cyst wall to involve surrounding structures. On section, papillary projections are grossly apparent, and the histology in the vast majority is that of a serous tumor of LMP. In some cases, the cellular growth is solid and there is stromal invasion, so that at least histologically it must be recognized as a serous cystadenocarcinoma (254).

A few patients with endometrioid, clear cell, and mucinous carcinoma of the broad ligament have been reported (256), but follow-up was too short to indicate the degree of biologic malignancy. Brenner tumors have been described in the broad ligament, but thus far all have been benign (257).

Paraovarian tumors of probable wolffian origin (258,259) are usually benign, but rare cases may behave in a malignant fashion, with omental, lung, and liver metastasis (260,261). Tumors originating from the rete ovarii are usually benign cysts or cystadenomas, but one carcinoma has been described (262). Histologically, it had a transitional cell appearance.

Peritoneal Papillary Tumors

Peritoneal serous papillary tumors, because of their clinical presentation and strong histologic resemblance to ovarian serous carcinomas, are briefly considered here. Peritoneal serous papillary carcinoma (PSPC), also known as serous surface papillary carcinoma (263) and by other similar names, was first described by Swerdlow in 1959 as a peritoneal mesothelioma resembling ovarian papillary cystadenocarcinoma and may be of LMP or frankly malignant (264). They are histologically and immunohistochemically different from mesotheliomas but virtually indistinguishable from ovarian primaries (265).

Peritoneal Serous Papillary Carcinoma of Low Malignant Potential (Borderline Tumors)

Two series of cases describe an entity of LMP (borderline) serous tumors of the peritoneum. These are important because of their markedly better prognosis compared with ordinary PSPCs (57,58). These tumors, which have on occasion also have been termed atypical endosalpingiosis or serous micropapillomatosis (20), tend to occur in younger women (mean age, 33 years; range 16 to 67 years); most patients are under 40. At operation, which is often for another condition such as caesarian section but may be for chronic pelvic pain, the tumor is seen to form small miliary nodules on peritoneal surfaces, especially those of the pelvis. Microscopically these growths are identical to the implants seen with primary ovarian serous tumors of LMP. Psammoma bodies are common. With or without removal of the internal genitalia, and with or without chemotherapy, patients observed for a mean period of 7 to 8 years have done surprisingly well (57,58). Small bowel obstruction or invasive low-grade peritoneal serous carcinoma may eventually lead to complications in a few patients.

Peritoneal Serous Papillary Carcinoma

We now recognize PSPC as a generally highly malignant tumor originating from pelvic peritoneum and manifesting with signs and symptoms similar to those of ovarian carcinoma (263,266,267). On pelvic exploration, a papillary serous tumor is seen to form nodules or a velvety surface growth on omentum and pelvic and abdominal serosal surfaces, similar to that of a stage III or IV ovarian carcinoma, but the ovaries typically have only surface involvement with minimal if any stromal invasion. By definition the volume of tumor that involves the ovarian stroma is no larger than 5 mm in extent; tumor merely adherent to the surface is not considered. If the intraovarian tumor is greater than 5 mm, it is considered primary there. PSPC has been termed, rather appropriately, the "normal-sized ovary carcinoma syndrome" (268). These tumors are relatively frequent, comprising about

8% to 15% of lesions presenting as stage III or IV serous carcinoma. PSPC patients are similar in age and other factors to patients with serous ovarian primary tumors (263,269), with a mean age of 56 years (270) to 68 years (271) and a range from 25 to 85 years. Histologically, the tumors appear identical to primary ovarian serous carcinomas, forming papillae with one or more layers of epithelial cells with marked nuclear atypia and varying numbers of psammoma bodies. There is also definite invasion of underlying connective tissue. Molecular studies indicate that one quarter of the cases have multifocal origin of the tumor, especially those with BRCA1 germline mutations (272). This may relate to the finding of peritoneal primaries in women with a family history of ovarian carcinoma who have had prophylactic oophorectomy (273). Positive immunohistochemical staining for Leu M1 (diffuse), B72.3, PLAP, or CEA helps separate this tumor from diffuse peritoneal mesothelioma (274). Survival, despite debulking and adjuvant chemotherapy or radiation therapy, is poor; some find it similar to that of stage III or IV ovarian carcinoma, about 1 year (269,271), while others find PSPC worse (263,275). An S phase percentage of less than 10% on flow cytometric study may indicate a better prognosis (276). Longer survival times are seen when lesions are included that may perhaps be better categorized as serous tumors of LMP (269,277).

REFERENCES

1. Scully RE. *Histological typing of ovarian tumors,* 2nd ed. New York: World Health Organization, Springer, 1999.
2. Scully RE, Young RH, Clement PB. Tumors of the ovary, maldeveloped gonads, fallopian tube, and broad ligament. In: *Atlas of tumor pathology,* Fascicle 23, Series 3. Washington, DC: Armed Forces Institute of Pathology, 1998.
3. Tyler CW, Lee NC, Robboy SJ, et al. The diagnosis of ovarian cancer by pathologists: how often do diagnoses by contributing pathologists agree with a panel of gynecologic pathologists? *Am J Obstet Gynecol* 1991;164:65–70.
4. Baak JPA, Langley FA, Talerman A, et al. Interpathologist and intrapathologist disagreement in ovarian tumor grading and typing. *Anal Quant Cytol Histol* 1986;8:354–357.
5. Cramer SF, Roth LM, Ulbright TM, et al. Evaluation of the reproducibility of the World Health Organization classification of common ovarian cancers with emphasis on methodology. *Arch Pathol Lab Med* 1987;111:819–829.
6. Sevelda P, Vavra N, Schemper M, et al. Prognostic factors for survival in stage I epithelial ovarian carcinoma. *Cancer* 1990;65:2349–2352.
7. Baak JPA, Wisse-Brekelmans EC, Langley FA, et al. Morphometric data to FIGO stage and histological type and grade for prognosis of ovarian tumours. *J Clin Pathol* 1986;39:1340–1346.
8. Hernandez E, Rosenshein NB, Bhagavan BS, et al. Tumor heterogeneity and histopathology in epithelial ovarian cancer. *Obstet Gynecol* 1984;63:330–334.
9. Malkasian GD, Melton LJ, III, O'Brien PC, et al. Prognostic significance of histologic classification and grading of epithelial malignancies of the ovary. *Am J Obstet Gynecol* 1984;149 274–284.
10. Duplat J, et al. Changes in the histocytologic grading of epithelial ovarian carcinoma following treatment. *Int J Gynecol Pathol* 1988;7:12–22.
11. Shimizu Y, Kamoi S, Amada S, et al. Toward the development of a universal grading system for ovarian epithelial carcinoma. *Cancer* 1998;82:893–901.
12. Silverberg SG. Histopathologic grading of ovarian carcinoma: a review and proposal. *Int J Gynecol Pathol* 2000;19:7–15.
13. Iversen O-E. Prognostic value of the flow cytometric DNA index in human ovarian carcinoma. *Cancer* 1988;61:971–975.
14. Kallioniemi O-P, Funnonen R, Mattila J, et al. Prognostic significance of DNA index, multiploidy, and S-phase fraction in ovarian cancer. *Cancer* 1988;61:334–339.
15. Kuhn W, Kaufmann M, Feichter GE, et al. DNA flow cytometry, clinical and morphological parameters as prognostic factors for advanced malignant and borderline ovarian tumors. *Gynecol Oncol* 1989;33:360–367.
16. Harding M, Cowan S, Mole D, et al. Estrogen and progesterone receptors in ovarian cancer. *Cancer* 1990;65:486–491.
17. Slotman BJ, Nauta JJP, Rao BR. Survival of patients with ovarian cancer: apart from stage and grade, tumor progesterone receptor content is a prognostic indicator. *Cancer* 1990;66:740–744.
18. Gramlich T, Austin RM, Lutz M. Histologic sampling requirements in ovarian carcinoma: a review of 51 tumors. *Gynecol Oncol* 1990;38:249–256.
19. Puls L, Heidtmann E, Hunter JE, et al. The accuracy of frozen section by tumor weight for ovarian epithelial neoplasms. *Gynecol Oncol* 1997;67:16–19.
20. Blaustein A. Peritoneal mesothelium and ovarian surface cells-shared characteristics. *Int J Gynecol Pathol* 1984;3:361–375.
21. Blaustein A, et al. Inclusions in ovaries of females aged day 1–30 years. *Int J Gynecol Pathol* 1982;1:145–153.
22. Chen L, et al. Proliferative activity and BRCA1 expression in ovarian epithelial inclusions. *Mod Pathol* 2000;13:22A(abs).
23. Werness BA, et al. p53, c-erbB, and Ki-67 expression in ovaries removed prophylactically from women with a family history of ovarian cancer. *Int J Gynecol Pathol* 1999;18:338–343.
24. Sherman ME, Lee JS, Banks RT, et al. Histopathologic features of ovaries at increased risk for carcinoma: a case-control analysis. *Int J Gynecol Pathol* 1999;18:151–157.

25. Deligdisch L, Gill J, Kenner H, et al. Ovarian dysplasia in prophylactic oophorectomy specimens: cytogenetic and morphometric correlations. *Cancer* 1999;86:1544–1550.
26. Werness BA, et al. Loss of heterozygosity in ovarian epithelial and related neoplasms. *Mod Pathol* 2000;13:134A(abst).
27. Caduff RF, et al. Comparative analysis of histologic homologues of endometrial and ovarian carcinoma. *Am J Surg Pathol* 1998;22:319–326.
28. Feldman GB, Knapp RC. Lymphatic drainage of the peritoneal cavity and its significance in ovarian cancer. *Am J Obstet Gynecol* 1974;11:991–994.
29. Burghardt E, Girardi F, Lahousen M, et al. Patterns of pelvic and paraaortic lymph node involvement in ovarian cancer. *Gynecol Oncol* 1991;40:103–106.
30. Piver MS, Barlow JJ, Lele SB. Incidence of subclinical metastasis in stage I and II ovarian carcinoma. *Obstet Gynecol* 1978;52:100–104.
31. Petru E, Pickel H, Tamussino K, et al. Pretherapeutic scalene lymph node biopsy in ovarian cancer. *Gynecol Oncol* 1991;43:262–264.
32. Bell DA, Scully R. Clinicopathologic features of lymph node (LN) involvement with ovarian serous borderline tumors (OSBT). *Lab Invest* 1992;66:61A(abst).
33. Leake JF, Rader JS, Woodruff JD, et al. Retroperitoneal lymphatic involvement with epithelial ovarian tumors of low malignant potential. *Gynecol Oncol* 1991;42:124–130.
34. Dauplat J, Hacker NF, Nieberg RK, et al. Distant metastases in epithelial ovarian carcinoma. *Cancer* 1987;60:1561–1566.
35. Barrow MV. Metastatic tumors of the umbilicus. *J Chron Dis* 1966;19:1113–1117.
36. Rose PG, Piver MS, Tsukada Y, et al. Metastatic patterns in histologic variants of ovarian cancer: an autopsy study. *Cancer* 1989;64:1508–1513.
37. Dvoretsky PM, Richards KA, Angel C, et al. Distribution of disease at autopsy in 100 women with ovarian cancer. *Hum Pathol* 1988;19:57–63.
38. Dauplat J, Nieberg RK, Hacker NF. Central nervous system metastases in epithelial ovarian cancer. *Cancer* 1987;60:2559–2562.
39. Kerr VE, Cadman E. Pulmonary metastases in ovarian cancer: analysis of 357 patients. *Cancer* 1985;56:1209–1213.
40. Young RH, Scully RE. Endocrine tumors of the ovary. *Curr Top Pathol* 1992;85:113–164.
41. Scully RE, Richardson GS. Luteinization of the stroma of metastatic cancer involving the ovary and its endocrine significance. *Cancer* 1961;14:827–840.
42. Clement PB, Young RH, Scully RE. Clinical syndromes associated with tumors of the female genital tract. *Semin Diagn Pathol* 1991;8:204–233.
43. SaterziWake N, Hireshchy shyn MM, Piver SM, et al. Specific cytogenetic changes in ovarian cancer involving chromosomes 6 and 14. *Cancer Res* 1980;40:4512–4518.
44. Aure JC, Hoeg K, Kolstad P. Clinical and histologic studies of ovarian carcinoma: long term follow-up of 990 cases. *Obstet Gynecol* 1971;37:1–9.
45. Russell P. The pathological assessment of ovarian neoplasms: II. The proliferating "epithelial" tumours. *Pathology* 1979;11:251–282.
46. Russell P, Merkur H. Proliferating ovarian "epithelial" tumours: a clinico-pathological analysis of 144 cases. *Aust N Z J Obstet Gynecol* 1979;19:45–51.
47. Taylor HC. Malignant and semi-malignant tumors of the ovary. *Surg Gynecol Obstet* 1929;48:204–230.
48. Barnhill D, Heller P, Brzozowski P, et al. Epithelial ovarian carcinoma of low malignant potential. *Obstet Gynecol* 1985;65:53–59.
49. Hopkins MP, Kumar NB, Morley GW. An assessment of pathologic features and treatment modalities in ovarian tumors of low malignant potential. *Obstet Gynecol* 1987;70:923–929.
50. Segal GH, Hart WR. Ovarian serous tumors of low malignant potential (serous borderline tumors): the relationship of exophytic tumors to peritoneal "implants." *Am J Surg Pathol* 1992;16:577–583.
51. Lim-Tan SK, Cajigas HE, Scully RE. Ovarian cystectomy for serous borderline tumors: a follow-up study of 35 cases. *Obstet Gynecol* 1988;72:775–781.
52. Tazelaar HD, Bostwick DG, Ballon SC, et al. Conservative treatment of borderline ovarian tumors. *Obstet Gynecol* 1985;66:417–422.
53. Karp LA, Czernobilsky B. Glandular inclusions in pelvic and abdominal para-aortic lymph nodes: a study of autopsy and surgical material in males and females. *Am J Clin Pathol* 1969;52:212–218.
54. Moore WF, et al. Some mullerian inclusion cysts in lymph nodes may sometimes be metastases from serous borderline tumors of the ovary. *Am J Surg Pathol* 2000;24:710–718.
55. Kliman L, Rome RM, Fortune DW. Low malignant potential tumors of the ovary: a study of 76 cases. *Obstet Gynecol* 1986;68:338–344.
56. Lin PS, Gershenson DM, Bevers MW, et al. The current status of surgical staging of ovarian serous borderline tumors. *Cancer* 1999;85:905–911.
57. Bell DA, Scully RE. Serous borderline tumors of the peritoneum. *Am J Surg Pathol* 1990;14:230–239.
58. Biscotti CV, Hart WR. Peritoneal serous micropapillomatosis of low malignant potential (serous borderline tumors of the peritoneum): a clinicopathologic study of 17 cases. *Am J Surg Pathol* 1992;16:467–475.
59. Lu KH, Bell DA, Welch WR, et al. Evidence for the multifocal origin of bilateral and advanced human serous borderline ovarian tumors. *Cancer Res* 1998;58:2328–2330.
60. Kupryjanczyk J, et al. Ovarian, peritoneal, and endometrial serous carcinoma: clonal origin of multifocal disease. *Mod Pathol* 1996;9:166–173,1996.
61. Malpica A, et al. Serous tumors involving extra-abdominal/pelvic sites after the diagnosis of an ovarian serous neoplasm of low malignant potential. *Mod Pathol* 2000;13:128A(abst).
62. Bostwick DG, Tazelaan MD, Ballon SC, et al. Ovarian epithelial tumors of borderline malignancy: a clinical and pathologic study of 109 cases. *Cancer* 1986;58:2052–2065.
63. Kao GF, Norris HJ. Cystadenofibromas of the ovary with epithelial atypia. *Am J Surg Pathol* 1978;2:357–363.
64. Katzenstein A-LA, Mazur MT, Morgan TE, et al. Proliferative serous tumors of the ovary: histologic features and prognosis. *Am J Surg Pathol* 1978;2:339–355.
65. Burks RT, Sherman ME, Kurman RJ. Micropapillary serous carcinoma of the ovary: a distinctive low-grade carcinoma related to serous borderline tumors. *Am J Surg Pathol* 1996;20:1319–1330.

66. Eichhorn JH, Bell DA, Young RM, et al. Ovarian serous borderline tumors with micropapillary and cribriform patterns: a study of 40 cases and comparison with 44 cases without these patterns. *Am J Surg Pathol* 1999;23:397–409.
67. Komitowski D, et al. Quantitative nuclear morphology in the diagnosis of ovarian tumors of low malignant potential (borderline). *Cancer* 1989;64:905–910.
68. Bell DA, Scully RE. Ovarian serous borderline tumors with stromal microinvasion: a report of 21 cases. *Hum Pathol* 1990;21:397–403.
69. Campo E, Merino MJ, Tauassoli FA, et al. Evaluation of basement membrane components and the 72 kDa type IV collagenase in serous tumors of the ovary. *Am J Surg Pathol* 1992;16:500–507.
70. Tavassoli FA. Serous tumor of low malignant potential with early stromal invasion (serous LMP with microinvasion). *Mod Pathol* 1988;1:407–414.
71. Deavers M, et al. Microinvasion in ovarian serous tumors of low malignant potential: a study of 100 high stage cases. *Mod Pathol* 2000;13:124A(abst).
72. McCaughey WTE, Kirk ME, Lester W, et al. Peritoneal epithelial lesions associated with proliferative serous tumors of the ovary. *Histopathology* 1984;8:195–208.
73. Zinsser KR, Wheeler JE. Endosalpingiosis in the omentum: a study of autopsy and surgical material. *Am J Surg Pathol* 1982;6:109–117.
74. Copeland LJ, Silva EG, Gershenson DM, et al. The significance of mullerian inclusions found at second-look laparotomy in patients with epithelial ovarian neoplasms. *Obstet Gynecol* 1988;71:763–770.
75. DeNardi FG, McCaughey WTE. *Peritoneal neoplastic and metaplastic lesions associated with serous ovarian tumors of low malignant potential.* XVII International Congress of the International Academy of Pathology, Dublin, 9 Sept. 1988(abst).
76. Gershenson DM, Silva EG. Serous ovarian tumors of low malignant potential with peritoneal implants. *Cancer* 1990;65:578–585.
77. Michael H, Roth LM. Invasive and non-invasive implants in ovarian serous tumors of low malignant potential. *Cancer* 1986;57:1240–1247.
78. Bell DA, Weinstock MA, Scully RE. Peritoneal implants of ovarian serous borderline tumors: histologic features and prognosis. *Cancer* 1988;62:2212–2222.
79. Seidman JD, Kurman RJ. Ovarian serous borderline tumors: a critical review of the literature with emphasis on prognostic indicators. *Hum Pathol* 2000;31:539–557.
80. Bell KA, Smith AE, Kurman RJ. Refinement of criteria for diagnosis of implants associated with ovarian atypical proliferative serous tumors (APT) and micropapillary serous carcinomas (MPSC). *Mod Pathol* 2000;13:121A(abst).
81. Padberg B-C, Arps H, Franke U, et al. DNA cytomorphometry and prognosis in ovarian tumors of borderline malignancy: a clinicomorphologic study of 80 cases. *Cancer* 1992;69:2510–2514.
82. Kotylo PK, Michael H, Fineberg N, et al. Flow cytometric analysis of DNA content and RAS P21 oncoprotein expression in ovarian neoplasms. *Int J Gynecol Pathol* 1992;11:30–37.
83. Lai CH, Hsueh S, Tsao KC, et al. DNA aneuploidy in benign tumors and normal tissues of the female genital tract. *Int J Gynecol Pathol* 1996;15:63–68.
84. Khattech A, Spatz A, Prade M, et al. Nucleolar organizer regions in ovarian tumors: discrimination between carcinoma and borderline tumor. *Int J Gynecol Pathol* 1992;11:11–14.
85. Demopoulos RI, Bigelow B, Blaustein A, et al. Characterization and survival of patients with serous cystadenocarcinoma of the ovaries. *Obstet Gynecol* 1984;64:557–563.
86. Ferenczy A, Talens M, Zoghby M, et al. Ultrastructural studies on the morphogenesis of psammoma bodies in ovarian serous neoplasia. *Cancer* 1977;39:2451–2459.
87. Aure JC, Hoeg K, Kolstad P. Psammoma bodies in serous carcinoma of the ovary. *Am J Obstet Gynecol* 1971;109:113–118.
88. Clarke TJ. Sarcoma-like mural nodules in cystic serous ovarian tumours. *J Clin Pathol* 1987;40:1443–1448.
89. Bichel P, Jakobsen A. A new histologic grading index in ovarian carcinoma. *Int J Gynecol Pathol* 1989;8:147–155.
90. Gocneratne S, Sassone M, Blaustein A, et al. Serous surface papillary carcinoma of the ovary: a clinicopathologic study of 16 cases. *Int J Gynecol Pathol* 1982;1:258–269.
91. Gilks CB, Bell DA, Scully RE. Serous psammocarcinoma of the ovary and peritoneum. *Int J Gynecol Pathol* 1990;9:110–121.
92. Menuck L. Intraabdominal calcification in treated disseminated carcinoma of the ovary. *Obstet Gynecol* 1977;49[Suppl]:56s–58s.
93. Fenoglio CM, Ferenczy A, Richart RM. Mucinous tumors of the ovary: ultrastructural studies of mucinous cystadenomas with histogenetic considerations. *Cancer* 1975;36:1709–1722.
94. Teh M, Lee Y-S. Lectin histochemistry of ovarian mucinous cystadenomas. *Int J Gynecol Pathol* 1991;10:170–176
95. Hart WR, Norris HJ. Borderline and malignant mucinous tumors of the ovary: histologic criteria and clinical behavior. *Cancer* 1973;31:1031–1045.
96. Chaitin BA, Gershenson DM, Evans HL. Mucinous tumors of the ovary: a clinicopathologic study of 70 cases. *Cancer* 1985;55:1958–1962.
97. Radii M, et al. Mucinous neoplasms of the ovary: a clinicopathological study of 270 cases and a proposed clinicopathologic re-definition of the LMP category. *Lab Invest* 1988;58: 74A(abst).
98. Sumithran E, Susil BJ, Looi L-M. The prognostic significance of grading in borderline mucinous tumors of the ovary. *Hum Pathol* 1988;19:15–18.
99. Baak JPA, Blanco AA, Kurver PH, et al. Quantitation of borderline and malignant mucinous ovarian tumors. *Histopathology* 1981;5:353–360.
100. Baak JPA, Van Der Ley G. Borderline or malignant ovarian tumour? A case report of decision making with morphometry. *J Clin Pathol* 1984;37:1110–1113.
101. Hart WR. Ovarian epithelial tumors of borderline malignancy (carcinoma of low malignant potential). *Hum Pathol* 1977;8:541–549.
102. Kempson RL. *Case 4.* United States-Canadian Academy of Pathology, Gynecologic Pathology Specialty Conference, Atlanta, GA, March 17, 1992.
103. Watkin W, Silva EG, Gershenson DM. Mucinous carcinoma of the ovary: pathologic prognostic factors. *Cancer* 1992;69:208–212.

104. Rutgers JL, Scully RE. Ovarian mullerian mucinous papillary cystadenomas of borderline malignancy. *Cancer* 1988;61:340–348.
105. Young RH, Scully RE. Mucinous ovarian tumors associated with mucinous adenocarcinomas of the cervix: a clinicopathological analysis of 16 cases. *Int J Gynecol Pathol* 1988;7:99–111.
106. Prat J, Scully RE. Ovarian mucinous tumors with sarcoma-like mural nodules: a report of seven cases. *Cancer* 1979;44:1332–1344.
107. Czernobilsky B, Dgani R, Roth LM. Ovarian mucinous cystadenocarcinoma with mural nodule of carcinomatous derivation: a light and electron microscopic study. *Cancer* 1983;51:141–148.
108. Prat J, Young RH, Scully RE. Ovarian mucinous tumors with foci of anaplastic carcinoma. *Cancer* 1982;50:300–304.
109. Sondergaard G, Kaspersen P. Ovarian and extraovarian mucinous tumors with solid mural nodules. *Int J Gynecol Pathol* 1991;10:145–155.
110. Prat J, Scully RE. Sarcomas in ovarian mucinous tumors: a report of two cases. *Cancer* 1979;44:1327–1331.
111. Woodruff JD, Perry H, Gevaday R, et al. Mucinous cystadenocarcinoma of the ovary. *Obstet Gynecol* 1978;51:483–489.
112. Campbell JS, Lou P, Ferguson JP, et al. Pseudomyxoma peritonei et ovarii with occult neoplasms of appendix. *Obstet Gynecol* 1973;42:897–902.
113. Michael H, Sutton G, Roth LM. Ovarian carcinoma with extracellular mucin production: reassessment of "pseudomyxoma ovarii et peritonei." *Int J Gynecol Pathol* 1987;6:298–312.
114. Prayson RA, Hart WR, Petras RE. Pseudomyxoma peritonei: a clinicopathologic study of 19 cases with emphasis on site of origin and nature of associated ovarian tumors. *Am J Surg Pathol* 1994;18:591–603.
115. Young RH, Gilks CB, Scully RE. Mucinous tumors of the appendix associated with mucinous tumors of the ovary and pseudomyxoma peritonei: a clinicopathological analysis of 22 cases supporting an origin in the appendix. *Am J Surg Pathol* 1991;15:415–429.
116. Kahn MA, Demopoulos RI. Mucinous ovarian tumors with pseudomyxoma peritonei: a clinicopathologic study. *Int J Gynecol Pathol* 1992;11:15–23.
117. Cuatrecasas M, Matias-Guiu X, Prat J. Synchronous mucinous tumors of the appendix and ovary associated with pseudomyxoma peritonei: a clinicopathologic study of six cases with comparative analysis of c-Ki-ras mutations. *Am J Surg Pathol* 1996;20:739–746.
118. Chuaqui RF, Zhuang Z, Emmert-Buck MR, et al. Genetic analysis of synchronous mucinous tumors of the ovary and appendix. *Hum Pathol* 1996;27:165–171.
119. Mann WF, et al. The management of pseudomyxoma peritonei. *Cancer* 1990;66:1635–1640.
120. Beller FK, Zimmerman RE, Nienhaus H. Biochemical identification of the mucus of pseudomyxoma peritonei as the basis for mucolytic treatment. *Am J Obstet Gynecol* 1986;155:970–973.
121. Sampson JA. Endometrial carcinoma of the ovary arising in endometrial tissue in that organ. *Arch Surg* 1925;19:1–72.
122. Long ME, Taylor HC Jr. Endometrioid carcinoma of the ovary. *Am J Obstet Gynecol* 1964;90:936–950.
123. Aure JC, Hoeg K, Kolstad P. Carcinoma of the ovary and endometriosis. *Acta Obstet Gynecol Scand* 1971;50:63–67.
124. Kline RC, Wharton JT, Atkinson EN, et al. Endometrioid carcinoma of the ovary: retrospective review of 145 cases. *Gynecol Oncol* 1990;39:337–349.
125. Kurman RJ, Craig JM. Endometrial and clear cell carcinoma of the ovary. *Cancer* 1972;29:1653–1664.
126. Schueller EF, Kirol PM. Prognosis in endometrioid carcinoma of the ovary. *Obstet Gynecol* 1966;27:850–858.
127. Czernobilsky B, Morris WJ. A histologic study of ovarian endometriosis with emphasis on hyperplastic and atypical changes. *Obstet Gynecol* 1979;53:318–323.
128. Bell DA, Scully RE. Atypical and borderline endometrioid adenofibromas of the ovary: a report of 27 cases. *Am J Surg Pathol* 1985;9:205–214.
129. Kao GF, Norris HJ. Unusual cystadenofibromas: endometrioid, mucinous, and clear cell types. *Obstet Gynecol* 1979;54:729–736.
130. Roth LM, Czernobilsky B, Langley FA. Ovarian endometrioid adenofibromatous and cystadenofibromatous tumors: benign, proliferating, and malignant. *Cancer* 1981;48:1838–1845.
131. Snyder RR, Norris HJ, Tavassoli F. Endometrioid proliferative and low malignant potential tumors of the ovary: a clinicopathologic study of 46 cases. *Am J Surg Pathol* 1988;12:661–671.
132. Lu D, Hedrick Ellenson L, Isacson C. Endometrioid borderline tumors of the ovary: a clinicopathologic study of 17 cases. *Mod Pathol* 2000;13:127A(abst).
133. Bell KA, Kurman RJ. A clinicopathologic analysis of proliferative (well differentiated) endometrioid tumors of the ovary. *Mod Pathol* 2000;13:121A(abst).
134. Czernobilsky B, Silverman BB, Mikuta JJ. Endometrioid carcinoma of the ovary: a clinicopathologic study of 75 cases. *Cancer* 1970;26:1141–1152.
135. Tidy J, Mason WP. Endometrioid carcinoma of the ovary: a retrospective study. *Br J Obstet Gynaecol* 1988;95:1165–1169.
136. Fu YS, et al. Significance of squamous components in endometrioid carcinoma of the ovary. *Cancer* 1979;44:614–616.
137. Brescia RJ, Dubin N, Demopoulos RI. Endometrioid and clear cell carcinoma of the ovary: factors affecting survival. *Int J Gynecol Pathol* 1989;8:132–138.
138. Tornos C, Silva EG, Burke TW. Endometrioid carcinoma of the ovary: pure versus mixed histologic pattern. *Lab Invest* 1992; 66:69A(abst).
139. Young RH, Prat J, Scully RE. Ovarian endometrioid carcinomas resembling sex cord–stromal tumors: a clinicopathological analysis of 13 cases. *Am J Surg Pathol* 1982;6:513–522.
140. Roth LM, Liban E, Czernobilsky B. Ovarian endometrioid tumors mimicking Sertoli and Sertoli-Leydig cell tumors: sertoliform variant of endometrioid carcinoma. *Cancer* 1982;50:1322–1331.
141. Ordi J, et al. Sertoliform endometrioid carcinomas of the ovary: a clinicopathologic and immunohistochemical study of 13 cases. *Mod Pathol* 1999;12:933–940.
142. Aguirre P, Thor AD, Scully RE. Ovarian endometrioid carcinomas resembling sex cord-stromal tumors: an immunohistochemical study. *Int J Gynecol Pathol* 1989;8:364–373.
143. Tornos C, et al. Endometrioid carcinoma of the ovary with a prominent spindle-cell component, a source of

144. Eifel P, Hendrickson M, Ross J, et al. Simultaneous presentation of carcinoma involving the ovary and uterine corpus. *Cancer* 1982;50:163–170.
145. Zaino RJ, Unger RE, Whitney C. Synchronous carcinoma of the uterine corpus and ovary. *Gynecol Oncol* 1984;19:329–335.
146. Ulbright T, Roth LM. Metastatic and independent cancers of the endometrium and ovary: a clinicopathologic study of 34 cases. *Hum Pathol* 1985;16:28–34.
147. Daya D, Nazerali L, Frank GL. Metastatic ovarian carcinoma of large intestinal origin simulating primary ovarian carcinoma: a clinicopathologic study of 25 cases. *Am J Clin Pathol* 1992;97:751–758.
148. Lash RH, Hart WR. Intestinal adenocarcinomas metastatic to the ovaries: a clinicopathologic evaluation of 22 cases. *Am J Surg Pathol* 1987;11:114–121.
149. Clement PB, Scully RE. Extrauterine mesodermal (mullerian) adenosarcoma: a clinicopathologic analysis of five cases. *Am J Clin Pathol* 1978;69:276–283.
150. Kao GF, Norris HJ. Benign and low grade variants of mixed mesodermal tumor (adenosarcoma) of the ovary and adnexal region. *Cancer* 1978;42:1314–1324.
151. Cooper P. Malignant mixed mesodermal tumor and clear cell carcinoma arising in ovarian endometriosis. *Cancer* 1978;42:2827–2831.
152. Barwick KW, LiVolsi VA. Malignant mixed mesodermal tumor of ovary. *Am J Surg Pathol* 1980;4:37–42.
153. Dictor M. Malignant mixed mesodermal tumor of the ovary: a report of 22 cases. *Obstet Gynecol* 1985;65:720–724.
154. Hernandez W, DiFaria PJ, Marrow CP, et al. Mixed mesodermal sarcoma of the ovary. *Obstet Gynecol* 1977;49(Suppl 1):59–63.
155. Masuda A, Taked A, Fukami N, et al. Characteristics of cell lines established from a mixed mesodermal tumor of the human ovary: carcinomatous cells are changeable to sarcomatous cells. *Cancer* 1987;60:2696–2703.
156. Dehner LP, Norris HJ, Taylor HB. Carcinosarcomas and mixed mesodermal tumors of the ovary. *Cancer* 1971;27:207–216.
157. Dictor M. Ovarian malignant mixed mesodermal tumor: the occurrence of hyaline droplets containing α_1-antitrypsin. *Hum Pathol* 1982;13:930–933.
158. George E, et al. Malignant mixed mullerian tumor versus high grade endometrial carcinoma and aggressive variants of endometrial carcinoma: a comparative analysis of survival. *Int J Gynecol Pathol* 1995;14:39–44.
159. Gruskin P, Osborne NG, Morley GW, et al. Primary endometrial stromatosis of ovary: report of a case. *Obstet Gynecol* 1970;36:702–707.
160. Young RH, Prat J, Scully RE. Endometrioid stromal sarcomas of the ovary: a clinicopathologic analysis of 23 cases. *Cancer* 1984;53:1143–1155.
161. Peham H. Aus accessorischen nebennieren-anlagen entandene ovarial-tumoren. *Monatsschr f Geburtsh u Gynaek* 1899;10:685–694.
162. Schiller W. Mesonephroma ovarii. *Am J Cancer* 1939;35:1–21.
163. Teilum G. Histogenesis and classification of mesonephric tumors of the female and male genital systems and relationship to benign so-called adenomatoid tumor (mesotheliomas): a comparative histologic study. *Acta Path Microbiol Scand* 1954;34:431–481.
164. Scully RE, Barlow JF. "Mesonephroma" of ovary: tumor of mullerian nature related to the endometrioid carcinoma. *Cancer* 1967;20:1405–1417.
165. Shevchuk MM, Winkler-Monsanto B, Fenoglio CM, et al. Clear cell carcinoma of the ovary: a clinicopathologic study with review of the literature. *Cancer* 1981;47:1344–1351.
166. Bell DA, Scully RE. Benign and borderline clear cell adenofibromas of the ovary. *Cancer* 1985;56:2922–2931.
167. Roth LM, et al. Ovarian clear cell adenofibromatous tumors: benign, of low malignant potential, and associated with invasive clear cell carcinoma. *Cancer* 1984;53:1156–1163.
168. Ohkawa K, et al. Clear cell carcinoma of the ovary: light and electron microscopic studies. *Cancer* 1977;40:3019–3029.
169. Eastwood J. Mesonephroid (clear cell) carcinoma of the ovary and endometrium: a comparative prospective clinico-pathological study and review of literature. *Cancer* 1978;41:1911–1928.
170. Montag AG, Jenison EL, Griffiths CT, et al. Ovarian clear cell carcinoma: a clinicopathologic analysis of 44 cases. *Int J Gynecol Pathol* 1989;8:85–96.
171. Jenison EL, et al. Clear cell adenocarcinoma of the ovary: a clinical analysis and comparison with serous carcinoma. *Gynecol Oncol* 1989;32:65–71.
172. Yoonessi M, Weldon D, Satchiand SK, et al. Clear cell ovarian adenocarcinoma. *J Surg Oncol* 1984;27:289–297.
173. Czernobilsky B, Silverman BB, Enterline HT. Clear-cell carcinoma of the ovary: a clinicopathologic analysis of pure and mixed forms and comparison with endometrioid carcinoma. *Cancer* 1970;25:762–772.
174. Fine G, Clarke HD, Horn RC Jr. Mesonephroma of the ovary: a clinical, morphological, and histogenetic appraisal. *Cancer* 1973;31:398–410.
175. Silverberg SG. Ultrastructure and histogenesis of clear cell carcinoma of the ovary. *Am J Obstet Gynecol* 1973;115:394–400.
176. Young RH, Scully RE. Oxyphilic clear cell carcinoma of the ovary: a report of nine cases. *Am J Surg Pathol* 1987;11:661–667.
177. Wade-Evans T, Langley FA. Mesonephric tumors of the female genital tract. *Cancer* 1961;14:711–725.
178. Crozier MA, Copeland LJ, Silva EG, et al. Clear cell carcinoma of the ovary: a study of 59 cases. *Gynecol Oncol* 1989;35:199–203.
179. Hitti IF, Glasberg SS, Lubicz S. Clear cell carcinoma arising in extraovarian endometriosis: report of three cases and review of the literature. *Gynecol Oncol* 1990;39:314–320.
180. Doshi N, Tobon H. Primary clear cell carcinoma of the ovary: an analysis of 15 cases with review of the literature. *Cancer* 1977;39:2658–2664.
181. Listinsky CM, Bonfiglio TA, Leary J. Variable ploidy of ovarian clear cell carcinomas: implications for adequacy of tissue sampling. *Anal Quant Cytol Histol* 1988;10:21–27.
182. Atkin NB. Model DNA value and chromosome number in ovarian neoplasia: a clinical and histopathologic assessment. *Cancer* 1971;27:1064–1073.
183. Friedlander ML, et al. The influence of cellular DNA content on survival in advanced ovarian cancer. *Cancer Res* 1984;44:397–400.

184. Rodenberg CJ, et al. Tumor ploidy as a major prognostic factor in advanced ovarian cancer. *Cancer* 1987;59:317–323.
185. Young RH, Hart WR. Renal cell carcinoma metastatic to the ovary: a report of three cases emphasizing possible confusion with ovarian clear cell adenocarcinoma. *Int J Gynecol Pathol* 1992;11:96–104.
186. Klemi PJ, et al. Clear cell (mesonephroid) tumors of the ovary with characteristics resembling endodermal sinus tumor. *Int J Gynecol Pathol* 1982;1:95–100.
187. Nozawa S, et al. Cancer-associated galactosyltransferase as a new tumor marker for ovarian clear cell carcinoma. *Cancer Res* 1990;50:754–759.
188. Gersell DJ. Primary ovarian transitional cell carcinoma: diagnostic and prognostic considerations [Editorial]. *Am J Clin Pathol* 1990;93:586–588.
189. Santini D, Gelli MC, Mazzoleni G, et al. Brenner tumor of the ovary: a correlative histologic, histochemical, immunohistochemical, and ultrastructural investigation. *Hum Pathol* 1989;20:787.
190. Arey LB. The origin and form of the Brenner tumor. *Am J Obstet Gynecol* 1961;81:743–751.
191. Lauchlan SC. Histogenesis and histogenetic relationships of Brenner tumors. *Cancer* 1966;19:1628–1634.
192. Shevchuk MM, Fenoglio CM, Richart RM. Histogenesis of Brenner tumors: I. Histology and ultrastructure. *Cancer* 1980;46:2607–2616.
193. Shevchuk MM, Fenoglio CM, Richart RM. Histogenesis of Brenner tumors: II. Histochemistry and CEA. *Cancer* 1980;46:2617–2622.
194. Roth LM, Dallenbach-Hellweg G, Czernobilsky B. Ovarian Brenner tumors: I. Metaplastic, proliferating, and of low malignant potential. *Cancer* 1985;56:582–591.
195. Svenes KB, Eide J. Proliferative Brenner tumor or ovarian metastases? A case report. *Cancer* 1984;52:2692–2697.
196. Austin RM, Norris HJ. Malignant Brenner tumor and transitional cell carcinoma of the ovary: a comparison. *Int J Gynecol Pathol* 1987;6:29–39.
197. Miles PA, Norris HJ. Proliferative and malignant Brenner tumors of the ovary. *Cancer* 1972;30:174–186.
198. Roth LM, Czernobilsky B. Ovarian Brenner tumors: II. Malignant. *Cancer* 1985;56:592–601.
199. Seldenrijk CA, Willig AP, Baak JP, et al. Malignant Brenner tumor. A histologic, morphometrical, immunohistochemical, and ultrastructural study. *Cancer* 1986;58:754–760.
200. Trebeck CE, et al. Brenner tumours of the ovary: a study of the histology, immunohistochemistry, and cellular DNA content in benign, borderline, and malignant ovarian tumours. *Pathology* 1987;19:241–246.
201. Silva EG, Robey-Cafferty SS, Smith TL, et al. Ovarian carcinomas with transitional cell carcinoma pattern. *Am J Clin Pathol* 1990;93:457–465.
202. Robey SS, Silva EG, Gershenson DM, et al. Transitional cell carcinoma in high-grade high-stage ovarian carcinoma: an indication of favorable response to chemotherapy. *Cancer* 1989;63:839–847.
203. Lele SB, Piver MS, Barlow JJ, et al. Squamous cell carcinoma arising in ovarian endometriosis. *Gynecol Oncol* 1978;6:290–293.
204. Yetman TJ, Dudzinski MR. Primary squamous carcinoma of the ovary: a case report and review of the literature. *Gynecol Oncol* 1989;34:240–243.
205. Nogales FF, Silverberg SG. Epidermoid cysts of the ovary: a report of five cases with histogenetic considerations and ultrastructural findings. *Am J Obstet Gynecol* 1976;124:523–528.
206. Young RH, Prat J, Scully RE. Epidermoid cyst of the ovary: a report of three cases with comments on histogenesis. *Am J Clin Pathol* 1980;73:272–276.
207. Rutgers JL, Scully RE. Ovarian mixed-epithelial papillary cystadenomas of borderline malignancy of mullerian type: a clinicopathologic analysis. *Cancer* 1988;61:546–554.
208. Silva EG, et al. Undifferentiated carcinoma of the ovary. *Arch Pathol Lab Med* 1991;115:377–381.
209. Casper S, van Nagrell Jr, Powell DF, et al. Immunohistochemical localization of tumor markers in epithelial ovarian cancer. *Am J Obstet Gynecol* 1984;149:154–158.
210. Dickersin GR, Kline IW, Scully RE. Small cell carcinoma of the ovary with hypercalcemia: a report of eleven cases. *Cancer* 1982;49:188–197.
211. Aguirre P, Thor AD, Scully RE. Ovarian small cell carcinoma: histogenetic considerations based on immunohistochemical and other findings. *Am J Clin Pathol* 1989;92:140–149.
212. Ulbright TM, Roth CM, Stehman FB, et al. Poorly differentiated (small cell) carcinoma of the ovary in young women: evidence supporting a germ cell origin. *Hum Pathol* 1987;18:175–184.
213. Eichhorn JH, Young RH, Scully RE. Primary ovarian small cell carcinoma of pulmonary type: a clinicopathologic, immunohistologic, and flow cytometric analysis of 11 cases. *Am J Surg Pathol* 1992;16:926–938.
214. Young RH, Oliva E, Scully RE. Small cell carcinoma of the ovary, hypercalcemic type: a clinicopathologic analysis of 150 cases. *Am J Surg Pathol* 1994;18:1102–1116.
215. Jensen ML, et al. Ovarian small cell carcinoma: a case report with histologic, immunohistochemical, and ultrastructural findings. *Acta Pathol Microbiol Immunol Scand Suppl* 1991;23:126–131.
216. Matias-Guiu X, et al. Human parathyroid hormone-related protein in ovarian small cell carcinoma: an immunohistochemical study. *Cancer* 1994;73:1878–1881.
217. McMahon JT, Hart WR. Ultrastructural analysis of small cell carcinomas of the ovary. *Am J Clin Pathol* 1988;90:523–529.
218. Young RH, Eichhorn JH, Dickersin GR, et al. Ovarian involvement by the intra-abdominal desmoplastic small round cell tumor with divergent differentiation: a report of three cases. *Hum Pathol* 1992;23:454–464.
219. Aguirre P, Scully RE. Malignant neuroectodermal tumor of the ovary–a distinctive form of monodermal teratoma: report of five cases. *Am J Surg Pathol* 1982;6:282–291.
220. Young RH, Scully RE. Alveolar rhabdomyosarcoma metastatic to the ovary: a report of two cases and a discussion of the differential diagnosis of small cell malignant tumors of the ovary. *Cancer* 1989;64:899–904.
221. Eichhorn JH, et al. DNA content and proliferative activity in ovarian small cell carcinomas of the hypercalcemic type: implications for diagnosis, prognosis and histogenesis. *Am J Clin Pathol* 1992;98:579–586.

222. Prat J, Scully RE. Cellular fibromas and fibrosarcomas of the ovary: a comparative clinicopathologic analysis of seventeen cases. *Cancer* 1981;47:2663–2670.
223. Nogales FF, Ayale A, Rhiz Avila J, et al. Myxoid leiomyosarcoma of the ovary: analysis of three cases. *Hum Pathol* 1991;22:1268–1273.
224. Ongkasuwan C, Taylor JE, Tang CK, et al. Angiosarcomas of the uterus and ovary: clinicopathologic report. *Cancer* 1982;49:1469–1475.
225. Talerman A. Nonspecific tumors of the ovary, including mesenchymal tumors and malignant lymphoma. In: Kurman RJ, ed: *Blaustein's pathology of the female genital tract,* 3rd ed. Philadelphia: Springer-Verlag, 1987:722–741.
226. Petru E, et al. Nongenital cancers metastatic to the ovary. *Gynecol Oncol* 1992;44:83–86.
227. Ulbright TM, Roth LM, Stehman FB. Secondary ovarian neoplasia: a clinicopathologic study of 35 cases. *Cancer* 1984;53:1164–1174.
228. Johansson H. Clinical aspects of metastatic ovarian cancer of extragenital origin. *Acta Obstet Gynecol Scand* 1960;39:681–697.
229. Mazur MT, Hsueh S, Gersell DJ. Metastases to the female genital tract: analysis of 325 cases. *Cancer* 1984;53:1978–1984.
230. Dollar JR, Orr JW, Shingleton HM, et al. Metastatic tumors mimicking gynecologic cancer. *Obstet Gynecol* 1987;69:865–867.
231. Hale RW. Krukenberg tumors of the ovaries: a review of 81 records. *Obstet Gynecol* 1968;32:221–225.
232. Harcourt KF, Dennis DL. Laparotomy for "ovarian tumors" in unsuspected carcinoma of the colon. *Cancer* 1968;21:1244–1245.
233. Young RH, Hart WR. Metastatic intestinal carcinomas simulating primary ovarian clear cell carcinoma and secretory endometrioid carcinoma: a clinicopathologic and immuno-histochemical study of five cases. *Am J Surg Pathol* 1998;22:805–815.
234. Ji H, Kurman RJ, Ronnett BM. Gastric (MUC5AC) mucin immunostaining is superior to cytokeratins in differentiating primary from metastatic mucinous ovarian tumors. *Mod Pathol* 2000;13:126A(abst).
235. Gagnon Y, Tetu B. Ovarian metastases of breast carcinoma: a clinicopathologic study of 59 cases. *Cancer* 1989;64:892–898.
236. Harris M, Howell A, Chrissohan M, et al. A comparison of the metastatic pattern of infiltrating lobular carcinoma and infiltrating duct carcinoma of the breast. *Br J Cancer* 1984;50:23–30.
237. Young RH, Scully RE. Metastatic tumors in the ovary: a problem-oriented approach and review of the recent literature. *Semin Diagn Pathol* 1991;8:250–276.
238. Holtz F, Hart WR. Krukenberg tumors of the ovary: a clinicopathologic analysis of 27 cases. *Cancer* 1982;50:2438–2447.
239. Connor TB, Ganis FM, Levin HS, et al. Gonadotropin-dependent Krukenberg tumor causing virilization during pregnancy. *J Clin Endocrinol Metab* 1968;28:198–214.
240. Krukenberg F. Ueber des fibrosarcoma ovarii mucocellulare (carcinomatodes). *Arch Gynakol* 1896;50:287–321.
241. Paget J. *Lectures on surgical pathology,* 3rd Am ed. Philadelphia: Lindsay & Blakiston, 1865:540–541.
242. Jolles CJ, Beeson JH, Abbott T. Progesterone production in adenocarcinoma of the colon metastatic to the ovaries. *Obstet Gynecol* 1985;65:853–857.
243. Young RH, Scully RE. Sarcomas metastatic to the ovary: a report of 21 cases. *Int J Gynecol Pathol* 1990;9:231–252.
244. Fitzgibbons PL, Martin SE, Simmons TJ. Malignant melanoma metastatic to the ovary. *Am J Surg Pathol* 1987;11:959–964.
245. Young RH, Scully RE. Malignant melanoma metastatic to the ovary: a clinicopathologic analysis of 20 cases. *Am J Surg Pathol* 1991;15:849–860.
246. Chorlton I, Norris HJ, King FM. Malignant reticuloendothelial disease involving the ovary as a primary manifestation: a series of 19 lymphomas and 1 granulocytic sarcoma. *Cancer* 1974;34:397–407.
247. Morgan ER, Labotka RS, Gonzalez-Crussi F, et al. Ovarian granulocytic sarcoma as the primary manifestation of acute infantile myelomonocytic leukemia. *Cancer* 1981;48:1819–1824.
248. Osborne BM, Robboy SJ. Lymphomas or leukemia presenting as ovarian tumors: an analysis of 42 cases. *Cancer* 1983;52:1933–1943.
249. Park U, et al. A primary mucinous cystadenocarcinoma of the retroperitoneum. *Gynecol Oncol* 1991;42:64–67.
250. Ulbright TM, Morley DJ, Roth LM, et al. Papillary serous carcinoma of the retroperitoneum. *Am J Clin Pathol* 1983;79:633–637.
251. Evans H, et al. Clear cell carcinoma of the sigmoid mesocolon: a tumor of the secondary mullerian system. *Am J Obstet Gynecol* 1990;162:161–163.
252. Gardner GH, Green RR, Peckham BM. Normal and cystic structures of the broad ligament. *Am J Obstet Gynecol* 1948;55:917–939.
253. Gardner GH, Greene RR, Peckham B. Tumors of the broad ligament. *Am J Obstet Gynecol* 1957;73:536–555.
254. Altaras MM, Jaffer R, Carduba A, et al. Primary paraovarian cystadenocarcinoma: clinical and management aspects and literature review. *Gynecol Oncol* 1990;38:268–272.
255. Aslani M, Ahn G-H, Scully RE. Serous papillary cystadenoma of borderline malignancy of broad ligament: a report of 25 cases. *Int J Gynecol Pathol* 1988;7:131–138.
256. Aslani M, Scully RE. Primary carcinoma of the broad ligament: report of four cases and review of the literature. *Cancer* 1989;64:1540–1545.
257. Hampton HL, Huffman HT, Meeks GR. Extraovarian Brenner tumor. *Obstet Gynecol* 1992;79:844–846.
258. Kariminejad MH, Scully RE. Female adnexal tumor of probable wolffian origin. *Cancer* 1973;31:671–677.
259. Devouassoux-Shisheboran M, Silver SA, Tavassoli FA. Wolffian adnexal tumor, so-called female adnexal tumor of probable wolffian origin (FATWO): immunohistochemical evidence in support of a wolffian origin. *Hum Pathol* 1999;30:856–863.
260. Young RH, Scully RE. Ovarian tumors of probable wolffian origin: a report of 11 cases. *Am J Surg Pathol* 1983;7:125–135.
261. Daya D. Malignant female adnexal tumor of probable wolffian origin with review of the literature. *Arch Pathol Lab Med* 1994;118:310–312.
262. Rutgers JL, Scully RE. Cysts (cystadenomas) and tumors of the rete ovarii. *Int J Gynecol Pathol* 1988;7:330–342.

263. Mills SE, et al. Serous surface papillary carcinoma: a clinicopathologic study of 10 cases and comparison with stage III and IV ovarian serous carcinoma. *Am J Surg Pathol* 1988;12:827–834.
264. Swerdlow M. Mesothelioma of the pelvic peritoneum resembling papillary cytoadenocarcinoma of the ovary. *Am J Obstet Gynecol* 1959;77:197–200.
265. Ordonez NG. Role of immunohistochemistry in distinguishing epithelial peritoneal mesotheliomas from peritoneal and ovarian serous carcinomas. *Am J Surg Pathol* 1998;22:1203–1214.
266. Altaras MM, et al. Primary peritoneal papillary serous adenocarcinoma: clinical and management aspects. *Gynecol Oncol* 1991;40:230–236.
267. Fromm G-L, Gershenson DM, Silva EG. Papillary serous carcinoma of the peritoneum. *Obstet Gynecol* 1990;75:89–95.
268. Feuer GA, Shevchuk M, Calanog A. Normal-sized ovary carcinoma syndrome. *Obstet Gynecol* 1989;73:786–792.
269. Dalrymple JC, Bannatyne P, Russell P, et al. Extraovarian peritoneal serous papillary carcinoma: a clinicopathologic study of 31 cases. *Cancer* 1989;64:110–115.
270. Truong LD, et al. Serous surface carcinoma of the peritoneum: a clinicopathologic study of 22 cases. *Hum Pathol* 1990;21:99–110.
271. Schorge JO, et al. Molecular evidence for multifocal papillary serous carcinoma of the peritoneum in patients with germline BRCA1 mutations. *J Nat Cancer Inst* 1998;90:841–845.
272. Foyle A, Al-Jabi M, McCaughey WTE. Papillary peritoneal tumors in women. *Am J Surg Pathol* 1981;5:241–249.
273. Tobacman JK, Greene MH, Tucker MA, et al. Intraabdominal carcinomatosis after prophylactic oophorectomy in ovarian-cancer-prone families. *Lancet* 1982;2:795–797.
274. Bollinger DJ, Wick MR, Dehner LP, et al. Peritoneal malignant mesothelioma versus serous papillary adenocarcinoma: a histochemical and immunohistochemical comparison. *Am J Surg Pathol* 1989;13:659–670.
275. Chu C, Menzin AW, Leonard DG, et al. Primary peritoneal carcinoma: a review of the literature. *Obstet Gynecol Surv* 1999;54:323–335.
276. Bonin D, et al. Serous surface papillary carcinoma, a clinicopathologic and DNA flow cytometric study with emphasis on prognostic indicators. *Lab Invest* 1992;66:61A(*abst*).
277. Raju U, Fine G, Greenwald KA, et al. Primary papillary serous neoplasia of the peritoneum: a clinicopathologic and ultrastructural study of eight cases. *Hum Pathol* 1989;20:426–436.

6

Pathology of Ovarian Germ Cell Tumors

Helen Michael and Lawrence M. Roth

The current edition of *Histological Typing of Ovarian Tumors,* published by the World Health Organization (1), subclassifies ovarian germ cell tumors into the following categories: dysgerminoma, yolk sac tumor (endodermal sinus tumor), embryonal carcinoma, polyembryoma, choriocarcinoma, teratoma (immature, mature, and monodermal), and mixed germ cell tumors. Tumors composed of both germ cells and sex cord-stromal elements are also described in this chapter; they include gonadoblastoma and the mixed germ cell-sex cord-stromal tumor of nongonadoblastoma type (1).

DYSGERMINOMA

Dysgerminoma is the most common ovarian malignant germ cell tumor (2–6). It occurs primarily in adolescent girls and young women before the age of 30 years, although it has been reported in patients who range from 7 months to 70 years of age . Five percent to 10% of dysgerminomas occur in sexually maldeveloped patients; most dysgerminomas in this clinical setting arise from gonadoblastomas. The majority of dysgerminomas are seen in normally developed phenotypic and genotypic females. Most patients present with abdominal enlargement, a mass, or pain caused by torsion. Endocrine symptoms, including isosexual pseudoprecocity and menstrual abnormalities, may occur if tumors contain syncytiotrophoblastic giant cells, luteinized ovarian stromal cells, or coexisting choriocarcinoma (7).

About 10% of dysgerminomas are bilateral on gross examination of the ovary, and another 10% have microscopic foci of tumor in a contralateral ovary that appears normal on gross examination (2). In contrast, other germ cell tumors are almost always unilateral. Grossly, dysgerminomas are usually large, round or lobulated masses that have smooth, glistening external surfaces, unless the tumor has extended outside or ruptured through the ovary. On cut section, dysgerminomas are well-circumscribed neoplasms that are gray to tan in color (Figure 6.1). They often have a fluctuant, fleshy consistency, but abundant fibrous tissue in some tumors can cause increased firmness. Large tumors may have focal hemorrhage or necrosis, and small cystic areas may be present. The possibility of a mixed malignant germ cell tumor should be considered if abundant hemorrhage, necrosis, or substantial cystic areas are present.

Microscopically, pure dysgerminoma is identical to testicular seminoma. Nests or cords of tumor cells are separated by fibrous septa that contain variable numbers of lymphocytes, mostly T cells (8) and sometimes plasma cells. Granulomas that contain Langhans or foreign-body giant cells may also be present. Tumor cells are large, round or polygonal, and they display well-demarcated cell borders (Figure 6.2). The cytoplasm is clear to eosinophilic, and nuclei are enlarged and round to oval, with clumped chromatin and one or two eosinophilic nucleoli. Numerous mitoses are often present. Approximately 3% of ovarian dysgerminomas contain syncytiotrophoblastic giant cells (7). They must be distinguished from Langhans giant cells, foreign-body giant cells, and choriocarcinoma. In contrast to choriocarcinoma, dysgerminoma with syncytiotrophoblastic giant cells does not display admixed cytotrophoblast. The presence of syncytiotrophoblastic giant cells alone does not alter treatment or prognosis. Likewise, no evidence indicates that cellular anaplasia, high mitotic rate, degree of lymphoid infiltrate, or the amount of fibrous tissue affects prognosis.

II. HISTOPATHOLOGY OF OVARIAN CANCER

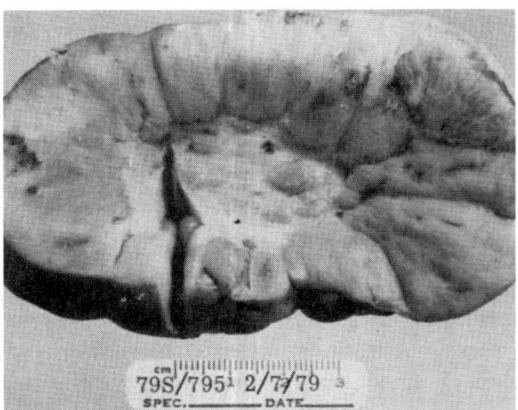

FIG. 6.1. Dysgerminoma showing a lobulated fleshy tumor without significant hemorrhage or necrosis.

Tumor cells in dysgerminoma contain glycogen that can be demonstrated by a periodic acid-Schiff (PAS) stain with and without prior diastase digestion. A rim of placental-like alkaline phosphatase beneath the cell membrane may be demonstrated immunohistochemically. Tumors are generally cytokeratin negative, although occasional cells may stain positively for low-molecular-weight cytokeratins. Epithelial membrane antigen and carcinoembryonic antigen are not present (10). Human chorionic gonadotropin (hCG) is present in admixed syncytiotrophoblastic giant cells. Some cases of dysgerminomas associated with elevated hCG and not containing syncytiotrophoblast cells have displayed cytoplasmic hCG in dysgerminoma cells (9). Overexpression of p53 is often seen in dysgerminomas (11). Most dysgerminomas are not diploid, and DNA ploidy has not been a useful prognostic indicator (12,13).

Thorough sectioning of the neoplasm is essential to exclude the presence of other malignant germ cell tumor components that can drastically affect therapy and prognosis. Dysgerminoma is a malignant tumor that metastasizes first to abdominal lymph nodes. Because of its sensitivity to chemotherapy and radiotherapy, survival rates are high.

YOLK SAC TUMOR

Yolk sac tumor (endodermal sinus tumor) is the second most common ovarian germ cell tumor, accounting for 22% of ovarian germ cell tumors studied at the Armed Forces Institute of Pathology (AFIP) (3). It occurs mainly in adolescent and young adult women. Reported age ranges are from 14 to 45 years, with the median age in the late teens (14–16). Most patients are younger than 30 years of age. The most frequent presenting symptom is abdominal pain, which may be accompanied by an abdominal or pelvic mass and abdominal enlargement (3,14–16). Most patients do not display endocrine symptoms, but a few cases associated with hirsutism have been described (17,18). Yolk sac tumor is a very rapidly growing tumor; almost half of patients have a duration of symptoms of 1 week or less (3), and some have had normal pelvic examinations only 4 weeks before discovery of their tumors (14).

Ovarian yolk sac tumors are typically large, unilateral neoplasms, although metastasis to the opposite ovary may occur. On gross examination, the tumor is round, oval, or lobulated, with a smooth external surface, unless rupture or invasion into surrounding structures has occurred. On cut section, these neoplasms are tan or gray, with abundant hemorrhage and necrosis (Figure 6.3). They are partially solid, but they contain cysts

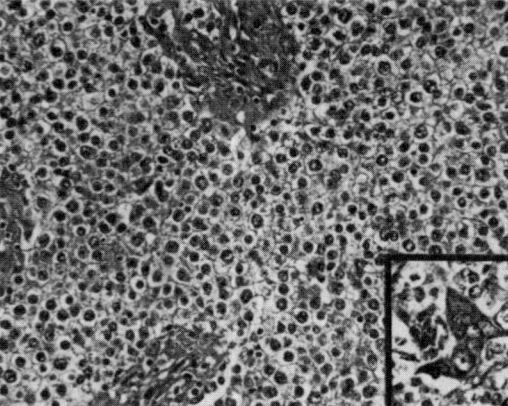

FIG. 6.2. Dysgerminoma displaying cells with large nuclei, clear cytoplasm, and prominent cell borders. Fibrous trabeculae containing lymphocytes are present. Inset shows syncytiotrophoblastic giant cell (hematoxylin and eosin stain, ×250).

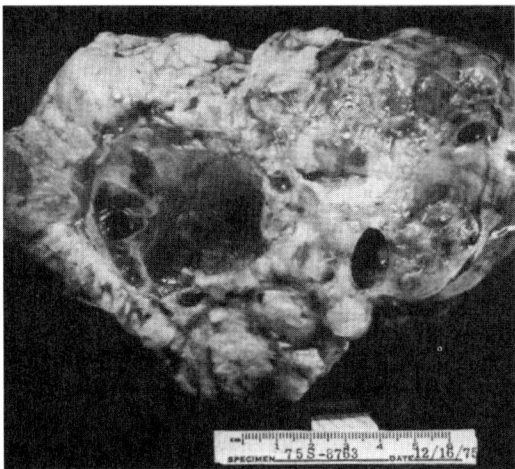

FIG. 6.3. Yolk sac tumor composed of fleshy and myxoid tissue with scattered cysts as well as hemorrhage and necrosis.

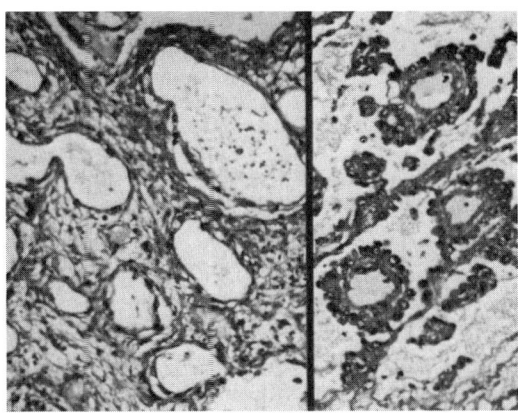

FIG. 6.5. Yolk sac tumor. The polyvesicular vitelline pattern *(left)* is characterized by cysts lined by flattened epithelium and sometimes containing central constrictions. Perivascular formations (Schiller-Duvall bodies, *right*) have a central blood vessel surrounded by connective tissue and cuboidal cells (hematoxylin and eosin stain, ×160).

that vary in size from a few millimeters to several centimeters in diameter. The cut surface appears mucoid, slimy, or gelatinous.

Yolk sac tumors may display a large variety of histologic patterns (3,14,18–25). The most common is the reticular pattern (Figure 6.4), in which the tumor displays a loose network of spaces lined by flattened or cuboidal cells with eosinophilic cytoplasm, indistinct cell borders, and round to oval, hyperchromatic nuclei.

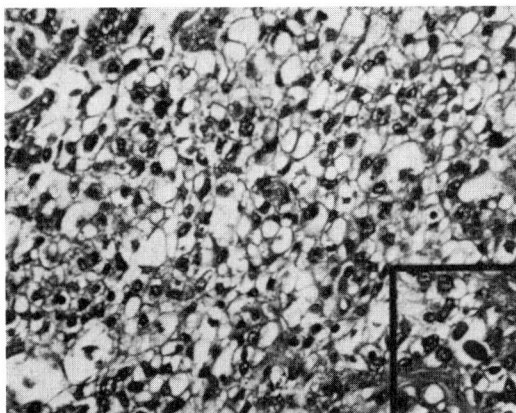

FIG. 6.4. Yolk sac tumor with reticular pattern. There is a loose network of spaces lined by cuboidal cells. Hyaline globules are present in the inset (hematoxylin and eosin stain, ×250).

The festoon (pseudopapillary) pattern contains Schiller-Duvall bodies; when present, they are diagnostic of yolk sac tumor. A central capillary is surrounded by connective tissue and a layer of cuboidal to columnar cells with eosinophilic cytoplasm and relatively large nuclei that contain prominent eosinophilic nucleoli (Figure 6.5). This vascular structure is surrounded by a space lined by flattened cells. The polyvesicular vitelline pattern is characterized by a dense spindle cell stroma that contains cysts lined by mucinous columnar, cuboidal, or flattened epithelium, often with a central constriction (Figure 6.5). The polyvesicular vitelline pattern is almost always admixed with other yolk sac tumor patterns (19). The solid pattern of yolk sac tumors contains cells with eosinophilic cytoplasm, hyperchromatic nuclei, and, sometimes, prominent nucleoli. Eosinophilic hyaline extracellular material with the immunohistochemical (laminin-positive, type IV collagen-positive) and ultrastructural characteristics of basement membrane characterize parietal yolk sac tumors (20,21). Enteric yolk sac tumor consists of glands lined by mucinous epithelium that sometimes contains goblet or Paneth cells (21,22,24). Hepatoid yolk sac tumors (18) display large, polygonal epithelial cells with prominent cell borders, abundant eosinophilic cytoplasm, and round, central nuclei with prominent nucleoli. This type of yolk sac tumor displays histologic, immunohistochemical, and ultrastructural similarities to hepatocellular carcinoma. Endometrioid-like yolk sac tumor (23) is characterized by glands lined by columnar cells, often with subnuclear or supranuclear vacuoles and eosinophilic luminal material. A variant of yolk sac tumor resembling the mesenchyme of the primitive yolk sac has been described (25). It may contain striated muscle and cartilage and may be the source of some sarcomas arising from germ cell tumors. Recently, the histologic features of late recurrences of germ cell tumors after initial response to cisplatin-based chemotherapy have been studied (26). Unusual variants of yolk sac tumor, including clear cell, glandular, hepatoid, parietal, and pleomorphic tumors appear to be especially common in patients with late recurrences of germ cell tumors after chemotherapy.

All histologic patterns of yolk sac tumor may contain, in various numbers, intracellular and extracellular, round, eosinophilic, hyaline globules that are PAS-positive and diastase resistant. These bodies are helpful when other features of yolk sac tumor are present, but they also occur in many other neoplasms and are not by themselves diagnostic of yolk sac tumor. Some globules contain α-fetoprotein (AFP), but many do not. AFP positivity is usually characterized by granular cytoplasmic staining and is sometimes limited to a few cells. Laminin may stain eosinophilic, basement membrane-like material between cells (21). Yolk sac tumors stain positively for cytokeratin but are generally negative for epithelial membrane antigen. Tumors with enteric differentiation may display apical cytoplasmic staining for carcinoembryonic antigen.

Most patients with an ovarian yolk sac tumor have significantly elevated serum levels of AFP, which is useful in monitoring results of therapy and the possibility of recurrence or metastases. However, normal serum levels of AFP do not exclude the possibility of the disease; the parietal variant of yolk sac tumor does not produce AFP. Chemotherapy has induced alteration of an AFP-producing yolk sac tumor to an AFP-negative, widely metastatic, recurrent yolk sac tumor with parietal differentiation (20).

Yolk sac tumors are rapidly growing neoplasms that metastasize early via lymphatics to regional lymph nodes and hematogenously to the lungs, liver, and other organs. Extensive intraabdominal disease is often present when the tumor is discovered. The fact that most patients with apparent stage Ia neoplasms died before modern combination chemotherapy became available indicates that occult metastases are often present (3). The most common sites of metastases at autopsy are the liver, abdominal and pelvic peritoneum, lymph nodes, bowel, and lungs (3). The prognosis of this neoplasm has improved markedly with the advent of cisplatin-based chemotherapy.

EMBRYONAL CARCINOMA

Embryonal carcinoma is a rare ovarian germ cell tumor, in contrast to its relatively high incidence among testicular tumors (3,27). Fourteen cases of ovarian embryonal carcinoma were seen during a 30-year time span at the AFIP (27). These tumors occurred in girls and young women between the ages of 4 and 28 years; seven were prepubertal. Eighty percent of the patients presented with an abdominal mass. Abdominal pain was the next most common symptom, occurring in about half of the patients. Sixty percent exhibited precocious pseudopuberty. For the majority of patients, the duration of symptoms was about 3 weeks.

On gross examination, these tumors are large and predominantly solid, with color that varies from tan to yellow-white. Areas of hemorrhage and necrosis are typically present. Microscopically, embryonal carcinoma is characterized by sheets of large, primitive, epithelial-appearing cells. Clefts, gland-like areas, and papillary structures may be present. Cells are large and round, with amphophilic to eosinophilic cytoplasm. Cell borders are not well visualized. Nuclei are large and irregular, with vesicular chromatin and a tendency to overlap other nuclei in paraffin sections. One or two very large eosinophilic nucleoli are present. Numerous mitoses, including abnormal forms, are present. Necrosis is frequently present.

Syncytiotrophoblastic giant cells are commonly seen in ovarian embryonal carcinoma, and they stain positively for hCG. Some tumors contain intracellular and extracellular hyaline globules similar to those associated with yolk sac tumors. Both hyaline globules and mononuclear tumor cells may stain positively for AFP. These findings may indicate yolk sac differentiation within the tumor.

The diagnosis of embryonal carcinoma is usually straightforward, but it must be distinguished from other germ cell tumors. Embryonal carcinoma lacks the compartmentalized architecture of dysgerminomas. The fibrous septa that contain lymphocytes and that separate nests of tumor cells in dysgerminoma are not seen in embryonal carcinoma. Dysgerminoma also has better defined cell borders and less nuclear pleomorphism. Cytokeratin stains are negative or only focally positive in dysgerminomas and diffusely positive in embryonal carcinoma. Embryonal carcinoma can also be distinguished histologically from yolk sac tumor; it does not display the reticular, festoon, or vitelline patterns of yolk sac tumors. The nuclei of yolk sac tumors are smaller and do not tend to overlap. Syncytiotrophoblastic cells, which stain positively for hCG, are frequently present in embryonal carcinoma. However, they are scattered, and the tumor does not display the biphasic pattern of choriocarcinoma. Embryonal carcinoma also stains positively for placental-like alkaline phosphatase. It is generally negative for epithelial membrane antigen (10). The clinical behavior of embryonal carcinoma is similar to that of yolk sac tumor.

POLYEMBRYOMA

Polyembryoma is a very rare malignant ovarian tumor (2,3). In the few cases reported, the embryoid bodies have frequently coexisted with other germ cell tumor types, often teratoma (28–30). These neoplasms occur in children and young adults; the oldest reported patient was 38 years old (28). Symptoms include isosexual precocious pseudopuberty (29), increasing abdominal girth, and abnormal bleeding (30).

Polyembryomas, like most other ovarian germ cell tumors, are unilateral neoplasms. Dimensions of up to 34 cm have been reported (28). They are gray-white on cross section and may display small, barely visible, cystic areas (28). Hemorrhage and necrosis may be present. Microscopically, embryoid bodies are present in various stages of differentiation, and atypical forms may be present (30). Well-developed embryoid bodies display a yolk sac and an amnionic cavity that are separated by an embryonic disk composed of ectoderm (tall, columnar cells), mesoderm, and endoderm (cuboidal cells). Cells lining the yolk sac have been shown to contain AFP (29). The embryoid body may be partially or completely surrounded by primitive extraembryonic mesenchyme. Atypical embryoid bodies may have more than one yolk sac or amnionic cavity and may exhibit discrepancies of size and shape (30). Syncytiotrophoblastic giant cells may be present in the surrounding tumor tissue and produce hCG. Teratoma, mature or immature, is often present (28,29). Polyembryomas behave like other primitive malignant germ cell tumors.

CHORIOCARCINOMA

Pure, primary, nongestational choriocarcinoma is extremely rare. Most cases cited in the literature represent isolated reports (31–36). Like other malignant germ cell neoplasms, nongestational ovarian choriocarcinoma occurs in girls, adolescents, and young adult women. Prepubertal girls may present with isosexual precocious pseudopuberty or abdominal discomfort. After puberty, menorrhagia, metrorrhagia, and signs suggesting ectopic gestation are present.

Nongestational choriocarcinoma of the ovary is a unilateral neoplasm, but it may metastasize to the opposite ovary. Most examples have been large, gray-white masses with abundant hemorrhage and necrosis. Microscopically, cytotrophoblast and/or intermediate trophoblast cells are admixed with syncytiotrophoblast cells (Figure 6.6). Syncytiotrophoblastic giant cells have abundant eosinophilic or amphophilic cytoplasm that contains several relatively small, dark, hyperchromatic nuclei. Cytotrophoblastic and intermediate trophoblast cells are round and often have fairly well-defined cell borders and clear

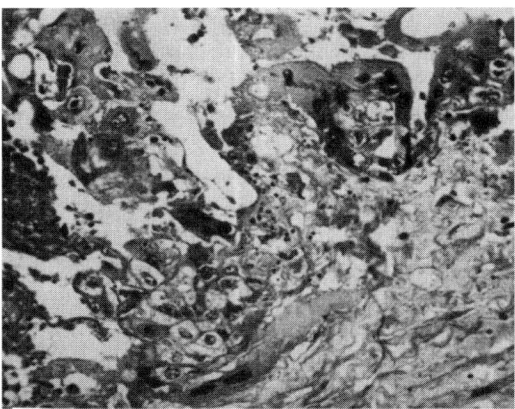

FIG. 6.6. Choriocarcinoma displaying admixture of syncytiotrophoblast and cytotrophoblast (hematoxylin and eosin stain, ×250).

or lightly eosinophilic, vacuolated cytoplasm. Nuclei are centrally located and hyperchromatic, with irregular nuclear membranes. A biphasic pattern is usually present in which aggregates of cytotrophoblast are surrounded by larger syncytiotrophoblastic giant cells in a manner that produces a plexiform pattern. Substantial hemorrhage and necrosis are seen, and tumor cells may line vascular spaces. Cytotrophoblast is the most primitive element of the tumor. It does not produce hCG. Syncytiotrophoblast is formed from cytotrophoblast and produces hCG. Intermediate trophoblast stains for human placental lactogen. All types of trophoblast are cytokeratin positive. Choriocarcinoma may also stain for placental-like alkaline phosphatase, epithelial membrane antigen, and carcinoembryonic antigen (10).

Nongestational ovarian choriocarcinoma occurs more often as a component of malignant mixed germ cell tumors than in pure form, but even then it is among the least common of all germ cell tumor types (37,38). Nongestational ovarian choriocarcinoma must be distinguished from gestational choriocarcinoma because the former has a worse prognosis and requires more aggressive, multiagent chemotherapy (36). Occurrence before menarche and coexistence with other malignant germ cell tumor types provide evidence that an ovarian choriocarcinoma is nongestational in origin (36).

TERATOMAS

Teratomas, as defined in the WHO classification of ovarian tumors (1), are neoplasms composed of tissue that is derived from two or three embryonic layers. They are subclassified according to whether the tumor elements are immature, mature, or monodermal and highly specialized.

Immature Teratomas

Immature teratomas are uncommon. They represent 3% of all ovarian teratomas (2). However, pure immature teratoma is the third most common form of malignant ovarian germ cell tumor. It represented 15% of these tumors in one study done at the AFIP (37). Immature teratoma can also occur as part of a mixed malignant germ cell tumor in the ovary (37). The age of patients with ovarian immature teratomas ranges from 14 to 40 years, with a median age of 19 years (39). The young age of these patients contrasts with the higher mean age of patients with mature teratomas. Most patients present with a pelvic or abdominal mass or with pain (39–41).

Virtually all immature ovarian teratomas are unilateral, although they may metastasize to the opposite ovary and can be associated with a synchronous or metachronous mature teratoma in the opposite ovary (39,40). These tumors are large, round or oval masses whose external surfaces are usually smooth and glistening. On cut section, they are predominantly solid but may contain scattered cystic areas (Figure 6.7). The cut surface is soft and fleshy or encephaloid in appearance, and areas of hemorrhage and necrosis are common.

Microscopically, these tumors contain a variety of mature and immature tissue elements (Figure 6.8). There is a correlation between prognosis and the degree of immaturity (39,40); the immature elements are often neural. The grading system devised by Norris and colleaues (39) is currently used. Grade 1 neoplasms display some immaturity, but immature neural tissue does not exceed in aggregate the area of one low-power field (×40) in any slide. Grade 2 teratomas display more immaturity, but immature neural tissue occupies no more than an area equal to three

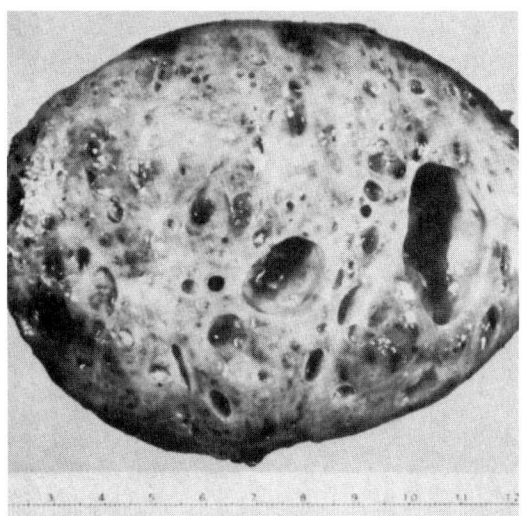

FIG. 6.7. Immature teratoma mainly composed of solid, fleshy tissue but also containing cysts of various sizes.

low-power fields in any slide. Immaturity is prominent in grade 3 neoplasms, with immature neural tissue occupying an area greater than three low-power fields in at least one slide. Mature tissue elements are easily identified in grade 1 lesions, are present to a lesser extent in grade 2 neoplasms, and may be absent altogether in grade 3 immature teratomas (36). The amount of mitotic

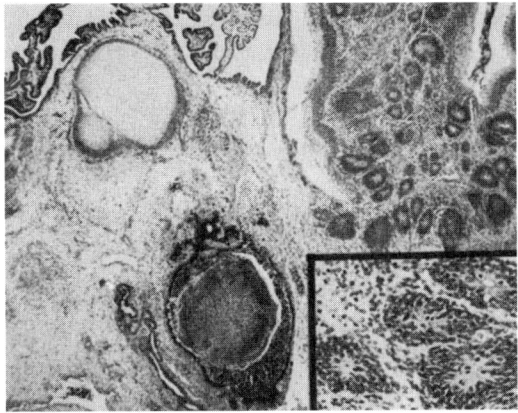

FIG. 6.8. Immature teratoma with immature neural tissue forming rosettes (right top and inset). Cartilage and choroid plexus-like structures (top left) are also present (hematoxylin and eosin stain, ×40; inset ×160).

activity and immature neural tissue with rosettes also increases with increasing grade. It is clinically important to distinguish grade 1 tumors from higher-grade neoplasms, because the latter require chemotherapy even in patients with stage I disease. Although some authors (42) have proposed a two-grade system that combines grades 2 and 3 into one category, the three-grade system is generally preferred (2). Dermoid cysts containing only microscopic foci of immature neural tissue should not be classified as immature teratomas (43).

Immature teratomas invade adjacent adnexal structures and seed the peritoneal surfaces. They may metastasize to retroperitoneal and paraaortic lymph nodes and to more distant sites (39). A good correlation is seen between the degree of immaturity (grade) of the ovarian tumor and prognosis. However, in patients whose neoplasm has disseminated beyond the ovary, the grade of the tumor metastases is more important in predicting survival and determining treatment (39). Occasionally, patients have implants that contain only mature tissue; these implants should be well sampled to exclude the possibility of small areas of immature tissue. Many of the mature implants associated with immature teratomas are composed of mature glial tissue (gliomatosis peritonei) (44,45), but mature epithelial elements or cartilage may also be present (2). Rare cases have been reported with transformation of mature glial implants into lesions resembling glioblastoma multiforme (46–48). Mature implants have been associated with endometriosis in some cases (49,50).

The prognosis of immature teratoma has improved markedly with cisplatin-based chemotherapy. We have, however, seen a case of grade 3 immature teratoma treated with combination chemotherapy that recurred as a primitive neuroectodermal tumor.

Mature Teratomas

Mature (grade 0) solid teratomas are rare. The few cases that have been reported have all occurred in young women (51). Thorough sampling of solid teratomas is essential to identify small foci of immature elements that would change the tumor classification to immature teratoma (2) and may affect treatment and prognosis.

Mature cystic teratoma is the most common type of ovarian teratoma and the most common ovarian germ cell tumor. It has a wide age distribution, ranging from young girls to elderly women; however, most mature cystic teratomas occur in women of reproductive age (2,52,53). Many mature cystic teratomas are asymptomatic. They may be found during routine physical examination, radiographic studies, or operations for other conditions. Patients may also present with symptoms of ovarian enlargement, including pain or a mass.

Most mature cystic teratomas are unilateral, but 15% to 20% are bilateral (52,54). On gross examination, these neoplasms are round or oval, with smooth, glistening capsules. The cut section reveals one or more cystic cavities that are usually filled with malodorous, greasy, yellow material that is liquid at body temperature but solid at room temperature. Hair and teeth may be present in the cysts (Figure 6.9). A protuberance on the inner wall of the cyst (Rokitansky's

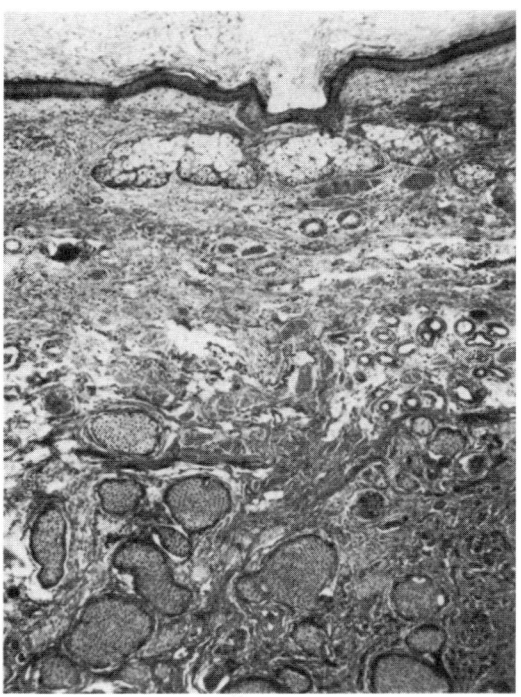

FIG. 6.10. Mature cystic teratoma lined by squamous epithelium with adnexal structures. An insular carcinoid tumor (bottom half of picture) has nests of uniform cells with round nuclei (hematoxylin and eosin stain, ×63).

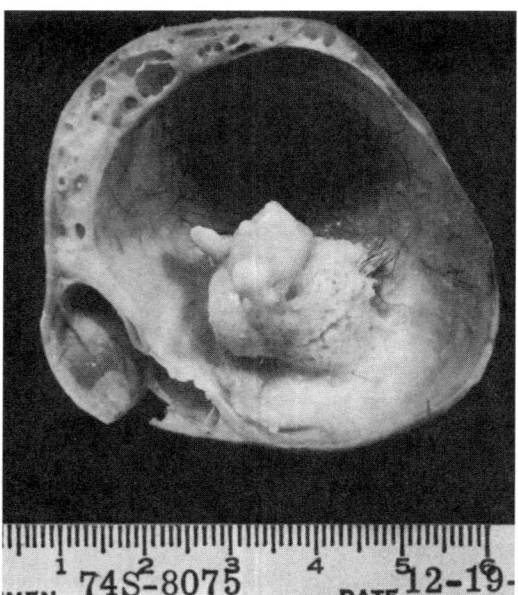

FIG. 6.9. Mature cystic teratoma. The cyst contains hair; teeth protrude from Rokitansky's tubercle.

protuberance) contains a wider variety of tissue types than the surrounding cyst wall and should be thoroughly sectioned. The cystic portion of the neoplasm is usually lined by stratified squamous epithelium with underlying skin adnexal structures (Figure 6.10). Other tissues likely to be identified in Rokitansky's protuberance include fat, cartilage, bone, glia, muscle, respiratory and gastrointestinal epithelium, and thyroid. Virtually any tissue found in the body may occur in mature cystic teratomas.

Complications of mature cystic teratomas include torsion, rupture, infection, hemolytic anemia, benign implants of mature glia in the peritoneal cavity (gliomatosis peritonei), and malignant transformation (44,45,52–55). Malignant transformation occurs in about 2% of mature cystic teratomas (54,55). Most patients with malignant transformation of mature cystic teratoma are postmenopausal. Any tissue component can become malignant, but squamous carcinoma is the most frequent malignancy to develop in mature cystic teratomas (55–58). Other malignancies reported rarely in mature cystic teratomas include adenocarcinoma and adenosquamous carcinoma, Paget disease, various sarcomas, malignant melanoma, lymphoma, and basal cell carcinoma (59–66). The malignant element may be apparent only on microscopic examination or may exist as a nodule or mass grossly identifiable in the cyst wall. Malignancies that arise in mature cystic teratomas spread by direct extension and peritoneal implantation; lymphatic and hematogenous spread is less common (55,58). The prognosis is poor, although patients in whom the malignant element is squamous carcinoma or adenocarcinoma that has no vascular invasion and is limited to a cystic teratoma that is removed without tumor rupture have a better prognosis than patients with sarcoma (55).

Monodermal Teratomas

Struma Ovarii

Struma ovarii represents a one-sided development of teratoma. Thyroid tissue is relatively common in mature cystic teratomas, but the term "struma ovarii" is reserved for tumors composed predominantly or entirely of thyroid tissue. The age range and clinical presentation are usually similar to those of mature cystic teratoma, although some patients have had symptoms suggesting thyrotoxicosis (67). On gross examination, the tumors usually measure less than 10 cm in diameter. The capsule is most often intact, and the tumor may be partially cystic if other teratomatous elements are present (67). Thyroid tissue is grossly identifiable as reddish-tan tissue with glistening colloid. Microscopically, thyroid follicles vary in size and contain variable amounts of colloid. Both the cells lining the thyroid follicles and the colloid stain for thyroglobulin; this stain may be useful if the struma has an unusual histologic appearance. In most cases, the appearance is that of mature thyroid tissue, but some cases have patterns mimicking oxyphil or clear cell carcinoma, or Sertoli or granulosa cell tumors (68). Features of hyperplasia may occur. Rare examples of papillary or follicular carcinoma arising in struma ovarii have been reported (67,69). However, most histologically malignant thyroid lesions in struma ovarii are not associated with a malignant clinical course, even in the presence of extraovarian disease (69). Features that may be associated with increased likelihood of recurrent disease include tumor size, adhesions, ascites, and a solid pattern (70). In "benign strumosis" (71,72), benign thyroid tissue may spread to the abdominal cavity.

Carcinoid Tumors

Ovarian carcinoid tumors may be primary or metastatic. Primary neoplasms represent variants of monodermal teratomas and are designated as insular, trabecular, strumal, or goblet cell (mucinous) types (1).

The most common primary ovarian carcinoid tumor is insular in type. It usually occurs in perimenopausal or postmenopausal women, and one third of patients have clinical manifestations of the carcinoid syndrome (73). Liver metastases are not necessary for the occurrence of the carcinoid syndrome, because the ovarian vein bypasses the portal circulation and enters the systemic circulation directly. Primary insular carcinoid tumor of the ovary is a unilateral neoplasm, although the contralateral ovary may contain a mature cystic teratoma. On gross examination, the carcinoid tumor may be part of a mature cystic teratoma, or it may exist as a solid, gray to yellow, firm nodule. Microscopically, the tumor resembles the midgut carcinoid tumor and is characterized by nests of cells with abundant cytoplasm and round to oval, uniform nuclei with few mitoses (Figure 6.11). An acinar pattern is sometimes present. Neuroendocrine granules are evident on argentaffin or argyrophil stains, immunohistochemical stains (neuron-specific enolase, synaptophysin, and chromogranin), and electron micrographs. A direct and significant relationship exists between tumor size and the presence of the carcinoid syndrome (73). Tumors with an acinar pattern are more likely to be associated with the carcinoid syndrome. Metastases are uncommon (73).

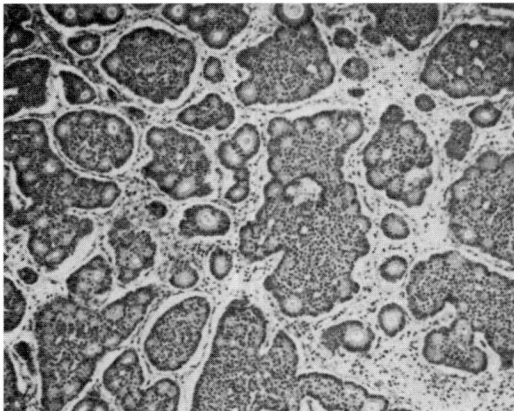

FIG. 6.11. Insular carcinoid tumor with acinar pattern. Cells are uniform, with small round nuclei (hematoxylin and eosin stain, ×63).

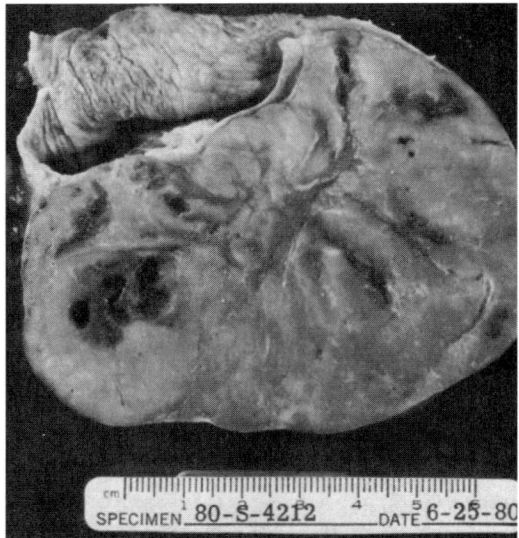

FIG. 6.12. Strumal carcinoid. Areas of glistening colloid are apparent in the partially cystic, tan neoplasm.

Primary trabecular carcinoid tumors of the ovary are less common than primary insular carcinoid tumors. Most patients are postmenopausal. They usually present with symptoms of an ovarian mass or are asymptomatic (74,75). Most primary trabecular carcinoid tumors occur in mature cystic teratomas, but rare examples of pure ovarian trabecular carcinoid tumors have been reported (74,75). Almost all trabecular carcinoid tumors are unilateral, but the opposite ovary may contain mature cystic teratoma. On gross examination, the carcinoid tumor is firm, gritty, and tan to yellow. Microscopically, trabecular carcinoid tumors display ribbons of cells separated by fibrous stroma. The cells contain eosinophilic cytoplasm and oval, uniform nuclei with few mitoses. Neurosecretory granules are present. Primary trabecular carcinoid tumor of the ovary has a favorable prognosis; extraovarian spread has been rare (74).

Struma ovarii and carcinoid ("strumal carcinoid") tumors represent monodermal teratomas composed of thyroid follicles that are intimately associated with ribbons and islands of carcinoid tumor (1). Most strumal carcinoid tumors occur in association with other teratomatous elements. The age incidence in one large series ranged from 21 to 77 years (76). Strumal carcinoid tumor is not associated with the carcinoid syndrome. It is a unilateral neoplasm, but 10% are associated with mature cystic teratoma in the opposite ovary (76). Grossly, the tumor may occur as part of a mature cystic teratoma or in pure form (Figure 6.12). Microscopically, colloid-containing thyroid follicles are intimately admixed with carcinoid tumor, which may have both trabecular and insular areas (Figure 6.13). Neurosecretory

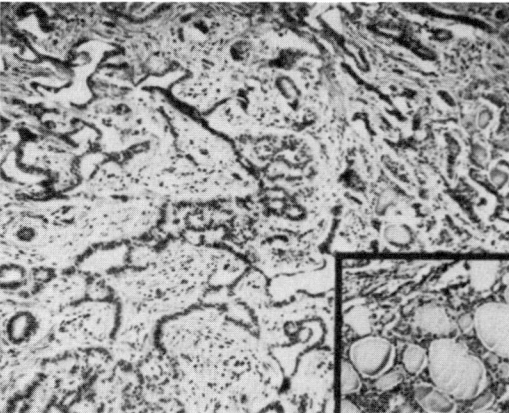

FIG. 6.13. Strumal carcinoid. Trabecular carcinoid displays anastomosing ribbons of uniform cuboidal cells. Admixed thyroid follicles are present *(right center* and *inset)* (hematoxylin and eosin stain, ×100).

granules are present in the carcinoid tumor but may also occur in cells around the follicles, which has led some authors to postulate that these neoplasms represent pure carcinoid tumors (77–79). However, immunohistochemical demonstration of thyroglobulin (80,81) and thyroxine (82) has proved the existence of a thyroid component. Strumal carcinoid tumors generally behave in a benign manner, but rare patients have had extraovarian disease (76,83) and one patient died of the disease (76).

Primary mucinous carcinoid tumors of the ovary, which are analogous to mucin-producing appendiceal carcinoid tumors (84), are rarely seen. They display an organoid pattern, with nests of cells whose round to oval nuclei may show more variation in nuclear size and more mitoses than are normally seen in insular carcinoid tumors. Variable numbers of goblet cells contain mucin, while other cells contain neurosecretory granules; some cells may contain both mucin and neurosecretory granules. These tumors behave in a more malignant manner than other types of primary ovarian carcinoid. They spread via lymphatic channels, and metastases may be present at the time of diagnosis (84).

Carcinoid tumors of the ovary may be metastatic (usually from an intestinal primary neoplasm). The importance of distinguishing primary from metastatic carcinoid tumors of the ovary is underscored by the fact that most patients with carcinoid tumors metastatic to the ovaries die within 4 years after ovarian tumor diagnosis, whereas patients with primary carcinoid tumors of the ovary have a favorable prognosis (85). Carcinoid tumors metastatic to the ovary are typically bilateral, multinodular, and not associated with teratomas. Microscopic features are similar to those of primary ovarian carcinoid tumors.

Other Teratomas

Neuroectodermal tumors of the ovary are considered variants of monodermal teratoma (1). They resemble tumors of the central nervous system. Differentiated neoplasms resemble ependymomas, are usually not associated with other teratomatous elements, and often behave in an indolent manner (86,87). Primitive tumors (86,88) are composed of small round blue cells with necrosis and numerous mitoses; rosettes, pseudorosettes and structures resembling primitive neural tubes may be seen. These neoplasms may have features of neuroblastoma, medulloepithelioma, ependymoblastoma, or medulloblastoma. They may be associated with other teratomatous elements, but they do not display the variety of neural tissue types or the intermingling with other teratomatous elements seen in immature teratoma. A rare case has arisen in a mature cystic teratoma (89). Anaplastic neuroectodermal tumors resemble glioblastoma multiforme (86). The prognosis is grave for patients with extraovarian involvement by primitive or anaplastic neuroectodermal tumors. They do not respond to cisplatin-based germ cell tumor chemotherapy. Treatment is surgical excision and radiation and chemotherapy designed for similar neoplasms occurring in other locations of the body.

Other monodermal teratomas encountered more rarely include sebaceous tumors, retinal anlage tumors, and pituitary neoplasms. These neoplasms are reviewed in a more comprehensive discussion of ovarian germ cell tumors (2).

MALIGNANT MIXED GERM CELL TUMORS

Malignant mixed germ cell tumors contain two or more different types of germ cell neoplasm, either intimately admixed or as separate foci within the tumor. Malignant mixed germ cell tumors are much less common in the ovary than in the testis, and they accounted for only 8% of malignant ovarian germ cell tumors accessioned at the AFIP over a period of 30 years (37). Patients in that series ranged from 5 to 33 years of age, and more than one third were prepubertal. Most patients had a palpable abdominal or pelvic mass, and more than half presented with lower abdominal pain. Some prepubertal patients had isosexual precocious pseudopuberty, and the tumors caused positive pregnancy tests in several patients. The average duration of symptoms before diagnosis was 4 weeks.

Malignant mixed germ cell tumors are usually large, unilateral neoplasms, but the gross appearance on cut surface depends on the particular types of germ cell tumor present. Microscopically, various combinations of dysgerminoma, yolk sac tumor, embryonal carcinoma, choriocarcinoma, and immature teratoma are present. The most common germ cell element in the AFIP series was dysgerminoma (80%), followed by yolk sac tumor (70%), teratoma (53%), choriocarcinoma (20%), and embryonal carcinoma (13%) (37). The most frequent combination reported has been dysgerminoma and yolk sac tumor (37,38). Syncytiotrophoblast may occur either as a component of choriocarcinoma or as isolated cells in other germ cell tumor types. The diagnosis and prognosis of malignant mixed germ cell tumors depend on adequate tumor sampling in order to reveal small foci of different types of germ cell neoplasms, which may alter therapy and prognosis. Smaller tumors have been associated with a better prognosis, as have tumors in which less than one third of the neoplasm consisted of endodermal sinus tumor, choriocarcinoma, or grade 3 immature teratoma (37). However, with modern chemotherapy, the International Federation of Gynecology and Obstetrics (FIGO) stage alone may be the most important prognostic factor (38).

Gonadoblastoma

Gonadoblastoma, a rare tumor with admixed sex cord elements and germ cells, was first described by Scully in 1953 (90). This tumor occurs in young patients, most frequently in the second decade of life. Eighty percent of patients are phenotypic females who are often virilized, and 20% are phenotypic males with cryptorchidism, hypospadias, and female internal secondary sex organs (91). Eighty-nine percent are sex-chromatin negative, and the most common karyotypes are 46,XY and 45,XO/46,XY (mosaic) (91). Patients usually present with primary amenorrhea, virilization, or developmental abnormalities of the genitalia; they may also present with gonadal tumors. Rare gonadoblastomas occur in normal ovaries (92).

The gross appearance of gonadoblastomas depends on the degree of hyalinization, calcification, and overgrowth by malignant germ cell

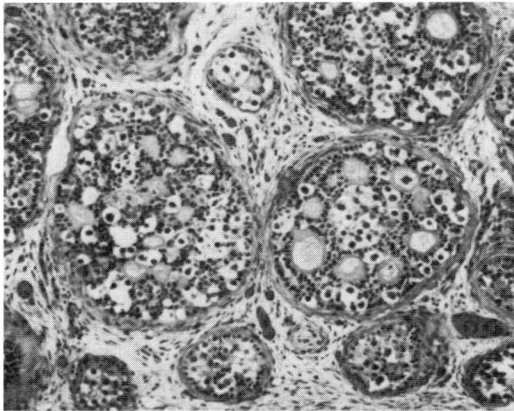

FIG. 6.14. Gonadoblastoma with tumor nests containing large germ cells, smaller sex cord cells, and rounded masses of hyaline material (hematoxylin and eosin stain, ×160).

tumors. Typically, gonadoblastomas are small, yellow-brown or gray, partially calcified tumors that range in size from microscopic to several centimeters (91). They are often bilateral. Microscopically, gonadoblastomas are characterized by cellular nests surrounded by connective tissue stroma (Figure 6.14). The nests of cells contain both large, mitotically active germ cells (93) with pale cytoplasm and large, round nuclei and smaller, mitotically inactive, epithelial-like cells with oval, dark nuclei that sometimes possess nuclear grooves (91). These smaller cells resemble immature Sertoli and granulosa cells and are seen at the periphery of the cell nests. They surround the germ cells as well as eosinophilic, hyaline, PAS-positive material, the latter forming structures resembling Call-Exner bodies (91). Immunohistochemical and electron-microscopic evidence suggests Sertoli cell derivation (94). Luteinized or Leydig cells may be present in the connective tissue stroma (91). The cell nests may undergo progressive hyalinization and calcification.

Half of gonadoblastomas are associated with dysgerminomas, and another 10% have been associated with other malignant germ cell tumors, including embryonal carcinoma, yolk sac tumor, teratoma, and choriocarcinoma (90,91,95). Scully regards gonadoblastoma as an *in situ* germ cell tumor (1).

Other Mixed Germ Cell-Sex Cord-Stromal Tumors

Few cases of mixed germ cell-sex cord-stromal tumors other than gonadoblastoma have been reported. They occur most often in young, phenotypically normal female children with a 46,XX karyotype (96–100). Most patients have symptoms of an abdominal mass, which may undergo torsion. Isosexual precocious pseudopuberty has occurred rarely (96). Mixed germ cell-sex cord-stromal tumors are large and almost always unilateral neoplasms associated with normal contralateral ovaries, although one case has been bilateral (101). They are composed of an intimate admixture of germ cells and smaller sex cord-stromal elements (primitive Sertoli and granulosa cells) and sometimes luteinized cells. The tumor cells may be arranged in long trabeculae, tubules without lumina, or large, structureless masses (98). Both germ cell and sex cord components may display mitotic activity. These tumors are distinguished microscopically from gonadoblastoma by the lack of a nesting pattern, hyalinization, and calcification. In contrast to gonadoblastoma, most mixed germ cell-sex cord-stromal tumors are not associated with malignant germ cell neoplasms, and most patients have a benign clinical course after excision (2), although rare tumors have behaved aggressively (97).

REFERENCES

1. Scully RE, Sobin LN. Histological typing of ovarian tumors. In: *World Health Organization International Classification of Tumors,* 2nd ed. Berlin: Springer-Verlag, 1999;28–36.
2. Scully RE, Young RH, Clement PB. Tumors of the ovary, maldeveloped gonads, fallopian tube, and broad ligament. In: *Atlas of Tumor Pathology,* 3rd ser., fascicle 23. Washington, DC: Armed Forces Institute of Pathology, 1998:239–312.
3. Kurman RJ, Norris HJ. Malignant germ cell tumors of the ovary. *Hum Pathol* 1977;8:551–564.
4. Talerman A, Huyzinga WT, Kuipers T. Dysgerminoma: clinicopathologic study of 22 cases. *Obstet Gynecol* 1973;41:137–147.
5. Burkons DM, Hart WR. Ovarian germinomas (dysgerminomas). *Obstet Gynecol* 1978;51:221–224.
6. Asadourian LA, Taylor HB. Dysgerminoma: an analysis of 105 cases. *Obstet Gynecol* 1969;33:370–379.
7. Zaloudek CJ, Tavassoli FA, Norris HJ. Dysgerminoma with syncytiotrophoblastic giant cells: a histologically and clinically distinctive subtype of dysgerminoma. *Am J Surg Pathol* 1981;5: 361–367.
8. Stewart CJ, Farquharson MA, Foulis AK. Characterization of the inflammatory infiltrate in ovarian dysgerminoma: an immunocytochemical study. *Histopathology* 1992;20:491–497.
9. Mullin TJ, Lankerani MR. Ovarian dysgerminoma: immunochemical localization of human chorionic gonadotropin in the germinoma cell cytoplasm. *Obstet Gynecol* 1986;68 80S–83S.
10. Niehans GA, Manivel JC, Copland GT, et al. Immunohistochemistry of germ cell and trophoblastic neoplasms. *Cancer* 1988; 62:1113–1123.
11. Dietl J, Horny HP, Kaiserling E. Frequent overexpression of p53 in dysgerminoma of the ovary. *Gynecol Obstet Invest* 1994; 37:141–142.
12. Oud PS, Soeters RP, Pahlplatz MM, et al. DNA cytometry of pure dysgerminoma of the ovary. *Int J Gynecol Pathol* 1988;7: 258–267.
13. Palmquist MB, Webb MJ, Lieber MM, et al. DNA ploidy of ovarian dysgerminomas: correlation with clinical outcome. *Gynecol Oncol* 1992;44:281–283.
14. Kurman RJ, Norris HJ. Endodermal sinus tumor of the ovary: a clinical and pathologic analysis of 71 cases. *Cancer* 1976;38: 2404–2419.
15. Jimerson GK, Woodruff JD. Ovarian extraembryonic teratoma: 1. Endodermal sinus tumor. *Am J Obstet Gynecol* 1979;127: 73–79.
16. Langley FA, Govan AD, Anderson MC, et al. Yolk sac and allied tumors of the ovary. *Histopathology* 1981;5:389–401.
17. Stewart KR, Casey MJ, Gondos B. Endodermal sinus tumor of the ovary with virilization: light- and electron-microscopic study. *Am J Surg Pathol* 1981;5:385–391.
18. Prat J, Bhan AK, Dickersin GR, et al. Hepatoid yolk sac tumor of the ovary (endodermal sinus tumor with hepatoid differentiation). A light-microscopic, ultrastructural, and immunohistochemical study of seven cases. *Cancer* 1982;50:2355–2368.
19. Nogales FF Jr, Matilla A, Nogales-Ortiz F, Galera-Davidson HL. Yolk sac tumors with pure and mixed polyvesicular vitelline patterns. *Hum Pathol* 1978;9:553–566.
20. Damjanov L, Amenta PS, Zarghami F. Transformation of an AFP-positive yolk sac carcinoma into an AFP-negative neoplasm. *Cancer* 1984;53:1902–1907.
21. Ulbright TM, Roth LM, Brodhecker CA. Yolk sac differentiation in germ cell tumors: a morphologic study of 60 cases with emphasis on hepatic, enteric, and parietal yolk sac features. *Am J Surg Pathol* 1986;10:151–164.
22. Cohen MB, Mulchahey KM, Molnar JJ. Ovarian endodermal sinus tumor with intestinal differentiation. *Cancer* 1986;57:1580–1583.
23. Clement PB, Young RH, Scully RE. Endometrioid-like variant of ovarian yolk sac tumor: a clinicopathological analysis of eight cases. *Am J Surg Pathol* 1987;11:767–778.
24. Kim CR, Hsiu JG, Given FT. Intestinal variant of ovarian endodermal sinus tumor. *Gynecol Oncol* 1989;33:379–381.
25. Michael H, Ulbright TM, Brodhecker CA. The pluripotential nature of the mesenchyme-like component of yolk sac tumor. *Arch Pathol Lab Med* 1989;113:1115–1119.

26. Michael H, Lucia J, Foster RS, Ulbright TM. The pathology of late recurrence of testicular germ cell tumors. *Am J Surg Pathol* 2000;24:257–273.
27. Kurman RJ, Norris HJ. Embryonal carcinoma of the ovary: a clinicopathologic entity distinct from endodermal sinus tumor resembling embryonal carcinoma of the adult testis. *Cancer* 1976;38:2420–2433.
28. Simard LC. Polyembryonic embryoma of the ovary of parthenogenetic origin. *Cancer* 1957;10:215–223.
29. Takeda A, Ishizuka T, Goto T, et al. Polyembryoma of ovary producing alpha-fetoprotein and HCG: immunoperoxidase and electron microscopic study. *Cancer* 1982;49:1878–1889.
30. Beck JS, Fulmer HF, Lee ST. Solid malignant ovarian teratoma with "embryoid bodies" and trophoblastic differentiation. *J Pathol* 1969;99:67–73.
31. Oliver HM, Horne EO. Primary teratomatous chorionepithelioma of the ovary: report of a case. *N Engl J Med* 1948;239:14–16.
32. Marrubini G. Primary chorionepithelioma of the ovary: report of two cases. *Acta Obstet Gynecol* 1949;28:251–284.
33. Turner HB, Douglas WM, Gladding TC. Choriocarcinoma of the ovary. *Obstet Gynecol* 1964;24:918–920.
34. DeHaan QC. Nongestational choriocarcinoma of the ovary: report of a case. *Obstet Gynecol* 1965;26:708–709.
35. Jacobs AJ, Newland JR, Green RK. Pure choriocarcinoma of the ovary. *Obstet Gynecol Surv* 1982;37:603–609.
36. Vance RP, Geisinger KR. Pure nongestational choriocarcinoma of the ovary: report of a case. *Cancer* 1985;56:2321–2325.
37. Kurman RJ, Norris HJ. Malignant mixed germ cell tumors of the ovary: a clinical and pathologic analysis of 30 cases. *Obstet Gynecol* 1976;48:579–589.
38. Gershenson DM, Del Junco G, Copeland LJ, Rutledge FN. Mixed germ cell tumors of the ovary. *Obstet Gynecol* 1984;64:200–206.
39. Norris HJ, Zirkin HJ, Benson WL. Immature (malignant) teratoma of the ovary: a clinical and pathologic study of 58 cases. *Cancer* 1976;37:2359–2372.
40. Wisniewski M, Deppisch LM. Solid teratomas of the ovary. *Cancer* 1973;32:440–446.
41. Thurlbeck WM, Scully RE. Solid teratomas of the ovary: a clinicopathologic analysis of 9 cases. *Cancer* 1960;13:804–811.
42. O'Connor DM, Norris HJ. The influence of grade of the outcome of stage I ovarian immature (malignant) teratomas and the reproducibility of grading. *Int J Gynecol Pathol* 1994;13:283–289.
43. Yanai-Inbar I, Scully RE. Relation of ovarian dermoid cysts and immature teratomas: an analysis of 350 cases of immature teratoma and 10 cases of dermoid cyst with microscopic foci of immature tissue. *Int J Gynecol Pathol* 1987;6:203–212.
44. Robboy SJ, Scully RE. Ovarian teratoma with glial implants on the peritoneum: an analysis of 12 cases. *Hum Pathol* 1970;1:643–653.
45. Truong LD, Jurco S III, McGavran MH. Gliomatosis peritonei: report of two cases and review of literature. *Am J Surg Pathol* 1982;6:443–449.
46. Dadmanesh F, Miller DM, Swenerton KD, Clement PB. Gliomatosis peritonei with malignant transformation. *Mod Pathol* 1997;10:597–601.
47. Nielsen SN, Scheithauer BW, Gaffey TA. Gliomatosis peritonei. *Cancer* 1985;56:2499–2503.
48. Shefren G, Collin J, Soreiro O. Gliomatosis peritonei with malignant transformation: a case report and review of the literature. *Am J Obstet Gynecol* 1991;164:1617–1620.
49. Calder CJ, Light AM, Rollason TP. Immature ovarian teratoma with mature peritoneal metastatic deposits showing glial, epithelial, and endometrioid differentiation: a case report and review of the literature. *Int J Gynecol Pathol* 1994;13:279–282.
50. Dworak O, Knopfle G, Varchmin-Schultheiss K, Meyer G. Gliomatosis peritonei with endometriosis externa. *Gynecol Oncol* 1988;29:263–266.
51. Peterson WF. Solid histologically benign teratomas of the ovary: a report of four cases and review of the literature. *Am J Obstet Gynecol* 1956;72:1094–1102.
52. Peterson WF, Prevost EC, Edmunds FT, et al. Benign cystic teratomas of the ovary: a clinicostatistical study of 1007 cases with review of the literature. *Am J Obstet Gynecol* 1955;70:368–382.
53. Caruso PA, Marsh MR, Minkowitz S, Karten G. An intense clinicopathologic study of 305 teratomas of the ovary. *Cancer* 1971;27:343–348.
54. Malkasian GD Jr, Dockerty MB, Symmonds RE. Benign cystic teratomas. *Obstet Gynecol* 1967;29:719–725.
55. Peterson WF. Malignant degeneration of benign cystic teratomas of the ovary: a collective review of the literature. *Obstet Gynecol Surv* 1957;12:793–830.
56. Hirakawa T, Tsuneyoshi M, Enjoji M. Squamous cell carcinoma arising in mature cystic teratoma of the ovary: clinicopathologic and topographic analysis. *Am J Surg Pathol* 1989;13:397–405.
57. Pins MR, Young RH, Daly WJ, Scully RE. Primary squamous cell carcinoma of the ovary: report of 37 cases. *Am J Surg Pathol* 1996;20:823–833.
58. Pantoja E, Rodriguez-Ibanez I, Axtmayer RW, et al. Complications of dermoid tumors of the ovary. *Obstet Gynecol* 1975;45:89–94.
59. Manson CM, Cross PA, Herd ME, Wake CR. Mixed adeno- and squamous carcinoma in a mature cystic teratoma in a young woman. *Histopathology* 1993;23:481–482.
60. Ueda G, Fujita M, Ogawa H, et al. Adenocarcinoma in a benign cystic teratoma of the ovary: report of a case with a long survival period. *Gynecol Oncol* 1993;48:259–263.
61. Randall BJ, Ritchie C, Hutchison RS. Paget's disease and invasive undifferentiated carcinoma occurring in a mature cystic teratoma of the ovary. *Histopathology* 1991;18:469–470.
62. Shimizu S, Kobayashi H, Suchi T, et al. Extramammary Paget's disease arising in mature cystic teratoma of the ovary. *Am J Surg Pathol* 1991;15:1002–1006.
63. Ngwalle KE, Hirakawa T, Tsuneyoshi M, Enjoji M. Osteosarcoma arising in a benign dermoid cyst of the ovary. *Gynecol Oncol* 1990;37:143–147.
64. Carlson JA Jr, Wheeler JE. Primary ovarian melanoma arising in a dermoid stage IIIC: long-term disease-free survival with aggressive surgery and platinum therapy. *Gynecol Oncol* 1993;48:397–401.
65. Davis GL. Malignant melanoma arising in mature ovarian cystic teratoma (dermoid cyst): report of two

cases and literature analysis. *Int J Gynecol Pathol* 1996;15:356–362.
66. Seifer DB, Weiss LM, Kempson RL. Malignant lymphoma arising within thyroid tissue in a mature cystic teratoma. *Cancer* 1986;58:2459–2461.
67. Woodruff JD, Rauh JT, Markley RL. Ovarian struma. *Obstet Gynecol* 1966;27:194–201.
68. Szyfelbein WM, Young RH, Scully RE. Struma ovarii simulating ovarian tumors of other types: a report of 30 cases. *Am J Surg Pathol* 1995;19:21–29.
69. Devaney K, Snyder R, Norris HJ, Tavassoli FA. Proliferative and histologically malignant struma ovarii: a clinicopathologic study of 54 cases. *Int J Gynecol Pathol* 1993;12:333–343.
70. Robboy SJ, Krigman HR, Donohue J, Scully RE. Prognostic indices in malignant struma ovarii: clinicopathologic analysis of 36 patients with 20+ year followup. *Mod Pathol* 1995;8: 95A.
71. Karseladze AI, Kulinitsch SI. Peritoneal strumosis. *Pathol Res Pract* 1994;190:1086–1088.
72. Kragel PJ, Devaney K, Merino MJ. Struma ovarii with peritoneal implants: a case report with lectin histochemistry. *Surg Pathol* 1991;4:274–281.
73. Robboy SJ, Norris HJ, Scully RE. Insular carcinoid primary in the ovary: a clinico-pathologic analysis of 48 cases. *Cancer* 1975;36:404–418.
74. Robboy SJ, Scully RE, Norris HJ. Primary trabecular carcinoid of the ovary. *Obstet Gynecol* 1977;49:202–207.
75. Talerman A, Evans MI. Primary trabecular carcinoid tumor of the ovary. *Cancer* 1982;50:1403–1407.
76. Robboy SJ, Scully RE. Strumal carcinoid of the ovary: an analysis of 50 cases of a distinctive tumor composed of thyroid tissue and carcinoid. *Cancer* 1980;46:2019–2034.
77. Hart WR, Regezi JA. Strumal carcinoid of the ovary: ultrastructural observations and long term follow of study. *Am J Clin Pathol* 1978;69:356–359.
78. Livnat EJ, Scommegna A, Recant W, Jao W. Ultrastructural observations of the so-called strumal carcinoid of the ovary. *Arch Pathol Lab Med* 1977;101:585–589.
79. Ranchod M, Kempson RL, Dorgeloh JR. Strumal carcinoid of the ovary. *Cancer* 1976;37:1913–1922.
80. Ueda G, Sato SY, Yamasaki M, et al. Strumal carcinoid of the ovary: histological ultrastructural, and immunohistological studies with antihuman thyroglobulin. *Gynecol Oncol* 1978;6:411–419.
81. Greco MA, LiVolsi VA, Pertschuk LP, Bigelow B. Strumal carcinoid of the ovary: an analysis of its components. *Cancer* 1979;43:1380–1388.
82. Ulbright TM, Roth LM, Ehrlich CE. Ovarian strumal carcinoid: an immunocytochemical and ultrastructural study of two cases. *Am J Clin Pathol* 1982;77:622–631.
83. Armes JE, Ostor AG. A case of malignant strumal carcinoid. *Gynecol Oncol* 1993;51:419–423.
84. Warkel RL, Cooper PH, Helwig EB. Adenocarcinoid, a mucin producing carcinoid tumor of the appendix: a study of 39 cases. *Cancer* 1978;42:2781–2793.
85. Robboy SJ, Scully RE, Norris HJ. Carcinoid metastatic to the ovary: a clinicopathologic analysis of 35 cases. *Cancer* 1974;33:798–811.
86. Kleinman GM, Young RH, Scully RE. Primary neuroectodermal tumors of the ovary: a report of 25 cases. *Am J Surg Pathol* 1993;17:764–778.
87. Kleinman GM, Young RH, Scully RE. Ependymoma of the ovary: report of three cases. *Hum Pathol* 1984;15:632–638.
88. Aguirre P, Scully RE. Malignant neuroectodermal tumor of the ovary, a distinctive form of monodermal teratoma: report of five cases. *Am J Surg Pathol* 1982;6:283–292.
89. Kanbour-Shakir A, Sawady J, Kanbour AI, et al. Primitive neuroectodermal tumor arising in an ovarian mature cystic teratoma: immunohistochemical and electron microscopic studies. *Int J Gynecol Pathol* 1993;12:270–275
90. Scully RE. Gonadoblastoma: a gonadal tumor related to dysgerminoma (seminoma) and capable of sex hormone production. *Cancer* 1953;6:455–463.
91. Scully RE. Gonadoblastoma: a review of 74 cases. *Cancer* 1970;25:1340–1356.
92. Nakashima N, Nagasaka T, Fukata S, et al. Ovarian gonadoblastoma with dysgerminoma in a woman with two normal children. *Hum Pathol* 1989;20:814–816.
93. Jorgensen N, Mueller J, Jaubert F, et al. Heterogeneity of gonadoblastoma germ cells: similarities with immature germ cells, spermatogonia and testicular carcinoma in situ cells. *Histopathology* 1997;30:177–186.
94. Roth LM, Eglen DE. Gonadoblastoma: immunohistochemical and ultrastructural observations. *Int J Gynecol Pathol* 1989;8:72–81.
95. Talerman A. Gonadoblastoma associated with embryonal carcinoma. *Obstet Gynecol* 1974;43:138–142.
96. Talerman A, Van der Harten JJ. Mixed germ cell-sex cord stroma tumor of the ovary associated with isosexual precocious puberty in a normal girl. *Cancer* 1977;40:889–894
97. Lacson AG, Gillis DA, Shawwa A. Malignant mixed germ cell-sex cord-stromal tumors of the ovary associated with isosexual precocious puberty. *Cancer* 1988;61:2122–2133.
98. Talerman A. A distinctive gonadal neoplasm related to gonadoblastoma. *Cancer* 1972;30:1219–1224.
99. Talerman A. A mixed germ cell-sex cord stroma tumor of the ovary in a normal female infant. *Obstet Gynecol* 1972;40:473–478.
100. Bolen JW. Mixed germ cell-sex cord stromal tumor: a gonadal tumor distinct from gonadoblastoma. *Am J Clin Pathol* 1981;75:565–573.
101. Jacobsen GK, Braendstrup O, Talerman A. Bilateral mixed germ cell sex-cord stroma tumour in a young adult woman: case report. *APMIS Suppl* 1991;23:132–137.

7

Sex Cord-Stromal and Steroid Cell Tumors

Robert H. Young and Robert E. Scully

SEX CORD-STROMAL TUMORS

Sex cord-stromal tumors, which account for approximately 8% of all ovarian tumors (1,2), comprise those ovarian tumors that are derived ultimately from the sex cords and stroma (mesenchyme) of the embryonic ovary. They are composed of granulosa cells, fibroblasts, theca cells, Sertoli cells, and Leydig cells in varying proportions and in varying degrees of differentiation. The classification of these tumors used here is presented in Table 7.1. Most of the clinically malignant tumors are granulosa cell tumors.

Granulosa Cell Tumors

Granulosa cell tumors that occur most often in women in the reproductive age group and in older women (adult granulosa cell tumors) differ both clinically and pathologically from the much rarer tumors that are encountered most commonly in the first two decades (juvenile granulosa cell tumors).

Adult Granulosa Cell Tumor

Adult granulosa cell tumors account for approximately 1% of all ovarian tumors, approximately 5% of all ovarian cancers, and 95% of all granulosa cell tumors; they occur more often in postmenopausal than premenopausal women and have a peak age incidence between 50 and 55 years. Women in the reproductive age group typically present with irregular, excessive uterine bleeding, but amenorrhea may precede the abnormal bleeding by months or even years or may be the only hormonal manifestation. Postmenopausal bleeding is the most common endocrine symptom in older women. Rarely, the adult granulosa cell tumor is androgenic (3). Approximately 10% of the patients present with acute abdominal symptoms due to rupture of the tumor with hemoperitoneum.

Adult granulosa cell tumors vary in size from those that are too small to be felt on pelvic examination (10% to 15%) (4) to large abdominal masses. the average diameter is approximately 12 cm. At operation the tumor may appear predominantly solid or predominantly cystic and is unilateral in more than 95% of the cases; spread beyond the ovary at the time of presentation is uncommon. Most characteristically, the tumor is either predominantly cystic, with numerous locules that are filled with fluid or clotted blood and separated by solid tissue (Figure 7.1), or is solid with large areas of hemorrhage. The solid tissue may be gray-white or yellow, soft or firm. A rare cystic tumor is thin-walled and unilocular or oligolocular and is indistinguishable grossly from a serous cystadenoma (3).

Microscopic examination reveals an almost exclusive population of granulosa cells or, more often, an additional component of theca cells, fibroblasts, or both. The granulosa cells grow in a wide variety of patterns. The better-differentiated tumors usually have microfollicular, macrofollicular, insular, or trabecular patterns. The microfollicular pattern is characterized by numerous small cavities (Call-Exner bodies), which may contain eosinophilic fluid, one or a few degenerating nuclei, hyalinized basement membrane material (Figure 7.2), or, rarely, basophilic fluid. The microfollicles are separated typically by well differentiated granulosa cells that contain scanty cytoplasm and pale, angular or oval, often grooved nuclei arranged haphazardly in relation to one another and to the follicles (Figure 7.3). The macrofollicular pattern, which is relatively uncommon,

TABLE 7.1. *Classification of sex cord-stromal tumors and steroid cell tumors*

Granulosa-stromal cell tumors
  Granulosa cell tumor
    Adult type
    Juvenile type
  Tumors in the thecoma-fibroma group
    Thecoma
    Fibroma-fibrosarcoma
    Sclerosing stromal tumor
    Signet-ring stromal tumor
    Unclassified
Sertoli-stromal cell tumors
  Sertoli cell tumor
  Leydig cell tumor
  Sertoli-Leydig cell tumor
    Well differentiated
    Of intermediate differentiation
    Poorly differentiated
    With heterologous elements
    Retiform
    Mixed
Gynandroblastoma
Sex cord tumor with annular tubules
Unclassified sex cord tumors
Steroid cell tumors
  Stromal luteoma
  Leydig cell tumor
    Hilus cell tumor
    Leydig cell tumor, nonhilar type
  Steroid cell tumor, not otherwise specified

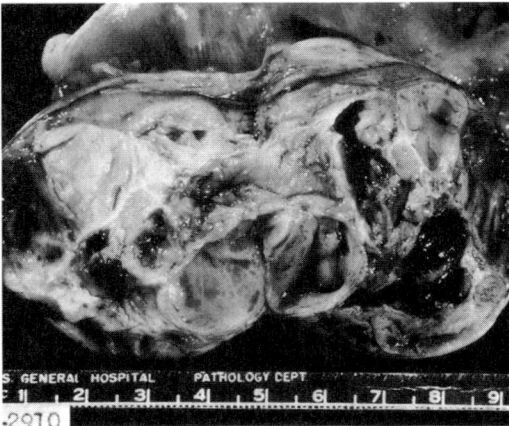

FIG. 7.1. Adult granulosa cell tumor. The sectioned surface of the tumor shows many cysts, some of which contain clotted blood.

(MFs) may be numerous but are rarely atypical. There is usually only mild nuclear atypia, but approximately 2% of tumors contain mononucleate and multinucleate cells with large, bizarre, hyperchromatic nuclei, the presence of which does not appear to worsen the prognosis (5).

is characterized by cysts lined by well differentiated granulosa cells, beneath which theca cells are usually present. The trabecular and insular forms of granulosa cell tumor are characterized by bands and islands of granulosa cells separated by a fibromatous or thecomatous stroma. The less well differentiated forms of the adult granulosa cell tumor typically have a watered silk (moire silk), gyriform, or diffuse (sarcomatoid) pattern, alone or in combination. The first two patterns are manifested by parallel undulating or zigzag rows of granulosa cells, usually in single file, whereas the diffuse form is characterized by a monotonous, patternless cellular growth. In some granulosa cell tumors the neoplastic cells have moderate to abundant quantities of dense or vacuolated cytoplasm; the term "luteinized granulosa cell tumor" is appropriate when such cells predominate. The cells in granulosa cell tumors usually have round to oval, pale, and often grooved nuclei (Figure 7.3), but rarely the cells are spindle shaped, resembling a cellular fibroma or low-grade fibrosarcoma; mitotic figures

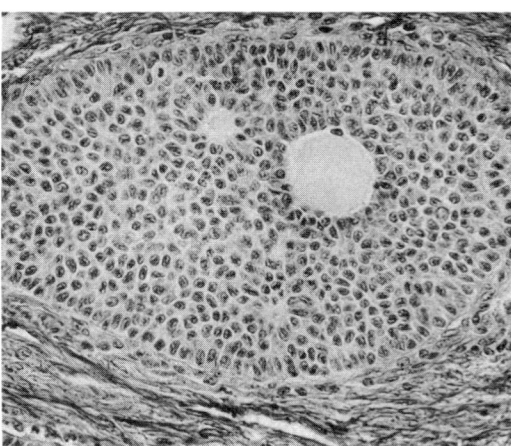

FIG. 7.2. Adult granulosa cell tumor. A nest of tumor contains two small follicles surrounded by haphazardly arranged granulosa cells. The microfollicles contained hyalinized basement membrane material (hematoxylin and eosin stain, ×400). (From Young RH, Scully RE: Ovarian sex cord-stromal tumors: recent advances in current status. *Clin Obstet Gynaecol* 1984;11:93–134, with permission.)

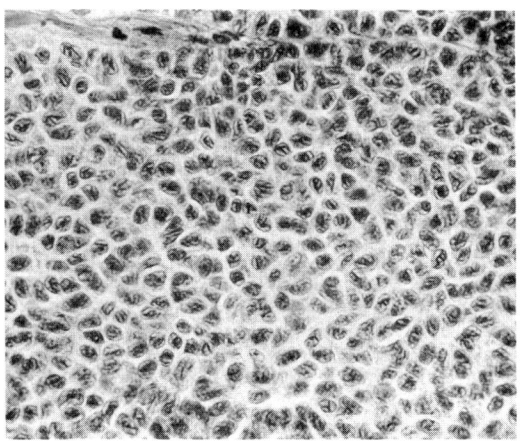

FIG. 7.3. Adult granulosa cell tumor. The tumor has a diffuse pattern. The granulosa cells have scant cytoplasm and pale, angular and oval nuclei with grooves (hematoxylin and eosin stain, ×520). (From Young RH, Scully RE: Ovarian sex cord-stromal and steroid cell tumors. In: Roth LM, Czernobilsky B, eds: *Tumors and tumor-like conditions of the ovary.* New York: Churchill Livingstone, 1985, with permission.)

Differential Diagnosis

An adult granulosa cell tumor with a diffuse pattern may be difficult to distinguish from a thecoma or cellular fibroma. In these cases a reticulum stain may be helpful, because the fibrils typically surround masses or groups of granulosa cells but invest individually the cells of fibromas and thecomas. Unlike thecomas and fibromas, adult granulosa cell tumors occasionally are positive for various cytokeratins on immunohistochemical staining (6). The misinterpretation of an undifferentiated carcinoma as a diffuse granulosa cell tumor is common. The single best criterion for distinguishing these two tumors is the appearance of the nuclei, which are hyperchromatic, usually of unequal size and shape, and rarely grooved in undifferentiated carcinomas; the latter with occasional exceptions have higher mitotic rates than diffuse granulosa cell tumors, and atypical MFs are often found as well.

Endometrioid carcinomas may have small glands that simulate Call-Exner bodies and result in misdiagnosis as a granulosa cell tumor. However, more typical endometrioid glands, squamous differentiation (sometimes only abortive), and in some cases an adenofibromatous background are clues to endometrioid carcinoma. Immunohistochemistry may help in a problem case (6). The small cell carcinoma of hypercalcemic type (7), which is associated with paraendocrine hypercalcemia in two thirds of the cases, may also be misdiagnosed as a granulosa cell tumor, particularly because it almost always contains follicle-like structures. However, other patterns of the granulosa cell tumor are not encountered, the nuclei are darker than granulosa cell nuclei and lack grooves, and MFs are usually much more numerous than in the adult granulosa cell tumor, which has never been reported to have an association with hypercalcemia. Conversely, small cell carcinomas are not accompanied by estrogenic manifestations. Unlike the typically indolent clinical course of the adult granulosa cell tumor, the small cell carcinoma is associated with a high mortality rate. Some macrofollicular adult granulosa cell tumors may be difficult to distinguish from follicle cysts, but, except during pregnancy and the puerperium (8), follicle cysts rarely exceed 8 cm in diameter. Other rare problems in differential diagnosis are discussed elsewhere (2).

The differentiation of AGCTs from tumors other than those in the sex cord-stromal category may be aided by immunohistochemical staining for inhibin, which is almost always positive in GCTs and most other sex cord-stromal tumors that have been studied to date and is typically negative, or at most weakly positive, in tumors that are not sex cord-stromal tumors (9). Furthermore, EMA and CK7, which give positive results in most surface epithelial carcinomas stain negative in GCTs (10). Desmin may aid in the distinction from an epithelioid smooth muscle tumor, a rare differential diagnosis.

A number of studies have concerned the relation of various clinical and pathologic features of adult granulosa cell tumors to prognosis (11-14). The stage of the tumor is the single most important prognostic feature, with the 10-year survival rate in one series falling from 86% in stage I cases to 49% when the tumor was present outside the ovary at the time of exploration (14). When only stage I tumors are considered, rupture is the major prognostic parameter, causing the 10-year survival rate to drop from 86% to 60% (11,12). Microscopic features have not been very helpful prognostically in the experience of most investigators, but two groups have found that stage I tumors with low-grade nuclear atypia have a better prognosis than those with high-grade atypia (11,12,14).

Juvenile Granulosa Cell Tumor

These tumors occur within the first two decades of life in almost 80% of the cases, and within the first three decades in 97% of the cases (15). In prepubertal girls they typically result in isosexual pseudoprecocity (15-17). When the juvenile granulosa cell tumor occurs after normal puberty it usually manifests with abdominal pain or swelling and sometimes is associated with menometrorrhagia or amenorrhea. Approximately 6% of the patients present with acute abdominal symptoms caused by rupture of the tumor and hemoperitoneum. An interesting clinical association of the juvenile granulosa cell tumor has been its occasional occurrence in patients with Ollier's disease (enchondromatosis) or Maffucci syndrome (enchondromatosis and hemangiomatosis) (15).

The juvenile granulosa cell tumor is bilateral in only about 2% of the cases. It appears ruptured at operation in approximately 10% of cases, and ascites is present in a similar percentage. Spread beyond the ovary is unusual; in a series of 125 cases, only three tumors were stage II (15) and none were stage III. The diameter of the tumor ranges from 3.0 to 32.0 cm, with an average of 12.5 cm. Because of the usual moderate to large size of the tumor, an adnexal mass is almost always detectable clinically. Rarely, however, a mass is not palpable preoperatively on bimanual rectal examination.

The range in gross appearance of the juvenile granulosa cell tumor is similar to that of the adult form. The single most common presentation is as a solid and cystic neoplasm; the cysts may contain hemorrhagic fluid. Uniformly solid and uniformly cystic neoplasms are also encountered; the latter may be multilocular or, rarely, unilocular. The solid component is typically

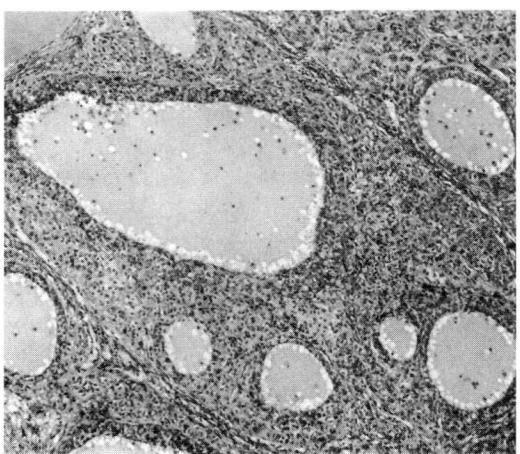

FIG. 7.4. Juvenile granulosa cell tumor. The tumor has a solid and follicular pattern. The follicles vary in size and contain fluid that was eosinophilic (hematoxylin and eosin stain, ×100).

yellow-tan or gray and occasionally exhibits extensive necrosis, hemorrhage, or both.

Microscopic examination typically reveals a predominantly solid cellular tumor with focal follicle formation (Figure 7.4), but occasionally a uniformly solid or uniformly follicular pattern is seen. In the solid areas the neoplastic cells may be arranged diffusely or as multiple nodules of various sizes. The follicles typically vary in size and shape (Figure 7.4); Call-Exner bodies are rarely encountered, and the follicles rarely reach the large size of those in the macrofollicular adult granulosa cell tumor. The follicular lumens in the juvenile tumor contain eosinophilic or basophilic fluid, which stains with mucicarmine in approximately two thirds of the cases.

The two characteristic cytologic features of neoplastic juvenile granulosa cells that distinguish them from those of the adult granulosa cell tumor are their generally rounded, hyperchromatic nuclei, which almost always lack grooves, and the almost invariable presence of moderate to abundant eosinophilic or vacuolated (luteinized) cytoplasm (Figure 7.5). Nuclear atypicality in juvenile granulosa cell tumors varies from minimal to marked; in approximately 13% of the cases severe degrees of atypia are present. The mitotic rate also varies greatly, but it is generally higher

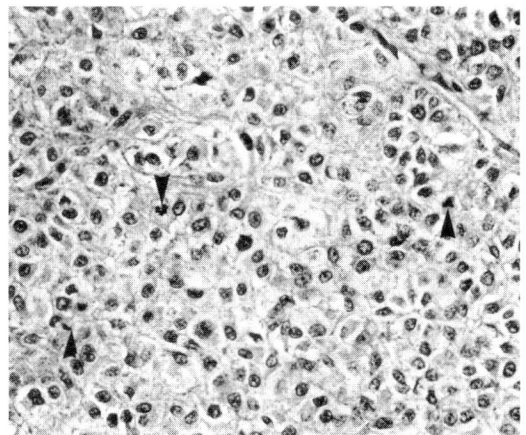

FIG. 7.5. Juvenile granulosa cell tumor. The tumor cells have abundant cytoplasm that was eosinophilic to pale. The nuclei lack grooves, and several mitotic figures are visible *(arrows)* (hematoxylin and eosin stain, ×400).

than that seen in adult granulosa cell tumors, often being 5 or more per 10 high-power fields (hpf) (15,17). The stage of the tumor is the best indicator of prognosis. The survival rate for patients with stage I tumors is greater than 90%.

Differential Diagnosis

The distinctive appearance of the follicles and the rarity of Call-Exner bodies in juvenile granulosa cell tumors, their cytologic features (i.e. dark, round, ungrooved nuclei and luteinized cytoplasm), and their usual content of mucin in the follicular lumens almost always allows differentiation of these tumors from adult granulosa cell tumors. When the juvenile granulosa cell tumor is characterized by moderate to severe nuclear atypicality it may be mistaken for a yolk sac tumor or the exceptionally rare embryonal carcinoma. Rarely, the diagnosis of yolk sac tumor is further suggested by the presence of hyaline bodies in a juvenile granulosa cell tumor. The variety of patterns seen in yolk sac tumors—reticular, endodermal sinus with Schiller-Duval bodies, papillary and polyvesicular, and embryonal carcinomas, granular and papillary—are not encountered in juvenile granulosa cell tumors, nor are the follicular patterns of the latter present in the germ cell tumors. Immunohistochemical staining for α-fetoprotein (AFP) and for chorionic gonadotropin is negative in juvenile granulosa cell tumors.

The young age at which the small cell carcinoma occurs and its content of follicle-like structures often leads to a misdiagnosis of juvenile granulosa cell tumor. The follicles of the former, however, are typically round and contain eosinophilic fluid that rarely stains with mucicarmine. The solid areas of the tumor are usually characterized by a monotonous proliferation of uniformly small cells that typically have scanty cytoplasm, in contrast to the abundant cytoplasm of the cells in juvenile granulosa cell tumors.

The juvenile granulosa cell tumor is sometimes misinterpreted as a thecoma because of the occasional absence or rarity of follicles. Thecomas almost always lack significant mitotic activity, occur before 30 years of age in fewer than 10% of the cases, rarely if ever occur in children, and lack follicles. However, juvenile granulosa cell tumors may contain a large theca cell component.

The juvenile granulosa cell tumor may be confused with clear cell or undifferentiated carcinoma. The tubulocystic variant of clear cell carcinoma may be suggested by the occasional lining of follicles of a juvenile granulosa cell tumor by hobnail cells. The young age of the patient, the presence of follicles, and focal presence of more characteristic areas of juvenile granulosa cell tumor, as well as the absence of other features of clear cell carcinoma, should facilitate the differential diagnosis. Similar features should also eliminate the diagnosis of undifferentiated carcinoma.

The juvenile granulosa cell tumor may be confused with malignant melanoma metastatic to the ovary when the latter is characterized by cells with abundant cytoplasm and the formation of spaces simulating follicles (18). The presence of melanin granules and intranuclear cytoplasmic inclusions suggests melanoma, and staining for melanin granules or HMB-45 confirm the diagnosis. Staining for inhibin may help establish the diagnosis of juvenile granulosa cell tumor in particularly problematic cases (9).

Malignant Tumors in the Thecoma-Fibroma Group

The vast majority of thecomas and fibromas are benign. Exceptionally, a thecoma that exhibits conspicuous mitotic activity and nuclear atypicality pursues a malignant course (19) and merits the diagnosis of malignant thecoma, but most of the so-called malignant thecomas in the literature appear to be misdiagnosed diffuse granulosa cell tumors or fibrosarcomas. Occasional fibromatous tumors have malignant cytologic features and merit designation as fibrosarcomas. They typically pursue a rapid course and have a poor prognosis. Atypical cellular fibromatous tumors with three or four MFs and no more than mild nuclear atypicality are usually clinically benign and are designated "cellular fibromas" (20). These tumors have a tendency to recur if incompletely removed or ruptured; when an intact tumor appears to be completely removed, it still may recur more than 10 years after its removal.

SERTOLI-STROMAL CELL TUMORS

Sertoli Cell Tumors

Sertoli cell tumors account for only 4% of Sertoli-stromal cell tumors (21,22). Microscopic examination shows hollow or solid tubules lined by cells that almost always have relatively bland cytologic features. Rare tumors exhibit moderate nuclear atypicality, and one tumor in a sexually precocious child was focally poorly differentiated, metastasized distantly, and was rapidly fatal (21).

Sertoli-Leydig Cell Tumors

Sertoli-Leydig cell tumors account for the great majority of Sertoli-stromal cell tumors but for fewer than 0.5% of all ovarian tumors (23-29). They are now divided into six categories: well differentiated (26), of intermediate differentiation, poorly differentiated, with heterologous elements (27,28), retiform (29), and admixtures of these patterns. Sertoli-Leydig cell tumors may be encountered in all age groups but are diagnosed most often in young women, with an average age of 25 years; 75% of the patients are 30 years of age or younger, and only about 10% are older than 50 years of age (23). The well differentiated tumors occur on average a decade later than Sertoli-Leydig cell tumors in general, and tumors with a retiform pattern are encountered on average a decade earlier, occurring more commonly in the first decade than any other subtype.

Although the most striking mode of presentation of Sertoli-Leydig cell tumors is virilization, it develops in only about one third of the cases. Most patients complain of abdominal swelling or pain. Virilizing Sertoli-Leydig cell tumors are typically associated with increased levels in the plasma of testoserone, but weaker androgens may also be present in increased amounts. Occasional tumors are accompanied by estrogenic manifestations. Twenty-one Sertoli-Leydig cell tumors have been associated with elevated plasma levels of AFP, but values as high as those accompanying yolk sac tumors are rare (30).

Sertoli-Leydig cell tumors are stage Iai in about 80% of the cases; in 12% the tumor has either ruptured or involved the external surface of the ovary; and 1% to 2% are bilateral. Ascites is present in 4% of the cases. Only 2% to 3% of the tumors have spread beyond the ovary at the time of operation, usually within the pelvis and rarely in the upper abdomen. All of the well differentiated tumors in one large series were stage Iai; the poorly differentiated tumors were more often ruptured or were of higher stage at presentation than the tumors of intermediate differentiation (23).

Sertoli-Leydig cell tumors vary as greatly in their gross appearance as granulosa cell tumors do, but they less often contain cysts filled with blood and almost never have the appearance of a unilocular thin-walled cyst. They vary in size from microscopic to huge masses, but most are between 5 and 15 cm in diameter (Figure 7.6). Poorly differentiated tumors tend to be larger than those of better differentiation, and they more frequently contain areas of hemorrhage and necrosis. Tumors with heterologous or retiform components are more often cystic than other tumors in this category. The heterologous tumors occasionally simulate mucinous cystic tumors on gross examination; retiform tumors may contain large, edematous intracystic papillae, resembling

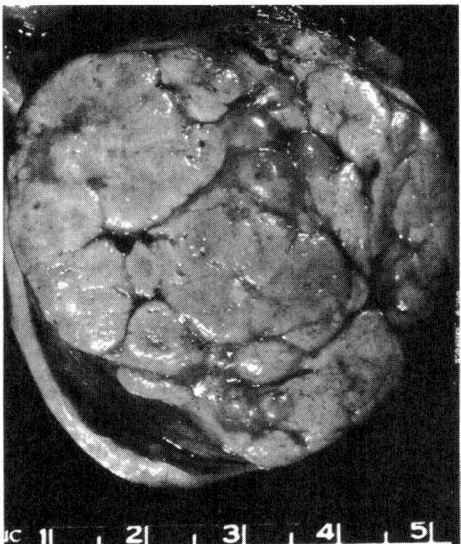

FIG. 7.6. Sertoli-Leydig cell tumor. The sectioned surface of the tumor is lobulated and was yellow in the fresh state.

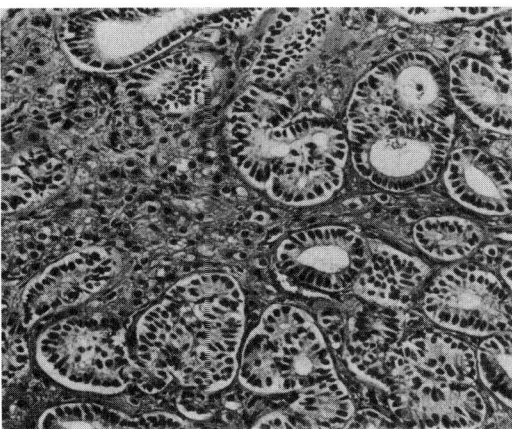

FIG. 7.7. Sertoli-Leydig cell tumor, well differentiated. Hollow tubules are separated by Leydig cells in the intervening stroma. (From Young RH, Scully RE: Well differentiated ovarian Sertoli-Leydig cell tumors: a clinicopathological analysis of 23 cases. *Int J Gynecol Pathol* 1984;3:277–290, with permission.)

serous papillary tumors, or they may be soft and spongy with varying degrees of cystification (29).

Well-differentiated Sertoli-Leydig cell tumors are characterized by a predominantly tubular pattern (26). On low-power examination a nodular architecture is often conspicuous, with fibrous bands intersecting lobules composed of small, round, hollow or less often solid tubules lined by well differentiated cells and separated by variable numbers of Leydig cells (Figure 7.7). These tumors are clinically benign.

Sertoli-Leydig cell tumors of intermediate and poor differentiation form a continuum characterized by a variety of patterns (Figure 7.8) and combinations of cell types. Some tumors exhibit intermediate differentiation in some areas and poor differentiation in others; less commonly, tumors of intermediate differentiation contain well differentiated foci. Both the Sertoli cells and Leydig cells may exhibit varying degrees of immaturity. In the tumors of intermediate differentiation, immature Sertoli cells have small, round, oval or angular nuclei and generally scanty cytoplasm and are arranged typically in ill-defined masses, often creating a lobulated appearance on low power; solid and hollow tubules, nests, broad columns of Sertoli cells, and, most characteristically, thin cords resembling the sex cords of the embryonic testis are often present. These structures are separated by stroma, which ranges from fibromatous to densely cellular to edematous (Figure 7.8) and typically contains

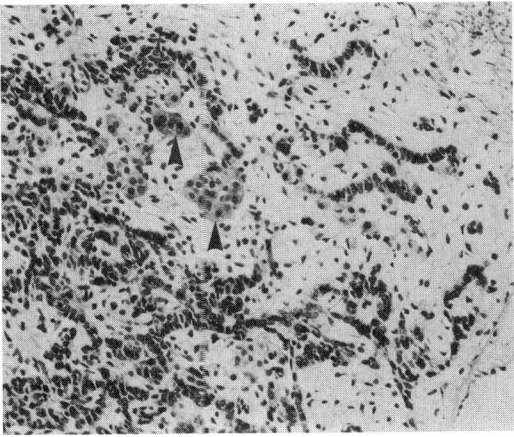

FIG. 7.8. Sertoli-Leydig cell tumor of intermediate differentiation. Small cords of darkly staining Sertoli cells are separated by an edematous stroma containing clusters of Leydig cells and single Leydig cells with abundant cytoplasm that was eosinophilic *(arrows)* (hematoxylin and eosin stain, ×200).

clusters of well differentiated Leydig cells. Cysts containing eosinophilic secretion may be present and create a thyroid-like appearance, and follicle-like spaces are encountered rarely. The Sertoli and Leydig cell elements, singly or in combination, may contain varying and sometimes large amounts of lipid in the form of small or large droplets. When a significant amount of the stromal component is made up of immature, cellular mesenchymal tissue with high mitotic activity resembling a nonspecific sarcoma, the tumor is poorly differentiated.

Fifteen percent of Sertoli-Leydig cell tumors have a substantial retiform component; they are designated retiform because they are composed of a network of elongated tubules and cysts, both of which may contain papillae (Figure 7.9), resembling the rete testis (29,31,32). This pattern is usually accompanied by other patterns of Sertoli-Leydig cell tumor, but sometimes an entire tumor has a retiform pattern.

Heterologous elements occur in approximately 20% of Sertoli-Leydig cell tumors (27,28). In one series of these tumors, 18% contained glands and cysts lined by mode-rately differentiated to well differentiated intestinal-type epithelium (27). Mesenchymal heterologous elements, encountered in 5% of Sertoli-Leydig cell tumors, include islands of cartilage arising on a sarcomatous background, areas of embryonal rhabdomyosarcoma, or both (28).

Differential Diagnosis

Sertoli-Leydig cell tumors are often difficult to differentiate from tumors outside the sex cord-stromal category and from granulosa cell tumors. The small, hollow, tubular glands; solid tubular structures; and cords that are occasionally seen in endometrioid carcinomas may closely mimic similar structures in Sertoli-Leydig cell tumors (33,34). At least some of the glands of endometrioid carcinomas, however, are usually larger than the tubules of Sertoi-Leydig cell tumors and are lined by epithelium that is often less well differentiated. In addition, mucin secretion; areas of squamous differentiation that range from nests of uniform, immature, spindle-shaped epithelial cells to morules to keratinizing foci; and an adenofibromatous component of common epithelial type are present in many endometrioid carcinomas, facilitating their diagnosis. Clinical features, such as the postmenopausal status of the patient and the almost invariable absence of androgenic manifestations, support the diagnosis of endometrioid carcinoma.

Krukenberg tumors with a tubular pattern (35) may mimic Sertoli-Leydig cell tumors, especially if luteinization of the stroma is present; further confusion arises in the rare tubular Krukenberg tumor associated with virilization as a result of luteinization of its stroma. However, Krukenberg tumors have been reported to be bilateral in approximately 80% of the cases, and they contain markedly atypical cells, including signet-ring cells that contain mucin.

Carcinoid tumors, especially those of the trabecular type, may be confused with intermediate Sertoli-Leydig cell tumors. The ribbons of the former, however, are longer, thicker, and more uniformly distributed than the sex cord-like formations of the latter. Also, rare carcinoid tumors with a solid tubular pattern can be difficult to distinguish from well differentiated Sertoli cell tumors. Examination of the stroma of carcinoid tumors may be helpful in the differential diagnosis. It is typically less cellular and more fibromatous than that of Sertoli-Leydig cell tumors and

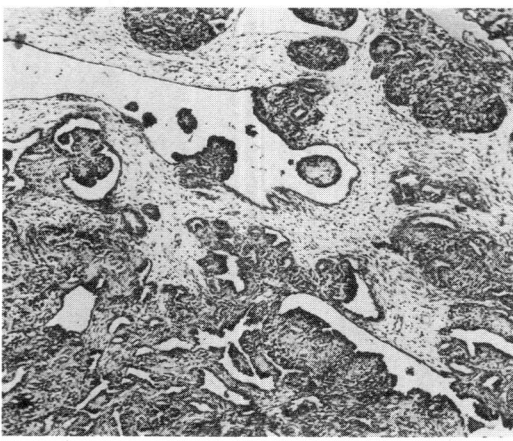

FIG. 7.9. Sertoli-Leydig cell tumor with retiform pattern. The tumor contains elongated tubules, cysts, a few papillae, and solid clusters of immature Sertoli cells (hematoxylin and eosin stain, ×79).

does not contain Leydig cells. The most specific diagnostic criterion is the presence of argyrophil granules in almost all carcinoid tumors and of argentaffin granules in many of them; in contrast, only heterologous Sertoli-Leydig cell tumors with glands and cysts lined by gastrointestinal-type epithelium contain such granules. Finally, primary carcinoid tumors are associated with teratomatous elements in 70% of the cases, and metastatic carcinoids are usually bilateral and associated with a primary tumor of the intestine and metastases elsewhere in the abdomen.

A retiform Sertoli-Leydig cell tumor may be misdiagnosed as a yolk sac tumor because of the young age of the patient and the presence of papillae, which may be mistaken for Schiller-Duval bodies. The association of androgenic manifestations with about one quarter of retiform Sertoli-Leydig cell tumors contrasts with their very rare association with yolk sac tumors. The presence of other distinctive patterns of either tumor and immunohistochemical staining for AFP in the yolk sac tumor almost always facilitates the diagnosis. The papillary pattern and cellular stratification in retiform tumors may cause them to mimic a serous cystadenoma of borderline malignancy or a serous or endometrioid carcinoma. A variety of clinical and pathologic features, including the young age of the patient, the occasional association with virilization, and the presence of other more easily recognizable patterns of Sertoli-Leydig cell tumor, are helpful clues to the correct diagnosis. Staining for inhibin may help in the differential diagnosis as it does for the granulosa cell tumor (9).

The prognosis of Sertoli-Leydig cell tumors is closely related to their stage and degree of differentiation. The rare tumors that are higher than stage I have a poor prognosis. The survival rates of patients with stage I tumors correlate with the degree of differentiation. In one large series of cases, none of the well differentiated tumors, 11% of those of intermediate differentiation, 59% of the poorly differentiated tumors, and 19% of those with heterologous elements were clinically malignant (23). The homologous component of the tumor was poorly differentiated in all eight clinically malignant tumors in the heterologous category, and in seven of them the heterologous elements included skeletal muscle, cartilage, or both. Other investigations have supported the findings in this series. The only clinically malignant tumor in the series of Roth and colleagues (25) was poorly differentiated, and 4 of the 20 poorly differentiated tumors reported by Zaloudek and Norris (24) were malignant, in contrast to only 1 of the 44 tumors of intermediate differentiation and none of the 7 well differentiated tumors. In our experience the presence of a retiform pattern also has an adverse effect on the prognosis: 25% of stage I retiform tumors were malignant, as opposed to only 10% of tumors of similar grade without a retiform component (23). In two other reports of retiform Sertoli-Leydig cell tumors, metastases occurred in 4 of 15 patients, and 3 of them died from their disease, suggesting a somewhat more aggressive behavior than that of nonretiform Sertoli-Leydig cell tumors.

SEX CORD TUMOR WITH ANNULAR TUBULES

Sex cord tumors with annular tubules (SCTATs) vary both clinically and pathologically depending on whether the patient has the Peutz-Jeghers syndrome (36,37). Most female patients with this syndrome whose ovaries have been examined microscopically have had sex cord tumorlets with annular tubules, which have been multifocal and bilateral in at least two thirds of the cases; the largest reported lesion in a patient with this syndrome was 3 cm in diameter. All the tumorlets associated with the Peutz-Jeghers syndrome have been benign. In patients without the Peutz-Jeghers syndrome, the tumors are almost always unilateral and usually form large palpable masses. At least one fifth of these tumors have been clinically malignant; in contrast to other tumors in the sex cord-stromal category, the SCTAT tends to metastasize to lymph nodes. The malignant tumors may have an indolent clinical course.

This tumor is characterized microscopically by the presence of simple and complex annular tubules (Figure 7.10). The simple tubules have the shape of a ring, with the nuclei oriented around the periphery and around a central

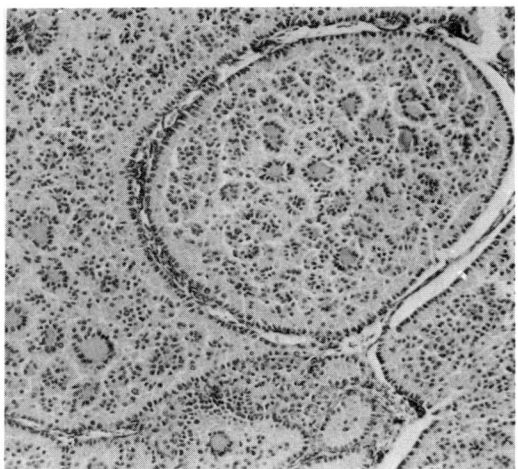

FIG. 7.10. Sex cord tumor with annular tubules. Numerous rounded tubules encircle multiple hyaline bodies (hematoxylin and eosin stain, ×125).

hyalinized body composed of basement membrane material; an intervening anuclear cytoplasmic zone forms the major component of the ring. The much more numerous complex tubules are rounded structures made up of intercommunicating rings revolving around multiple hyaline bodies. In patients with the Peutz-Jeghers syndrome, the tumors are typically multifocal and exhibit calcification. These tumors are intermediate morphologically between granulosa cell tumor and Sertoli cell tumors and exhibit focal differentiation in the direction of both of these tumors (22,38). Like them, the SCTATs may have estrogenic and rarely androgenic manifestations; a few tumors produce progesterone.

SEX CORD-STROMAL TUMORS, UNCLASSIFIED

This ill-defined group of tumors, which accounts for fewer than 10% of those in the sex cord-stromal category, comprises those in which a predominant pattern of testicular or ovarian differentiation is not clearly recognizable. The boundary lines between these tumors and those of ovarian and testicular cell types are vague because interpretations of intermediate patterns of growth and closely similar cell types are inevitably subjective. Talennan and associates (37) segregated from within this category a group of tumors for which they proposed the designation "diffuse nonlobular androblastoma." The six ovarian tumors they reported were mostly estrogenic and had a predominant diffuse proliferation of cells resembling theca cells, granulosa cells, or both but also contained steroid-type cells in all of the cases and tubules typically of Sertoli cell neoplasia in five of the six cases.

Sex cord-stromal tumors may be particularly difficult to subclassify when they occur in pregnant patients because of alterations in their usual clinical and pathologic features (40). Their nature is rarely suggested clinically, because during pregnancy estrogenic manifestations are not recognizable and androgenic manifestations are rare. In one study 17% of 36 sex cord-stromal tumors that were removed during pregnancy were placed in the unclassified group, and many of those that were classified in the granulosa cell or Sertoli-Leydig cell category had large areas with an indifferent appearance (40).

STEROID CELL TUMORS

These neoplasms, formerly called lipid or lipoid cell tumors, are composed entirely, or almost entirely, of cells resembling typical steroid hormone-secreting cells. Steroid cell tumors account for only 0.1% of all ovarian neoplasms. They are subclassified into three major categories: stromal luteoma, Leydig (hilus) cell tumor, and steroid cell tumor not otherwise specified (NOS) (41–43). Only tumors in the last group may be clinically malignant.

Steroid cell tumors NOS may occur at any age, with the average age in the largest reported series being 43 years (39). Tumors that occur in children may cause heterosexual pseudoprecocity, or less commonly, isosexual pseudoprecocity. The tumors are androgenic in about half of the cases. Eight percent of them are estrogenic, and occasional examples are progestagenic. Four tumors have caused Cushing's syndrome (41,44,45), and three others have been accompanied by elevated cortisol concentrations without clinical manifestations of the syndrome. Hormone studies performed in patients with androgenic changes, Cushing's syndrome,

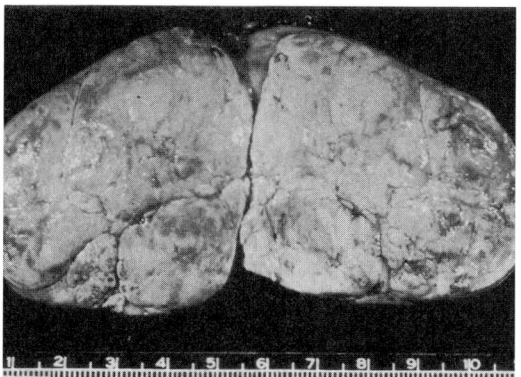

FIG. 7.11. Steroid cell tumor unclassified. The sectioned surface of the tumor is lobulated and was yellow-orange in the fresh state. This tumor was from a 9-year-old girl who presented because of virilization.

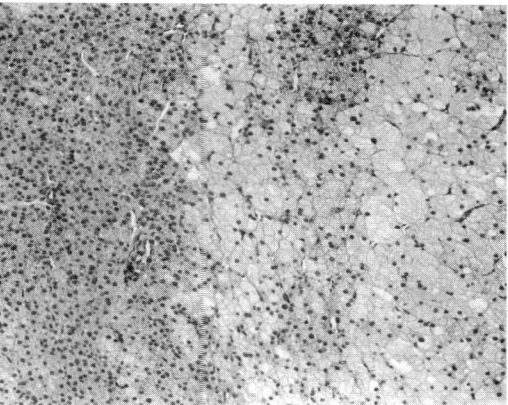

FIG. 7.12. Steroid cell tumor, not otherwise specified. This illustration shows the two characteristic cell types that may be seen in these tumors, cells with abundant eosinophilic cytoplasm *(left)* and cells with abundant pale vacuolated cytoplasm *(right)* (hematoxylin and eosin stain, ×125).

or both typically show increased urinary levels of 17-ketosteroids and 17-hydroxycorticosteroids, as well as increased serum levels of testosterone and androstenedione. In 20% of the cases, extraovarian spread of tumor is apparent at the time of operation.

The tumors are typically solid, well circumscribed, and occasionally lobulated (Figure 7.11); they average 8.4 cm in diameter, and approximately 5% of them are bilateral. They are typically yellow or orange but occasionally red to brown or black. Necrosis, hemorrhage, and cystic degeneration are occasionally observed. On microscopic examination, the tumor cells are typically arranged diffusely (Figure 7.12), but occasionally they grow in nests, irregular clusters, thin cords, or columns.

The polygonal to rounded tumor cells have distinct cell borders, central nuclei, and moderate to abundant amounts of cytoplasm that varies from eosinophilic and granular to vacuolated and spongy (Figure 7.12). In approximately 60% of the cases nuclear atypia is absent or minimal, and mitotic activity is low (fewer than 2 MFs per 10 hpf). In the remaining cases, grade 1 to 3 nuclear atypia (Figure 7.13) is present, usually associated with an increase in mitotic activity (up to 15 MFs per 10 hpf).

Twenty-five percent to 40% of these tumors are clinically malignant. Such a behavior is more frequent in older patients, and all of the reported tumors from patients in the first two decades have been benign. The best pathologic correlates with a malignant behavior in one series were as follows: 2 or more MFs per 10 hpf, 92% malignant; necrosis, 86% malignant; diameter of 7 cm or greater, 78% malignant; hemorrhage, 77% malignant; and grade 2 or 3 nuclear atypia, 64%

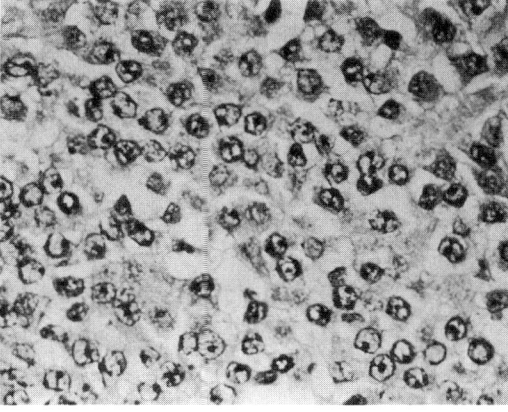

FIG. 7.13. Steroid cell tumor, not otherwise specified. The nuclei exhibit moderate nuclear atypicality. This tumor, which was responsible for Cushing's syndrome, was clinically malignant (hematoxylin and eosin stain, ×500).

malignant. Rare tumors that appear cytologically benign are clinically malignant (41).

Differential Diagnosis

These tumors may be confused with numerous other neoplasms, particularly extensively luteinized granulosa cell tumors and thecomas, and clear cell carcinomas, particularly those of the oxyphil type (46). Other, less common problems in diagnosis are reviewed elsewhere (2). The focal presence of nonluteinized areas in luteinized granulosa cell tumors and luteinized thecomas, as well as the characteristic cytologic features and patterns of these neoplasms and the finding of abundant reticulum in thecomas, facilitates the identification of these tumors. The clear cells of the clear cell carcinoma and metastatic renal cell carcinoma, unlike those of steroid cell tumors, have glycogen-rich cytoplasm and eccentric nuclei. Also, other patterns of clear cell carcinoma (e.g., tubulocystic, glandular, papillary) are inconsistent with a steroid cell tumor. Similar features help in the differentiation from oxyphilic clear cell carcinomas. As is the case with tumors of sex cord-stromal type, staining for inhibin occasionally may assist in the differential diagnosis, steroid cell tumors being positive and tumors that mimic them being negative (9).

REFERENCES

1. Young RH, Scully RE. Ovarian sex cord-stromal tumors: recent advances and current status. *Clin Obstet Gynecol* 1984;11:93–134.
2. Young RH, Scully RE. Sex cord-stromal tumors, steroid cell tumors and other ovarian tumors with endocrine, paraendocrine and paraneoplastic manifestations. In: Kurman RJ (ed). *Blaustein's pathology of the female genital tract,* 4th ed. New York: Springer-Verlag, 1994:783–847.
3. Nakashima N, Young RH, Scully RE. Androgenic granulosa cell tumors of the ovary: a clinicopathological analysis of seventeen cases and review of the literature. *Arch Pathol Lab Med* 1984;108:786–791.
4. Fathalla MF. The occurrence of granulosa and theca tumors in clinically normal ovaries: a study of 25 cases. *J Obstet Gynaecol Brit Cmwlth* 1967;74:279–282.
5. Young RH, Scully RE. Ovarian sex cord-stromal tumors with bizarre nuclei: a clinicopathologic analysis of seventeen cases. *Int J Gynecol Pathol* 1983;1:325–335.
6. Aguirre P, Thor AD, Scully RE. Ovarian endometrioid carcinomas resembling sex cord-stromal tumors: an immunohistological study. *Int J Gynecol Pathol* 1989;8:364–373.
7. Young RH, Oliva E, Scully RE. Small cell carcinoma of the ovary, hypercalcemic type: a clinicopathologic analysis of 150 cases. *Am J Surg Pathol* 1996;18:1102–1116.
8. Clement PB, Scully RE. Large solitary luteinized follicle cyst of pregnancy and puerperium. *Am J Surg Pathol* 1980;4:431–438.
9. McCluggage WG. Value of inhibin staining in gynecological pathology. *Int J Gynecol Pathol* 2001;20:79–85.
10. Guerrieri C, Franlund B, Malmstrom H, et al. Ovarian endometrioid carcinomas simulating sex cord-stromal tumors: a study using inhibin and cytokeratin. *Int J Gynecol Pathol* 1998;17:266–271.
11. Bjorkholm E, Pettersson F. Granulosa-cell and theca-cell tumors: the clinical picture and long term outcome for the Radiumhemmet series. *Acta Obstet Gynecol Scand* 1980;59:361–365.
12. Bjorkholm E, Silfversward C. Prognostic factors in granulosa cell tumors. *Gynecol Oncol* 1981;11:261–274.
13. Fox H, Agrawal K, Langley FA. A clinicopathologic study of 92 cases of granulosa cell tumor of the ovary with special reference to the factors influencing prognosis. *Cancer* 1975;35:231–241.
14. Stenwig JT, Hazekamp JT, Beecham JB. Granulosa cell tumors of the ovary: a clinicopathological study of 118 cases with long-term follow-up. *Gynecol Oncol* 1979;7:136–152.
15. Young RH, Dickersin GR, Scully RE. Juvenile granulosa cell tumor of the ovary: a clinicopathologic analysis of 125 cases. *Am J Surg Pathol* 1984;8:575–596.
16. Lack EE, Perez-Atayde AR, Murthy ASK, et al. Granulosa theca cell tumors in premenarchal girls: a clinical and pathologic study of ten cases. *Cancer* 1981;48:1846–1854.
17. Zaloudek C, Norris HJ. Granulosa tumors of the ovary in children: a clinical and pathologic study of 32 cases. *Am J Surg Pathol* 1982;6:503–512.
18. Young RH, Scully RE. Malignant melanoma metastatic to the ovary: a clinicopathologic analysis of 20 cases. *Am J Surg Pathol* 1991;15:849–860.
19. Waxman M, Vuletin JC, Urcuyo R, Belling CG. Ovarian low-grade stromal sarcoma with thecomatous features: a critical reappraisal of the so-called "malignant thecoma." *Cancer* 1979;44:2206–2217.
20. Prat J, Scully RE. Cellular fibromas and fibrosarcomas of the ovary: a comparative clinicopathologic analysis of seventeen cases. *Cancer* 1981;47:2663–2670.
21. Young RH, Scully RE. Ovarian Sertoli cell tumors: a report of ten cases. *Int J Gynecol Pathol* 1984;2:349–363.
22. Tavassoli FA, Norris HJ. Sertoli tumors of the ovary: a clinicopathologic study of 28 cases with ultrastructural observations. *Cancer* 1980;46:2281–2297.
23. Young RH, Scully RE. Ovarian Sertoli-Leydig cell tumors: a clinicopathologic analysis of 207 cases. *Am J Surg Pathol* 1985;9:543–569.
24. Zaloudek C, Norris HJ. Sertoli-Leydig tumors of the ovary: a clinicopathologic study of 64 intermediate and poorly differentiated neoplasms. *Am J Surg Pathol* 1984;8:405–418.
25. Roth LM, Anderson MC, Govan ADT, et al. Sertoli-Leydig cell tumors: a clinicopathologic study of 34 cases. *Cancer* 1981;48:187–197.
26. Young RH, Scully RE. Well-differentiated ovarian Sertolli-Leydig cell tumors: a clinicopathological analysis of 23 cases. *Int J Gynecol Pathol* 1984;3:277–290.

27. Young RH, Prat J, Scully RE. Ovarian Sertoli-Leydig cell tumors with heterologous elements: I. Gastrointestinal epithelium and carcinoid: a clinicopathologic analysis of thirty-six cases. *Cancer* 1982;50:2448–2456.
28. Prat J, Young RH, Scully RE. Ovarian Sertoli-Leydig cell tumors with heterologous elements: II. Cartilage and skeletal muscle: a clinicopathologic analysis of twelve cases. *Cancer* 1982;50:2465–2475.
29. Young RH, Scully RE. Ovarian Sertoli-Leydig cell tumors with a retiform pattern: a problem in histopathologic diagnosis. A report of 25 cases. *Am J Surg Pathol* 1983; 7:755–771.
30. Gagnon S, Tetu B, Silva EG, McCaughey WTE. Frequency of α-fetoprotein production by Sertoli-Leydig cell tumors of the ovary: an immunohistochemical study of eight cases. *Mod Pathol* 1989;2:63–67.
31. Roth LM, Slayton RE, Brady LW, et al. Retiform differentiation in ovarian Sertoli-Leydig cell tumors: a clinicopathologic study of six cases from a gynecologic oncology study group. *Cancer* 1985;55:1093–1098.
32. Talerman A. Ovarian Sertoli-Leydig cell tumor (androblastoma) with retiform pattern: a clinicopathologic study. *Cancer* 1987;60:3056–3064.
33. Young RH, Prat J, Scully RE. Ovarian endometrioid carcinomas resembling sex cord-stromal tumors: a clinicopathological analysis of 13 cases. *Am J Surg Pathol* 1982; 6:513–522.
34. Roth LM, Liban E, Czemobilsky B. Ovarian endometrioid tumors mimicking Sertoli and Sertoli-Leydig cell tumors: sertoliform variant of endometrioid carcinoma. *Cancer* 1982;50:1322–1331.
35. Bullon A, Arseneau J, Prat J, et al. Tubular Krukenberg tumor: a problem in histopathologic diagnosis. *Am J Surg Pathol* 1981;5:225–232.
36. Scully RE. Sex cord tumor with annular tubules: a distinctive ovarian tumor of the Peutz-Jeghers syndrome. *Cancer* 1970;25:1107–1121.
37. Young RH, Welch WR, Dickersin GR, Scully RE. Ovarian sex cord tumor with annular tubules: review of 74 cases including 27 with Peutz-Jeghers syndrome and 4 with adenoma malignum of the cervix. *Cancer* 1982; 50:1384–1402.
38. Hart WR, Kumar N. Crissman JD. Ovarian neoplasms resembling sex cord tumors with annular tubules. *Cancer* 1980;45:2352–2363.
39. Talerman A, Hughesdon PE, Anderson MC. Diffuse nonlobular ovarian androblastoma usually associated with feminization. *Int J Gynecol Pathol* 1982;1:155–171.
40. Young RH, Dudley AG, Scully RE. Granulosa cell, Sertoli-Leydig cell and unclassified sex cord-stromal tumors associated with pregnancy: a clinicopathological analysis of thirty-six cases. *Gynecol Oncol* 1984;18:181–205.
41. Hayes MC, Scully RE. Ovarian steroid cell tumor (not otherwise specified): a clinicopathological analysis of 63 cases. *Am J Surg Pathol* 1987;11:835–845.
42. Hayes MC, Scully RE. Stromal luteoma of the ovary: a clinicopathological analysis of 25 cases. *Int J Gynecol Pathol* 1987;6:313–321.
43. Paraskevas M, Scully RE. Hilus cell tumor of the ovary: a clinicopathological analysis of 12 Reinke-crystal-positive and 9 crystal-negative cases. *Int J Gynecol Pathol* 1989;3:299–310.
44. Marieb HJ, Spangler S, Kashgarian M, et al. Cushing's syndrome secondary to ectopic cortisol production by an ovarian carcinoma. *J Clin Endocrinol Metab* 1983;57:737–740.
45. Young RH, Scully RE. Ovarian steroid cell tumors associated with Cushing's syndrome: a report of three cases. *Int J Gynecol Pathol* 1987;6:40–48.
46. Young RH, Scully RE. Oxyphilic clear cell carcinoma of the ovary: a report of nine cases. *Am J Surg Pathol* 1987;11: 661–667.

PART III

Clinical Aspects of Ovarian Cancer

8
Epidemiology, Etiology, and Screening of Ovarian Cancer

Katherine Y. Look

EPIDEMIOLOGY

The National Cancer Institute's Surveillance, Epidemiology, and End Results (SEER) program estimated that 25,400 new cases of epithelial ovarian carcinoma occurred in the United States in 1998 and led to 14,500 deaths (1). By 1998 ovarian cancer had become the fifth most common cancer in this country, and it is the fifth most common cause of female cancer deaths, ranking behind lung, colon, breast, and pancreas cancer (1).

The incidence of ovarian epithelial cancer is influenced by country of origin, race, and age. The highest rates are found in industrialized countries, with the exception of Japan, and the lowest rates are seen in the nonindustrialized world (Table 8.1). Based on SEER data from 1973 to 1977, the age-adjusted rate of ovarian cancer for the white population in the United States was 14.2 per 100,000, and for the African-American population it was 9.3 per 100,000 (2). In more recent SEER data from 1988 to 1992, the incidence rates per 100,000 were 15.8 for white Americans, 17.5 for American Indians, and 9.3 for Chinese-Americans (3). In comparison, the rate per 100,000 for European-born Jews is 17.2, and for native-born Japanese in the Fukuoka prefecture it is 3.2 (2). Beral and coworkers (4) postulated that the international differences in average completed family size are the most likely explanation for the variation in incidence rates between industrialized and nonindustrialized nations. After living in the United States for one to two generations, immigrants from low-incidence countries such as Japan develop a risk similar to that of native-born Americans (5). In 1994 the incidence of ovarian cancer in America per 100,000 was 41.4 for women older than 50 years of age, compared with only 5.3 for younger women (6). Dos Santos and Swerdlow (7) postulated that a unifying explanation for the various rates between countries and over time might be secondary to the changes in family size before the introduction of oral contraceptives with their recognized protective effect.

Ovarian cancer *mortality* rates are also influenced by country of origin, race, and age. The age-adjusted mortality rate calculated from 1973–1977 SEER data was 8.7 per 100,000 for the white population in the United States and 6.9 per 100,000 for the African-American population (2). In the 1988–1992 SEER data, the ovarian cancer mortality rate per 100,000 population was 8.1 for whites, 7.3 for American Indians, 4.8 for Hispanics, and 3.4 for Filipinos (3). SEER data from 1997 revealed an overall ovarian cancer mortality ratio of 7.8 per 100,000; however, the rate was 25.5 per 100,000 among women older than 50 years of age and only 1.0 per 100,000 among younger women (6). Beral and coworkers (4) proposed that mean completed family size between birth cohorts and between countries best explains the difference in mortality ratios over time and between different countries (Figure 8.1).

Five-year survival trends for patients with epithelial ovarian cancer have shown some improvement in the last 20 years. SEER data from 1997 show that in the past twenty years overall mortality rates decreased from 8.5 to 7.8 per 100,000 (6). The 5-year relative survival rate for all patients was 37% in 1974–1976 and 50% in 1989–1994, which represents a statistically

TABLE 8.1. Age–standardized average annual incidence rates per 100,000 population for all malignant neoplasms of the ovary, fallopian tube, and broad ligament in selected countries with population-based tumor registries[a]

Population	Incidence
Sweden	14.9
Israel (Jews born in United States or Europe)	14.3
Norway (urban)	14.2
Canada (British Columbia)	13.8
United States (San Francisco Bay area, white)	13.3
New Zealand (Maori)	12.8
United States (Iowa)	12.7
Norway (rural)	12.7
Israel (all Jews)	12.6
United States (Connecticut)	12.2
United States (New Mexico, white)	12.1
United States (Detroit, white)	12.0
German Democratic Republic	11.8
New Zealand (non-Maori)	11.3
Poland (Warsaw City)	11.2
United Kingdom (Birmingham)	11.1
Switzerland	10.6
United States (Detroit, black)	9.9
Canada (Alberta)	9.5
United States (Utah)	9.4
Canada (Quebec)	9.4
Israel (Jews born in Israel)	8.7
United States (San Francisco, black)	8.6
Finland	7.9
United States (New Mexico, American Indian)	7.5
United States (San Francisco, Chinese)	6.7
Brazil (São Paulo)	6.1
Israel (Jews born in Africa or Asia)	5.8
India (Bombay)	4.6
Japan (Miyagi)	2.7

[a] Neoplasms of the fallopian tube and broad ligament are so infrequent that they can be disregarded for statistical purposes. From Lingeman CH: Environmental factors and etiology of carcinoma of the human ovary. *Am J Indust Med* 1983;4:365–379, with permission.

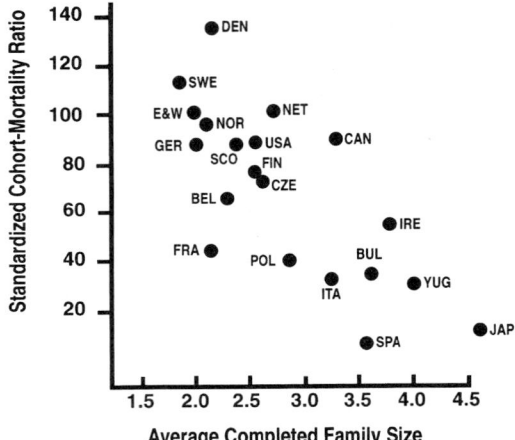

FIG. 8.1. Age-standardized mortality ratio from ovarian cancer plotted against the average completed family size from women in 20 countries whose midyear of birth was 1901. (From Beral V, Fraser P, Chilvers C: Does pregnancy protect against ovarian cancer? *Lancet* 1978;1:1084, with permission.)

significant increase ($p < .05$) (8). When analyzed by race, the 5-year relative survival rates for whites showed the same improvement as that for the overall population; for African-Americans, the rate improved from 41% in 1974–1976 to 46% in 1989–1994, also a statistically significant difference (8). The improvement may be the result of stage migration, with better staging being done, wider availability of aggressive cytoreductive surgery, and introduction of multiagent cytotoxic regimens, including platinum and now paclitaxel. However, most of the 60% of patients diagnosed with advanced-stage disease will experience recurrences, even though the progression-free interval has been lengthened by contemporary cytotoxic regimens. Advanced stage of the disease at the time of diagnosis is associated with cellular mutations leading to drug resistance to current active drugs. Nonmyelosuppressive dose-limiting toxicities that occur with some agents (e.g., cisplatin) used to treat ovarian carcinoma limit any clinically meaningful increase in dose intensity. Further improvement in survival rates may occur as screening methods are developed for the populations thought to be at highest risk for ovarian cancer so that the disease can be discovered when at an early stage and most amenable to cure.

ETIOLOGY

The precise cause of epithelial ovarian carcinoma is not known. However, numerous authors have reported associations between ovarian cancer and environmental factors, including exposure to dietary, viral, and industrial agents. An increased risk of ovarian cancer is seen with particular reproductive history and endocrinologic

TABLE 8.2. *Purported risk factors for the development of ovarian neoplasms*

Risk factor	Reference nos.
Environmental	
Radiation	19, 30
Talc/asbestos exposure	18–22, 24–29
Viral	
Rubella exposure as an adolescent	34
Mumps parotitis	32, 33
Dietary	
Coffee consumption	12, 15, 16
Fat consumption	10–14
Diet low in fiber or vitamin A	17
Reproductive/hormonal	
Nulliparity	26, 34–36, 39
Menopausal estrogen replacement	26, 35, 43–44
Oral contraceptives	26, 40–42
Tubal ligation	45, 46
Hysterectomy	45–47
Genetic familial	
Positive family history	38–43
BRCA1, BRCA2 mutations	58, 60–68
Replication error repair mutations	69, 70

profiles, familial syndromes, and mutations in the tumor suppressor genes BRCA1 and BRCA2 on chromosome 17 and 13, respectively. In addition, there is evidence that some familial clusters of epithelial ovarian cancer may be secondary to mutations in the replication error repair genes of MSH2 and MLH1 on chromosomes 2 and 3. A summary of references for the various risk factors is given in Table 8.2. Daly and Abrams have published a through review of the various factors that are thought to modify lifetime risk for development of ovarian cancer (9).

Dietary Factors

Excessive dietary intake of animal fat or red meat has been reported to increase the risk of epithelial ovarian cancer. Countries such as Sweden, with higher *per capita* animal fat consumption, have a higher incidence of epithelial ovarian malignancy than countries such as Japan and China, which have low *per capita* fat consumption (10–13). Cramer and associates (14) hypothesized that an increased risk for the development of ovarian cancer may be seen in populations that consume a high fat-galactose diet but lack the enzyme galactose-1-phosphate uridyltransferase to break the galactose down to glucose. In these cases, the ovary is exposed over a long period to increased concentrations of galactose.

Conflicting reports exist in the literature regarding the increased risk of ovarian cancer that has been correlated with coffee consumption. An early report by Stocks (15) suggested a link, based on the observation that Swedes, with the highest *per capita* coffee consumption in the world, have the highest rates of incidence and mortality from ovarian cancer. Trichopoulos and associates (16), in a case-control study, noted that patients with ovarian cancer consumed more coffee than did matched controls. However, a later report by Cramer and colleagues (12) was unable to confirm any association between coffee consumption and the risk of ovarian carcinoma. Byers and associates (17) also failed to find a significant increase in risk associated with coffee consumption in their case-control study, but they did report an increased risk in the group that consumed diets low in fiber and vitamin A. Vitamin A may offer a protective effect because of its antioxidant mechanism, which prevents the formation of free radicals that might initiate DNA damage. Vitamin A is also useful in the maintenance of normal cellular differentiation (17).

Industrial Agents

Asbestos and the related compound talc (hydrous magnesium trisilicate) have been implicated as possible causative agents for epithelial ovarian/peritoneal neoplasms. In 1960, Keal (18) noted an excess of abdominal neoplasms and/or carcinomatosis peritoneii that histologically resembled epithelial ovarian cancer in women with significant occupational exposure to asbestos. This observation was later confirmed by Newhouse and coworkers (19). Laboratory investigations undertaken by Graham and Graham (20) and later by Henderson and associates (21) revealed that atypical ovarian epithelial changes can be incited in guinea pigs and rabbits exposed to asbestos, and talc particles can be found in the epithelium of normal, cystic, and malignant ovaries. The work of Longo and Young (22) supported a causative role for talc. They hypothesized that talc could be introduced into the upper genital tract in the presence of patent fallopian tubes if it were used as a dusting powder on diaphragms or sanitary napkins. Using technetium Tc 99m–labeled human albumin microspheres, Venter (23) demonstrated that the upward migration of particles placed in the lower genital tract enabled them to reach the ovarian epithelium. In a case-control study, Cramer and colleagues (24) noted a relative risk of 1.9 associated with the use of talc on the perineum or on sanitary napkins. A more recent report by Cook and colleagues (25) found a similar relative risk of 1.6 (95% confidence interval [CI], 1.1 to 2.3) for the development of ovarian cancer in women who performed perineal dusting with talcum powder compared with those without such exposure. Purdie and coworkers (26) also were able to find a positive association between use of talc and the risk of ovarian cancer in an Australian case-control study. The causative role of asbestos and talc is not universally accepted, because other reports have failed to find any increased risk of ovarian cancer associated with the use of talc (27–29).

Radiation

Case-control studies have provided conflicting data regarding radiation exposure and the risk of subsequent ovarian cancer. Annegers and associates (30) noted a relative risk of 1.8 associated with radiation exposure. However, Newhouse and coworkers (19) did not find such an association.

Viruses

The role of viruses as putative causative agents in epithelial ovarian cancer has been debated. West (31) noted that patients with ovarian cancer are less likely to have a history of mumps parotitis and theorized that the mumps virus may be protective. Two subsequent analyses, however, reported that ovarian cancer patients may have had subclinical mumps; they had less clear recall of mumps infection and lower complement fixation titers (32,33). Both of these reports postulated that exposure to the mumps virus might be associated with subsequent development of ovarian cancer. The suggestions were that the virus might cause oocyte depletion in the gonad or altered immunocompetence, followed by early ovarian failure with an associated elevation of gonadotropins that could stimulate epithelial proliferation and lead to malignancy (32,33).

The possible roles of other viruses in the development of ovarian carcinoma have prompted an occasional report. Peripubertal rubella infection has been cited as a risk factor (34). McGowan and coworkers (34) also noted that patients with ovarian cancer have had fewer bouts of influenza.

As can be seen, the reports in the literature do not agree about the roles of various environmental agents as definitive causative factors for epithelial ovarian cancer.

Reproductive, Hormonal, and Endocrinologic Factors

In contrast, most opinions are in accord regarding the reproductive profile of women at high risk for this disease. Three analyses, dating from 1974 to 1981, independently reported that women with a history of involuntary infertility or low parity had an increased risk of epithelial ovary cancer (34–36). This association with infertility was confirmed in two more recent studies by Mosgaard and associates (37,38), which reported odds ratios of 2.7 and 1.9 when comparing infertile women with parous women. Furthermore, these authors were unable to detect any further increase in risk with exposure to ovulation induction agents. Rather, it was the nulliparity that conferred the increased risk. The odds ratio of ovarian cancer was 0.8 among treated nulliparous women (95% CI, 0.4 to 2.0) compared with nontreated nulliparous women (37). Conversely, the protective effect of increasing parity was confirmed in two studies, one from Australia and the other from Norway (26,39). Other risk factors related to reproductive issues that were identified in these early reports include late menopause, prolonged ovulatory age, increased number of spontaneous abortions, and severe premenstrual symptomatology (34–36).

Hildreth and coworkers (35) also reported that postmenopausal hormonal replacement does not increase the risk of ovarian cancer and that the use of oral contraceptive pills halves the risk of this disease. Subsequent reports confirmed that the use of oral contraceptives is associated with a significantly decreased risk of ovarian carcinoma (26,40–42). The safety of menopausal hormonal replacement has been contested. Some authors have noted an increased risk of ovarian carcinoma in patients who use cyclic stilbestrol or estrogen during menopause (43,44). Neither Purdie et al. (26) nor Hildreth et al. (35) was able to confirm any increased risk with the use of menopausal estrogen replacement. The protective effect of prior tubal ligation, with odds ratios of 0.72 (95% CI, 0.48 to 1.08) and 0.69 (95% CI, 0.46 to 0.85), has been reported by groups working in Australia and in America (45,46). The Australian and American investigators also reported that hysterectomy was associated with a decreased risk of ovarian cancer, with odds ratios noted of 0.64 (95% CI, 0.48 to 0.95) and 0.58 (95% CI, 0.26 to 1.27) (45,46). In addition, Loft and colleagues (47) reported, based on the largest experience from the Danish registry, that hysterectomy conferred a protective effect with an odds ratio of 0.78 (95% CI, 0.60 to 0.96) and further noted that the protective effects diminished with the passage of time.

Genetic-Familial Ovarian Cancer Syndromes

Genetic components have been recognized as influential in the risk of ovarian cancer. An increased frequency of nonepithelial tumors is seen in several syndromes, including fibromas in basal cell nevus syndrome (48), granulosa cell tumors and serous cystadenomas in Peutz-Jeghers syndrome (49), and gonadoblastomas and dysgerminomas in patients with gonadal dysgenesis (50). Before the molecular techniques existed to allow precise "dissection" of the human genome, familial clusters of epithelial ovarian cancer were recognized and implied that there might be a genetic component. McGowan (34) and Hildreth (35) and their associates noted a strong correlation between family history of a gynecologic malignancy, either ovarian or endometrial, and later development of ovarian cancer. Hildreth's group estimated the odds ratio for development of ovarian cancer among patients with a positive family history to be 18 (95% CI, 4.8 to 69), compared with patients with a negative family history (35). Schildkraut and Thompson (51) reported the experience of the Centers for Disease Control and Prevention and the National Cancer Institute in a population-based case-control study, noting that the odds ratios for ovarian cancer in first- and second-degree relatives were 3.6 (95% CI, 1.8 to 7.1) and 2.9 (95% CI, 1.6 to 5.3), respectively, compared with the odds for women with no familial history of ovarian carcinoma (51).

Piver and colleagues (52) noted that only five familial clusters of epithelial ovarian carcinoma were reported before 1970. After that date, several institutions began describing families with multiple members affected with epithelial ovarian cancers (53–55). Piver and coworkers (56) established the Familial Ovarian Cancer Registry at Roswell Park Memorial Institute in 1981, and by 1998 it had recorded 1,451 families with two or more close relatives with ovarian cancer (56). Piver's group stated that analysis of the available pedigrees supported an autosomal dominant pattern of inheritance with variable penetrance, with some pedigree members having an approximately 50% chance of developing ovarian cancer (51). Lynch and colleagues (57) reported the existence of the site-specific ovarian cancer syndrome, the breast ovarian cancer syndrome, and the Lynch II syndrome. These three familial syndromes are associated with a significantly earlier onset of disease than is usually seen in patients with negative family histories.

The increasing sophistication of molecular biology techniques such as positional cloning revolutionized the understanding of hereditary ovarian carcinoma syndromes when in 1994 the BRCA1 gene was located on the long arm of chromosome 17 in families with susceptibilities to breast and ovarian cancer (58). Sharan and coworkers (59) hypothesized that mutations in BRCA1, as well as the later recognized BRCA2 on chromosome 13, lead to impaired ability to repair double-stranded DNA breaks, resulting in increased susceptibility to breast and ovarian cancer.

TABLE 8.3. *Modeled probabilities that women with breast cancer before 50 years of age carry a mutation in BRCA1 or BRCA2*

Any relative with BrCa at <50 y	Any relative with OvCa	Proband bilateral BrCa or OvCa	Proband with BrCa at <40 y	Modeled probability of mutation in BRCA1 (%)	Modeled probability of mutation in BRCA2 (%)	Modeled probability of mutation in BRCA1 or BRAC2 (%)
•				10.1	14.5	25
•			•	28.2	11.6	40
•		•	•	41.5	9.5	51
•	•	•	•	71.1	4.7	76
		•		22.9	12.5	35
		•	•	22.9	12.5	35
	•	•		65.0	5.7	71
	•	•	•	65.0	5.7	71
•	•			22.9	12.5	35
•	•		•	50.9	7.9	59
•	•	•		65.0	5.7	71
•	•	•	•	86.7	2.2	89

BrCa, breast cancer; OvCa, ovarian cancer.
From Frank TS, Manley SA: Correlation of mutations with family history and ovarian cancer risk. *J Clin Oncol* 1998;16:2423, with permission.

Approximately 10% of ovarian cancers are thought to be caused by mutations in BRCA1 and BRCA2 (60). Each offspring has a 50% chance to inherit the mutation from an affected parent; however, for as yet incompletely understood reasons, the gene is variably penetrant, with some mutations resulting in ovarian cancer–dominated family clusters and others in breast cancer–dominated family clusters.

In early linkage studies (61) with highly penetrant mutations it was estimated that there was 44% risk for development of epithelial ovarian cancer by 70 years of age. In more recent studies of less penetrant mutations, which are likely to be more reflective of the "average" risk associated with BRCA1 mutations, the risk before 70 years of age was estimated to be 28% by Whittemore and colleagues (62) and 16% by Streuwing and associates (63). Ford and associates (64) reported that the risk of developing ovarian cancer before age 70 associated with BRCA2 mutations is 27%. Data have also been generated that examine the question of whether a family carries the mutation based on the age at onset of breast and/or ovarian carcinoma in the family. Frank and Manley (65) reported a 40% chance of a BRCA1 or BRCA2 mutation if the proband had breast cancer before 40 years of age and there was a family history of breast cancer among women younger than 50 years; however, in families with a proband with breast cancer before age 40, bilateral breast or ovarian cancer, and a family history of breast and ovarian cancer, the risk of mutation was as high at 89% (Table 8.3). They suggested that anyone diagnosed with breast cancer before age 50 or with ovarian cancer should inquire of other family members whether similar events have occurred. In those families with breast *and* ovarian cancer, the potential to find a BRCA1 or BRCA2 mutation is great enough to merit consideration of evaluation for the same (65). The likelihood that a BRCA1 mutation will be found is influenced by the nature of the cancer cluster noted within the clinic families, ranging from 7% if only breast cancer is noted, to 13% if there is early-onset breast cancer (before 40 years of age), to 40% if both ovarian and breast cancer are found within the family (66). Newman and colleagues (67) reported that the risk of finding a BRCA1 mutation was 23% if only ovarian cancer was extant within the family, 13% if at least four breast cancer cases were noted, and 33% if both breast and ovarian cancer were present within the family. The clinical and pathologic features of the epithelial ovarian carcinomas associated with these BRCA1 mutations include a predominance of papillary serous cell type and a longer median survival that compared with those without BRCA1 mutations (68). However, this observation has been questioned by others, who believe that the survival differences may be secondary to degree of residual cancer, percentage of patients optimally debulked, and better surveillance because of heightened awareness of the entity within these patients, who may then gravitate to centers with special expertise in ovarian carcinoma.

Boyd (69) reported that approximately 3% of hereditary ovarian carcinomas are caused by mutations in the mismatch repair mechanisms located on the hMSH2 and hMLH1 genes on short arms of chromosomes 2 and 3, respectively. These mutations are more widely associated with hereditary non-polyposis colon cancer (HNPCC), but the affected kindreds have an increased risk of endometrial, upper urologic tract, and ovarian cancer in addition to colon cancer (70).

Clinicians faced with patients at increased risk for epithelial ovarian carcinoma have long recognized that patients seek opinions as to what they can do to minimize or eliminate their risk. Narod and associates (71) reported in a case-control study that any past use of oral contraceptives decreased the risk of developing ovarian cancer by half in women from families with hereditary ovarian cancer syndromes. The number of life years added in these hereditary kindreds by prophylactic oophorectomy was estimated to be 0.3 to 1.7 years by Schrag and coworkers (72) and 0.4 to 2.6 years by Grann and colleagues (73). However, several authors (74,75) have reported peritoneal carcinomatosis in 2% to 10% of patients after prophylactic oophorectomy. Not all geneticists support the recommendation of prophylactic surgery, but they may hold it out as an option for patients after completion of childbearing (76). In addition to its potential to greatly reduce the risk of ovarian cancer in BRCA1 families, there is now evidence that prophylactic oophorectomy significantly reduces the risk of breast cancer in these families, to a hazard ratio of 0.53 (95% CI, 0.33 to 0.84), and even lower to 0.28 (95% CI, 0.08 to 0.94) in those monitored for 5 to 10 years (77). This protective effect, given the perceived cosmetic impact of choosing between prophylactic mastectomy and prophylactic oophorectomy, may make the latter operation, after childbearing is completed, relatively more attractive to some patients in an era when the oophorectomy may be undertaken with minimally invasive surgical technology.

The implications that these recognized hereditary BRCA1, BRCA2, and HNPCC syndromes have for screening are addressed later in this chapter

PATHOGENESIS

Despite the lack of evidence for a single causative agent in epithelial ovarian carcinoma, circumstantial evidence suggested by the reproductive profile of women at highest risk indicates that repetitive ovulation is involved in the pathophysiology of the disease. The fact that pregnancy and the use of the oral contraceptive pill seem to have a protective effect is further evidence that persistent ovulation is involved in the development of ovarian cancer (34–36,40–42). In 1971, Fathalla (78) first proposed that repeated, purposeless ovulation might lead to minor trauma of the surface epithelium, which would then be exposed to the high estrogen content of the follicular fluid which had been shown to induce mitoses and proliferation in rats and mice. Cramer and Welch (79) postulated that the physiologic states that lead to elevated gonadotropin secretion (e.g., radiation, exposure to toxic chemicals or metabolites, mumps) may cause stromal proliferation and increased steroid production, which in turn would act to stimulate the entrapped epithelium seen with incessant ovulation (79). In addition to the incessant ovulation and elevated gonadotropin, Joly and associates (36) proposed that a third factor indirectly associated with infertility might contribute to the development of ovarian cancer. They cited the observation that married nulligravidas have a higher risk of ovarian carcinoma than single nulligravidas. Both populations might theoretically ovulate incessantly. However, in the married population, with its presumed repetitive exposure to pregnancy risk, involuntary infertility is a likely explanation for the lack of pregnancy in some cases. More recently, elegant work by Schildkraut and Berchuck (80) showed that the duration of "ovulatory life" is associated with an increase in p53 mutations, suggesting that the more opportunities there are to require postovulation proliferative repair of the ovarian epithelium, the greater the chance of a p53 mutation which might act as a first or second "hit" and lead to the eventual malignant phenotype.

SCREENING

As surgical staging has improved, the 5-year survival rate for patients with stage I disease (confined to the ovary) has been shown to be greater than 90% (81). However, for the great majority of patients who present with advanced stage III and IV disease, survival to 5 years remains disappointingly low, 15% to 20%, despite the use of aggressive cytoreductive surgery, multiagent cisplatin-based chemotherapy, and salvage therapy (82). The identification of a subset of patients thought to have highly curable disease has intensified the search for an appropriate screening strategy to identify early-stage disease.

Before the use of ideal surgical staging and ultrasonography, patients with the findings of ascites or large abdominal pelvic masses were recognized as being unlikely to do well. Many clinicians advocated a high index of suspicion and recommended pelvic examinations, including thorough assessment of the rectovaginal septum for the presence of nodularity (83). However, it has since been estimated that the finding of one truly asymptomatic ovarian carcinoma would necessitate as many as 10,000 bimanual examinations (84). Piver and Barlow (85), reporting the Roswell Park Memorial Institute experience, found that only 15% of patients with ovarian cancer were diagnosed at the time of a routine pelvic examination. Earlier, Graham and coworkers (86) had proposed that, because of the frequent finding of malignant cytology in ascites fluid, it might be possible to detect ovarian carcinoma before the development of a palpable mass by screening patients with routine culdocentesis and cytology. They reported 8 positive specimens in a series of 576 volunteers and claimed that a 70% satisfactory specimen yield could be achieved. Subsequent work by McGowan (87) and Funkhouser (88) and their associates refuted the routine use of culdocentesis cytology as a screening tool on the basis of very low yield of suspicious specimens, a high percentage of unsatisfactory specimens, and low patient acceptance of the invasive technique.

Realizing the limitations of bimanual examinations and cul-de-sac aspiration, investigators continued to look for other screening modalities. Serum markers with acknowledged usefulness in other malignancies—including α-fetoprotein, carcinoembryonic antigen, human chorionic antigen, and human placental lactogen—were evaluated as possible screening tests for epithelial carcinoma. However, all lacked sufficient specificity and/or failed to reflect stage or volume of disease (89–91). The refinement of protein purification and radioimmunoassay technology led to the development of new serum markers, such as the ovarian cancer antigen (OCA), which was proposed as a possible screening tool because of its elevation in approximately 75% of cases of stage I or stage II disease (92). Knauf and Urbach (92), the developers of OCA, acknowledged that a limitation of this marker was its failure to reflect volume of disease.

A breakthrough occurred in 1983, when Bast and associates reported on an immunoradiometric assay using a monoclonal antibody that recognized the müllerian-derived glycoprotein antigen designated CA 125. This marker is elevated in more than 80% of nonmucinous ovarian epithelial cancers, 30% of nonovarian malignancies, 6% of benign gynecologic disorders, and only 1% of normal cases (93). The majority of benign conditions that cause elevation of CA 125 include pregnancy, ovarian cysts, uterine leiomyomas, pelvic inflammatory disease, endometriosis, and menstruation. Because these conditions occur predominately in premenopausal women, CA 125 levels may be most useful in screening for ovarian cancer in the postmenopausal population (94). Jacobs and colleagues (94) reported on the use of CA 125 serum level as a screening test in 1,010 postmenopausal women and noted the detection of 1 malignancy. The sensitivity of the CA 125 assay was 100% and the specificity as 94.3%, but the predictive value of a positive result was only 1.72% (94). More recently, Jeyarajah and others (95) reported that asymptomatic postmenopausal women with a CA 125 concentration of 30 U/ml or higher had an odds ratio of 30.09 (95% CI, 4.0 to 221.59) for development of a subsequent gynecologic cancer. Einhorn and associates (96) used sequential serum CA 125 measurements in a population of 5,550 Swedish women older than 40 years of age in conjunction with pelvic examinations and transabdominal ultrasonography. They reported detection of six of nine malignancies in women older than 50 years of age but none of the three malignancies in women younger than 50. The sensitivity was 50%, the specificity was 96%, and the predictive value of a positive result was 3.43% (96). As can be seen in these two large, prospective studies of older women, serum CA 125 levels alone or in conjunction with transabdominal ultrasonography have such low positive predictive values that such a strategy is not practical for widespread screening. Too many women with nonmalignant disease would be subjected to the morbidity and possible mortality of invasive procedures, with very few benefiting from the removal of an early-stage ovarian cancer.

Concomitant with the development of serum markers, clinicians have sought radiologic means of assessing pelvic masses for malignancy. In the mid-1970s, transabdominal ultrasonography was found to be useful in discriminating between solid and cystic masses, in identifying papillary projections in otherwise cystic masses, and for guidance of needle biopsies of suspected metastases (97,98). Bowel gas or intestinal peristalsis sometimes interfered with interpretation of ultrasound images. Schaner and associates (99) reported on a series of 600 abdominal-thoracic malignancies that were assessed by computed axial tomography (CAT) scanning for the presence of hepatic, pulmonary, subcutaneous, and retroperitoneal metastases. The results were of sufficient accuracy that preoperative assessment with CAT scans became widespread. Lymphangiography has also been used to evaluate nodal involvement in cases of epithelial ovarian malignancy, with an overall accuracy of 91% in the assessment of enlarged nodes (100). Neither CAT scan imaging nor lymphangiography is ideally suited to screening in an asymptomatic population, because of the expense and the degree of invasiveness of the latter. Early use of ultrasound technology was limited to the evaluation of palpable masses, and it was not employed as a true screening tool. Finkler and coworkers (101) noted that in a symptomatic menopausal population the combination of ultrasonography and CA-125 measurement had great potential in the triage of women with pelvic masses to surgeons with expertise in malignant ovarian disease; in their series, the predictive value of a positive or negative result was 100% in the menopausal group. More recently, DePriest and colleagues (1994) used ultrasonographic characteristics to determine which masses were most likely to represent malignancy; they developed sufficient expertise with their morphometric index so that a predictive value of 45% was reached among menopausal patients with a score greater than, whereas none of these patients was found to have malignant disease if the index was less than 5 (102).

In the early 1980s, preliminary investigations were undertaken to determine whether transabdominal ultrasonography might offer sufficient sensitivity to quantify ovarian volume and/or detect subtle changes in ovarian morphology in patients before the onset of symptoms. Campbell and associates (103) described ultrasound volumetric assessment of the ovaries in climacteric patients who underwent laparotomy the following day, reporting a 97% correlation coefficient between volumes measured by ultrasound and those measured at the time of laparotomy. In addition, they were able to image 26 (84%) of 31 ovaries in these postmenopausal patients, suggesting that real-time sector scanning is accurate and reliable. The investigators stated that an ovary with twice the mean volume of the contralateral ovary should be regarded as suspicious and subjected to further evaluation (103).

In the middle to late 1980s, placement of a specialized transducer within the vaginal vault was shown to allow closer approximation to the ovaries than transabdominal scanning and to produce superior images (104). Rodriguez and associates (105) reported that 82% of postmenopausal ovaries were visualized, with 90% sensitivity and 100% specificity in the assessment of characteristics suggestive of malignancy. The technology appeared to be of sufficient accuracy and reliability for office use. In a large retrospective study, Granberg and colleagues (106) compared ovarian histologies found at laparotomy with preoperative transvaginal ultrasound characteristics and reported that the risk of malignancy was 0.3% in unilocular cysts, 2% in unilocular solid masses, 8% in multilocular cysts, and 66% in multilocular solid tumors. Masses of less than 5 cm had only a 6.9% chance of being malignant; the risk increased to 63% for masses larger than 10 cm (106). A weakness of the Granberg study was that more than 30% of the patients were younger than 40 years of age, representing a population that most investigators believe is unlikely to be screened in a cost-effective manner by any modality, given the low risk of ovarian cancer in premenopausal patients who are without any family history of ovarian cancer.

Higgins and colleagues (107) studied 506 asymptomatic women more than 40 years old and found that 85% of the postmenopausal patients' ovaries were identified. The use of the prolate ellipsoidal formula (width × height × thickness × 0.523) to calculate ovarian volume was proposed. They cited 18 cm^3 as the upper limit of normal size for premenopausal ovaries, and 8 cm^3 as the upper limit for postmenopausal ovaries, and reported that the incidence of abnormal scans was 2.4% (12/506). 10 of the 12 patients with abnormal scans agreed to laparotomy, and one was found to have a malignancy, a metastatic colon cancer (107). DePriest and coworkers (108), using the same criteria as in Higgins' earlier study, expanded the series and reported on the screening of 6,470 postmenopausal asymptomatic women. Ninety women (1.4%) had persistently abnormal scans and underwent surgery. Surgical findings included 37 serous cystadenomas, and 6 invasive ovarian cancers, including 5 that were stage IA; with 17,000 screened women-years, there were no deaths from ovarian cancer (108). As of 1999, with 12 years of experience, the University of Kentucky has screened 14,469 asymptomatic women [46,113 women-years] and explored 180 women with persistent ultrasound abnormalities, detecting 17 ovarian cancers (109). Of the 17 cancers detected, 14 were stage I–II, and all of these patients remained alive at a median of 4.5 years of follow-up. Three patients were found to have stage III disease, and two died of their disease. There were four false-negative scans in that four patients went on to develop ovary cancer within 12 months of a negative scan, and another four developed ovarian cancer more than 12 months since the last scan. The sensitivity was 81%, specificity 98.9%, positive predictive value 9.4%, and negative predictive value 99.97%. Of the patients in whom ovarian cancer was detected, 88% remained alive at 5 years, suggesting that such a screening strategy might decrease case-specific ovary cancer mortality (109).

Currently, Van Nagell and associates at the University of Kentucky are using transvaginal sonography in conjunction with serum CA 125 to screen women thought to be at significant risk for epithelial ovarian carcinoma, including postmenopausal women older than 50 years of age and women older than 25 years who have two relatives with a history of an epithelial ovarian malignancy. Their proposed algorithm is shown in Figure 8.2 (118).

Willson (110) pointed out that widespread population-based screening of even 50% of postmenopausal women would generate charges of 2.7 million dollars for every ovarian cancer that is found. This cannot be considered cost-effective. Sparks and Varner (111) reviewed the advances in sonographic imaging and serum markers and suggested that, in postmenopausal women, simple cysts with a diameter of less than 5 cm or a volume less than or equal to 8 cm^3 on transvaginal sonography should be clinically monitored, whereas surgical evaluation would be appropriate for masses of greater volume, masses of a complex nature, or masses associated with an increased CA 125 concentration. Transvaginal sonography should be considered as a screening tool for postmenopausal women whose pelvic examination is compromised by obesity or who have a family history of ovarian cancer (111).

In 1994 the National Institutes of Health Consensus Development Conference came out against a role for routine population-based screening, fearing that the lack of specificity

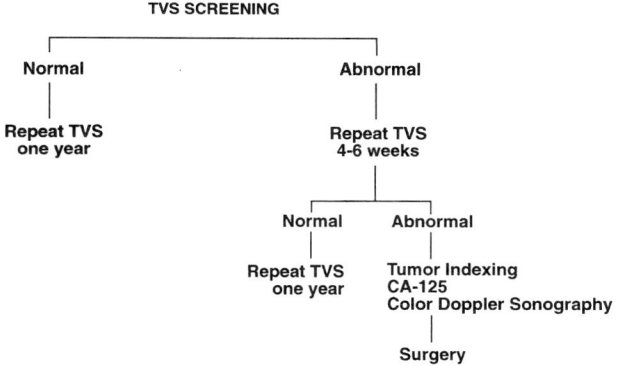

FIG. 8.2. Screening algorithm. To be used in women older than 50 years of age and women older than 30 years who have a family history with at least two relatives with epithelial ovarian cancer. TVS, transvaginal sonography (From DePriest PD, Gallion HH, Pavlik EJ, et al: Transvaginal sonography as a screening method for the detection of early ovarian cancer. *Gynecol Oncol* 1997;65: 409, with permission.)

of CA 125 and transvaginal sonography would lead to unnecessary surgery given the low prevalence of epithelial ovarian carcinoma in the general population; however, they did note that for patients with apparent familial ovarian cancer there might be a role for screening (112). Since that conference the BRCA1 and BRCA2 mutations were recognized (58), and in certain patients with recognized mutations who are unwilling to undergo prophylactic surgery or have not yet completed their families there is a role for screening (76). Although this development may have identified a population most likely to benefit from screening given its increased risk of ovarian cancer, it has raised new dilemmas as to who should be offered the screening. The American Society of Clinical Oncology has suggested that genetic susceptibility testing be offered only (a) to those women with a strong family history or very early age at onset, (b) at a location where the test can be interpreted correctly, and (c) when the results will influence management (113). Given the potential of insurance discrimination, employment discrimination, and psychologic vulnerability with mood disorder manifesting (114), testing should not be undertaken in the absence of rigorous informed consent procedures (115,116).

Van Nagell has proposed a prospective, randomized, controlled trial evaluating the utility of transvaginal sonography in combination with CA 125, compared with annual pelvic examination, to determine whether early-stage disease can be reliably identified in a population-based series of menopausal women. Such a study, if it accrued the expected 142,000 participants, would have a 99% power to determine whether screening can increase the percentage of ovarian cancers found in stage I from the current 20% to 80%, thereby cutting mortality from this disease in half (Van Nagell, personal communication). As of 1999 the National Cancer Institute's Prostate, Lung, Colon and Ovary (PLCO) screening trial has accrued 136,000 patients and is expected to complete accrual in 2001 (Gohagan and Trimble, personal communication, 2000).

Innovative strategies to improve the diagnosis of this epithelial ovarian cancer should be welcomed and supported by all who have ever cared for women with ovarian carcinoma.

REFERENCES

1. Landis SH, Murray T, Bolden S, Wingo P. Cancer statistics 1998. *CA Cancer J Clin* 1998;48:6–30.
2. Roush GC, Holford TR, Schymura MJ, White C. *Cancer risk and incidence trends: the Connecticut perspective.* New York: Hemisphere, 1987.
3. Parker SL, Davis KJ, Wingo PA, et al. Cancer statistics by race and ethnicity: Cancer statistics 1998. *CA Cancer J Clin* 1998;48:31–48.
4. Beral V, Fraser P, Chilvers C. Does pregnancy protect against ovarian cancer? *Lancet* 1978;1:1083–1087.
5. Buell P, Dunn JE. Cancer mortality among the Japanese Issei and Nisei of California. *Cancer* 1965;18:656–664.
6. Ries LAG, Kosary CL, Hankey BF, et al., eds. *Cancer statistics review 1973–1994.* National Institutes of Health Publication No. 97-2789. Bethesda, MD: National Cancer Institute, 1997:370.
7. Dos Santos SI, Swerdlow AJ. Recent trends in incidence and mortality from breast, ovarian and endometrial cancers in England and Wales and their relation to changing fertility and oral contraceptive use. *Br J Cancer* 1995;72:485–492.

8. Ries LAG, Kosary CL, Hankey BF, et al., eds. Cancer statistics review, 1973–1995. National Institutes of Health Publication No. 98-xxx. Bethesda MD: National Cancer Institute, 1998.
9. Daly M, Obrams GI. Epidemiology and risk assessment for ovarian cancer. Semin Oncol 1998;25:255–264.
10. Waterhouse J, et al. Cancer incidence in five continents, vol 3. Lyons: International Agency for Research on Cancer, 1976:453–485.
11. Li FP, Shiang EL. Cancer mortality in China. J Natl Cancer Inst 1980;65:217–221.
12. Cramer DW, Welch WR, Hutchinson GB, et al. Dietary animal fat in relation to ovarian cancer risk. Obstet Gynecol 1984;63:833–837.
13. Rose DP, Boyar AP, Wynder EL. International comparisons of mortality rates for cancer of the breast, ovary, prostate, and colon and per capita food consumption. Cancer 1986;58:2363–2371.
14. Cramer DW, Harlow BL, Willett WC, et al. Galactose consumption and metabolism in relation to the risk of ovarian cancer. Lancet 1989;2:66–71.
15. Stocks P. Cancer mortality in relation to national consumption of cigarettes, solid fuel, tea and coffee. Br J Cancer 1970;24:215–225.
16. Trichopoulos D, Papapostolou M, Polychronopoulou A. Coffee and ovarian cancer. Int J Cancer 1981;28:691–693.
17. Byers T, Marshall J, Graham S, et al. A case-control study of dietary and nondietary factors in ovarian cancer. J Natl Cancer Inst 1983;71:681–686.
18. Keal EE. Asbestosis and abdominal neoplasms. Lancet 1960;2:1211–1216.
19. Newhouse ML, Pearson RM, Fullerton JM, et al. A case control study of the ovary. Br J Prev Soc Med 1977;31:148–153.
20. Graham J, Graham R. Ovarian cancer and asbestos. Environ Res 1967;1:115–128.
21. Henderson WJ, Hamilton TC, Griffiths K. Talc in normal and malignant ovarian tissue. Lancet 1979;1:499.
22. Longo DL, Young RC. Cosmetic talc and ovarian cancer. Lancet 1979;2:349–351.
23. Venter PF. Ovarian epithelial cancer and chemical carcinogenesis. Gynecol Oncol 1981;12:281–285.
24. Cramer DW, Welch WR, Scully RE, Wojciechowski CA. Ovarian cancer and talc: a case control study. Cancer 1982;50: 372–376.
25. Cook LS, Kamb ML, Weiss NS. Perineal powder exposure and the risk of ovarian cancer. Am J Epidemiol 1997;145:459–465.
26. Purdie D, Green A, Bain C, et al. Reproductive and other factors and risk of epithelial ovarian cancer: an Australian case-control study. Survey of Women's Health Study Group. Int J Cancer 1995;62:678–684.
27. Hartge P, Hoover R, Lesher LP, McGowan L. Talc and ovarian cancer. JAMA 1983;250:1844.
28. Roe FJ. Controversy: cosmetic talc and ovarian cancer. Lancet 1979;2:744.
29. Whittemore AS, Wu ML, Paffenbarger RS Jr, et al. Personal and environmental characteristics related to epithelial ovarian cancer: II. Exposure to talcum powder, tobacco, alcohol, and coffee. Am J Epidemiol 1988;128:1228–1240.
30. Annegers JF, Strom DH, Decker DG, et al. Ovarian cancer incidence and case control study. Cancer 1979; 43:723–729.

31. West TO. Epidemiologic study of malignancies of the ovaries. Cancer 1966;19:1001–1007.
32. Menczer J, Modan M, Ranon L, Golan A. Possible role of mumps virus in the etiology of ovarian cancer. Cancer 1979;43:1375–1379.
33. Cramer DW, Welch WR, Cassels S, Scully RE. Mumps, menarche, menopause and ovarian cancer. Am J Obstet Gynecol 1983;147:1–6.
34. McGowan L, Parent L, Lednur W, Norris HJ. The woman at risk for developing ovarian cancer. Gynecol Oncol 1979;7:325–344.
35. Hildreth NG, Kelsey JL, LiVolsi VA, et al. An epidemiologic study of ovarian carcinoma of the ovary. Am J Epidemiol 1981;114:398–405.
36. Joly DJ, Lilienfeld AM, Diamond EL, Bross AD. An epidemiologic study of the relationship of reproductive experience to cancer of the ovary. Am J Epidemiol 1974;99:190–209.
37. Mosgaard BJ, Lidegaard O, Kjaer SK, et al. Infertility, fertility drugs, and invasive ovarian cancer: a case-control study. Fertil Steril 1997;67:1005–1012.
38. Mosgaard BJ, Lidegaard O, Kjaer SK, et al. Ovarian stimulation and borderline ovarian tumors: a case-control study. Fertil Steril 1998;70:1049–1055.
39. Albrektsen G, Heuch I, Kvale G. Reproductive factors and incidence of epithelial ovarian cancer: a Norwegian prospective study. Cancer Causes Control 1996;7:421–427.
40. Centers for Disease Control: Cancer and steroid hormone study: oral contraceptive use and the risk of ovarian cancer. JAMA 1983;249:1596–1599.
41. Rosenbergh L, Shapiro S, Slone D, et al. Epithelial ovarian cancer and combination oral contraceptives. JAMA 1982;247:3210–3212.
42. Risch HA, Weiss NS, Lyon JL, et al. Events of reproductive life and the incidence of epithelial ovarian cancer. Am J Epidemiol 1983;117:128–139.
43. Hoover R, Gray LA, Fraumeni JF. Stilbestrol (diethylstilbestrol) and the risk of ovarian cancer. Lancet 1977;2:533–534.
44. Cramer DW, Hutchinson GB, Welch WR, et al. Determinants of ovarian cancer risk: I. Reproductive experience and family history. J Natl Cancer Inst 1983; 71:711–716.
45. Green A, Purdie D, Bain C, et al. Tubal sterilisation, hysterectomy and decreased risk of ovarian cancer. Survey of Women's Health Study Group. Int J Cancer 1997;71:948–951.
46. Rosenblatt KA, Thomas DB. Reduced risk of ovarian cancer in women with a tubal ligation or hysterectomy. The World Health Organization Collaborative study of Neoplasia and Steroid Contraceptives. Cancer Epidemiol Biomarkers Prev 1996;5:933–935.
47. Loft A, Lidegaard O, Tabor A. Incidence of ovarian cancer after hysterectomy: a nationwide controlled follow up. Br J Obstet Gynaecol 1997;104:1296–1301.
48. Berlin NI, Van Scott EJ, Clendenning WE, et al. Basal cell nevus syndrome: combined clinical staff conference at the National Institutes of Health. Ann Intern Med 1966;64:403–421.
49. Dozois RR, Kempers RD, Dahlin RC, Bartholomeew LG. Ovarian tumors associated with the Peutz-Jeghers syndrome. Ann Surg 1970;172:233–238.
50. Troche V, Hernandez E. Neoplasia arising in dysgenetic gonads. Obstet Gynecol Surv 1986;41:74–79.

51. Schildkraut JM, Thompson WD. Familial ovarian cancer: a population-based case-control study. *Am J Epidemiol* 1988;128:456–466.
52. Piver MS, Baker TS, Piedmonte M, Sandecki AM. Epidemiology and etiology of ovarian cancer. *Semin Oncol* 1991;18:177–185.
53. Fraumeni JF Jr, Grundy GW, Creagan ET, Everson RB. Six families prone to ovarian cancer. *Cancer* 1975;36:364–369.
54. Lurain JR, Piver MS. Familial ovarian cancer. *Gynecol Oncol* 1979;8:185–192.
55. Franceschi S, LaVecchia C, Mangioni C. Familial ovarian cancer: eight more families. *Gynecol Oncol* 1982;13:31–36.
56. Piver MS. *The Gilda Radner Familial Ovarian Cancer Registry Newsletter* 1998:1.
57. Lynch HT, Watson P, Bewtra C, et al. Hereditary ovarian cancer heterogeneity in age at diagnosis. *Cancer* 1991;67:1460–1466.
58. Miki Y, Swensen J, Shattuck-Edens D, et al. A strong candidate for the breast and ovarian cancer susceptibility gene BRCA1. *Science* 1994;266:66–71.
59. Sharan SK, Morimatsu M, Albrecht U, et al. Embryonic lethality and radiation hypersensitivity mediated by Rad 51 in mice lacking BRCA2. *Nature* 1997;386:804–810.
60. Claus EB, Schildkraut J, Thompson WD, Risch NJ. The genetic attributable risk of breast and ovarian cancer. *Cancer* 1996;77:2318–2324.
61. Easton DF, Ford D, Bishop DT. Breast Cancer Linkage Consortium: breast and ovarian cancer incidence in BRCA1 mutations. *Am J Hum Genet* 1995;56:265–271.
62. Whittemore AS, Gong G, Itnyre J. Prevalence and contribution of BRCA1 mutation in breast cancer and ovarian cancer: results from three U.S. population based case-control studies of ovarian cancer. *Am J Hum Genet* 1997;60:496–504.
63. Struewing JP, Hartge P, Wacholder S, et al. The risk of cancer associated with specific mutations of BRCA1 and BRCA2 among Ashkenazi Jews. *N Engl J Med* 1997;336:1401–1408.
64. Ford D, Easton DF, Stratton M, et al. Genetic heterogeneity and penetrance analysis of the BRCA1 and BRCA2 genes in breast cancer families. *Am J Hum Genet* 1998;62:676–689.
65. Frank TS, Manley SA. Correlation of mutations with family history and ovarian cancer risk. *J Clin Oncol* 1998;16:2417–2425.
66. Couch FJ, DeShano ML, Blackwood A, et al. BRCA1 mutations in women attending clinics that evaluate the risk of breast cancer. *N Engl J Med* 1997;336:1409–1415.
67. Newman B, Mu H, Butler LM, et al. Frequency of breast cancer attributable to BRCA1 in a population-based series of American women. *JAMA* 1998;279:915–921.
68. Rubin SC, Benjamin I, Behbakht K, et al. Clinical and pathologic features of ovarian cancer in women with germ-line mutations of BRCA1. *N Engl J Med* 1996;335:1413–1416.
69. Boyd J. Molecular genetics of hereditary ovarian cancer. *Oncology* 1998;12:399–406.
70. Watson P, Lynch HT. Extracolonic cancer in hereditary nonpolyposis colorectal cancer. *Cancer* 1993;71:677–685.
71. Narod SA, Risch H, Moslehi R. Oral contraceptives and the risk of hereditary ovarian cancer. *N Engl J Med* 1998;339:424–428.
72. Schrag D, Kuntz KM, Garber JE, Weeks JC. Decision analysis: effects of prophylactic mastectomy and oophorectomy on life expectancy among women with BRCA1 or BRCA2 mutations. *N Engl J Med* 1997;336:1465–1471.
73. Grann VR, Panageas V, Whang W, et al. Decision analysis of prophylactic mastectomy and oophorectomy in BRCA1-positive or BRCA2-positive patients. *J Clin Oncol* 1998;16:979–985.
74. Piver MS, Jishi JF, Tsukada Y, Nava G. Primary peritoneal carcinoma after prophylactic oophorectomy in women with a family history of ovarian cancer. *Cancer* 1993;71:2751–2755.
75. Tobacman JK, Tucker MA, Costa J, et al. Intraabdominal carcinomatosis after prophylactic oophorectomy in ovarian cancer-prone families. *Lancet* 1982;2:795–797.
76. Burke W, Daly M, Garber J, et al. Recommendations for follow-up care of individuals with an inherited predisposition to cancer: II. BRCA1 and BRCA2. *JAMA* 1997;277:997–1003.
77. Rebbeck TR, Levin AM, Eisen A. Breast cancer risk after bilateral prophylactic oophorectomy in BRCA1 mutation carriers. *J Natl Cancer Inst* 1999;91:1475–1479.
78. Fathalla MF. Incessant ovulation: a factor in ovarian neoplasia? *Lancet* 1971;2:163.
79. Cramer DW, Welch WR. Determinants of ovarian cancer risk: II. Inferences regarding pathogenesis. *J Natl Cancer Inst* 1983;71:717–721.
80. Schildkraut JM, Berchuck A. Relationship between lifetime ovulatory cycles and overexpression of mutant p53 in epithelial ovarian cancer. *J Natl Cancer Inst* 1997;89:1726–1727.
81. Young RC, Walton LA, Ellenberg SS, et al. Adjuvant therapy in stage I and stage II epithelial ovarian cancer: results of two prospective randomized trials. *N Engl J Med* 1990;322:1021–1027.
82. DiSaia PJ, Creasman WT, eds. Advanced epithelial ovarian cancer. In: *Clinical gynecologic oncology*, 5th ed. St. Louis: CV Mosby, 1997, 300.
83. DeVita VT, Hellman S, Rosenberg SA, eds. *Cancer principles and practice of oncology*. Philadelphia: JB Lippincott, 1989, 166.
84. Knapp RC, Berkowitz RS, eds. *Gynecologic oncology*. New York: Macmillan, 1986.
85. Piver MS, Barlow JJ. Preoperative and intraoperative evaluation in ovarian malignancy. *Obstet Gynecol* 1976;148:312–315.
86. Graham JB, Graham RM, Schueller EF. Pre-clinical detection of ovarian cancer. *Cancer* 1964;17:1414–1432.
87. McGowan L, Stein DB, Miller W. Cul de sac aspiration for diagnostic cytologic study. *Am J Obstet Gynecol* 1966;96:413–417.
88. Furkhouser JW, Hunter KK, Thompson NJ. The diagnostic value of cul de sac aspiration in the detection of ovarian carcinoma. *Acta Cytol* 1975;19:538–541.
89. Masopust J, Kithier K, Radl J, et al. Occurrence of fetoprotein in patients with neoplasms and non-neoplastic disease. *Int J Cancer* 1968;3:364–373.
90. Van Nagell JR Jr, Meeker WR, Parker JC Jr, Harrelson JD. Carcinoembryonic antigen in patients with gynecologic malignancy. *Cancer* 1975;35:1372–1376.

91. Samaan NA, Smith JP, Rutledge FN, Schultz PN. The significance of measurement of human placental lactogen, human chorionic gonadotropin, and carcinoembryonic antigen in patients with ovarian carcinoma. *Am J Obstet Gynecol* 1976;123:186–189.
92. Knauf S, Urbach GI. A study of ovarian cancer patients using a radioimmunoassay for human ovarian tumor-associated antigen OCA. *Am J Obstet Gynecol* 1980;138:1222–1223.
93. Bast RC, Klug TL, St. John E, et al. A radioimmunoassay using a monoclonal antibody to monitor the course of epithelial ovarian cancer. *N Engl J Med* 1983;309:883–887.
94. Jacobs I, Stabile I, Bridges S, et al. Multimodal approach to screening for ovarian cancer. *Lancet* 1988;2:268–271.
95. Jeyarajah AR, Ind TE, Skates S, et al. Serum CA125 elevation and risk of clinical detection of cancer in asymptomatic postmenopausal women. *Cancer* 1999;85:2068–2072.
96. Einhorn N, Sjovall K, Knapp RC, et al. Prospective evaluation of serum CA 125 levels for early detection of ovarian cancer. *Obstet Gynecol* 1992;80:14–18.
97. Cochrane WJ, Thomas MA. Ultrasound diagnosis of gynecologic pelvic masses. *Radiology* 1974;110:649–654.
98. Samuels BI. Usefulness of ultrasound in patients with ovarian cancer. *Semin Oncol* 1975;2:229–233.
99. Schaner EG, Head GL, Kalman MA, et al. Whole-body computed tomography in the diagnosis of abdominal-thoracic malignancy: a review of 600 cases. *Cancer Treat Rep* 1977;61:1537–1560.
100. Musumeci R, ePalo G, Kenda R, et al. Retroperitoneal masses from ovarian carcinoma: reassessment of 365 patients studied with lymphangiography. *AJR Am J Roentgenol* 1980;134:449–452.
101. Finkler NJ, Benacerraf B, Lavin PT, et al. Comparison of serum 125, clinical impression and ultrasound in the preoperative evaluation of ovarian masses. *Obstet Gynecol* 1988;72:659–664.
102. DePriest PD, Varner E, Powell J, et al. The efficacy of sonographic morphology index in identifying ovarian cancer: a multi-institutional investigation. *Gynecol Oncol* 1994;55:174–178.
103. Campbell S, Goessens L, Goswamy R, Whitehead M. Real-time ultrasonography for determination of ovarian morphology and volume: a possible early screening test for ovarian cancer? *Lancet* 1982;1:425–426.
104. Guy RL, King E, Ayers AB. The role of transvaginal ultrasound in the assessment of the female pelvis. *Clin Radiol* 1988;39:669–672.
105. Rodriguez MH, Platt LD, Medearis AL, et al. The use of transvaginal sonography for evaluation of postmenopausal ovarian size and morphology. *Am J Obstet Gynecol* 1988;159:810–814.
106. Granberg S, Wikland M, Jansson I. Macroscopic characterization of ovarian tumors and the relation to the histologic diagnosis: criteria to be used for ultrasound evaluation. *Gynecol Oncol* 1989;35:139–144.
107. Higgins RV, Van Nagell JR Jr, Donaldson ES, et al. Transvaginal sonography as a screening method for ovarian cancer. *Gynecol Oncol* 1989;34:402–406.
108. DePriest PD, Gallion HH, Pavlik EJ, et al. Transvaginal sonography as a screening method for the detection of early ovarian cancer. *Gynecol Oncol* 1997;65:408–414.
109. Reedy M, DePriest PD, Van Nagell JR Jr. The efficacy of transvaginal sonographic screening in asymptomatic women at risk for ovarian cancer. *Gynecol Oncol* 2000;77:350–356.
110. Willson JR. Ultrasonography in the diagnosis of gynecologic disorders. *Am J Obstet Gynecol* 1991;164:1064–1071.
111. Sparks JM, Varner RE. Ovarian cancer screening. *Obstet Gynecol* 1991;77:787–792.
112. NIH Consensus Development Panel on Ovarian Cancer: Ovarian cancer screening, treatment and follow-up. *JAMA* 1995;273:491–497.
113. Statement of the American Society of Clinical Oncology: Genetic testing for cancer susceptibility. *J Clin Oncol* 1996;14:1730–1736.
114. Lerman C, Daly M, Masney A, Balshem A. Attitudes about genetic testing for breast-ovarian cancer susceptibility. *J Clin Oncol* 1994;12:843–850.
115. Geller G, Botkin J, Green MK, et al. Genetic testing for susceptibility to adult-onset cancer: the process and content of informed consent. *JAMA* 1997;277:1467–1474.
116. Audrain J, Rimer B, Cella D, et al. Genetic counselling and testing for breast-ovarian cancer susceptibility: what do women want? *J Clin Oncol* 1998;16:133–138.

9

Hereditary Ovarian Cancer: Clinical Syndromes and Management

Jeanne M. Schilder, Dawn V. Holladay, and Holly H. Gallion

EPIDEMIOLOGIC EVIDENCE FOR THE EXISTENCE OF HEREDITARY OVARIAN CANCER

In the United States the lifetime risk for developing ovarian cancer is approximately 1 in 70, or 1.4%. Although reproductive, demographic, and lifestyle factors affect the risk for ovarian cancer, the greatest ovarian cancer risk factor is a family history of the disease (Table 9.1) (1,2). In 1988, Schildkraut and Thompson performed a population-based case-control study to evaluate the degree of aggregation of epithelial ovarian cancer in families (3). In this study of almost 3,000 ovarian cancer cases and controls, a familial clustering of ovarian cancer was noted. The odds ratio for ovarian cancer in relatives of women with ovarian cancer compared with controls was 3.6 for first-degree relatives and 2.9 for second-degree relatives, clearly confirming that ovarian cancer runs in families.

In order to better estimate ovarian cancer risk for a woman with a family history of ovarian cancer, Kerlikowske and coworkers derived pooled estimates of relative risk from seven case-control studies, including the Cancer and Steroid Hormone Study (CASH) (4). The estimated odds ratio for ovarian cancer was 3.1 (95% confidence interval [CI], 2.1 to 4.5) for a woman with a single first-degree relative with ovarian cancer and 4.6 (95% CI, 1.1 to 18.4) for a woman with two or three relatives with ovarian cancer. These odds ratios translate into lifetime probabilities for ovarian cancer of 5.0% and 7.2%, respectively, compared to the incidence of just 1.4% observed in the general population.

Stratton and colleagues also performed an analysis of published case-control and cohort studies in ovarian cancer that included almost 18,000 women (5). In this series, the relative risk of ovarian cancer for women with a first-degree family history of ovarian cancer was 3.1, which is consistent with that reported by other investigators. However, the relative risk to mothers of women with ovarian cancer was substantially lower than the relative risk to sisters and daughters. Although germline transmission of the cancer-predisposing trait through the paternal side and possibly higher parity among the mothers (which is protective) may account for some of the difference, the lower cancer risk to mothers is not easily explained. Therefore, barring some unaccounted artifact associated with the data, other, as yet unidentified factors probably influence ovarian cancer risk in the familial setting.

The association between breast and ovarian cancer in families was described by Claus and associates, who used data from the CASH study to calculate the risk of developing breast cancer based on family history of ovarian cancer (6). The lifetime risk of developing breast cancer for a woman with one or two first-degree relatives with ovarian cancer was 13% and 31%, respectively, compared with the population risk of just 11%. A first-degree family history of ovarian cancer, in conjunction with a first-degree family history of breast cancer, increased the breast cancer risk even more dramatically, depending on the age at breast cancer diagnosis. Breast cancer risk ranged from a low of 16.3% if the relative affected with breast cancer was diagnosed between 80 and 90 years of age to a high of 43.4% when the relative with breast cancer was

TABLE 9.1. *Ovarian cancer risk factors*

Factor	Relative risk
Parity	
Nulliparous	1.0
1 FT pregnancy	0.6
2 FT pregnancies	0.53
≥6 FT pregnancies	0.29
Use of oral contraceptive prophylaxis	
Never	1.0
Ever	0.75
3 mo–4 y	0.6–0.7
5–9 y	0.4
≥10 y	0.2
History of breast cancer	
None	1.0
First-degree relative	2.1
Personal history	10
History of ovarian cancer	
None	1.0
1 first-degree relative	3.1
≥2 first-degree relatives	4.6–15
Hereditary ovarian cancer syndrome	12–30

FT, full term.
From Whittemore AS, Harns R, Intyre J, and the Collaborative Ovarian Cancer Group: Characteristics relating to ovarian cancer risk: collaborative analysis of 12 U.S. case control studies. IV: padiogenesis of epithelial ovarian cancer. *Am J Epidemiol* 1992;136:1212–1220. Cancer and Steroid Hormone Study of the Centers for Disease Control and the National Institute of Child Health and Human Development: The reduction in risk of ovarian cancer associated with oral-contraceptive use. *N Engl J Med* 1987;316:650–655, with permission.

diagnosed in her twenties. No such association was noted for age at diagnosis of ovarian cancer.

Risk Factors for Ovarian Cancer

Age

Risk for ovarian cancer increases as a woman gets older. Before 30 years of age, the risk of developing epithelial ovarian cancer is remote, and even in hereditary cancer families epithelial ovarian cancer is virtually nonexistent before age 20. However, ovarian cancer incidence rises in a linear fashion between age 30 and 50 years, and it continues to increase, although at a slower rate, thereafter. The highest incidence is found in the eighth decade of life, with a rate of 57 cases per 100,000 women in the 75- to 79-year-old age group, compared with 16 cases per 100,000 women in the 40- to 44-year-old age group (7).

Demographic Factors

Ovarian cancer incidence varies significantly depending on country of birth, ranging from a high of 14.9 per 100,000 in Sweden to a low of 2.7 per 100,000 in Japan (8). Incidence in the United States is 13.3 per 100,000. Immigration alters the risk to match that of the host country. For example, offspring of Japanese immigrants to the United States have an increased risk of ovarian cancer that approaches the rate among women born in the United States. Theories to explain this effect argue against a major role for ethnicity; rather, they support of a possible role for dietary and environmental factors. Conflicting data implicate animal fat, meat, obesity, and alcohol (9).

Reproductive Factors

Nulliparity, early age at menarche, and late menopause are associated with increased ovarian cancer risk. These all increase the number of lifetime ovulatory cycles, leading to the currently accepted "incessant ovulation" hypothesis of ovarian cancer development (10). Conversely, factors that suppress ovulation, such as pregnancy, lactation, and use of oral contraceptives (OCs), confer a protective effect, providing further credence to this hypothesis. The disruption and subsequent repair of the ovarian epithelium resulting from ovulation leads to cell division, increasing the opportunity for cancer-causing mutations to occur.

Surgical History

Bilateral tubal ligation and hysterectomy have also been reported to reduce ovarian cancer risk, but the mechanism for this effect is unknown (1,11). Among the possible explanations, the creation of a physical barrier that prevents potential carcinogens from reaching the ovaries via the lower genital tract seems the most likely.

Family History

The single greatest risk factor for development of ovarian cancer is a family history of the disease. Lifetime risk is dependent on the number of family members affected, the degree of their relationship, and even which family members among first-degree relatives are affected (4). Estimates of ovarian cancer risk for a carrier of a mutation in the breast cancer susceptibility gene BRCA1 range from 16% to 60% (12,13).

HEREDITARY OVARIAN CANCER SYNDROMES

Epidemiologic studies have provided indisputable proof that family history of disease is an important risk factor for ovarian cancer. In addition, descriptive studies of large, multiple-case families have revealed that ovarian cancer may occur in three, partially overlapping cancer syndromes. These are as follows, in order of highest frequency: breast/ovarian cancer syndrome (HBOC), which is typified by multiple cases of early-onset (before 50 years of age) breast and ovarian cancer; hereditary site-specific ovarian cancer, in which the excess cancer cases are strictly ovarian; and hereditary nonpolyposis colon cancer syndrome (HNPCC) or Lynch syndrome type II, in which there is a predominance of early-onset proximal colon cancer as well as extracolonic adenocarcinomas including cancers of the endometrium and ovary. Together, these cancer syndromes are responsible for almost all known cases of hereditary epithelial ovarian cancer.

Each of the ovarian cancer family syndromes is characterized by autosomal dominant transmission of the cancer-predisposing trait. Children of an affected parent (either mother or father) have a 50% chance of inheriting a mutated copy of the susceptibility gene. Because penetrance of the disease trait in large, multicase ovarian cancer families is relatively high, the majority of the individuals in these families who inherit a predisposing gene eventually develop cancer. In addition, these syndromes often display the classic features of hereditary cancer syndromes, including early age at onset of disease and the occurrence of bilateral or metachronous cancers.

HBOC accounts for 75% to 90% of all hereditary ovarian cancer cases and 30% to 70% of all hereditary breast cancer cases (14). Fifty percent of breast cancer cases associated with this syndrome are diagnosed by the age of 41 years, compared with 63 years in the general population. Although not as striking as the early age at onset for breast cancer, ovarian cancer in at least some HBOC families manifests at a younger age compared to ovarian cancer in the general population. As with most hereditary cancer syndromes, multiple primary tumors may be seen among members of these families. For example, breast and ovarian cancer or bilateral breast cancer in the same individual is not an uncommon finding and frequently indicates the presence of a genetic predisposition. There also appears to be an increased incidence of prostate cancer and possibly colon cancer in HBOC families (14). Papillary serous adenocarcinoma of the ovary is the predominant histologic type, but endometrioid and mucinous carcinomas have also been observed. One series reported serous histology in 83% of patients with familial ovarian cancer, compared with 49% of matched controls (15). Mucinous adenocarcinomas are found in only 1.4% of familial ovarian cancer cases, compared with 12.7% of sporadic cases. Most tumors occurring in BRCA1 and BRCA2 families are invasive; however, tumors of low malignant potential have been reported as well. The vast majority of these families are due to mutations in the BRCA1 gene located on chromosome 17q; a smaller percentage are due to a second gene, BRCA2, located on chromosome 13q.

Site-specific ovarian cancer, which was initially described as a separate syndrome, is now considered to be a variant of HBOC. The absence of breast cancer cases in site-specific ovarian cancer families may be the result either of chance or of variability in the specific cancer risks with a particular mutation. Alternatively, the absence of breast cancer in these families may simply result from incomplete or inaccurate family history information. Disease in these families is almost universally associated with BRCA1 and BRCA2 mutations. Overall, site-specific ovarian cancer syndrome probably accounts for only a small percentage (less than 5%) of hereditary ovarian cancer.

HNPCC, also known as Lynch syndrome II, is the third known hereditary ovarian cancer syndrome. Although there are no definitive estimates, HNPCC probably accounts for no more than 2% of hereditary ovarian cancer and 5% of all colorectal cancer (CRC). As mentioned earlier, families with HNPCC are characterized by an increased incidence of predominantly early-onset proximal nonpolyposis CRC in conjunction with adenocarcinomas at other sites including the endometrium, ovary, stomach, urinary tract, small bowel, and bile ducts and sebaceous skin tumors. HNPCC is the result of germline mutations in the DNA mismatch repair (MMR) genes. Mutations in five different MMR genes have been recognized to result in HNPCC. Two of these are found on chromosome 2 (MSH2 and PMS1), and one each on chromosomes 3 (MLH1) and 7 (PMS2). MLH1 and MSH2 mutations account for 45% and 49% of HNPCC families, respectively (16). The remaining 6% are due largely to PMS2, with germline mutations in PMS1 and MSH6 being reported only rarely.

THE GENES THAT CAUSE HEREDITARY OVARIAN CANCER

BRCA1 and BRCA2

Isolation and Structure

In 1990, genetic linkage between a polymorphism within chromosome segment 17q12-q21 and breast cancer cases was discovered in large, multicase breast cancer families (17). Linkage to the BRCA1 region was present in almost all families in which the mean age at onset of disease was less than 50 years, whereas families that had an older mean age at disease onset appeared unlinked. This finding heralded a tremendous breakthrough in the search for genes responsible for hereditary breast and ovarian cancer and marked the beginning of a 5-year struggle that resulted in the identification of two genes that cause most, if not all, cases of HBOC and site-specific ovarian cancer. The gene within chromosome segment 17q12-q21 was named BRCA1 for *br*east *ca*ncer gene number 1 and was soon found to account for 45% to 50% of breast cancer families and for most HBOC families. The BRCA1 gene itself was finally cloned in 1994 (18). Within the same year, genetic linkage between a second chromosomal locus and hereditary breast cancer was reported (19). This chromosomal region, 13q12, was found to harbor another gene, BRCA2, that was responsible for the remaining approximately 50% of breast cancer families and 10% to 20% of HBOC families not linked to BRCA1. The BRCA2 gene was isolated in 1995 (20).

Much has been learned about the molecular structure and function of BRCA1 and BRCA2 since their discovery. BRCA1 is a large gene, encoding a protein of 1,863 amino acids, with 24 coding exons distributed over about 100 kb of genomic DNA. To date, more than 600 different disease-associated mutations in BRCA1 have been identified spread throughout the entire coding sequence of this very large gene. BRCA1 is a tumor suppressor gene, and most of the mutations cause loss of BRCA1 protein function because they result in truncated, presumably inactive proteins. Many other sequence changes in BRCA1 have been reported that change only a single amino acid; because the functional significance of these changes is not yet known or determinable, they have been called "unclassified variants."

BRCA2 is also a large gene. Encoding some 3,418 amino acids, the coding sequence of BRCA2 is nearly twice the size of BRCA1. Like BRCA1, BRCA2 has many coding exons, 27 in total, spanning about 80 kb of genomic DNA. The structural organization of the BRCA1 and BRCA2 genes is also very similar: both have a large exon 11, and the coding sequence of each begins in exon 2. The tally of disease-associated mutations in BRCA2 is at about 450. As with BRCA1, the mutations in BRCA2 are expected to cause premature termination of translation, producing truncated protein products.

Tumor Suppressor Genes

Evidence suggests that BRCA1 and BRCA2 are tumor suppressor genes that have an important role in the regulation of normal cell growth and proliferation. Tumor suppressor genes act to inhibit cell proliferation, counteracting the stimulatory effect of oncogenes. Each person inherits two copies of a tumor suppressor gene, one from the maternal line and one from the paternal line. Because only one normally functioning copy (wild type) of a tumor suppressor gene is adequate to control cell growth, the function of both the maternal and the paternal copies of a tumor suppressor gene must be lost in order to initiate carcinogenesis. This is consistent with the so called "two-hit" theory of carcinogenesis, which proposes that two genetic "hits," or alterations, are required to result in carcinogenesis (21). In hereditary cancer families, an inactivating inherited germline mutation is present in one copy of a tumor suppressor gene. Because this is a germline mutation, it is present in all the cells of a mutation carrier and represents the "first hit." These individuals are phenotypically normal until a second mutation occurs in a somatic tissue (e.g., breast or ovary) and inactivates the remaining wild-type copy: the so-called "second hit." Individuals who inherit two normal copies of a tumor suppressor gene must undergo somatic mutations in both copies of the same tumor suppressor gene in the same tissue in order to develop cancer. With loss of both copies of the tumor suppressor gene, the normal constraints to cell proliferation are lost and carcinogenesis is initiated. Individuals who inherit a germline mutation have a "head start," accounting for a higher cancer incidence as well as earlier age at disease onset and multiple primary tumors compared with the general population.

Functions of BRCA1 and BRCA2

Although their exact function is not yet known, a wealth of evidence now suggests that products of BRCA1 and BRCA2 play a role in DNA repair. Evidence supporting such a role includes the following: (a) BRCA1 and BRCA2 proteins interact with RAD51, a known DNA repair protein; (b) after exposure of cells to DNA-damaging radiation, BRCA1 protein becomes phosphorylated and disperses from "nuclear dots" to proliferating cell nuclear antigen (PCNA) containing complexes, possibly at the site of DNA damage; (c) mice that are genetically lacking Brca1 and Brca2, the murine homologs of the human BRCA1 and BRCA2 genes, die early in embryogenesis owing to growth arrest apparently caused by activation of the p53 DNA-damage response pathway; and (d) murine embryonic fibroblasts that are null for BRCA1 are defective in the repair of oxidative DNA damage, a type of DNA repair that corrects oxidative lesions in the bases of DNA (22).

A role for BRCA1 and BRCA2 proteins in the repair of DNA damage is consistent with the function of BRCA1 and BRCA2 as so-called caretaker genes. In their landmark paper, Kinzler and Vogelstein described how loss of tumor suppressor function may contribute to tumor formation along two partially overlapping pathways: a "gatekeeper" pathway and a "caretaker" pathway (23). Tumors form along the gatekeeper pathway when both alleles of a tumor suppressor gene that directly regulates cell division are lost or inactivated, allowing the cell to proliferate, free of the previously inhibitory action of the gatekeeper protein. An example of a gatekeeper tumor suppressor gene is RB1, which is mutated in hereditary and sporadic retinoblastoma. Tumors form along the caretaker pathway when both alleles of a tumor suppressor gene that encodes a protein involved in DNA repair become inactivated, followed by loss or inactivation of two gatekeeper gene alleles. In the caretaker pathway, loss of both copies of a DNA repair gene causes a mutation phenotype, speeding up the process by which mutations are accumulated in other cancer-related genes. An example of a caretaker gene, other than BRCA1 and BRCA2, is MLH1, which encodes a protein involved in DNA mismatch repair; it is mutated in about half of all HNPCC cases and frequently is inactivated by methylation in sporadic colon cancers.

The finding that BRCA1 and BRCA2 are likely caretaker genes is consistent with the reported cancer risks associated with BRCA1 and BRCA2 germline mutations and the observation that these genes are rarely mutated in sporadic breast and ovarian cancers. Four mutations (or "hits") are required for tumors to form along the caretaker pathway, whereas only two mutations are necessary along the gatekeeper pathway. Patients with an inherited mutation in BRCA1 or BRCA2 therefore need three further somatic mutations for a tumor to occur, one in the wild-type copy of the relevant BRCA gene and one in each of both alleles of a gatekeeper gene. Because the likelihood of three additional mutations (falling in the same cell) is low, cancer-predisposing mutations in BRCA1 and BRCA2 are not fully penetrant. In comparison, loss-of-function mutations in RB1 are fully penetrant because retinal cells are only one mutation away from tumor formation. It also follows that sporadic tumors form along the caretaker pathway infrequently, since four mutations are required for tumor formation. In keeping with this prediction, BRCA1 and BRCA2 are rarely, if at all, mutated in sporadic breast tumors, but about 10% of ovarian tumors have mutations in BRCA1 and BRCA2.

Prevalence and Founder Effects

It is estimated that 1 in 800 individuals in the general population carry a potentially disease-causing mutation in BRCA1. However, the prevalence of BRCA1 and BRCA2 mutations is higher in certain individuals (Table 9.2) (24,25). For example, in certain ethnic groups or geographically isolated populations, mutations are much more common due to a phenomenon known as the founder effect. A founder mutation is a specific mutation that has entered an isolated population only once or a few times and becomes more frequent as the population grows. A number of different founder mutations have been documented in individuals of Ashkenazi Jewish descent whose ancestors are from central and eastern Europe. These include the BRCA1 185delAG mutation, the BRCA1 5382insC mutation, and the BRCA2 6174delT mutation, which have carrier frequencies of 1%, 0.155%, and 1.5%, respectively, in this population, or approximately 2.5% (1 in 40) overall (13,26). Together, these three founder mutations account for hereditary breast and ovarian cancer in up to 90% of Ashkenazi Jewish families, which represent the majority of Jewish individuals in the United States. It is important to bear in mind that mutations other than BRCA1 and BRCA2 may cause disease in the remaining 10% of these families, so genetic screening for these three mutations alone will not detect all predisposing mutations in Ashkenazi Jewish families. Additional founder mutations in BRCA1 and BRCA2 have also been observed in geographically isolated populations including the Netherlands and Iceland (27).

As would be expected, the prevalence of BRCA1 and BRCA2 mutations is also higher in women with ovarian cancer compared with the general population. In a large series of ovarian cancer patients unselected for family history of disease, Rubin and coworkers detected BRCA1 and BRCA2 mutations in approximately 10%. More than half of the patients with BRCA1 mutations had unremarkable family histories for breast and ovarian cancer, indicating that family history alone does not identify all mutation carriers (28). In a study by the Gynecologic Oncology Group, Smith and colleagues determined the frequency of BRCA1 mutations in an unselected, clinic-based series of ovarian cancer cases to be 12 of 258, or 4.6 percent. The frequency of BRCA2 mutations is likely to be similar, with an overall frequency of BRCA mutations consistent with Rubin's findings (29).

The prevalence of mutations is even higher in women with both a personal history of cancer and a family history of disease. Frank and coworkers evaluated the prevalence of BRCA1 and BRCA2 mutations in 238 women with breast cancer diagnosed before age 50, or ovarian cancer at any age (30). All of these women had a family history of at least one first- or second-degree relative with either cancer. Deleterious mutations were detected in 39% of women, including 50% of women from families with ovarian cancer and 29% of women from families without ovarian cancer. Ten out of 11 of the women in this series who had a personal history of both breast and ovarian cancer had a BRCA1 or BRCA2 mutation.

TABLE 9.2. *Prevalence of BRCA mutations*

Population	Prevalence (%)
General population	.00125
Ashkenazi Jewish population	2.5
Personal history of breast cancer	
Age at diagnosis <50 y	20
Age at diagnosis ≥50 y	7
Family history of breast cancer	
1 first-degree relative	3.8
≥3 relatives	20
Family history of bilateral breast cancer	18
Family history of both breast and ovarian cancer	40

From Couch FJ, Hartmann LC: BRCA1 testing: advances and retreats. *JAMA* 1998;279:955–957. Malone KE, Daling JR, Thompson JD, et al: BRCA1 mutations and breast cancer in the general population: analyses in women before age 35 years and in women before age 45 years with first-degree family history. *JAMA* 1998:279(12):922–929, with permission.

Penetrance

Inheriting a mutation associated with a hereditary cancer syndrome does not necessarily mean the individual will ultimately develop cancer during his or her lifetime. The actual risk of cancer depends on the penetrance of the inherited susceptibility gene. Penetrance, which refers to the percentage of individuals with a given mutation who will actually develop the disease, is highly variable and can depend on such factors as age, gender, and the specific mutation. Initial estimates of BRCA1 penetrance were based on the large, multicase families used to first identify linkage to chromosome 17q by the Breast Cancer Linkage Consortium (BCLC) (14). In these families, it was estimated that more than half of BRCA1 mutation carriers would develop breast cancer by age 50 years and that 82% to 87% would develop the disease by age 70. By comparison, approximately 11% of women in the general population will develop breast cancer by age 70. BRCA1 mutation carriers in these large families were estimated to have a 44% to 63% chance of developing ovarian cancer by 70 years of age, compared with a lifetime risk of only 1.4% in the general population. Penetrance was extremely high in these severely affected families, with a almost 95% lifetime risk of developing either breast or ovarian cancer.

BRCA2 penetrance was also estimated from data derived from the BCLC families (31). The overall risk of developing either breast or ovarian cancer by 70 years of age was estimated to be 88%, with most of this risk being attributed to breast cancer. The cumulative risk of breast cancer for a BRCA2 carrier was estimated to be 28% by age 50 and 84% by age 70. The risk of ovarian cancer was only 0.4% by age 50, but rose substantially to 27% by age 70. The cumulative risk of breast cancer in male carriers of BRCA2 was 6% by age 70, or 100 times the baseline population risk. The BCLC data represent the largest collection of breast cancer families in the world. Even so, this BRCA2 penetrance data is derived from only 32 families and, as such, are likely to be revised as more mutation carriers are identified.

Lower penetrance estimates have come from studies of BRCA1 and BRCA2 mutation carriers in the general population. The high prevalence of mutations in the Ashkenazi Jewish population makes this an ideal population to estimate prevalence in the general population (compared to high-risk multicase families.) In a study of Ashkenazi Jewish individuals in the Washington D.C. area unselected for family history of disease, carriers of one of the three previously described founder mutations in BRCA1 or BRCA2 had much lower breast and ovarian cancer risks compared with those observed in the BCLC multicase families (13). In this study, penetrance by 70 years of age was estimated to be 56% for breast cancer and 16% for ovarian cancer. In this large series of 120 carriers, there was no difference in breast/ovarian cancer risk between individuals who carried a BRCA1 or a BRCA2 mutation. Although the most accurate way to determine penetrance is to prospectively compare cancer incidence in carriers and noncarriers, these studies provide the current best estimates of BRCA1 and BRCA2 penetrance.

In addition to breast and ovarian cancer, BRCA1 and BRCA2 mutation carriers appear to be at an increased risk for other cancers as well. Specifically, the BCLC reported that mutation carriers were at increased risk for colon and prostate cancer, with relative risks of 4 and 3.3, respectively. A similar increased risk of prostate cancer was detected in men carrying BRCA1 and BRCA2 mutations. However, neither male nor female carriers were at risk of colon cancer. The BCLC data is currently being evaluated to determine the possible association of additional cancers in BRCA mutation carriers.

Factors That Modify BRCA1 and BRCA2 Penetrance

The penetrance of BRCA1 and BRCA2 may also be influenced by other genetic, hormonal, or environmental factors. The HRAS1 variable number of tandem repeat (VNTR) locus on chromosome 11 has been suggested as a possible genetic modifier of ovarian cancer risk in BRCA1 carriers (32). Five "common" HRAS1 VNTR alleles account for 88% of this allele; the remainder are considered "rare" and have been associated with an increased risk of certain types of cancers. Phelan and associates reported a 2.11 greater risk of ovarian cancer in BRCA1 carriers who also carried one or two of these rare alleles, compared with BRCA1 carriers who carried only common alleles ($p = .015$) (32).

Other genes that may influence BRCA1 penetrance include those involved in endocrine signaling pathways. The CAG repeat-length polymorphism found in exon 1 of the androgen-receptor gene (AR-CAG) has been proposed by Rebbeck and coworkers to have this function (33). AR alleles contain a variable number of CAG repeats. As the number of repeats increases, the function of the gene decreases, which appears to correlate with an increased risk of breast cancer. For example, in their study, they found that women who carried at least one AR allele with 28 or more CAG repeats were at significantly increased risk of developing breast cancer compared with women who carried only shorter alleles. In addition, 100% of the women in this study who had at least one allele with 29 or more CAG repeats developed breast cancer. There also appeared to be a direct correlation between size of the CAG repeat and age at breast cancer diagnosis. Women with CAG repeat lengths of more than 28, more than 29, and more than 30 were diagnosed with breast cancer at a mean of 0.8, 1.8, and 6.3 years earlier, respectively, than women who carried only alleles of shorter length.

The DNA Mismatch Repair Genes

Function

At about the same time that BRCA1 and BRCA2 were linked to autosomal dominant breast and ovarian cancer, a totally new class of genes, the MMR genes, were found to play a role in disease occurring in HNPCC families (34,35). One of the functions of the MMR genes is to "proofread" DNA for mismatched nucleotides, thus helping to maintain the integrity of the genome. Mutation in these genes results in loss of this proofreading function or destabilization of the genome, resulting in a phenomenon known as microsatellite instability (MSI). Tumors displaying MSI have been recognized in a small subset of sporadic CRCs, and in 85% to 90% of tumors in patients with HNPCC (36). This loss of replication fidelity results in the accumulation of errors within tumor suppressor genes and oncogenes, ultimately resulting in tumorigenesis.

Prevalence and Founder Effects

Very little is known about the prevalence of MMR gene mutations, but it is estimated that 5% of all cases of CRC in the United States are familial, the vast majority of which can be attributed to mutations in the MMR genes. The largest study to date to estimate MMR mutation contribution to CRC was a prospective study of consecutive CRC tumors in the Finnish population (37). More than 1,000 of these individuals were affected with CRC, and 28 of them had germline mutations in MLH1 and MSH2. The overall carrier frequency for mutations in these two MMR genes in Finland was estimated to be 3% to 5%, or 1 in 660.

Founder mutations have also been well described for HNPCC (37). A deletion of exon 16 in MLH1 accounts for half of HNPCC families in Finland. Similarly, a splicing mutation affecting exon 5 is detected in approximately 5% of HNPCC families in Newfoundland. To date, there have been three additional HNPCC founder mutations described, all affecting MLH1 and resulting in 10% to 25% of HNPCC cases in the affected Finnish or Danish population. Tests for these specific founder mutations may be used as an initial screen for HNPCC mutations in individuals of Finnish or Danish descent.

Penetrance

The average age at CRC diagnosis in HNPCC carriers is 45 years, with a penetrance of 68% to 75% by age 65 (38,39). The cumulative lifetime risks for the most common extracolonic cancers in HNPCC families are as follows: endometrium, 43% to 60%; stomach, 13% to 19%; biliary tract, 18%; urinary tract, 10%; and ovary, 9% to 12% (38). For HNPCC families, the types of cancers observed vary greatly among families, with gynecologic cancers being much more common in some HNPCC families than in others. Pedigree analyses of 40 families from The Finnish HNPCC Registry found that, as with most hereditary cancer syndromes, cancer frequently occurred at a younger age compared with sporadic tumors of the same type. In the Finnish study, the median age at disease onset was 42 years for CRC, 47 years for ovarian cancer, and 49 years for endometrial cancer. Almost 90% of MMR mutation carriers with CRC will develop a second primary, most commonly colorectal or endometrial cancer. The identification of HNPCC has important clinical implications, because cancer screening should encompass all sites known to be associated with the syndrome.

GENETIC SUSCEPTIBILITY TESTING

Identification of Individuals Most Likely to Benefit from Testing

Because of the low prevalence of BRCA1 or BRCA2 mutations and the high cost of clinical testing, it is not appropriate to screen unaffected individuals in the general population. According to the 1996 Statement of the American Society of Clinical Oncology (ASCO), genetic testing should be recommended when (a) the person has a strong family history of cancer or very early age at onset of disease; (b) the test can be adequately interpreted; and (c) the results will influence the medical management of the patient or family member (40). The consensus panel suggested that genetic susceptibility testing is most likely to be of clinical value for individuals who have a greater than 10% probability of carrying the mutation (Table 9.3). An individual has a 10% or greater risk of a BRCA1 mutation if he or she has a family history of any one of the following: (a) more than two breast cancer cases and more than one ovarian cancer case diagnosed at any age; (b) more than three cases of premenopausal (before 50 years of age) breast cancer; or (c) sister pairs with two cases of breast cancer, two cases of ovarian cancer, or a breast and an ovarian cancer, all diagnosed before age 50.

In addition to these very specific guidelines, numerous risk assessment models are available that can be used to evaluate whether risk is sufficient to warrant genetic testing. The Couch model predicts the probability of a BRCA1 mutation based on the average age at breast cancer diagnosis in the family and on whether the family history includes breast cancer only or both breast and ovarian cancer (26). The likelihood of a BRCA1 mutation is increased if the family history includes even one case of ovarian cancer, and the risk rises even more dramatically in families of Ashkenazi Jewish ancestry. This model is most useful for multicase breast cancer families and may not be predictive in families with few cases. It is limited by the small number of families from which the data were derived, thus resulting in wide confidence intervals. In addition, it does not provide information about BRCA2 mutations.

Frank and colleagues developed a model to predict the probability of detecting a BRCA1 or BRCA2 mutation in a woman diagnosed with breast cancer before age 50 (30). This model takes into account the patient's (proband's) personal or family history of breast or ovarian cancer. Again, any history of ovarian cancer dramatically increases the chance that she is a mutation carrier. Bilateral breast cancer in the proband is also highly predictive of carrier status. This model can be applied to family members based on their relationship to the proband. For example, a first-degree relative of the proband would have 50% of the proband's predicted risk, her second-degree relative would have 25% of her risk of being a mutation carrier, and so on.

The Amsterdam and Bethesda criteria are useful in identifying families at increased risk for HNPCC association (Table 9.4). In addition, several characteristic features of the syndrome have been well described, including (a) autosomal dominant transmission; (b) gene penetrance for

TABLE 9.3. *Factors identifying individuals most likely to benefit from BRCA1 and BRCA2 testing*

1. Personal or family history of premenopausal breast cancer (age <50 y) and ovarian cancer at any age
2. First-degree relative with BRCA1 or BRCA2 mutation
3. Family history of two or more cases of premenopausal breast cancer
4. Family history of two or more cases of ovarian cancer
5. Personal or family history of bilateral breast cancer
6. Family history of male breast cancer, especially in the context of other risk factors
7. Ashkenazi Jewish ancestry in the setting of a personal or family history of breast or ovarian cancer

From Easton DR, Ford D, Bishop DT, and the Breast Cancer Linkage Consortium: Breast and ovarian cancer incidence in BRCA1-mutation carriers, *Am J Hum Genet* 1995;56:265–271. Struewing JP, Hartge P, Wacholder S, et al: The risk of cancer associated with specific mutations of BRCA1 and BRCA2 among Ashkenazi Jews. *N Engl J Med* 1997;336:1401–1408. Statement of the American Society of Clinical Oncology: Genetic testing for cancer susceptibility. *J Clin Oncol* 1996;14:1730–1736, with permission.

TABLE 9.4. *Criteria to identify families at high risk for colon cancer*

Amsterdam Criteria

1. At least two successive generations with colorectal cancer
2. Diagnosis of at least one individual before 50 years of age
3. Histologically verified colon cancer in at least three relatives, one of whom is a relative of the other two
4. Increased incidence of other cancers within the family, especially cancer of the ovary, uterus, stomach, urinary tract, small bowel, and bile duct

Bethesda Criteria

1. Very small families with two cases of colon cancer OR two first-degree relatives with colon cancer, AND
2. A third relative with early-onset cancer or endometrial cancer

From Burke W, Petersen G, Lynch P, et al: Recommendations for follow-up care of individuals with an inherited predisposition to cancer: I. Hereditary nonpolyposis colon cancer. *JAMA* 1997;277:915–919, with permission.

CRC of approximately 90%; (c) early age at CRC onset (mean, 45 years); (d) preponderance of proximal CRC tumors (approximately 70% proximal to the splenic flexure); (e) increased frequency of synchronous and metachronous CRCs; (f) better prognosis for CRC compared to sporadic cases; (g) characteristic, but not pathognomonic, pathologic features of CRC, including increased signet cells, medullary features, and peritumoral lymphocytic infiltration; and (h) increased risk for extracolonic malignancies, including endometrial, ovarian, gastric, small bowel, and pancreatic tumors (37). When the personal or family history is suggestive of these features, surveillance and prevention strategies, genetic counseling, and possibly genetic testing should be discussed with the family.

Obtaining a Family History of Cancer

The most important tool in risk assessment is the family history, which remains a cost-effective, crucial tool to identify individuals at high risk of breast and ovarian cancer (41). In order to adequately assess risk, the pedigree should include a three-generation family history with evaluation of the patient's children, siblings, parents, aunts, uncles, cousins, and grandparents and should include race, ethnic background, current age, all types of cancers, age at diagnosis of cancer, and age at death. Information should be gathered for both maternal and paternal relatives, because familial cancer genes can be inherited from either the father or the mother.

The family history should be updated at each visit, because a familial cancer syndrome may become apparent as other cancers are diagnosed in the family. An example is a single case of ovarian cancer in a family that may not initially appear striking. In time, if a close relative develops ovarian, breast, uterine, or colon cancer, HBOC or HNPCC may be considered, and screening and risk management of the initial patient and family members may be heightened. In addition, the diagnosis of cancer within a family often leads to increased discussion about other family members that may have had cancer or died of cancer. The family history should be confirmed with medical records and pathology reports whenever possible. It is well recognized that a verbally reported family history is not entirely accurate and may change once the pathology and medical records are actually reviewed. Commonly reported misdiagnoses include stomach rather than ovarian cancer and liver or bone metastasis reported as primary liver or bone cancer. In many cases, accurate information changes the predicted probability of carrying a mutation.

A hereditary breast or ovarian cancer syndrome should also be suspected if the family history includes individuals who have had both breast and ovarian cancer or bilateral breast cancer; similar cancers in two or more relatives on the same side of the family; premenopausal breast cancer; or male breast cancer, especially in the context of other cases of breast or ovarian cancer in the family. Individuals of Ashkenazi Jewish ancestry in conjunction with a personal or family history of premenopausal breast cancer, or ovarian cancer at any age, are also at considerable risk of being mutation carriers. The younger the age at diagnosis and the more relatives affected, the higher the likelihood that a disease-causing mutation is responsible.

Although many families with a cancer predisposition display these features, a predisposing condition can be present in the absence of these features. In some pedigrees, cancer may appear to "skip" a generation. The predisposing gene does not actually skip a generation; rather, the gene may not be expressed in every generation because it affects sex-specific organs (breast or ovary) and there are not many females in the family, because it has incomplete penetrance, or simply because the kindred size is small. When a family history does show features consistent with an inherited predisposition, the patient may well benefit from a consultation with a cancer genetics program. These programs have cancer genetic professionals usually including a team of physicians, nurses, and genetic counselors who are specially trained in hereditary cancer risk assessment, genetic testing protocols, and psychosocial support.

Testing for BRCA1 and BRCA2 Gene Mutations

Direct DNA sequencing of the entire coding portion of the BRCA1 and BRCA2 genes is the most sensitive method for detecting mutations and is considered the "gold standard" (42). Because of the overwhelming number of different BRCA1 and BRCA2 mutations spread throughout the entire coding portion of the genes and the large size of the genes, this approach is highly labor intensive and costly. Although the majority of disease-causing mutations should be detected with this technique, it is important to note that false-negative results can occur. False-negative results will occur if there are large deletions removing one or several exons, which will be missed by a polymerase chain reaction (PCR) sequencing approach. Also, mutations outside of the coding exons within the 5′ and 3′ untranslated portion of the genes which affect transcription or mRNA stability will not be detected with sequencing, because only the coding portion of the gene is sequenced. Once a specific disease causing mutation has been identified in a particular family, other family members can be tested for the presence of that specific mutation only; this is technically an easier task and much less costly.

Allele-specific oligonucleotide (ASO) analysis is used to screen for the presence of specific mutations that may be present in a patient's DNA. Radioactive oligonucleotides are able to bind specific mutations by complementary hybridization base pairing and are fast and relatively easy to use. Because of the high frequency of the three founder mutations in the Ashkenazi Jewish population, ASO analysis for these "ethnic-specific" mutations is a useful screening test for women of Ashkenazi Jewish descent. If positive, this test can obviate the need for the more expensive, direct sequencing. However, if the test is negative, direct sequencing must be performed to detect mutations other than the three common founder mutations.

Less expensive and more rapid screening tests are available and are used primarily for research purposes because they are associated with a higher false-negative rate. The protein truncation assay analyzes the DNA indirectly by using RNA to produce the protein product. By comparing the size of this protein to that of the normal protein, premature termination of protein synthesis can be detected. This method is highly sensitive for the many frameshift and nonsense mutations that result in shortened or truncated proteins. However, because not all BRCA1 and BRCA2 mutations result in truncated proteins, this test lacks the necessary sensitivity for clinical testing. Other gel-based methods, such as single-strand conformation polymorphism analysis and heteroduplex analysis, rely on the fact that a change in DNA sequence results in alteration of the shape or size of the DNA, thus changing the speed of migration through the gel when compared with normal DNA. Once an abnormality on gel migration has been identified, that region must then be sequenced to identify the specific mutation.

Tests for HNPCC Mutations

To date, more than 200 disease-causing mutations have been identified in the MMR genes responsible for HNPCC families. In general, mutation detection in HNPCC families is relatively insensitive due to technical limitations of screening assays and the genetic heterogeneity of the disease. A protein truncation assay for mismatched repair gene mutations is commercially available, but has a very high false-negative rate. Likewise, denaturing gel electrophoresis followed by sequencing of mutations detected is hampered by a high false-negative rate. Direct sequencing of the entire coding portion of the gene is considered the gold standard, but this is available only for MSH2 and MLH1.

Interpretation of Genetic Susceptibility Testing Results

A positive test result indicates that a disease-causing mutation has been detected in the individual tested. If an affected individual tests positive for a disease-causing mutation, then the clinical significance of test results in blood relatives is clear. Individuals in such families who test positive for the mutation are at high risk for cancer and should begin heightened surveillance and prevention measures. When the disease-causing mutation in the family is known, relatives who test negative for the mutation can be reassured that their cancer risk is the same as in the general population. This is one of the few situations in genetic testing when an individual can be assured of a "true-negative" result. However, these individuals should be counseled that although they have not inherited the mutation, their cancer risk has not fallen to zero; rather, their risk is the same as that of the general population.

A negative test result in an affected individual must be interpreted with caution. False-negative test results can occur for a variety of reasons, including the presence of a mutation in a noncoding region of the gene or a large deletion, both of which will not be picked up by PCR-based gene sequencing. Alternatively, the disease may result from a mutation in a disease in a susceptibility gene that was not tested. Finally, there is the chance occurrence of sporadic cancer in the individual selected for testing. In this situation, if possible, other affected blood relatives should be tested to rule out the possibility that the initial affected person tested was merely a sporadic case. If testing of an affected relative is not possible, then testing of an unaffected individual can be performed, but the results must be interpreted with extreme caution. In the absence of a known familial mutation, positive results are informative but negative results are not; high-risk management strategies should be continued in patients with negative results.

Another possible outcome of genetic testing is obtaining an indeterminate result. In this case, gene alterations are identified that have unknown functional significance and may or may not confer an increased risk of cancer. This is not unexpected because of the large size of these genes and the large number of mutations of unknown functional significance detected thus far. Again, high-risk management regimens should be employed for individuals with a family history of disease.

Risks, Benefits and Limitations of Testing

It is critical to completely counsel individuals considering genetic susceptibility testing regarding the potential benefits and risks before any decision is made to proceed (43). The pretest discussion must be done by knowledgeable professionals and should include a thorough discussion of the risks, benefits, and limitations of testing, as well as the availability and effectiveness of management options. The results of genetic testing may have an impact on blood relatives, and this should be discussed as well. Careful consideration must be given to the content and process of informed consent because of the complexity of the issues and potential ramifications of the results (Table 9.5).

In families where the mutation is known, there is a clear benefit to testing. When the specific deleterious mutation in the family is known,

TABLE 9.5. *Elements of informed consent for genetic testing*

1. Information on the genetic test performed
2. Implications of positive, negative, and indeterminate results
3. Risk of passing mutation to children
4. Option of risk estimation using tables rather than genetic testing
5. Technical accuracy of the test
6. Cost of testing and counseling
7. Emotional ramifications
8. Risk of genetic discrimination
9. Confidentiality issues
10. Options for medical screening after testing

From Statement of the American Society of Clinical Oncology: Genetic testing for cancer susceptibility. *J Clin Oncol* 1996;14:1730–1736, with permission.

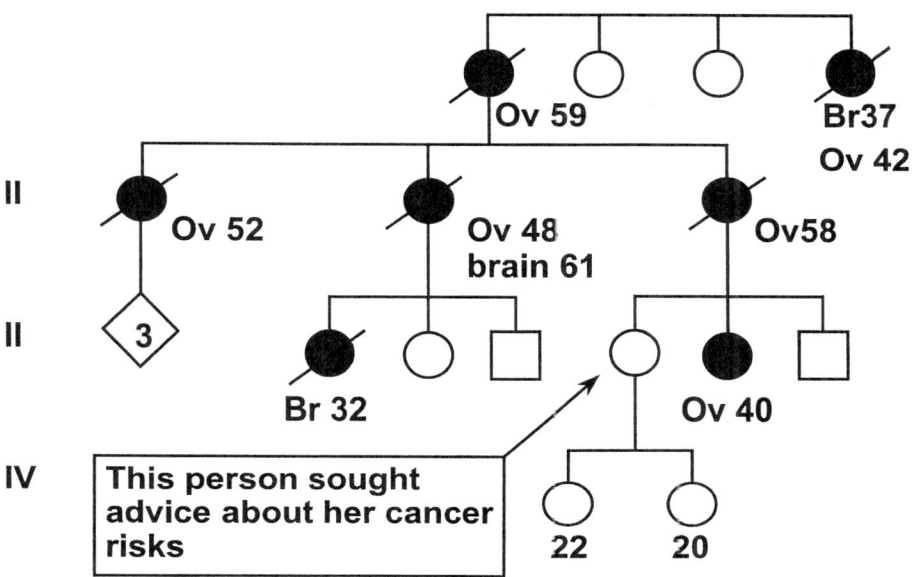

FIG. 9.1. Based on pedigree analysis, this individual has a 50:50 chance of inheriting a disease-causing mutation from her mother. With genetic susceptibility testing, her carrier status can be determined. Either she has inherited a disease-causing mutation and therefore is at high risk for ovarian and breast cancer or she has not, in which case her cancer risk would be the same as in the general population. Without the benefit of genetic testing, this individual could only be counseled that her risk of carrying a hereditary susceptibility mutation is 50%. Genetic testing could potentially identify her as a carrier (100%) or noncarrier (0%). Her risk of developing ovarian cancer, as well as her clinical management (screening), would be significantly different depending on the result. Ov, ovarian cancer; Br, breast cancer, followed by age at diagnosis.

the carrier status of family members can be determined with certainty. Based on family history alone, first-degree blood relatives of a mutation carrier can be advised that they have a 50% chance of having inherited the disease gene (Figure 9.1). With genetic susceptibility testing, the exact status of each of these individuals can be determined. In other words, it can determine whether they have inherited the mutation or not. This is particularly useful information for women considering prophylactic oophorectomy or mastectomy. In this situation, an individual with a negative test result can be reassured that her cancer risk is the same as in the general population, and prophylactic surgery can be avoided. In contrast, if the result is positive the woman must be advised that her risk of cancer is high, and appropriate screening and prevention measures should be implemented.

Frequently, identification of noncarrier status results in alleviation of fear and anxiety. On the other hand, a phenomenon known as survivor guilt has been described in family members who are identified as noncarriers, particularly in late-onset disorders such as hereditary cancer. Survivor guilt describes the uneasiness an individual experiences when a sibling (or other close relative) tests positive for the mutation and she or he does not. Survivor guilt can be surprising to the physician in light of what is thought to be "good news" for the patient. Thus, knowledge of negative carrier status may be considered a "benefit" to some patients and a "risk" to others, and these potential outcomes should be discussed before testing.

It is important that individuals considering testing be aware of all the possible outcomes of testing in the context of their family history and that the genetic testing results may not provide them a clear answer. If a test result is negative for an individual from a family with a known deleterious mutation, he or she can be reassured that their cancer risk is similar to that of the general population. However, a negative test in families in which the disease causing mutation is not known must be interpreted with extreme caution. A false-negative test result can occur because even direct gene sequencing cannot detect all disease-causing mutations. Also, increased cancer risk in these families may be caused by mutations in other genes that were not tested, including as yet unidentified cancer-causing genes. In the situation of a negative test result in a multicase cancer family without a known disease-causing mutation, family members must be advised they are still at high risk for cancer and encouraged to avail themselves of screening and prevention measures for the cancers observed in their family. If a person has a negative result from an ASO screening test for specific founder mutations, complete BRCA1 and BRCA2 sequencing should be performed, because a deleterious mutation may be present in another portion of the gene. Finally, a test may be reported as a "variant of uncertain significance." That is, there is an abnormality in gene sequence detected but its impact on cancer risk is unclear.

Numerous studies have shown the range of emotions in cancer genetic testing, and pretest counseling should be tempered with an understanding of the underlying psychological issues. In addition to survival guilt, other psychological issues include depression, grief, and fear of disfigurement or loss of body image when a disease-causing mutation is identified. Some particularly concerning issues are unwillingness of family members to share results and inadvertent discovery that one is an obligate carrier of the condition when a first-degree relative is found to be a carrier. Changes in family dynamics related to these issues have been well described. Anxiety and fear are also common, because most patients are aware of the many potential adverse implications of a cancer diagnosis. This may even result in avoidance of routine follow-up or seeking medical attention for symptoms of disease.

The process of genetic testing has also unveiled ethical issues for the patient and physician (44). For the physician, upholding patient autonomy is the most important consideration. It is critical that a patient be presented with the option of genetic testing in a neutral environment. Although it is always best to begin genetic testing on a relative with a history of cancer, that relative should never feel coerced into testing. The choice to undergo testing must remain an individual decision, because motivation and readiness for testing vary.

Many patients fear genetic discrimination from employers, as well as health insurance companies, after testing. Although federal legislation has been passed to protect individuals, discrimination remains a significant concern. The Americans with Disabilities Act (ADA) includes legislation to stop employers from discriminating against individuals based on genetic information. More recently, the Health Insurance Portability and Accountability Act (HIPAA), effective in 1997, was enacted to protect individuals from having genetic information considered as a preexisting condition and from having insurance rates increased based on this information. Yet, breach of confidentiality and potential discrimination remain threats and should be discussed, because federal legislation does not cover all aspects of discrimination and state legislation varies.

Genetic testing should be considered only when the physician is certain that the individual has been adequately counseled; understands the potential ramifications of positive, negative, and indeterminate results; and has adequate psychosocial support to cope with potentially unfavorable results.

MANAGEMENT OPTIONS FOR HIGH-RISK INDIVIDUALS

Surveillance Options for Ovarian Cancer

Transvaginal ultrasonography (TVS) is currently the preferred screening test for ovarian cancer (45). TVS is relatively sensitive in providing an accurate morphologic image of the ovary and has been proven to be safe, time-efficient, and well tolerated by patients (46). Large-scale screening studies in the general population and in women with a family history of the disease indicate that TVS can be useful in detecting small, potentially curable early-stage tumors. Recently, van Nagell and coworkers evaluated the efficacy of annual TVS in more than 14,000 asymptomatic women who were at least 50 years of age, or 25 years of age if they had a family history of ovarian cancer (47). A total of 17 ovarian cancers were detected, of which 14 were potentially curable stage I or II cancers. Clearly, this study illustrates that TVS, when performed annually, is associated with a decrease in stage at detection of ovarian cancer compared with detection in an unscreened population. However, TVS cannot reliably distinguish between benign and malignant tumors, leading to potentially unnecessary operative intervention. Moreover, TVS can fail to detect primary peritoneal malignancies or ovarian cancer in which the size of the ovary is normal. Karlan and associates performed TVS, CA 125, and CD1 analysis on more than 1,200 women with a family history of ovarian cancer (48). Three ovarian cancers, all stage I, were detected by TVS. Seven women in this population were found to have papillary serous peritoneal carcinoma. Of these, two were detected by TVS, two by CA 125, and the remaining three were undetected by screening. Of the tumor markers available, CA 125 is the serum marker used most extensively in ovarian screening trials (49). Although serum CA 125 is elevated in 80% of all epithelial ovarian cancers, serum levels are directly related to tumor volume, and small, potentially curable, early-stage tumors may not be detected by this technique. In fact, serum CA-125 is elevated in only half of patients with clinically detectable stage I tumors and in a much smaller percentage of asymptomatic ovarian malignancies detected by TVS (50). As with TVS, the high rate of falsely elevated serum levels in benign disease may lead to unnecessary intervention.

Despite their limitations, TVS and CA 125 have become widely accepted as screening tests for women with a family history of ovarian cancer. The 1994 National Cancer Institute (NCI) Consensus Statement on Ovarian Cancer recommended annual pelvic examination, TVS evaluation of the ovaries, and a serum CA 125 determination for women who are members of hereditary ovarian cancer families (51) (Table 9.6). This evaluation should begin at age 20 to 25 years, or 5 years earlier than the age at which the youngest relative was diagnosed with ovarian cancer, whichever is earlier. The NCI

TABLE 9.6. *Ovarian cancer screening and prevention for women at high risk for ovarian cancer*

1. Annual or semiannual bimanual pelvic examination
2. Annual or semiannual transvaginal ultrasonography
3. Annual or semiannual CA-125 measurement
4. Oral contraceptive pills
5. Prophylactic oophorectomy

From NIH Consensus Conference: Ovarian cancer screening, treatment, and follow-up. *JAMA* 1995;273: 491–497, with permission.

Consensus Statement recommends consultation with a genetic counselor or gynecologic oncologist for women with two or more first-degree relatives affected by ovarian cancer. Screening recommendations, including TVS and CA 125, should then be made on an individual basis, depending on patient and physician preference. The Consensus Statement acknowledges that these recommendations are made despite a lack of data demonstrating a survival benefit of screening modalities for ovarian cancer.

A task force convened by the Cancer Genetics Studies Consortium (CGSC) in 1997 likewise concluded that TVS timed to avoid ovulation was the single best modality for detecting ovarian cancer in high-risk women and was even better when combined with serum CA 125 testing (52). The task force recommended annual or semiannual TVS and CA 125 screening in BRCA1 or BRCA2 mutation-positive women beginning at age 25 to 35 years.

Ovarian Cancer Chemoprevention

In the general population, OC use reduces the risk of ovarian cancer by up to 60% with more than 5 years of use, with a protective effect evident even up to 10 years after discontinuation. Although this protective effect has been well established in the general population, many have questioned whether it would hold true in BRCA1 and BRCA2 mutation carriers. A 1997 case-control study that evaluated 207 BRCA1 and BRCA2 carriers demonstrated that any prior use of OCs was associated with a 50% reduction in ovarian cancer risk and continued to decrease with increasing length of OC use (53). Of note, in this study of BRCA1 and BRCA2 mutation carriers there was no difference noted in breast cancer risk between those who used OCs and those who did not. Although prospective clinical trials are needed, it appears that OC use can modify ovarian cancer risk in BRCA1 and BRCA2 mutation carriers without increasing breast cancer risk. Based on this data, OC prophylaxis can be recommended for women at high risk for ovarian cancer. Women who carry BRCA mutations and are interested in OC use for ovarian cancer prophylaxis should be encouraged to participate in ongoing clinical trials designed to address these issues.

Prophylactic oophorectomy is considered the definitive option for ovarian cancer prevention. In women who are proven to be BRCA1 and BRCA2 mutation carriers, the lifetime risk of ovarian cancer is sufficiently high to outweigh the potential risks of prophylactic oophorectomy, including the morbidity and mortality of the procedure, early menopause, the need for long-term hormone replacement therapy, and the risk of primary peritoneal carcinoma (4,51). In the past, this procedure was recommended solely on the basis of family history. However, now that BRCA testing can differentiate carriers from noncarriers in hereditary ovarian cancer families, prophylactic surgery can be offered to those who are identified as mutation carriers while sparing those who are noncarriers. For this reason, patients who are interested in prophylactic oophorectomy should be offered genetic counseling and testing before proceeding.

Although prophylactic removal of the ovaries was recommended by a National Institute of Health Consensus panel for women who are members of autosomal dominant ovarian cancer families. It is important for both the patient and the physician to understand that prophylactic oophorectomy is not completely protective. The occurrence of peritoneal carcinoma, clinically and histologically indistinguishable from epithelial ovarian cancer, has been well documented. It may occur in 2% to 11% of women with hereditary risk after prophylactic oophorectomy (54,55). For example, Tobacman and colleagues reported the occurrence of primary peritoneal carcinoma in 3 of 28 women from high-risk families between 1 and 11 years after prophylactic oophorectomy. The Gilda Radner Registry reported the occurrence of peritoneal carcinoma in 2% of high-risk women ranging from 1 to 27 years after the procedure (55). More recently, Struewing and coworkers, in an analysis of 12 families in which at least two women had ovarian cancer, estimated that prophylactic oophorectomy resulted in a 50% reduction in risk of serous carcinoma of the ovary or peritoneum (56). Prospective studies are ongoing to determine the actual incidence of peritoneal carcinomatosis in documented BRCA1 and BRCA2 mutation carriers.

Peritoneal carcinomas occurring after prophylactic oophorectomy may result from unrecognized microscopic metastasis at the time of the procedure or, more likely, from the development of cancer multifocally throughout the peritoneal cavity. Because the peritoneal lining originates from the same embryonic tissue as the ovary, it has the same potential to undergo carcinogenesis, and carcinomatosis can develop independent of ovarian involvement, arising either *de novo* in ectopic ovarian tissue or multifocally throughout the abdominal cavity after prophylactic oophorectomy. It is important to alert the pathologist to the indication for oophorectomy so that multiple sections of grossly normal-appearing ovaries can be obtained to rule out the presence of a microscopic primary ovarian cancer.

Initial recommendations for prophylactic oophorectomy included a midline incision, removal of the uterus, peritoneal biopsies, and even lymph node sampling to rule out micrometastases. More recent data suggest that laparoscopic oophorectomy without removal of the uterus, in the absence of other pathology, is acceptable and also reduces postoperative morbidity. In women who are proven mutation carriers, prophylactic oophorectomy should be considered after completion of childbearing or between the ages of 35 and 40 years. However, because evidence of benefit is lacking, the CGSC task force declined to make absolute recommendations for or against prophylactic oophorectomy (52).

Because bilateral oophorectomy induces surgical menopause, the risk of hypoestrogenemia and potential compliance with long-term estrogen replacement therapy should be discussed. Estrogen replacement is generally recommended after prophylactic oophorectomy to prevent side effects such as vasomotor symptoms, urogenital atrophy, osteoporosis, and heart disease. There is some concern, however, that administration of exogenous estrogen to mutation carriers may increase their risk of breast cancer. Studies investigating the potential link between hormone replacement therapy and breast cancer in the general population have yielded conflicting results, indicating that the association, if any, is likely to be small. The largest study to date, the Nurses' Health Study, found a relative risk of 1.46 for current users of 5 or more years, and no increased risk for past users of hormone therapy or for current users of less than 5 years (57). A large collaborative reanalysis of this data found that the occurrence of breast cancer in these women was unrelated to family history of the disease, suggesting that estrogen replacement can be given to women with strong family histories of breast cancer (58). As yet, however, there are no prospective data available on women with BRCA1 or BRCA2 mutations. Nevertheless, in the absence of a breast cancer diagnosis, BRCA mutation status should not preclude the use of hormone replacement therapy.

Breast Cancer Screening

The 1997 CGSC task force issued breast cancer surveillance recommendations for BRCA mutation carriers. These include self-breast examinations, clinical breast examinations, and mammography (52). Monthly self-breast examinations should begin at age 18, and annual mammography studies at age 25 to 35 years. Annual or semiannual clinical breast examinations are especially important in this population because of the technical difficulty in interpreting mammograms in women in this age group. Although there is some concern that mutation carriers may be particularly susceptible to the carcinogenic potential of radiation exposure, the task force concluded that the benefit of early detection is likely to outweigh any theoretic risk from early mammograms.

Breast Cancer Prophylaxis

Prophylactic mastectomy is another option for known mutation carriers. Simple mastectomy is preferred over subcutaneous mastectomy, which preserves the nipple, the areola, and a small amount of ductal tissue. However, even bilateral total mastectomy leaves some residual breast tissue under the skin and in the chest wall, so protection against breast cancer is not complete. A study of women with a family history suggestive of hereditary predisposition to breast cancer reported a significant reduction in the risk of breast cancer after prophylactic bilateral mastectomy. In women with a strong family history of breast cancer, prophylactic mastectomy was associated with a reduction in breast cancer of at least 90% (59). After mastectomy, continued surveillance with breast examinations is recommended.

Chemoprevention is another option for women at high risk for breast cancer. Tamoxifen has been shown to reduce the number of new primary cancers in the contralateral breast of breast cancer patients, stimulating interest in the drug as a means of prevention in high-risk women. In a randomized trial of tamoxifen versus no tamoxifen in women without cancer whose breast cancer risk was 1.67% or higher within the next 5 years, as calculated by the Gail model, the Breast Cancer Prevention Trial demonstrated a 45% reduction in invasive breast cancer in these high-risk women (60). Again, there are no definitive data regarding the efficacy of prophylactic mastectomy in BRCA mutation carriers.

Raloxifene has a pharmacologic effect on breast tissue similar to that of tamoxifen, with added cardioprotective effects and none of the additional endometrial cancer risk associated with tamoxifen. Raloxifene is currently being evaluated in the Study of Tamoxifen and Raloxifene (STAR) trial to determine whether this effect translates into protection against breast cancer. Mutation carriers who are interested in chemoprevention of breast cancer should be encouraged to enroll in clinical trials to evaluate the efficacy and safety of tamoxifen and raloxifene.

Management Options for HNPCC Carriers

The CGSC task force also made recommendations for follow-up care of individuals who are HNPCC-associated gene mutation carriers (39). Their consensus opinion, which was based on observational studies, recommends surveillance for colon and endometrial cancer, the two most prevalent cancers in these families. Colon cancer screening should include colonoscopy with the removal of adenomatous polyps every 1 to 3 years beginning at age 25 years. Screening sigmoidoscopy is not sufficient, because examination of the right side of the colon is necessary. Endometrial cancer screening should include either annual endometrial biopsy or TVS or both, beginning at age 25 to 35 years. The task force did not make any recommendations for or against prophylactic colectomy or hysterectomy because of their unproven efficacy. However, these are certainly reasonable options for HNPCC mutation carriers. If a female patient chooses to undergo prophylactic colectomy, simultaneous hysterectomy and possibly bilateral salpingo-oophorectomy should be considered. Although it was not addressed in the CGSC recommendations, heightened surveillance for ovarian cancer has also been suggested for female HNPCC-associated mutation carriers. Although the ovarian cancer risk is less than for members of HBOC families or BRCA1 and BRCA2 families, the 9% to 12% risk is substantially higher than the baseline population risk, and surveillance should be considered. Additional screening for other HNPCC-associated cancers should be based on the individual cancer family history.

SUMMARY

1. Ovarian cancer is the leading cause of death from gynecologic malignancy and the fourth most common cause of all cancer deaths among women in the United States. An estimated 23,100 new cases of ovarian cancer and 14,000 deaths are expected in the year 2000 (61). Unfortunately, the majority of women with ovarian cancer present with advanced disease, where prognosis is poor. The 5-year survival rate for stage III and IV ovarian cancer is only 14% to 29%, compared to approximately 85% to 90% when disease is confined to the ovary.
2. The strongest single risk factor for ovarian cancer is a family history of the disease. Lynch and coworkers first suggested that heredity plays an important role in ovarian cancer more than three decades ago (62). They described three distinct autosomal dominant ovarian cancer family syndromes: site-specific ovarian cancer, breast/ovarian cancer syndrome (HBOC), and hereditary nonpolyposis colon cancer syndrome (HNPCC), also known as Lynch syndrome type II. Extensive pedigree analyses, as well as epidemiologic studies, have confirmed the importance of heredity in the development of ovarian cancer. Currently it is estimated that inherited predisposition is responsible for at least 5% to 10% of all ovarian cancer cases.
3. In the 1990s, two breast cancer susceptibility genes, BRCA1 and BRCA2, were identified by positional cloning. Together, they are responsible for most hereditary breast cancer cases and at least 90% of HBOC and site-specific ovarian cancer, or hereditary ovarian cancer cases. Inherited mutations in DNA mismatch repair (MMR) genes were discovered soon after and are responsible for ovarian cancer occurring as part of HNPCC. Mutations in MLH1 and MSH2 account for disease in most HNPCC families.
4. In the initial very large multicase breast and ovarian cancer families used to establish linkage to the BRCA1 region, estimates of cancer risk penetrance by the age of 70 years for a BRCA1 mutation carrier was 82% to 87% for breast cancer and as high as 63% for ovarian cancer (12,14). However, more recent estimates of lifetime cancer risk for BRCA1 carriers unselected for family history are significantly lower; approximately 50% for breast cancer and 16% for ovarian cancer (13).
5. The ability to identify women who are at high risk for ovarian cancer by virtue of a genetic predisposition provides a unique opportunity to select women who are most likely to benefit from surveillance and prevention measures. Genetic testing for BRCA1 and BRCA2, as well as MLH1 and MSH2, is now commercially available, and public awareness of the importance of family history of disease in ovarian cancer has increased.
6. Currently, genetic testing for inherited mutations is recommended for individuals with at least a 10% probability of carrying a mutation based on family history of disease (40). Although we are now able to test for mutations

in these genes, genetic testing has created numerous dilemmas. These include difficulties in interpretation of test results, psychological implications, and potential ethical issues such as patient confidentiality and discrimination.

7. Prevention and surveillance options should be thoroughly discussed with women who are at increased risk for ovarian cancer by virtue of their family history or carrier status. Prevention options include chemoprevention with oral contraceptives or prophylactic oophorectomy. Currently, CA 125 and transvaginal ultrasound (TVS) are the most widely used screening methods for the early detection of ovarian cancer. Although they have not been shown to decrease mortality in the general population, it is recommended that women at high risk obtain annual or semiannual TVS and serum CA 125 studies obtained beginning at age 25 to 35 years (51).

REFERENCES

1. Whittemore AS, Harns R, Intyre J, and the Collaborative Ovarian Cancer Group. Characteristics relating to ovarian cancer risk: collaborative analysis of 12 U.S. case control studies. IV: pathogenesis of epithelial ovarian cancer. *Am J Epidemiol* 1992;136:1212–1220.
2. Cancer and Steroid Hormone Study of the Centers for Disease Control and the National Institute of Child Health and Human Development: The reduction in risk of ovarian cancer associated with oral-contraceptive use. *N Engl J Med* 1987;316:650–655.
3. Schildkraut JM, Thompson D. Familial ovarian cancer: a population-based case control study. *Am J Epidemiol* 1988;128: 456–466.
4. Kerlikowske K, Brown JS, Grady DG. Should women with familial ovarian cancer undergo prophylactic oophorectomy? *Obstet Gynecol* 1992;80:700–707.
5. Stratton JF, Pharoah P, Smith SK, et al. A systematic review and meta-analysis of family history and risk of ovarian cancer. *Br J Obstet Gynaecol* 1998;105:493–499.
6. Claus EB, Risch N, Thompson WD. The calculation of breast cancer risk for women with a first degree family history of ovarian cancer. *Breast Cancer Res Treat* 1993;28:115–120.
7. Amos CI, Struewing JP. Genetic epidemiology of epithelial ovarian cancer. *Cancer* 1993;71:566–572.
8. Heintz APM, Hacker NF, Lagasse LD. Epidemiology and etiology of ovarian cancer: a review. *Obstet Gynecol* 1985;66:127–135.
9. Mori M, Harabuchi I, Miyake H, et al. Reproductive, genetic, and dietary risk factors for ovarian cancer. *Am J Epidemiol* 1988; 128:771–777.
10. Casagrande JT, Louie EW, Pike MC, et al. Incessant ovulation and ovarian cancer. *Lancet* 1979;2:170–173.
11. Tortolero-Luna G, Mitchell MF. The epidemiology of ovarian cancer. *J Cell Biochem* 1995;23:200–207.
12. Easton DR, Ford D, Bishop DT, and the Breast Cancer Linkage Consortium. Breast and ovarian cancer incidence in BRCA1-mutation carriers. *Am J Hum Genet* 1995 56:265–271.
13. Struewing JP, Hartge P, Wacholder S, et al. The risk of cancer associated with specific mutations of BRCA1 and BRCA2 among Ashkenazi Jews. *N Engl J Med* 1997 336:1401–14C8.
14. Easton DR, Bishop DT, Ford D, et al., for the Breast Cancer Linkage Consortium: Genetic linkage analysis in familial breast and ovarian cancer: results from 214 families. *Am J Hum Genet* 1993;52:678–701.
15. Chang J, Fryatt I, Ponder B, et al. A matched control study of familial epithelial ovarian cancer: patient characteristics, response to chemotherapy and outcome. *Ann Oncol* 1995;6:80–82.
16. Bellacosa A, Genuardi M, Anti M, et al. Hereditary nonpolyposis colorectal cancer: review of clinical, molecular genetics, and counseling aspects. *Am J Med Genet* 1996 24:353–364.
17. Hall JM, Lee MK, Newman B, et al. Linkage of early-onset familial breast cancer to chromosome 17q21. *Science* 1990;250:1684–1689.
18. Miki Y, Swensen J, Schattuck-Eidens D, et al. Isolation of BRCA1, the 17q-linked breast and ovarian cancer susceptibility gene. *Science* 1994;266:66–71.
19. Wooster R, Neuhausen S, Manigion J, et al. Localisation of a breast cancer susceptibility gene (BRCA2) to chromosome 13q by genetic linkage analysis. *Science* 1994 265:2088–2090.
20. Wooster R, Bignell G, Lancaster J, et al. Identification of the breast cancer susceptibility gene BRCA2. *Nature* 1995 378:789–792.
21. Knudson AG. Hereditary cancer, oncogenes, and antioncogenes. *Cancer Res* 1985;45:1437–1443.
22. Brugarolas J, Jacks T. Double indemnity: p53, BRCA and cancer. p63 mutation partially rescues developmental arrest in Brca1 and Brca2 null mice, suggesting a role for familial breast cancer genes in DNA damage repair. *Nat Med* 1997;3:721–722.
23. Kinzler KW, Vogelstein B. Cancer-susceptibility genes: gatekeepers and caretakers. *Nature* 1997;386:761–763.
24. Couch FJ, Hartmann LC. BRCA1 testing: advances and retreats. *JAMA* 1998;279:955–957.
25. Malone KE, Daling JR, Thompson JD, et al. BRCA1 mutations and breast cancer in the general population: analyses in women before age 35 years and in women before age 45 years with first-degree family history. *JAMA* 1998;279(12):922–929.
26. Couch FJ, DeShano ML, Blackwood MA, et al. BRCA1 mutations in women attending clinics that evaluate the risk of breast cancer. *N Engl J Med* 1997;336:1409–1415.
27. Brody LC, Biesecker BB. Breast cancer susceptibility genes: BRCA1 and BRCA2. *Medicine (Baltimore)* 1998 77:208–226.
28. Rubin SC, Blackwood MA, Bandera C, et al. BRCA1, BRCA2, and hereditary nonpolyposis colorectal cancer gene mutations in an unselected ovarian cancer population: relationship to family history and implications for genetic testing. *Am J Obstet Gynecol* 1998;178:670–677.
29. Smith SA, Richards WE, Caito K, et al. BRCA1 germline mutations and polymorphisms in a clinic-based series of ovarian cancer cases: a Gynecologic Oncology Group study. *Am J Hum Genet* (submitted).
30. Frank TS, Manley SA, Olopade OI, et al. Sequence analysis of BRCA1 and BRCA2: correlation of mutations

with family history and ovarian cancer risk. *J Clin Oncol* 1998;16:2417–2425.
31. Ford D, Easton DR, Stratton M, et al. Genetic heterogeneity and penetrance analysis of the BRCA1 and BRCA2 genes in breast cancer families. *Am J Hum Genet* 1998;62:676–689.
32. Phelan, CM, Rebbeck TR, Weber BL, et al. Ovarian cancer risk in BRCA1 carriers is modified by the HRAS1 variable number of tandem repeat (VNTR) locus. *Nat Genet* 1996;12:309–311.
33. Rebbeck TR, Kantoff PW, Krithivas K, et al. Modification of BRCA1-associated breast cancer risk by the polymorphic androgen-receptor CAG repeat. *Am J Hum Genet* 1999;64:1371–1377.
34. Aaltonen LA, Peltomaki P, Leach FS, et al. Clues to the pathogenesis of familial colorectal cancer. *Science* 1993;260:812–816.
35. Leach FS, Nicolaides NC, Papadopoulos N, et al. Mutations of a mutS homolog in hereditary nonpolyposis colorectal cancer. *Cell* 1993;75:1215–1225.
36. Aaltonen LA, Peltomaki P, Mecklin JP, et al. Replication errors in benign and malignant tumors from hereditary nonpolyposis colorectal cancer patients. *Cancer Res* 1994;54:1645–1648.
37. Lynch HT, de la Chapelle. Genetic susceptibility to non-polyposis colorectal cancer. *J Med Genet* 1999;36:801–818.
38. Aarnio M, Mecklin JP, Aaltonen LA, et al. Life-time risk of different cancers in hereditary non-polyposis colorectal cancer (HNPCC) syndrome. *Int J Cancer* 1995;64:430–433.
39. Burke W, Petersen G, Lynch P, et al. Recommendations for follow-up care of individuals with an inherited predisposition to cancer: I. Hereditary nonpolyposis colon cancer. *JAMA* 1997;277:915–919.
40. Statement of the American Society of Clinical Oncology. Genetic testing for cancer susceptibility. *J Clin Oncol* 1996;14:1730–1736.
41. Tinley ST, Lynch HT. Integration of family history and medical management of patients with hereditary cancers. *Cancer* 1999;86:1705–1712.
42. Berchuck A, Cirisano F, Lancaster JM, et al. Role of BRCA1 mutation screening in the management of familial ovarian cancer. *Am J Obstet Gynecol* 1996;175:738–746.
43. Lynch HT, Watson P, Shaw TG, et al. Clinical impact of molecular genetic diagnosis, genetic counseling, and management of hereditary cancer: part I. Studies of cancer in families. *Cancer* 1999;86:1629–1636.
44. Weitzel JN. The current social, political, and medical role of genetic testing in familial breast and ovarian carcinomas. *Curr Opin Obstet Gynecol* 1999;22:65–70.
45. DePriest PD, Gallion HH, Pavlik EJ, et al. Transvaginal sonography as a screening method for the detection of early ovarian cancer. *Gynecol Oncol* 1997;65:408–414.
46. DePriest PD, Shenson D, Fried A, et al. A morphology index based on sonographic findings in ovarian cancer. *Gynecol Oncol* 1993;551:7–11.
47. van Nagell JR Jr, DePriest PD, Reedy MB, et al. The efficacy of transvaginal sonographic screening in asymptomatic women at risk for ovarian cancer. *Gynecol Oncol* 2000;77:350–356.
48. Karlan BY, Baldwin RL, Lopez-Luevanos E, et al. Peritoneal serous papillary carcinoma, a phenotypic variant of familial ovarian cancer: implications for ovarian cancer screening. *Am J Obstet Gynecol* 1999;4:917–928.
49. Berchuck A, Schildkraut JM, Marks JR, et al. Managing hereditary ovarian cancer risk. *Cancer* 1999;86:1697–1704.
50. van Nagell JR Jr, Gallion HH, Pavlik EJ, et al. Ovarian cancer screening. *Cancer* 1995;15:2086–2091.
51. NIH Consensus Conference. Ovarian cancer screening, treatment, and follow-up. *JAMA* 1995;273:491–497.
52. Burke W, Daly M, Garber J, et al. Recommendations for follow-up care of individuals with an inherited predisposition to cancer: II. BRCA1 and BRCA2. Cancer Genetics Studies Consortium. *JAMA* 1997;277:997–1003.
53. Narod SA, Risch H, Moslehi R, et al. Oral contraceptives and the risk of hereditary ovarian cancer. *N Engl J Med* 1998;339:424–428.
54. Tobacman JK, Tucker MA, Kase R, et al. Intra-abdominal carcinomatosis after prophylactic oophorectomy in ovarian cancer-prone families. *Lancet* 1982;2:795–797.
55. Piver MS, Jishi MF, Tsukada Y, et al. Primary peritoneal carcinoma after prophylactic oophorectomy in women with a family history of ovarian cancer: a report of the Gilda Radner Familial Ovarian Cancer Registry. *Cancer* 1993;71:2751–2755.
56. Streuwing JP, Watson P, Easton DF, et al. Prophylactic oophorectomy in inherited breast/ovarian cancer families. *Monogr Natl Cancer Inst* 1995;33–35.
57. Colditz GA, Hankinson SE, Hunter DJ, et al. The use of estrogens and progestins and the risk of breast cancer in postmenopausal women. *N Engl J Med* 1995;332:1589–1593.
58. Collaborative Group on Hormonal Factors in Breast Cancer. Breast cancer and hormone replacement therapy: collaborative reanalysis of data from 51 epidemiological studies of 52,705 women with breast cancer and 108,411 women without breast cancer. *Lancet* 1997;350:1047–1059.
59. Hartmann LC, Schaid DJ, Woods JE, et al. Efficacy of bilateral prophylactic mastectomy in women with a family history of breast cancer. *N Engl J Med* 1999;340:77–84.
60. Early Breast Cancer Trialists' Collaborative Study. Systemic treatment of early breast cancer by hormonal, cytotoxic, or immune therapy: 133 randomized trials involving 31,000 recurrences and 24,000 deaths among 75,000 women. *Lancet* 1992;339:1–15.
61. Greenlee RT, Murray T, Bolden S, Wingo PA. Cancer statistics, 2000. *CA Cancer J Clin* 2000;50:7–33.
62. Lynch HT, Shaw MW, Magnuson CW, et al. Hereditary factors in cancer: study of two large midwestern kindreds. *Arch Intern Med* 1966;117:206–212.

10

Primary Surgical Management of Early Epithelial Ovarian Carcinoma

David H. Moore

This chapter reviews the primary surgical management of early epithelial ovarian cancer. But what constitutes an "early" ovarian cancer? Certainly, any ovarian malignancy has the potential for widespread tumor dissemination and death. In this chapter, unless otherwise stated, an ovarian cancer is designated as "early" when, at the time of surgical exploration, all gross tumor is completely resected and the disease does not appear to extend beyond the true pelvis.

HISTORICAL PERSPECTIVES

In the 18th century, John Baptist Morgagni was chief professor of anatomy and president of the university in Padua, Italy. The English translation of his Treats of the Hydrops Ascites, Tympanites, of the Dropsy of the Peritonaeum, and of others that are call'd encysted Dropsies was published in 1769. Morgagni wrote: "Must we have no hopes then, you will say, of a cure in an internal encysted dropsy, because it is not possible, either to consume, or extirpate, the cyst?" (1).

Forty years later, Ephraim McDowell was credited with the first successful salpingo-oophorectomy for an ovarian neoplasm, although the first operative removal of an ovarian cyst was actually reported by Johannes Christian Anton Theden in 1771 (2). Born in Virginia, McDowell studied at the University of Edinburgh and practiced medicine in Kentucky. He was summoned to see a Mrs. Jane Todd Crawford, who was supposedly pregnant and experiencing severe abdominal pains. McDowell diagnosed an ovarian tumor and proposed surgical removal if she would travel to his office, a journey of 2 days on horseback. On Christmas Day, 1809, he evacuated 15 pounds of gelatinous material from an ovarian tumor and then excised the ovary through a left paramedian incision while the patient recited psalms. She returned home after 25 days, and 7 years later was in excellent health. McDowell performed two other successful abdominal procedures before reporting his results (3). By the mid-19th century, 22 American surgeons had attempted ovariotomy; of 36 completed operations, 21 women recovered (3).

Ovariotomy was unpopular in Europe because of much higher mortality rates than those achieved by American surgeons (4). Many years elapsed before the procedure was considered a primary therapeutic approach. Nonsurgical treatments for ovarian cysts ranged from medical (iodides, mercurials, emetics, purgatives, and leeches) to mechanical (abdominal binders) to palliative (repeated tappings of cyst fluid with a trocar, with or without instillation of foreign substances). Asymptomatic ovarian tumors were often left untreated.

There were many opponents to surgical intervention. Charles D. Meigs of Philadelphia tried to have oophorectomy prohibited by legal statute (5,6). Byford reported results of 59 women with ovarian tumors treated with ovariotomy, performed under chloroform anesthesia. All of the women died, 50% from peritonitis and 25% from hemorrhage or shock. "A small wound, two inches long, exposing but a small extent of the peritoneum, open but ten minutes, is as dangerous as an incision from sternum to pubis open for an hour" (7).

Despite many initial failures, the surgical advocates prevailed. Developments in anesthesia, surgical antisepsis, and antibiotics were primarily responsible for the eventual decline of operative mortality. Surgical intervention, in turn, facilitated study of the natural history of ovarian cysts and tumors. Lawson Tait wrote in 1883: "The conclusion from all this is that to which I have already pointed, that the growth of ovarian tumors is associated with a tendency toward malignant disease, which finds constant clinical expression, and which received its explanation in the marvellous changes we find produced in the epithelial linings of the cysts.... One thing I am certain it clearly establishes, and that is the absolute propriety of removing ovarian tumors at a very much earlier stage of their existence than has been, till recently, the accepted rule in practice" (8). By 1883, Tait had performed 101 consecutive operations for ovarian and paraovarian tumors with only 3 deaths.

During the early 20th century, surgical resection of ovarian neoplasms became standard practice. Alexander Skene wrote: "Ovariotomy is indicated when a neoplasm or tumor of the ovary is discovered, and the operation should be performed when the surgeon is satisfied that the tumor is growing and impairing the health or usefulness of the patient" (9). Surgical intervention was avoided in cases of poor general medical health or clinically advanced disease (flatulent distention of the bowels, adhesions, ascites, involvement of other organs) (10).

In Europe, Schauta and Martin removed ovarian masses through the vagina; however, the majority of surgeons preferred an abdominal approach. The operative technique consisted of exposing the ovarian tumor by a long midline incision, evacuating the cyst contents, excising the ovary, ligating the vascular pedicle, and cleansing the peritoneum prior to wound closure (11). By 1942, perioperative mortality was approximately 17% for malignant ovarian tumors and less than 5% for nonmalignant cases (12).

STAGING CRITERIA

When confronted with an ovarian mass, the surgeon must be prepared to perform an ovarian cancer staging operation. This requires knowledge of the procedures for assigning FIGO (International Federation of Gynecology and Obstetrics) stage. A cancer staging system must reflect the biologic behavior of the cancer by dividing patients into prognostic subgroups based on disease extent and other factors. Staging also facilitates treatment planning and the comparison of data between institutions.

Skene defined three cancer stages distinguished by symptoms and examination findings (9). The first FIGO staging system for ovarian cancer was also based on clinical examination (13). One of the earliest surgical staging systems was that of Munnell and Taylor, who divided ovarian cancer into four stages "according to extent of cancer as determined at operation" (14). In 1971, the FIGO committee adopted an ovarian cancer staging system based on surgical findings (15), a system that was modified in 1974 (16). The current FIGO ovarian cancer staging system, adopted in 1985, addresses multiple prognostic variables such as tumor distribution and volume, tumor rupture, malignant cytology, and lymph node metastases (Table 10.1) (17). Histologic type, tumor grade, DNA content, hormone receptor status, and residuum after cytoreductive surgery are prognostic factors that are not considered in FIGO staging.

INCIDENCE

The American Cancer Society estimated that 25,200 new cases of ovarian cancer would occur in the United States during 1999 (18). According to the National Cancer Data Base, approximately 25% of lesions are stage I and 22% are stage II (19). The stage distribution of ovarian cancer from several series published over recent decades is listed in Table 10.2 (20–25).

The frequency of early-stage epithelial ovarian cancer has not increased appreciably. The high mortality rate from ovarian cancer is a reflection of the large percentage of patients who present with advanced cancers. Cost-effective methods for the detection of early ovarian cancer must still be considered investigational. Developments in serum tumor markers (26), pelvic ultrasound (27,28), and Doppler flow studies (29) are encouraging, but at present these modalities are too nonspecific, insensitive, or

TABLE 10.1. *FIGO staging of ovarian cancer*

Stage	Characteristics
Stage I	Growth limited to the ovaries.
IA	Growth limited to one ovary; no ascites. No tumor on the external surface; capsule intact.
IB	Growth limited to both ovaries; no ascites. No tumor on the external surfaces; capsules intact.
IC	Tumor either stage IA or IB but with tumor on surface of one or both ovaries; or with capsule ruptured; or with ascites present containing malignant cells or with positive peritoneal washings.
Stage II	Growth involving one or both ovaries with pelvic extension.
IIA	Extension and/or metastases to the uterus and/or fallopian tubes.
IIB	Extension to other pelvic organs.
IIC	Tumor either stage IIA or IIB but with tumor on surface of one or both ovaries; or with capsule ruptured; or with ascites present containing malignant cells or with positive peritoneal washings.
Stage III	Tumor involving one or both ovaries with peritoneal implants outside the pelvis and/or positive retroperitoneal or inguinal nodes. Superficial liver metastasis equals stage III. Tumor is limited to the true pelvis but with histologically confirmed malignant extension to small bowel or omentum.
IIIA	Tumor grossly limited to the true pelvis with negative nodes but with histologically confirmed microscopic seeding of abdominal peritoneal surfaces.
IIIB	Tumor of one or both ovaries with histologically confirmed implants of abdominal peritoneal surfaces <2 cm in diameter. Nodes are negative.
IIIC	Abdominal implants >2 cm in diameter and/or positive retroperitoneal or inguinal nodes.
Stage IV	Growth involving one or both ovaries with distant metastases. If pleural effusion is present there must be positive cytology. Parenchymal liver metastasis equals stage IV.

FIGO, International Federation of Gynecology and Obstetrics.
From FIGO Cancer Committee. Staging announcement. *Gynecol Oncol* 1986;25:383, with permission.

costly for mass screening of asymptomatic populations.

IMPORTANCE OF ACCURATE SURGICAL STAGING

The surgical objective in advanced ovarian cancer is tumor cytoreduction, which optimizes the curative potential of adjunctive therapy by minimizing postoperative residual tumor volume. In cases of early ovarian cancer, the surgeon must perform a meticulous, systematic exploration to exclude the presence of occult metastases that not only would change stage and prognosis but would substantially change adjunctive treatment selection.

As recently as the mid-1970s, Griffiths and Tobias reported 5-year survival rates of 61% of patients with stage I and 40% with stage II ovarian cancer (30). Many of these women received no postoperative treatment. The Gynecologic Oncology Group (GOG) reported the

TABLE 10.2. *Frequency of early ovarian cancer*

Source (ref. no.)	No. patients	Stage I		Stage II	
		No.	%	No.	%
Burns et al., 1969 (20)	915	178	19	107	12
Munnell, 1970 (21)	235	78	33	21	9
Aure et al., 1971 (22)	829	220	27	242	29
Julian, 1974 (23)	256	101	39	54	21
Obel, 1976 (24)	297	105	35	46	15
Shepherd, 1985 (25)	145	17	12	11	8
Totals	2,677	699	26	481	18

results of protocol 1 in 1980. Women with stage IA or IB ovarian cancer after total abdominal hysterectomy and bilateral salpingo-oophorectomy (TAH/BSO) were randomly assigned to groups that received either no additional treatment, pelvic radiation therapy, or oral melphalan chemotherapy. Of the 168 randomized subjects, 49% were excluded from analysis, which left only 86 evaluable patients. Five-year survival rates were not calculated. Only 6% of patients treated with melphalan experienced a recurrence, compared with 17% of patients receiving no treatment and 30% of patients treated with pelvic radiation (31). A prospective, randomized trial comparing pelvic radiation therapy alone, pelvic plus abdominal radiation, and pelvic radiation plus chlorambucil chemotherapy was conducted at the Princess Margaret Hospital. After surgery—staging procedures not detailed—196 women with asymptomatic stages IB to III ovarian cancer were randomly assigned to the three treatment groups. Either chemotherapy or abdominal radiation plus pelvic radiation was superior to pelvic radiation therapy alone. The 5-year survival rate for patients treated by whole abdominal radiation after TAH/BSO was 81% and appeared to be independent of stage (32). Results from these two prospective studies suggest the following: (a) patients with early-stage ovarian cancer require postsurgical treatment; (b) pelvic radiation alone is insufficient therapy; and (c) optimal treatment must include the abdominal cavity (whole abdominal radiation or systemic chemotherapy).

Results from a prospective study conducted at the M.D. Anderson Hospital significantly influenced the postoperative management of early-stage ovarian cancer in favor of chemotherapy. A total of 149 women with stages I to III ovarian cancer and minimal residual disease were randomly assigned to receive either whole abdominal radiation or melphalan chemotherapy. After extended follow-up, survival in both groups was equivalent. Chemotherapy was deemed to be the preferred treatment because of its lower toxicity (33).

All of these investigations permitted less rigorous pretreatment surgical staging than what is advocated today. It is possible that there were many patients with more advanced disease than what was surgically appreciated. Furthermore, many important prognostic factors were not considered in the randomization processes or in data analyses. In 1982, Einhorn suggested that future adjuvant trials in early-stage ovarian cancer include only serous tumors and poorly differentiated tumors of other histologic types. She pointed out that only 5% of grade 1 tumors in GOG protocol 1 recurred (34). Others have substantiated the excellent prognosis for stage IA, well-differentiated ovarian cancer treated with surgery alone (35,36). In a prospective trial conducted by the GOG (protocol 7601), 92 women with stage IA or IB (well- or moderately-differentiated) ovarian cancer were randomly assigned to receive either melphalan or no further treatment. Five-year survival rates were equivalent in both groups and exceeded 90% (37). Therefore, selected patients with early-stage ovarian cancer, determined through comprehensive surgical staging, may be spared the toxicity of intensive multiagent chemotherapy without compromising survival.

In his review of patients with early-stage ovarian cancer treated on GOG protocols 7601 and 7602, Walton and colleagues noted that only 5% of patients who were asymptomatic before second-look surgery were found to have persistent disease at the reassessment operation (38). Therefore, asymptomatic patients with early-stage ovarian cancer, after comprehensive surgical staging and adjuvant therapy, need not undergo second-look surgery.

PATTERNS OF SPREAD

Direct Extension

Spread patterns are retrospective constructs from surgical observations and autopsy studies. Once the cancer penetrates the ovarian capsule, spread can occur by direct extension to surrounding organs such as the fallopian tube, uterus, bladder, cul-de-sac peritoneum, or rectosigmoid colon. The relative infrequency of stage II ovarian cancer implies that direct extension does not necessarily occur before, but rather simultaneously with, other spread patterns.

Intraperitoneal Dissemination

Perhaps the most common and widely recognized spread pattern is intraperitoneal dissemination. More than two centuries ago, Morgagni observed: "Finally, read over again what I have formerly written to you, of hard granules, or tubercles, being prominent on the internal surface of the peritoneum, or pleura; as water was even then extravasated in the great cavities" (1). Ovarian cancer implants may be found on the surface of any organ within the coelomic cavity (Figure 10.1). This process can occur in the absence of capsular rupture. Keettel and Pixley reported positive cytology in 33 (73%) of 45 patients with ovarian cancer; in 5 cases, cytology was positive without gross capsular penetration or rupture (39).

A clinical syndrome that is indistinguishable from ovarian cancer with peritoneal and mesenteric metastases has developed after prophylactic oophorectomy (40,41). This remarkable propensity for malignant transformation or involvement of the abdominal peritoneum raises the question of whether epithelial ovarian cancer is a malignancy of the ovary *per se,* or rather of the entire peritoneal cavity (42).

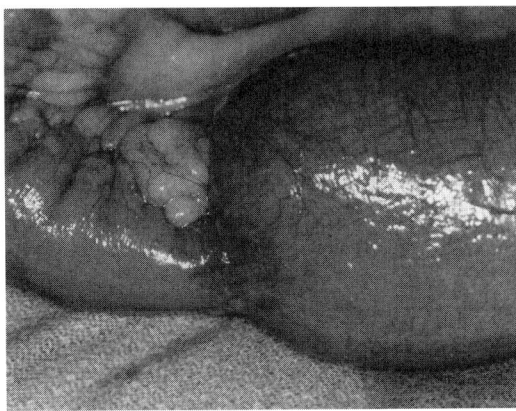

FIG. 10.1. The patient presented with a brief history of nausea, vomiting, and abdominal distention. An ovarian mass was palpable on pelvic examination. No ascites or abdominal metastases were readily apparent. Further study revealed a small tumor implant on the ileum, producing a partial small bowel obstruction. The involved ileum was resected, followed by primary side-to-side reanastomosis.

Ascites is a common manifestation in ovarian cancer; when present, it usually indicates advanced disease. Peritoneal fluid is continuously formed as a transudate from small blood vessels and is resorbed by subdiaphragmatic lymphatics. In cats, 1.5 times the plasma volume is absorbed each day by the diaphragmatic lymphatics (43). Schoenberger and coworkers demonstrated that in humans 75% of the total body albumin circulates each day through the peritoneal cavity (44). Ascites develops whenever equilibrium is shifted to favor formation over resorption. Peritoneal tumor implantation may lead to increased surface area, neovascularization, and increased plasma transudation. Using lymphoscintigraphy, Coates and associates demonstrated complete diaphragmatic lymphatic occlusion in 21 (91%) of 23 women with malignant ascites (45). The occasional presence of ascites in association with benign tumors such as fibromas (Meigs syndrome), or the absence of ascites in women with advanced ovarian cancer, underscores the fact that this process is poorly understood.

Retroperitoneal Dissemination

The tendency for ovarian cancer to metastasize to the retroperitoneal lymph nodes has been noted for many years. Autopsy studies by Abrams and associates (46) and by Bergman (47) demonstrated lymph node metastases in 65% to 80% of cases. Because these patients died of advanced cancer, it is important to assess the incidence of retroperitoneal lymph node dissemination at earlier points in the disease process. Burghardt and coworkers performed radical lymphadenectomy in 123 patients with stages IA to IV ovarian cancer. Except for 26 cases in which lymph node dissections were performed within 1 year after primary surgery and chemotherapy, lymph nodes were sampled at the primary operation. Pelvic lymph nodes were positive in 61.8% of the cases, and aortic lymph nodes were positive in 41.4% of the cases. Aortic lymph nodes were involved only in the presence of pelvic lymph node metastases (48). Wu and associates demonstrated the presence of retroperitoneal lymph node metastases in 42 (57%) of 74 cases. In his series, the aortic lymph nodes were positive in 6 patients

(19%) in the absence of pelvic lymph node metastases (49).

Distant Metastases

Widespread dissemination of ovarian cancer occurs late in the disease process. It rarely occurs in the absence of advanced intraperitoneal disease. The more common sites of distant metastases, particularly at initial presentation, are the lung and liver. Tumor implants on the liver capsule can directly invade the liver parenchyma. Tumor that involves the diaphragmatic lymphatics can invade the pleural space. Bergman identified metastases to the lung in 27% and metastases to the liver in 34% of patients who died of ovarian cancer (47). Other distant metastatic sites include bone, skin, and brain (50,51).

COMPREHENSIVE SURGICAL STAGING

The surgical objectives for suspected ovarian cancer are to confirm the diagnosis, determine the extent of disease, and excise gross tumor. Surgical staging is not merely an academic exercise. When the physician is confronted with cancer confined to the ovary and no apparent spread elsewhere within the pelvis or abdomen, a properly performed staging procedure is essential to rational treatment planning.

Preoperative Considerations

What preoperative studies are essential? Ovarian cancer is a surgical diagnosis, and preoperative studies should reduce the operative risk and provide some warning of what may be expected during the operation. Preoperative studies that do not fulfill either of these roles should be omitted. A minimum preoperative workup should include a chest radiograph, complete blood count, serum electrolytes, liver and renal chemistries, and blood typing and screening. Owing to tumor neovascularization, and particularly if tumor cytoreduction proves necessary, potential blood loss with ovarian cancer surgery is not trivial and transfusion with blood components is often required. Pleural effusions on chest radiographs should be aspirated for cytologic analysis.

Elevated serum tumor markers such as CA-125 should not influence whether surgery is performed when ovarian cancer is suspected but will prove useful in postoperative management if a cancer diagnosis is confirmed.

Patients with ovarian cancer are at increased risk for breast cancer and should undergo annual mammography. A preoperative mammogram, if breast cancer screening has not been performed in the preceding 12 months, is advisable. Occasionally, an ovarian mass proves to be metastatic breast or gastrointestinal cancer. Patients with bowel symptomatology may benefit from an upper gastrointestinal series, barium enema, or upper or lower gastrointestinal endoscopy (flexible sigmoidoscopy or colonoscopy). Evidence of bowel involvement suggests that bowel resection may be necessary. Under any circumstances, preoperative mechanical bowel preparation with antibiotics is strongly recommended.

Ultrasonography, computed tomography, and magnetic resonance imaging can provide a great deal of clinical information. However, inaccuracies in these expensive imaging procedures are recognized. Positive findings are far more useful in the prediction of metastatic disease than are negative findings in the prediction of early-stage ovarian cancer. Radiologic imaging is not a substitute for surgery in establishing the diagnosis of ovarian cancer. Clinical signs and symptoms are notoriously misleading and often underestimate the true extent of disease. Other cancers and nonmalignant conditions such as fibromas, endometriosis, or tuberculosis can mimic ovarian cancer, and surgery is required for proper diagnosis (Figure 10.2).

The Surgical Approach

Surgical requirements have changed dramatically as treatments for advanced disease have improved and the body of knowledge about metastatic spread patterns has increased. In 1970, Munnell stated that, for cancer limited to one or both ovaries, "maximal surgical effort is the indicated treatment and bilateral salpingo-oophorectomy and total hysterectomy should be carried out" (21). In 1977, Green recommended TAH/BSO and perhaps prophylactic

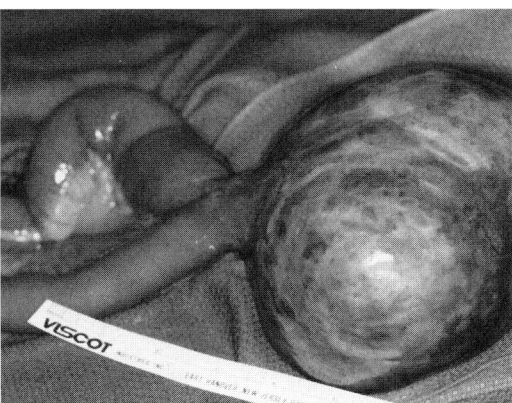

FIG. 10.2. The patient presented with abdominal cramping, intermittent distention, and a pelvic mass. Intraoperative findings included normal pelvic organs and a pedunculated mass arising from the mid-jejunum, which had fallen into the pelvis. Pathologic diagnosis was low-grade leiomyosarcoma of the small intestine.

TABLE 10.3. *Epithelial ovarian cancer: comprehensive surgical staging procedures*

Examination under anesthesia
Midline abdominal incision
Cytologic washings
    Ascites or peritoneal fluid
    Pelvic cul-de-sac
    Bilateral pericolic gutters
    Diaphragm
Total abdominal hysterectomy
Bilateral salpingo-oophorectomy
Omentectomy
Appendectomy
Meticulous intraabdominal inspection
    Small bowel from ligament of Treitz to terminal ileum
    Large bowel from cecum to rectum
    Peritoneal and mesenteric surfaces
    Liver, gall bladder, spleen, stomach, pancreas, kidneys
Biopsies of adhesions or any suspicious findings
Retroperitoneal lymph node biopsies
    Pelvic
    Aortic
Miscellaneous random biopsies
    Bladder peritoneum
    Pelvic cul-de-sac peritoneum
    Paracolic gutters
    Diaphragm

omentectomy (52). A year later, McGowan recommended TAH/BSO, omentectomy, and appendectomy for stage I ovarian cancer and TAH/BSO, omentectomy, appendectomy, and aspiration of peritoneal fluid for cytology for stage II disease (53). In 1984, no additions were suggested by Barber (54).

Comprehensive surgical staging for epithelial ovarian cancer should include all the procedures listed in Table 10.3. These procedures should be considered a minimum standard. Recently, the European Organization of Research and Treatment of Cancer (EORTC) adopted and published essentially identical guidelines for the surgical staging of ovarian cancer (55). Several studies have documented critical omissions in the staging of early ovarian cancer. As stated by Piver and coworkers in 1976: "The initial surgeon ordinarily has the best opportunity to establish the correct site of the primary malignancy and to delineate areas of metastases for proper staging prior to initiation of adjuvant therapy" (56). Unfortunately, Piver and associates found that out of 100 consecutive patients referred to Roswell Park Memorial Institute for the treatment of ovarian cancer who had undergone laparotomy before admission, the liver was not described in 59%, the stomach in 76%, the diaphragm in 84%, and the aortic nodes in 92%. No pelvic surgery was performed in 34% of patients (56). In 1983, Young and colleagues in the Ovarian Cancer Study Group reported results from 100 patients with presumed early-stage ovarian cancer who underwent restaging procedures. Despite the fact that only 4 patients were believed to have gross residual disease, 31% proved to have more extensive disease, and of these patients 23 (77%) of 31 had stage III ovarian cancer (57). Similarly, Helewa and coworkers detected more advanced disease in 25% of patients with apparent early-stage ovarian cancer (58).

We have not learned from past shortcomings in surgical staging accuracy. In 1990, Trimbos and associates reported a series of 86 women with early-stage ovarian cancer. After one or two laparotomies, surgical staging was complete in only 53% of cases. Staging performed at referring hospitals was complete in only 15% of cases. Reasons cited for incomplete surgical staging were equally divided between increased risk of difficulty of the procedure and lack of knowledge as to the sites at risk for metastases (59). In a review of the National Cancer Institute SEER

(Surveillance, Epidemiology, and End Results) database, Munoz and associates reported that only 10% of women with presumptive stage I ovarian cancer underwent appropriate surgical staging (60). Zanetta and colleagues reviewed the records of 351 patients with stage I ovarian cancer and performed multivariate analysis. Only tumor grade and thoroughness of surgical staging were significant prognostic factors for both disease-free and overall survival (61). Given the abundance of retrospective information, a prospective, randomized trial does not need to be conducted to verify the importance of accurate surgical staging for apparent early-stage ovarian cancer.

Choice of Incision

After the induction of general anesthesia, a bimanual pelvic examination should be performed. An "ovarian mass" may disappear with a mechanical bowel preparation, or a functional ovarian cyst may spontaneously resolve before surgical intervention. In general, the gynecologic surgeon should perform a pelvic examination with the patient under anesthesia regardless of the planned surgical intervention.

The dictum "the surgical incision should be tailored to fit the surgery and not the other way around" is particularly valid in the staging of epithelial ovarian cancer. A generous vertical incision that permits extirpation of pelvic organs and visual inspection, palpation, and biopsy of the abdominal viscera and diaphragmatic surfaces is needed. A lower transverse abdominal incision has definite cosmetic advantages, but these advantages are outweighed by the inability to adequately evaluate the upper abdominal cavity. When ovarian cancer is discovered unexpectedly through a lower transverse incision, the incision can be extended superiorly and parallel to the lateral border of the rectus abdominis to permit upper abdominal exposure. This extension often requires division of the inferior epigastric vessels and the hemilateral rectus muscle.

An inadequate surgical incision is a frequent cause of inadequate staging. In the series by Young and associates mentioned earlier, incisions used for the initial staging procedure included midline subumbilical (58%), Pfannenstiel (12%), McBurney (1%), and other (4%). Only 25% of patients had an adequate midline or paramedian incision extending above the umbilicus (57). In the series reported by Piver and coworkers, 83% of the incisions were considered inadequate (56). Failure to find a midline abdominal incision that extends above the umbilicus is the first sign that a staging procedure may have been unsatisfactory.

Cytologic Washings

If peritoneal fluid or ascites is present, it should be submitted for cytologic analysis. Otherwise, washings should be obtained from the pelvic cul-de-sac, the right and left pericolic gutters, and the right diaphragm. Keettel, Elkins, and associates reported the presence of malignant cells in peritoneal washings in the absence of ascites and later noted that 36% of patients with apparent stage IA ovarian cancer had positive peritoneal cytology (62,63). Others have reported positive cytology in 10% to 26% of stage I ovarian carcinomas (64,65). In the report by Young and colleagues, 14 (45%) of 31 patients found to have more advanced disease had malignant cytology, which was the most common positive finding in upstaged cases (57).

Removal of Pelvic Organs

Appropriate management of the reproductive organs in apparent early-stage ovarian cancer is one of the more difficult dilemmas facing the surgeon. The decision to remove pelvic organs may be complicated by many factors, including patient age and reproductive desire. The ovarian neoplasm should be removed intact and the presence of malignancy confirmed by frozen section analysis. Cyst rupture with spillage of tumor cells is believed to be an adverse prognostic factor and by FIGO staging criteria is equated with malignant ascites. Prognostic implications of cyst rupture are extremely important, because most ovarian neoplasms cannot be excised intact via laparoscopy and even needle aspiration and cyst drainage incur risks of intraperitoneal spillage.

In a series of 271 patients with stage I ovarian cancer treated at the Mayo Clinic, Webb and coworkers demonstrated a worsened prognosis with tumor rupture, capsular penetration, and adherence of the tumor to adjacent structures (66). Decker and coworkers, from the same institution, showed that survival could be improved with the postoperative administration of intraperitoneal radiation (^{198}Au) (67). In 1988, Sevelda and coworkers reported a series of 60 patients with stage I ovarian cancer treated with postoperative whole abdominal radiation. Tumor spillage had occurred in 30 patients. With mean follow-up of 75 months, cyst rupture did not appear to be an adverse prognostic factor (68). Dembo and colleagues conducted a large retrospective study of patients with stage I ovarian cancer treated at the Princess Margaret Hospital and the Norwegian Radium Hospital. Postoperative treatment was administered in 132 (26%) of 509 cases. Using multivariate analysis to control for tumor grade, dense adherence, and large-volume ascites (but not treatment), he was unable to demonstrate any prognostic significance for cyst rupture (69). Sjovall and colleagues reviewed 394 cases of early-stage ovarian cancer treated at the Radiumhemmet between 1974 and 1986. There was no difference in survival between patients whose tumors had intact capsules and patients in whom tumor rupture occurred during surgery. In contrast, patients in whom tumor rupture occurred before surgery had a significantly worse prognosis (70). In contrast, de la Cuesta and coworkers analyzed 79 patients with stage I epithelial ovarian cancer treated at Massachusetts General Hospital. Survival for patients with intraoperative cyst rupture was significantly worse than for patients with ovarian cancers removed intact but no different from survival for patients who had tumor rupture before surgery (71). In these studies, the vast majority of patients with cyst rupture received adjuvant treatment. Presently, no study has verified the inconsequence of cyst rupture without postoperative therapy. Pending further study, the surgical standard is to remove ovarian tumors without rupture and spillage of cyst contents. With tumor spillage, many patients may be subjected to adjunctive radiation or chemotherapy that otherwise would not have been administered.

Proper intraoperative management of ovarian cancer is contingent on the ability to obtain an accurate intraoperative diagnosis. The accuracy of frozen section analysis in the diagnosis of an ovarian tumor is a reflection of expertise of the pathologist, the histologic type, and the size of the ovarian tumor. The presence of a benign ovarian tumor or an invasive ovarian cancer may be determined with a high degree of accuracy, but frozen section analysis is often inaccurate in the diagnosis of ovarian tumors of low malignant potential (72–75) (Table 10.4). Menzin and colleagues found that, among 33 cases with a frozen section report of borderline or "at least borderline" tumor, no case later proved to have a benign tumor. However, 13 (27%) of 48 patients with a frozen section report of "rule out" borderline (3/15), borderline (3/16), or "at least" borderline (7/17) were found to have a focus of invasive cancer on final pathology review (76). Excluding the presence of invasive cancer within a large ovarian neoplasm is a daunting task (Figure 10.3). Puls and associates showed that, for serous ovarian tumors, the sensitivity of frozen section in detecting the presence of malignancy decreased from 96% to 94% to 75%, respectively, for tumors weighing 450 g or less, between 450 g and 1,360 g, and more than 1,360 g. For mucinous tumors, sensitivity also decreased from 92% to 87% to 67% (77). The distinction between primary and

TABLE 10.4. *Sensitivity of frozen section analysis in the diagnosis of ovarian tumors*

Source (ref. no.)	No. patients	Sensitivity (%)		
		Benign	LMP	Malignant
Slavutin and Rotterdam 1979 (72)	55	97	50	74
Twaalhoven et al., 1991 (73)	176	93	44	88
Obiakor et al., 1991 (74)	303	100	—[a]	93
Rose et al., 1994 (75)	383	99	45	93

LMP, low malignant potential.
[a] In this study low malignant potential tumors were classified as malignant.

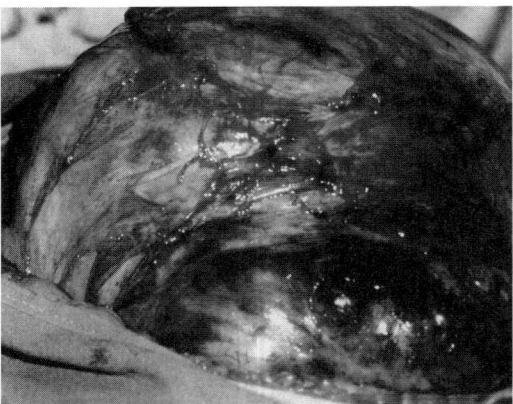

FIG. 10.3. The patient underwent surgery for a clinically obvious ovarian mass weighing in excess of 6,000 g. Frozen section diagnosis was mucinous cystadenoma, but the final pathologic diagnosis was mucinous cystadenocarcinoma of low malignant potential.

secondary ovarian cancer may also prove to be a diagnostic dilemma. In their study of patients with a history of breast or colorectal cancer who underwent surgical exploration for an adnexal mass, Abu-Rustum and colleagues found that frozen section analysis was able to determine the presence of malignancy in 36 (97%) of 37 cases, but in 17% of cases it was unable to identify the tumor as meta-static (78).

For a young patient who wishes to maintain fertility, it is prudent to defer hysterectomy and surgical staging to a second operation if the presence of malignancy is uncertain. At any age, TAH/BSO is considered standard treatment when the diagnosis of epithelial ovarian cancer is unequivocal. Preservation of reproductive function is acceptable treatment of nonepithelial ovarian cancers or tumors of low malignant potential, but only anecdotal data are available regarding conservative surgery for invasive epithelial ovarian cancer. In 1969, Munnell reported a 75% survival rate for patients treated with either unilateral salpingo-oophorectomy (USO) or hysterectomy with BSO (79). Similarly, Parker et al. reported no survival differences for patients treated with USO versus BSO (80). These early series lacked important pathology controls such as tumor grading and the possible inclusion of tumors of low malignant potential. More recently, Colombo and associates provided data on 56 women younger than 40 years of age who underwent conservative surgery for early-stage ovarian cancer. Recurrence was seen in only three patients, including one patient who relapsed in the contralateral ovary—and was effectively salvaged with surgery (81). Zanetta and colleagues compared patients with stage IA to IB ovarian cancer treated with USO versus BSO with or without hysterectomy. Only 2 of the 56 women treated conservatively experienced a recurrence in the contralateral ovary. The authors stated that tumor grade was the most important prognostic factor for recurrence and that even patients with stage IC disease could be considered for conservative surgery (82). Marchetti and associates treated 19 patients with epithelial ovarian cancer with USO; 8 patients also received postoperative cisplatin chemotherapy. Of these 19 women, 7 had tumors of low malignant potential and 12 had invasive cancers (stage I, 10 patients; stage III, 2 patients). One patient with stage III disease died from recurrent cancer. One patient was without evidence of recurrence when lost to follow-up at 3 years, and the other 10 patients were without evidence of recurrence with more than 5 years of follow-up. At the time of publication, 3 patients had conceived and delivered (4 children total), including 1 patient who had received chemotherapy (83).

Retention of the uterus and contralateral ovary theoretically leaves *in situ* potential sites for recurrence or second primary tumors. Based on the previously cited series, these risks appears small. Benjamin et al. reported that 9 (7.6%) of 118 women with stage I epithelial ovarian cancer had bilateral ovarian involvement, but in only 3 (2.5%) was the contralateral tumor clinically occult (84). If the patient is postmenopausal or if preservation of fertility is not an issue, the wisdom of conservative surgery must be questioned. If the patient strongly wishes to preserve reproductive potential and the tumor is stage I by rigorous criteria, this approach may be considered. More studies of conservative surgery are needed, because approximately 8% of all malignant stage I ovarian cancers occur in women younger than 35 years of age (85).

TABLE 10.5. Metastases in early epithelial ovarian carcinoma[a]

Source (ref. no.)	Diaphragm	Omentum	Cytology	Peritoneum
Knapp and Friedman, 1974 (89)	—	1/21	—	—
Rosenoff et al., 1975 (90)	7/16	—	—	2/16
Piver et al., 1978 (65)	1/31	0/5	8/31	—
Spinelli et al., 1979 (91)	2/33	—	2/28	—
Mangioni et al., 1979 (92)	2/13	—	3/10	—
Young et al., 1983 (57)	2/58	6/57	—	4/45
Buchsbaum and Lifshitz, 1984 (93)	3/72	7/79	—	—
Gynecologic Oncology Group, 1989 (94)	—	7/132	—	—
Totals	17/223 (7.6%)	21/294 (7.1%)	13/69 (18.8%)	6/61 (9.8%)

[a] Number of abdominal metastases per number of cases reported.

Abdominal Exploration: Pelvic and Abdominal Biopsies

The importance of a systematic surgical evaluation of abdominal contents cannot be overestimated. Subsequent to a meticulous visual and palpatory search for metastases, multiple biopsies are required to confirm the presence or absence of metastases. Omentectomy and appendectomy should be performed in all cases of ovarian cancer. The incidence of occult metastases to the omentum is 12% in apparent stage I disease (57). Studies by Malfetano (86) and by Fawzi and colleagues (87) suggested that metastasis to the appendix is common in advanced-stage ovarian cancer but rare with early-stage disease. However, Rose and coworkers discovered metastases to the appendix in 4.3% of patients with disease apparently confined to the pelvis. Noting that the frequency of metastasis to the appendix was similar to that to other sites in apparent early-stage ovarian cancer, the investigators recommended appendectomy at all primary staging procedures (88).

The frequency of occult metastases to various abdominal sites in early-stage ovarian cancer is shown in Table 10.5 (57,65,89–94). Many instances of extrapelvic metastasis in apparent early-stage ovarian cancer will be missed without a thorough abdominal exploration with biopsies.

Lymph Node Sampling

The reported frequency of lymph node metastasis in early-stage ovarian cancer is 8.9% for pelvic nodes and 12.3% for aortic nodes (48,49,57,89,94–97) (Table 10.6). The true incidence is unknown, because lymph node sampling is frequently omitted in primary staging operations. Furthermore, the prevalence of lymph node positivity depends on the number of lymph nodes removed and examined, suggesting that

TABLE 10.6. Lymph node metastases in apparent early-stage ovarian carcinoma[a]

Source (ref. no.)	Pelvic	Aortic	Overall
Knapp and Friedman, 1974 (89)	0/9	5/26	5/26
Musumeci et al., 1980 (95)	—	4/34	6/38
Knipscheer, 1982 (96)	—	5/20	5/20
Young et al., 1983 (57)	1/11	6/52	—
Averette et al., 1983 (97)	2/17	3/17	5/17
Wu et al., 1986 (49)	—	—	3/12
Burghardt et al., 1986 (48)	7/31	—	7/31
Gynecologic Oncology Group, 1989 (94)	8/134	12/136	—
Totals	18/202 (8.9%)	35/285 (12.3%)	31/144 (21.5%)

[a] Number of lymph node metastases per number of cases reported.

lymphadenectomy is preferred to lymph node sampling (98). Onda and colleagues performed systematic pelvic and aortic lymphadenectomy in 110 patients with epithelial ovarian cancer. Among the 48 women with positive lymph nodes, the incidence of metastasis to aortic lymph nodes above the inferior mesenteric artery was 79%, compared with 71% below the inferior mesenteric. The best results in sensitivity and negative predictive value were obtained when lymph node biopsies were obtained from the aortic lymph nodes above the inferior mesenteric artery along with sampling of the external iliac, internal iliac, and obturator lymph node groups (99). Ovarian cancers do not metastasize just to the ipsilateral lymph nodes. Flanagan and colleagues found no significant difference in the frequency of right-sided versus left-sided aortic node metastasis and recommended bilateral evaluation of the aortic lymph nodes (100). Walter and Magrina substantiated this recommendation with the report of a patient with apparent stage IA ovarian cancer, well encapsulated, arising from the left ovary. The peritoneal surfaces and omentum were grossly free of disease and there was no ascites. With further surgical exploration, the left aortic lymph nodes were found to be negative, but there was grossly metastatic cancer in the right aortic and common iliac lymph nodes (101). Aortic lymph node biopsies should include the precaval fat pad lateral to the aortic bifurcation (Figure 10.4). Pelvic lymph nodes should be sampled bilaterally, with specimens selected from the common iliac, external iliac, internal iliac (hypogastric), and obturator node groups (Figure 10.5).

Visualization/Palpation Versus Pathologic Findings

A grievous error in surgical staging is to assume that negative inspection and palpation indicate the absence of disease spread. The literature is replete with studies documenting inaccuracies of observation and palpation versus pathologic findings. Buchsbaum and colleagues reported surgical staging data from the GOG in 1989. In more than 50% of patients with histologically proven diaphragmatic metastases, and in 45% of patients

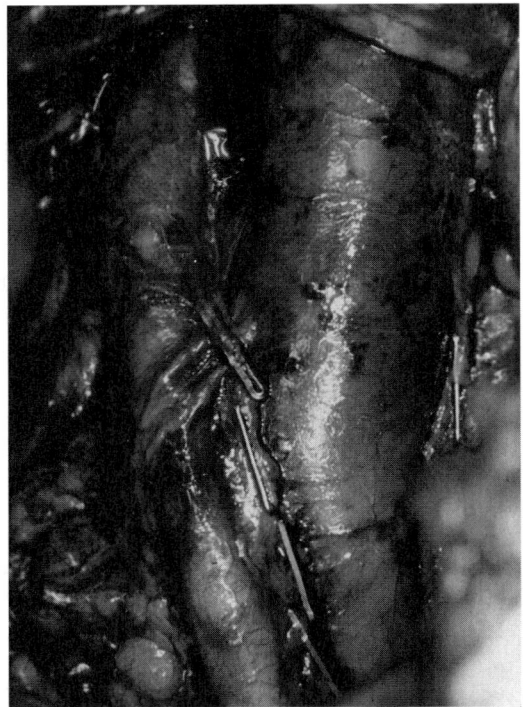

FIG. 10.4. The precaval fat pad, which contains the aortic lymph nodes, and the right common iliac lymph nodes have been excised. The lymph node dissection at this point has removed the aortic lymph nodes below the inferior mesenteric artery.

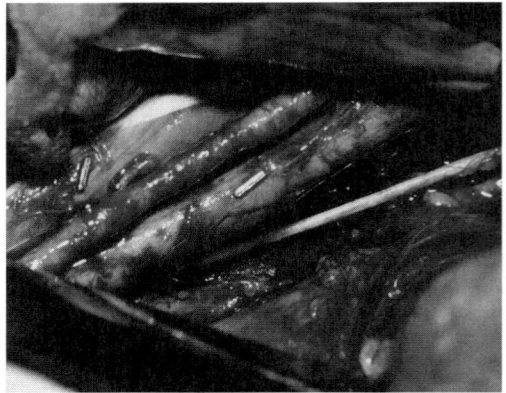

FIG. 10.5. The right external iliac, internal iliac (hypogastric), and obturator lymph nodes have been dissected, revealing (*top* to *bottom*) the psoas muscle, external iliac artery and vein, obturator nerve, and hypogastric vein. Lymph node sampling below the level of the obturator nerve usually is not performed.

with omental metastases, the metastases were not clinically evident by inspection and palpation (94). Wu and associates noted that 28 (87.5%) of 32 patients with suspicious lymph nodes proved to have nodal metastases on pathologic examination. However, microscopic metastases were also present in 14 (33%) of 42 of cases with palpably normal lymph nodes (49). Petru and colleagues at the University of Graz, Austria, performed systematic retroperitoneal lymphadenectomy in all patients with ovarian cancer and found positive lymph nodes in 23% of patients with stage I disease. Lymph nodes were clinically suspicious in only 33% of the patients with involved nodes; clinically suspicious nodes were present in 23% of patients with negative lymph nodes (102).

SURGICAL COMPLICATIONS

Extensive intraabdominal and pelvic exploration and retroperitoneal dissections can result in a number of intraoperative and postoperative complications proportional to the complexity of the operative procedure. Complications from comprehensive staging operations are more frequent and more severe than those from gynecologic surgeries for nonmalignant disease.

Trimbos and associates reported on a series of 86 women who underwent surgical staging for early ovarian carcinoma. Intraoperative complications occurred in approximately 15% of patients and included injuries to the vena cava (5 patients) and small bowel (2 patients), transection of the ureter (1 patient), splenic rupture (1 patient), and myocardial infarction (1 patient) (59). In the series reported by the GOG, 29% of patients had at least one operative complication. Visceral injuries occurred in 23 patients, including 11 to the intestine, 7 to the bladder, and 3 to the ureter. One vena caval injury occurred, and 1 patient sustained a pneumothorax secondary to diaphragmatic biopsy (94).

Surgeons must be skilled in the identification and repair of vascular, gastrointestinal, and genitourinary injuries when performing comprehensive surgical staging. It is not acceptable to avoid necessary procedures because of a lack of surgical expertise. In addition to vascular injuries, lymph node sampling can lead to postoperative lymphocysts, which are retroperitoneal collections of lymphatic fluid. A lymphocyst should be included in the differential diagnosis for any patient presenting with fever, flank pain, or a pelvic sidewall mass in the postoperative period. Closed suction drainage of the retroperitoneum and the meticulous application of hemoclips may reduce occurrence. The incidence of lymphocysts after radical pelvic surgery is less than 3% (103).

OTHER CONSIDERATIONS

Low Malignant Potential Ovarian Cancers

The diagnosis of low malignant potential (borderline) ovarian cancer is based on histologic features in the primary tumor: epithelial cellular proliferation and stratification, mitotic activity, and nuclear atypia in the absence of stromal invasion (104). These tumors account for 10% to 20% of all ovarian cancers. Low malignant potential tumors occur predominantly in younger women, and stage I disease is present in more than 80% of the cases (105,106). For these reasons, conservative surgery is appropriate in patients with apparent stage I disease who desire fertility preservation. For other patients, a comprehensive surgical staging procedure equivalent to that performed for invasive epithelial ovarian cancer has been advocated (107). Although information derived from comprehensive surgical staging is of undoubted prognostic importance, it is not clear how this information may otherwise be useful in treatment planning. To date, no study has demonstrated improved outcome with postoperative chemotherapy or radiation therapy (108). For patients with apparent early-stage low malignant potential tumors, the necessity of performing a comprehensive surgical staging operation is controversial.

Minimally Invasive Surgery: Laparoscopy

Morbidity, complications, and length of postoperative hospitalization are greatly reduced with laparoscopy compared to laparotomy. Inevitably, laparoscopy has been used for ovarian cancer staging (109). Pomel and associates performed laparoscopic surgical staging, including aortic and common iliac (but not pelvic) lymphadenectomy, infracolic omentectomy, cytology, and peritoneal biopsies in 10 women with apparent stage I ovarian cancer. Only one case was upstaged (presacral peritoneal biopsy). The average length of the procedure was 5 hours and 13 minutes, and the average postoperative stay was 4.75 days (110). Childers and colleagues performed laparoscopic surgical staging in 44 women with optimally debulked advanced stage ovarian cancer undergoing second-look procedures, and in 14 women with presumed early-stage ovarian cancer undergoing primary surgical staging. Laparoscopic second-look surgery was positive in 24 (56%) of the 44 patients, including 2 patients with microscopic positive residual disease in the aortic lymph nodes. Metastatic disease was found in 8 (57%) of 14 of patients with presumed early-stage ovarian cancer, including 3 patients with positive aortic lymph nodes. The average length of hospital stay was 1.6 days (range, 0 to 3 days). This study suggested that, when performed by experienced laparoscopic surgeons, staging laparoscopy for ovarian cancer is feasible and yields results similar to those obtained with laparotomy (111).

There are too few studies in the literature to consider laparoscopic surgery for ovarian cancer a standard operative approach. Considerable training, skill, and experience are prerequisites to laparoscopic surgery, particularly when sampling retroperitoneal lymph nodes. The experience of Dottino and colleagues is noteworthy in describing the increase in nodal yield with operator experience (112). Whereas obesity has been considered a relative contraindication to laparoscopic surgery, the authors found that it was the concentration of visceral fat—and not absolute body fat—that prohibited laparoscopic lymphadenectomy. When analyzing the mean number of pelvic or aortic lymph nodes obtained, they did not find a significant difference based on body mass index (112).

In addition to diagnostic yield, operative complications are a reflection of operator experience. See and associates surveyed a group of surgeons 3 and 12 months after their participation in a laparoscopic training course to determine complication rates. At 3 months, they found that surgeons who performed laparoscopic procedures without additional training were 3.39 times more likely to have an operative complication than were surgeons who received additional training, and at 12 months they were 4.85 times more likely to have operative complications. At both 3 and 12 months, laparoscopic complication rates were inversely correlated with the number of laparoscopic procedures performed (113). Laparoscopy, although minimally invasive, is not "minor" surgery. Possover and coworkers reported on a series of 150 patients undergoing laparoscopic pelvic and aortic lymphadenectomy, 7 of whom experienced major vessel injuries and 4 of whom required laparotomy (114). The majority of case series in the medical literature of laparoscopic surgery for gynecologic malignancies reflect the performance of only a few laparoscopic surgeons who have acquired considerable skill and expertise in operative procedures. It is unlikely that their results will be immediately duplicated by others who attempt these procedures. For the new laparoscopic surgeon, it is expected that operative complication rates will be higher and success rates in completing the desired operation will be lower. Early experiences with second-look laparoscopy for ovarian cancer were accompanied by both high false-negative rates and operative complications (115,116).

Faced with what appears to be an innocuous yet persistent ovarian cyst, the surgeon is tempted to excise the cyst via the laparoscope. Although the incidence of ovarian neoplasia in carefully selected patients is quite low (117), the implications of cyst rupture must be weighed against the morbidity of laparotomy. Cyst rupture cannot be considered inconsequential when malignant cells in peritoneal fluids can be grown in culture and form tumor implants at needle insertion and trocar sites (118,119) (Figure 10.6). The lengthy delays to definitive surgery that have occurred after laparoscopic diagnosis of ovarian cancer are distressing (120).

Laparoscopy is an exciting tool and should be studied for comprehensive ovarian cancer staging. Gynecologists and other surgeons must learn operative laparoscopy techniques in order to contribute to prospective, objective clinical evaluations of this developing surgical modality.

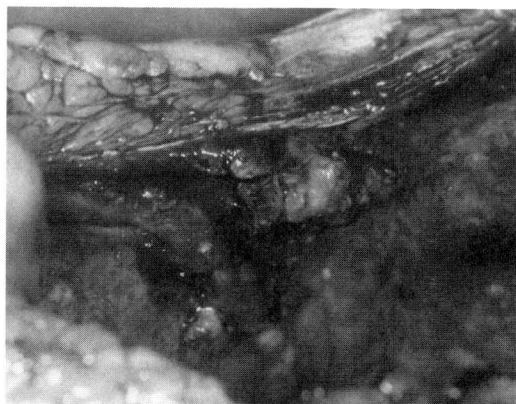

FIG. 10.6. The patient underwent diagnostic laparoscopy for an adnexal mass. Biopsy of a peritoneal nodule was positive for papillary serous adenocarcinoma. She was referred for gynecologic oncology consultation and 2 weeks later underwent surgical exploration. Intraoperative findings included an umbilical port site metastasis, which was resected.

REFERENCES

1. Morgagni JB. *The seats and causes of diseases.* Alexander B, trans. London: Millar and Cadell, 1769.
2. Ricci JV. *One hundred years of gynecology.* Philadelphia: Blakiston, 1945.
3. McDowell E. Three cases of extirpation of diseased ovaria. *Eclectic Repertory Annu Rev* 1817;7:242.
4. Leonardo RA. *History of gynecology.* New York: Froben Press, 1944.
5. Speert H. *Obstetrics and gynecology in America: a history.* Baltimore: Waverly Press, 1980.
6. Meigs CD. *Females and their diseases.* Philadelphia: Lea & Blanchard, 1848.
7. Byford WH. *The practice of medicine and surgery applied to the diseases and accidents incident to women.* Philadelphia: Lindsay & Blakiston, 1865.
8. Tait L. *The pathology and treatment of diseases of the ovaries,* 4th ed. Birmingham: Cornish Brothers, 1883.
9. Skene AJC. Ovariotomy. In: Kelly H, Noble CP, eds. *Gynecology and abdominal surgery.* Philadelphia: WB Saunders, 1907:565–590.
10. Curtis AH. *A text-book of gynecology.* Philadelphia: WB Saunders, 1930.
11. Gardner GH, Traut HF. Tumors of the ovaries. In: Kelly HA, ed. *Gynecology.* New York: Appleton, 1928:724–788.
12. Geist SH. *Ovarian tumors.* New York: Harper, 1942.
13. Kottmeier HL. Annual report of the results of treatment in carcinoma of the uterus and vagina, vol 14. Stockholm: Federation International of Gynecology and Obstetrics, 1967.
14. Munnell EW, Taylor HC. Ovarian carcinoma: a review of 200 primary and 51 secondary cases. *Am J Obstet Gynecol* 1949;48:943.
15. Classification and staging of malignant tumors in the female. *Acta Obstet Gynaecol Scand* 1971;50:1.
16. Kottmeier HL. Annual report on the results of treatment in carcinoma of the uterus, vagina, and ovary, vol 15. Stockholm: Federation International of Gynecology and Obstetrics, 1973.
17. FIGO Cancer Committee: Staging announcement. *Gynecol Oncol* 1986;25:383.
18. Landis SH, Murray T, Bolden S, Wingo PA. Cancer statistics, 1999. *CA Cancer J Clin* 1999;49:8–31.
19. Merck HR, Garfinkel L, Dodd GD. Preliminary report of the National Cancer Data Base. *Cancer* 1991;41:7.
20. Burns BC, Underwood PB, Rutledge FN. A review of carcinoma of the ovary at the University of Texas M.D. Anderson Hospital and Tumor Institute of Houston. In: *Cancer of the uterus and ovary.* Chicago: Year Book, 1969:123–147.
21. Munnell EW. Surgical treatment of ovarian carcinoma. In: Barber HRK, Graber EA, eds. *Gynecologic oncology.* Baltimore Williams & Wilkins, 1970:232–240.
22. Aure JC, Hoeg K, Kolstad P. Clinical and histologic studies of ovarian carcinoma: long term follow-up of 990 cases. *Obstet Gynecol* 1971;37:1.
23. Julian CG. Germinal epithelial neoplasia of the ovary. *Clin Obstet Gynecol* 1974;17:241.
24. Obel EB. A comparative study of patients with cancer of the ovary, who have survived more or less than 10 years. *Acta Obstet Gynecol Scand* 1976;55:429.
25. Shepherd JH. Surgical management of ovarian cancer. In: Shepherd JH, Monaghan MJ, eds. *Clinical gynaecological oncology.* Oxford: Blackwell, 1985:187–207.
26. Bast RC, Knauf S, Epenetos A, et al. Coordinate elevation of serum markers in ovarian cancer but not in benign disease. *Cancer* 1991;68:1758.
27. Campbell S, Bhan V, Royston P, et al. Transabdominal ultrasound screening for early ovarian cancer. *BMJ* 1989;299:1363.
28. DePriest PD, Gallion HH, Pavlik EJ, et al. Transvaginal sonography as a screening method for the detection of early ovarian cancer. *Gynecol Oncol* 1997;65:408.
29. Fleischer AC, Cullinan JA, Peery CV, Jones HW. Early detection of ovarian carcinoma with transvaginal color Doppler ultrasonography. *Am J Obstet Gynecol* 1996;174:101.
30. Griffiths CT, Tobias J. Management of ovarian carcinoma: current concepts and future prospects. *N Engl J Med* 1976;294:818.
31. Hreshchyshyn MM, Park RC, Blessing JA, et al. The role of adjuvant therapy in stage I ovarian cancer. *Am J Obstet Gynecol* 1980;138:139.
32. Dembo AJ, Bush RS, Beale FA, et al. Ovarian carcinoma: improved survival following abdominopelvic irradiation in patients with a completed pelvic operation. *Am J Obstet Gynecol* 1979;134:793.
33. Smith JP, Rutledge F, Delclos L. Postoperative treatment of early cancer of the ovary. *Natl Cancer Inst Monogr* 1975;42:149.
34. Einhorn N. The place of adjuvant chemotherapy in early stages. *Int J Radiat Biol Phys* 1982;8:257.
35. Dembo AJ, Bush RS. Radiation therapy of ovarian carcinoma 1983. In: Griffiths CT, Fuller AF, eds. *Gynecologic oncology.* Boston: Martinus Nijhoff, 1983:263–298.

36. Trimbos JB, Schueler JA, van der Burg M, et al. Watch and wait after careful surgical treatment and staging in well-differentiated early ovarian cancer. *Cancer* 1991;67:597.
37. Young RC, Walton LA, Ellenberg SS, et al. Adjuvant therapy in stage I and stage II epithelial ovarian cancer. *N Engl J Med* 1990;322:1021.
38. Walton L, Ellenberg SS, Major F, et al. Results of second-look laparotomy in patients with early-stage ovarian carcinoma. *Obstet Gynecol* 1987;70:770.
39. Keettel WC, Pixley EE. Diagnostic value of peritoneal washings. *Clin Obstet Gynecol* 1958;1:592.
40. Tobacman JK, Tucker MA, Kase R. Intra-abdominal carcinomatosis after prophylactic oophorectomy in ovarian cancer-prone families. *Lancet* 1982;2:795.
41. Chen KTK, Schooley JL, Flam MS. Peritoneal carcinomatosis after prophylactic oophorectomy in familial ovarian cancer syndrome. *Obstet Gynecol* 1985;66:93S.
42. Woodruff JD, TeLinde RW. The histology and histogenesis of ovarian neoplasia. *Cancer* 1976;37:411S.
43. Courtice FC, Steinbeck AW. The lymphatic drainage of plasma from the peritoneal cavity of the cat. *Aust J Exp Bio Med Sci* 1950;28:161.
44. Schoenberger JA, Kroll G, Sakamoto A, Kark RM. Investigation of the permeability factor in ascites and edema using albumin tagged with I-131. *Gastroenterology* 1952;22:607.
45. Coates G, Bush RS, Aspin N. A study of ascites using lymphoscintigraphy with 99mTc-sulfur colloid. *Radiology* 1973;107:577.
46. Abrams LA, Spiro R, Goldstein N. Metastases in carcinoma. *Cancer* 1950;3:74.
47. Bergman F. Carcinoma of the ovary: a clinicalpathological study of 86 autopsied cases with special reference to mode of spread. *Acta Obstet Gynecol Scand* 1966;45:211.
48. Burghardt E, Pickel H, Lahousen M, Stettner H. Pelvic lymphadenectomy in operative treatment of ovarian cancer. *Am J Obstet Gynecol* 1986;155:315.
49. Wu PC, Qu JY, Lang JH, et al. Lymph node metastasis of ovarian cancer: a preliminary survey of 74 cases of lymphadenectomy. *Am J Obstet Gynecol* 1986;155:1103.
50. LeRoux PD, Berger MS, Elliott JP, Tamimi HK. Cerebral metastases from ovarian carcinoma. *Cancer* 1991;67:2194.
51. Dauplat J, Hacker NF, Nieberg RK, et al. Distant metastases in epithelial ovarian carcinoma. *Cancer* 1987;60:1561.
52. Green TH. *Gynecology: essentials of clinical practice*, 3rd ed. Boston: Little, Brown, 1977.
53. McGowan L. *Gynecologic oncology*. New York: Appleton-Century-Crofts, 1978.
54. Barber HRK. Ovarian cancer: diagnosis and management. *Am J Obstet Gynecol* 1984;150:910.
55. Trimbos JB, Bolis G. Guidelines for surgical staging of ovarian cancer. *Obstet Gynecol Surv* 1994;49:814.
56. Piver MS, Lele SB, Barlow JJ. Preoperative and intraoperative evaluation in ovarian malignancy. *Obstet Gynecol* 1976;48:312.
57. Young RC, Decker DG, Wharton JT, et al. Staging laparotomy in early ovarian cancer. *JAMA* 1983;250:3072.
58. Helewa ME, Krepart GV, Lotocki R. Staging laparotomy in early epithelial ovarian carcinoma. *Am J Obstet Gynecol* 1986;154:282.
59. Trimbos JB, Schueler JA, Van Lent M, et al. Reasons for incomplete surgical staging in early ovarian carcinoma. *Gynecol Oncol* 1990;37:374.
60. Munoz KA, Harlan LC, Trimble EL. Patterns of care for women with ovarian cancer in the United States. *J Clin Oncol* 1997;15:3408.
61. Zanetta G, Rota S, Chiari S, et al. The accuracy of staging: an important prognostic determinant in stage I ovarian carcinoma. *Ann Oncol* 1998;9:1097.
62. Keettel WC, Elkins HB. Experience with radioactive colloidal gold in the treatment of ovarian carcinoma. *Am J Obstet Gynecol* 1956;71:553.
63. Keettel WC, Pixley EE, Buchsbaum HJ. Experience with peritoneal cytology in the management of gynecologic malignancies. *Am J Obstet Gynecol* 1974;120:174.
64. De Palo G, Musumeci R, Kenda R, et al. The reassessment of patients with ovarian carcinoma. *Eur J Cancer* 1980;16:1469.
65. Piver MS, Barlow JJ, Lele SB. Incidence of subclinical metastasis in stage I and II ovarian carcinoma. *Obstet Gynecol* 1978;52:100.
66. Webb MJ, Decker DG, Mussey E, Williams TJ. Factors influencing survival in stage I ovarian cancer. *Am J Obstet Gynecol* 1973;116:222.
67. Decker DG, Webb MJ, Holbrook MA. Radiogold treatment of epithelial cancer of the ovary: late results. *Am J Obstet Gynecol* 1973;114:751.
68. Sevelda P, Dittrich C, Salzer H. Prognostic value of the rupture of the capsule in stage I epithelial ovarian carcinoma. *Gynecol Oncol* 1989;35:321.
69. Dembo AJ, Davy M, Stenwig AE, et al. Prognostic factors in patients with stage I epithelial ovarian cancer. *Obstet Gynecol* 1990;75:263.
70. Sjovall K, Nilsson B, Einhorn N. Different types of rupture of the tumor capsule and the impact on survival in early ovarian carcinoma. *Int J Gynecol Cancer* 1994;4:333.
71. de la Cuesta RS, Goff BA, Fuller AF, et al. Prognostic importance of intraoperative rupture of malignant ovarian epithelial neoplasms. *Obstet Gynecol* 1994;84:1.
72. Slavutin L, Rotterdam H. Frozen section diagnosis of serous epithelial tumors of the ovary. *Am J Diagn Obstet Gynecol* 1979;1:89.
73. Twaalhoven FCM, Peters AAWB, Trimbos JB, Fleuren GJ. The accuracy of frozen section diagnosis of ovarian tumors. *Gynecol Oncol* 1991;41:189.
74. Obiakor I, Maiman M, Mittal K, et al. The accuracy of frozen section diagnosis of ovarian neoplasms. *Gynecology* 1991;43:61.
75. Rose PG, Rubin RB, Nelson BE, et al. Accuracy of frozen-section (intraoperative consultation) diagnosis of ovarian tumors. *Am J Obstet Gynecol* 1994;171:823.
76. Menzin AW, Rubin SC, Noumoff JS, LiVolsi VA. The accuracy of a frozen section diagnosis of borderline ovarian malignancy. *Gynecol Oncol* 1995;59:183.
77. Puls L, Heidtman E, Hunter JE, et al. The accuracy of frozen section by tumor weight for ovarian epithelial neoplasms. *Gynecol Oncol* 1997;676:16.
78. Abu-Rustum NR, Chi DS, Wiatrowska BA, et al. The accuracy of frozen-section diagnosis in metastatic

breast and colorectal carcinoma to the adnexa. *Gynecol Oncol* 1999;73:102.
79. Munnell EW. Is conservative therapy ever justified in stage IA cancer of the ovary? *Am J Obstet Gynecol* 1969;103:641.
80. Parker RT, Parker CH, Wilbanks GD. Cancer of the ovary: survival studies based upon operative therapy, chemotherapy, and radiotherapy. *Am J Obstet Gynecol* 1970;108:878.
81. Colombo N, Chiari S, Maggioni A, et al. Controversial issues in the management of early epithelial ovarian cancer: conservative surgery and role of adjuvant therapy. *Gynecol Oncol* 1994;55:47S–51S.
82. Zanetta G, Chiari S, Rota S, et al. Conservative surgery for stage I ovarian carcinoma in women of childbearing age. *Br J Obstet Gynaecol* 1997;104:1030.
83. Marchetti, Padovan P, Fracas M. Malignant ovarian tumors: conservative surgery and quality of life in young patients. *Eur J Gynaecol Oncol* 1998;19:297.
84. Benjamin I, Morgan MA, Rubin SC. Occult bilateral involvement in stage I epithelial ovarian cancer. *Gynecol Oncol* 1999;72:288.
85. Scully RE. Recent progress in ovarian cancer. *Hum Pathol* 1970;1:73.
86. Malfetano JH. The appendix and its metastatic potential in epithelial ovarian cancer. *Obstet Gynecol* 1987;69:396.
87. Fawzi HW, Robertshaw JK, Bolger BS, Monaghan JM. Role of appendicectomy in the surgical management of ovarian cancer. *Eur J Gynaecol Oncol* 1997;13:34.
88. Rose PG, Reale FR, Fisher A, Hunter RE. Appendectomy in primary and secondary staging operations for ovarian malignancy. *Obstet Gynecol* 1991;77:116.
89. Knapp RC, Friedman EA. Aortic lymph node metastases in early ovarian cancer. *Am J Obstet Gynecol* 1974;119:1013.
90. Rosenoff SH, DeVita VT, Hubbard S, Young RC. Peritoneoscopy in the staging and followup of ovarian cancer. *Semin Oncol* 1975;2:223.
91. Spinelli P, Pilotti S, Luini A, et al. Laparoscopy combined with peritoneal cytology in staging and restaging ovarian carcinoma. *Tumori* 1979;65:601.
92. Mangioni C, Bolis G, Molteni P, Bellonki C. Indications, advantages, and limits of laparoscopy in ovarian cancer. *Gynecol Oncol* 1979;7:47.
93. Buchsbaum HJ, Lifshitz S. Staging and surgical evaluation of ovarian cancer. *Semin Oncol* 11:227, 1984.
94. Buchsbaum HJ, Brady MF, Delgado G, et al. Surgical staging of carcinoma of the ovaries. *Surg Gynecol Obstet* 1989;169:226.
95. Musumeci R, DePalo G, Kenda R, et al. Retroperitoneal metastases from ovarian carcinoma: reassessment of 365 patients studied with lymphography. *AJR Am J Roentgenol* 1980;134:449.
96. Knipscheer RJJL. Para-aortal lymph node dissection in 20 cases of primary epithelial ovary carcinoma stage I (FIGO): influence on staging. *Eur J Obstet Gynecol Reprod Biol* 1982;13:303.
97. Averette HE, Lovecchio JL, Townsend PA, et al. Retroperitoneal lymphatic involvement by ovarian carcinoma. In: Grundmann E, ed. *Cancer campaign, vol 7: carcinoma of the ovary*. Stuttgart: Gustav Fischer Verlag, 1983:101–110.
98. Carnino F, Fuda G, Ciccone G, et al. Significance of lymph node sampling in epithelial carcinoma of the ovary. *Gynecol Oncol* 1997;65:467.
99. Onda T, Yoskikawa H, Yokota H, et al. Assessment of metastases to aortic and pelvic lymph nodes in epithelial ovarian carcinoma: a proposal for essential sites for lymph node biopsy. *Cancer* 1996;78:803.
100. Flanagan CW, Mannel RS, Walker JL, Johnson GA. Incidence and location of para-aortic lymph node metastases in gynecologic malignancies. *J Am Coll Surg* 1995;181:72.
101. Walter AJ, Magrina JF. Contralateral pelvic and aortic lymph node metastasis in clinical stage I epithelial ovarian cancer. *Gynecol Oncol* 1999;74:128.
102. Petru E, Lahousen M, Tamussino K, et al. Lymphadenectomy in stage I ovarian cancer. *Am J Obstet Gynecol* 1994;170:656.
103. Moore DH, Fowler WC, Walton LA, Droegemueller W. Morbidity of lymph node sampling in cancers of the uterine corpus and cervix. *Obstet Gynecol* 1989;74:180.
104. Scully RE. Tumors of the ovary and maldeveloped gonads. In: Hartman WH and Cowan WR, eds. *Atlas of tumor pathology*, 2nd series, fascicle 16. Washington, DC: Armed Forces Institute of Pathology, 1979, 55–91.
105. Trimble CL, Trimble EL. Management of epithelial ovarian tumors of low malignant potential. *Gynecol Oncol* 1994;55:52.
106. Hoskins PJ. Ovarian tumours of low malignant potential: borderline epithelial ovarian carcinoma. In: Lawton FG, Neijt JP, Swenerton KD, eds. *Epithelial cancer of the ovary*. London: BMJ Publishing Group, BMA House, 1995:112.
107. Lin PS, Gershenson DM, Bevers MW, et al: The current status of surgical staging of ovarian serous borderline tumors. *Cancer* 1999;85:905.
108. Trope C, Kaern J. Management of borderline tumors of the ovary: state of the art. *Semin Oncol* 1998;25:372.
109. Reich H, McGlynn F, Wilkie W. Laparoscopic management of stage I ovarian cancer: a case report. *J Reprod Med* 1990;35:601
110. Pomel C, Provencher D, Dauplat J, et al. Laparoscopic staging of early ovarian cancer. *Gynecol Oncol* 1995;58:301.
111. Childers JM, Lang J, Surwit EA, Hatch KD. Laparoscopic surgical staging of ovarian cancer. *Gynecol Oncol* 1995;59:25.
112. Dottino PR, Tobias DH, Beddoe A, et al. Laparoscopic lymphadenectomy for gynecologic malignancies. *Gynecol Oncol* 1999;73:383.
113. See WA, Cooper CS, Fisher RJ. Predictors of laparoscopic complications after formal training in laparoscopic surgery. *JAMA* 1993;270:2689.
114. Possover M, Krause N, Plaul K, et al. Laparoscopic para-aortic and pelvic lymphadenectomy: experience with 150 patients and review of the literature. *Gynecol Oncol* 1998;71:19.
115. Berek JS, Griffiths CT, Leventhal JM. Laparoscopy for second-look evaluation in ovarian cancer. *Obstet Gynecol* 1981;58 192.
116. Ozols RF, Fisher RI, Anderson T, et al. Peritoneoscopy in the management of ovarian cancer. *Am J Obstet Gynecol* 1981;140:611.

117. Peterson HB, Hulka JF, Phillips JM. American Association of Gynecologic Laparoscopists' 1988 membership survey on operative laparoscopy. *J Reprod Med* 1990;35:601.
118. Sinner WN, Zajecek J. Implantation metastasis after percutaneous needle aspiration biopsy. *Acta Radiol Diagn* 1976;17:473.
119. Hsiu JG, Given FT, Kemp GM. Tumor implantation after diagnostic laparoscopic biopsy of serous ovarian tumors of low malignant potential. *Obstet Gynecol* 1986;68:902.
120. Maiman M, Seltzer V, Boyce J. Laparoscopic excision of ovarian neoplasms subsequently found to be malignant. *Obstet Gynecol* 1991;77:563.

11

Laparoscopy in the Management of Ovarian Cancer

Tom P. Manolitsas, Parul Gupta, and Jeffrey M. Fowler

The introduction of laparoscopic surgery has the potential to revolutionize the practice of gynecologic oncology. In no other field of gynecology are the gains from the introduction of laparoscopic surgery likely to be so great or the pitfalls so profound. The conventional surgical approach to ovarian cancer has almost universally utilized a generous midline vertical incision of 15 to 30 cm, from above the umbilicus down to the pubis, in contrast to the 5- and 10-mm incisions created by a laparoscopic procedure. Patients with ovarian cancer tend to be older, undergo more extensive surgery, and remain as inpatients longer than patients with benign gynecologic conditions. Therefore, the introduction of laparoscopic surgery may be expected to have a proportionately greater positive impact on these patients than on those with benign conditions. But at what cost?

The most important outcome measures in oncology practice relate to cure rates, survival, and quality-of-life issues, and yet it is within these parameters that we have the least knowledge regarding the impact of laparoscopic surgery. Possible benefits of the minimally invasive approach include shorter hospitalization, decreased cost and time to recovery, and minimization of patient discomfort and analgesic requirements. However, in order to become a standard of care for the management of gynecologic malignancies, the procedure should be proven to be a safe alternative for the current standard, and it must not compromise accurate surgical staging and timely diagnosis of malignancy. Moreover, where the diagnosis of malignancy is confirmed, survival rates must be at least equivalent to those achieved with open surgery.

MANAGEMENT OF THE ADNEXAL MASS: EVALUATION OF CANDIDATES

Most adnexal masses are benign, yet the ability to accurately discriminate benign from malignant masses before surgery has proved elusive. Assessment of the risk of malignancy is important for patient counseling and consent and for selecting the optimal approach to surgery. In circumstances where surgical expertise or facilities are limited it may play a role in the triage of patients, so that they may receive optimal definitive management in the first instance and preferably at one operation.

It has long been held that clinical impression on pelvic examination has little predictive value in differentiating benign from malignant ovarian masses (1). Although some studies have shown that pelvic examination is considerably less sensitive than ultrasonography or measurement of the serum marker CA 125 (1,2), Schutter and colleagues (3) found that a suspicious pelvic examination was associated with a sensitivity of 93%, which, in their study of 228 postmenopausal women with a pelvic mass, was comparable to ultrasonography and better than CA 125 in predicting malignancy.

Pelvic ultrasonography is the single most important clinical test in predicting whether an adnexal mass is benign or malignant (2,4). Ultrasound features suggestive of a benign lesion include a thin cyst wall with no internal projections or papillarities, absent or thin septa, and overall low echogenicity. A thick-walled, complex mass (solid or cystic) with thick internal septae is more suggestive of a malignant lesion. Utilizing ultrasonography alone, estimation of the probability that an adnexal mass is malignant has been reported with 62% to 100% sensitivity, 73% to 95% specificity, 31% to 88% positive predictive value, and 81% to 100% negative predictive value (1,5–10). Results were superior with transvaginal ultrasonography compared with the abdominal method (9,10). A noteworthy finding in these studies was that the risk that a simple unilocular cyst is malignant is extremely low, at 0.3% (11), but may increase to as much as 6% in an exclusively postmenopausal population (12). In the postmenopausal setting, even simple unilocular cysts smaller than 5 cm in diameter have a significant risk of malignancy (12).

Scoring systems for defined ultrasound features such as inner wall structure, wall thickness, presence and nature of septa, and internal echogenicity provide a simple, rigidly defined, and easily reproducible method for prediction of malignancy in any adnexal mass (1,10). The scoring system proposed by Sassone and associates (10) achieved a 100% sensitivity, 83% specificity, 37% positive predictive value, and 100% negative predictive value in discriminating benign from malignant disease in a study population of 143 patients undergoing transvaginal ultrasonography before laparotomy for an adnexal mass, of whom 13 had malignant ovarian lesions.

The use of CA 125 in combination with ultrasonography and pelvic examination improves the accuracy of the estimation of risk of malignancy and provides improved discrimination compared with any one test alone (1–3,13). The gains in sensitivity and specificity afforded by the addition of CA 125 estimation to ultrasonography are much greater in postmenopausal patients (1,13) because of the relatively high prevalence of endometriosis, adenomyosis, fibroids, pelvic inflammatory disease, and pregnancy, which are common causes of elevated CA 125, in the premenopausal patient. In postmenopausal patients, the incidence of conditions, other than ovarian cancer, that can elevate the CA 125 is much lower. In a postmenopausal woman with an adnexal mass, even a small elevation in CA 125 above the normal cutoff value of 35 U/mL, may be associated with a 50% to 60% risk of malignancy; this risk rises to 98% if the CA 125 is greater than 65 U/mL (14).

Jacobs and associates (15) included menopausal status and formalized this panel of tests into an algorithm they termed the "risk of malignancy index" (RMI). The RMI is the product of the serum CA 125 level (in units per milliliter), the ultrasound scan result (0, 1, or 3), and the menopausal status (1 if premenopausal, 3 if postmenopausal). The ultrasound scan result includes 1 point for the presence of each of the following characteristics: multilocular cyst, solid areas, metastases, ascites, and bilateral lesions. These authors reported a sensitivity of 85% with a specificity of 97% in predicting malignancy if an RMI cutoff value of 200 is used. When the cutoff value was decreased to 50, then the sensitivity increased to 95% but the specificity fell to 76%. They then validated these results in a new population and reported an 87% sensitivity, 89% specificity, and 75% positive predictive value (given an RMI cutoff value of 200) (16).

Although initial reports were encouraging (17–20), the use of Doppler ultrasonography for discriminating benign from malignant ovarian lesions has not improved on the information provided by gray-scale ultrasonography. Neovascularization in ovarian cancers produces vessels lacking the normal muscular intima, resulting in low resistance to blood flow compared with the high flow resistance in benign tumors (21). This flow can be assessed and characterized as a resistive index (RI) and a pulsatility index (PI). However, there is considerable overlap in RI and PI between benign and malignant processes (22), and most studies have been unable to use these measures to distinguish between benign and malignant ovarian lesions (22–27). Somewhat more encouraging is a recent report by Schelling and coworkers (28), who studied 63 patients with an adnexal mass of unknown malignancy status and combined B-mode ultrasonography assessment of the presence of "solid areas" with Doppler assessment of "central vascularization" to achieve a sensitivity of 92% and a specificity of 94% in predicting malignancy.

Although some studies have reported that the combination of Doppler ultrasonography with serum CA 125 measurement improves the accuracy of the assessment (29–31), others have concluded that Doppler techniques provide no advantage (2,32–35). Doppler ultrasonography identifies a large number of false-positive results that reflect neovascularization in benign tumors (34). Therefore, the application of Doppler ultrasonography to the characterization of adnexal masses is at best controversial, and its routine use is not recommended (36).

Computed tomography (CT) and magnetic resonance imaging (MRI) are not widely used in the initial assessment of an adnexal mass, although at least one study showed a statistically significant increase in the sensitivity and specificity of contrast-enhanced MRI (91% and 93%, respectively) compared with transvaginal ultrasonography (89% and 84%) in the characterization of an adnexal mass as benign or malignant (37). CT has not been shown to be superior to transvaginal ultrasonography in distinguishing benign from malignant adnexal masses, and there have been no prospective trials comparing gray-scale transvaginal ultrasonography, CT, and contrast-enhanced MRI in this setting. We do not recommend that CT or MRI be used as a first-line investigation.

New technologies such as three-dimensional ultrasonography and power Doppler (38,39), positron emission tomography (40), and the use of artificial neural networks to enhance data interpretation (41,42) are all being investigated, but their roles in the assessment of the adnexal mass are yet to be defined.

In summary, the recommended assessment of an adnexal mass should include a pelvic examination, pelvic ultrasonography (preferably transvaginal), and, in most cases (always in the postmenopausal patient), a serum CA 125 estimation. In the younger patient, serum markers for germ cell tumors (β-human chorionic gonadotropin, α-fetoprotein, lactate dehydrogenase) should be measured (43,44). The results of these investigations can then be reviewed with reference to the patient's age and menopausal status (with or without a formal algorithm) and clinical impression, and the case can be categorized as either low risk or moderate/high risk for malignancy.

LAPAROSCOPIC MANAGEMENT OF THE ADNEXAL MASS AT LOW RISK FOR MALIGNANCY

If an adequate preoperative assessment has indicated that an adnexal mass is at low risk for malignancy, then the laparoscopic surgeon can, after careful inspection of the pelvis and abdomen, proceed to ovarian cystectomy, oophorectomy, or other procedure as clinically indicated. If an unforeseen malignancy is encountered, the procedure should be discontinued and definitive surgery rescheduled for a later date when a gynecologic oncologist is available. This should be an uncommon event in the patient with low risk factors for malignancy.

Laparoscopic aspiration of ovarian cysts should not be performed as an aid to diagnosis. A metaanalysis showed that aspiration cytology of ovarian cysts had a negative predictive value of 58% to 98% in the diagnosis of malignancy (45). Not only is it often falsely reassuring, but also the inadvertent aspiration of a malignant cyst may worsen the patient's prognosis. Cyst aspiration may result in the slow and continuous leak of malignant cells and increase the chance of peritoneal tumor cell implantation (46). If malignancy is not suspected, then there may be a considerable delay during which iatrogenic spread of tumor cells can occur. Trimbos and Hacker (46) reported two cases in which patients who had undergone laparoscopic aspiration of innocent-looking ovarian cysts that were negative on cytologic examination represented some weeks later with disseminated stage III ovarian cancer.

Aspiration of ovarian cysts is ineffective in achieving resolution, because 11% to 67% of cysts recur overall (45). Most of those that resolve are likely to be functional cysts. Although aspiration of functional cysts may be therapeutically effective, most functional cysts can be managed conservatively and disappear spontaneously within two cycles if managed with oral contraceptives (47). More recent evidence suggests that an observational period with no hormonal therapy is equally effective in causing functional cyst regression (48,49). Functional cysts never occur in postmenopausal women. Benign cystadenomas recur, because aspiration does not interrupt the neoplastic process. Likewise, endometriomas are likely to recur after aspiration, because the thick nature of the cyst contents hampers evacuation and the persistence of underlying endometriosis is a continuing source of new cyst formation (46).

LAPAROSCOPIC MANAGEMENT OF THE MASS AT MODERATE RISK FOR MALIGNANCY

In order to assess the role of laparoscopy in the management of the adnexal mass at moderate risk for malignancy a number of issues need to be addressed:

- Can laparoscopy reliably diagnose ovarian malignancy?
- Is it technically feasible to remove the adnexal mass without undue complications?
- Does rupture or spill from the cyst matter?
- If a malignancy is diagnosed at or after a laparoscopic procedure, does it matter if definitive surgical staging is delayed until a later date?
- Does laparoscopy cause acceleration of the spread of malignant cells?
- How does the survival of patients with ovarian cancer managed laparoscopically compare with that of patients whose disease is managed by the traditional approach of laparotomy and surgical staging?

There are no prospective, randomized trials comparing laparoscopy and laparotomy in this setting. Therefore, our knowledge is based on a small number of case series, case reports, and retrospective reviews.

Can Laparoscopy Reliably Diagnose Ovarian Malignancy?

Given that there is no way to preoperatively identify malignant adnexal masses with 100% sensitivity and 100% specificity, laparoscopy has been used to aid in the triage of patients and improve the accuracy of assessment. The risk of encountering a malignancy in the course of laparoscopy for an adnexal mass depends on the nature of the patient population and the exact criteria for ultrasonography and CA 125 findings that are used to define the group of adnexal masses at "moderate/high risk for malignancy." This risk ranges from 14% to less than 1% in published reports (Table 11.1) (50–59).

TABLE 11.1. *Laparoscopic diagnosis of malignant adnexal masses*

Source (ref. no.)	No. of cases	Menopausal status and risk factors	Malignancies diagnosed (no. [%])	LMP tumors
Mage et al., 1990 (53)	433	Premenopausal and postmenopausal	5 (1.1)	4
Parker and Berek, 1990 (50)	25	Postmenopausal	0 (0)	—
Mecke et al., 1992 (51)	773	Premenopausal	11 (1.4)	—
Nezhat et al., 1992 (52)	1011	Mostly premenopausal	4 (0.3)	—
Hulka et al., 1992 (55)	13,793	Mostly premenopausal	411 (2.9)	—
Wenzl et al., 1996 (54)	16,601	Premenopausal and postmenopausal	108 (0.65)	—
Canis et al., 1994 (59)	757	Premenopausal and postmenopausal	7 (0.9)	12
Dottino et al., 1999 (58)	160	Gynecologic oncology referrals	11 (7)	8
Childers et al., 1996 (57)	138	Suspicious ultrasound and/or CA-125	19 (14)	—
Canis et al., 1997 (56)	230	Suspicious ultrasound	15 (6)	10

LMP, low malignant potential.

Mage and colleagues reported that laparoscopic inspection of the pelvis and internal cyst wall correctly diagnosed all 5 ovarian cancers and 4 tumors of low malignant potential (LMP) in their series of 481 patients aged 9 to 88 years with cystic adnexal masses (53). Combining laparoscopic inspection of the ovarian mass and pelvis with inspection of the mass after excision, Canis and associates (59), in their series of 757 patients, were able to identify 6% of masses as suspicious for malignancy. Of these, 41% were frankly malignant or of LMP, and 59% were benign. No malignant masses were missed, but 7 of the 15 malignant tumors were punctured at the original laparoscopy.

In their follow-up study (56), Canis and colleagues reported on 558 adnexal masses, of which 247 were "suspicious" based on ultrasonography findings. Seventeen cases were immediately excluded because the mass was obviously malignant, larger than 12 cm, and predominately solid or because of medical contraindications to laparoscopic surgery. Of the remaining 230 "suspicious" cases, 62 were confirmed as suspicious on laparoscopic appearance alone. On excision, all suspicious cysts were sent for frozen section analysis. Forty percent were found to be malignant or LMP, and 60% were benign. Immediate staging was performed for malignant and LMP tumors. All malignancies and LMP tumors were identified as suspicious, but 3 of 15 malignant tumors and 5 of 10 LMP tumors had been punctured before the diagnosis was confirmed. In one 23-year-old patient, a mainly solid 12-cm mass identified by laparoscopy as being suspicious was thought to be a dermoid on frozen section. The tumor was morcellated before removal and was subsequently found to be an immature teratoma on permanent section. Three weeks later, stage IV peritoneal gliosis with mature and immature implants was found. The patient required chemotherapy followed by laparotomy with hysterectomy, contralateral adnexectomy, omentectomy, and excision of benign implants. In their discussion, the authors stated that morcellation of a solid tumor should be considered contraindicated.

In order to minimize the risk of intraperitoneal tumor dissemination, proponents of the use of laparoscopic assessment of "suspicious" adnexal masses advocate that this approach should be used only where there is availability of both frozen section analysis of specimens and the ability to perform immediate surgical staging (56,57,60). This would effectively limit this practice to surgeons skilled in the technique of surgical staging or to situations in which such a skilled person was immediately available.

Is It Technically Feasible to Remove the Adnexal Mass without Undue Complications?

A number of small studies have compared laparoscopic management of benign adnexal masses with management by laparotomy (61,62). The conclusions were that laparoscopic management is associated with similar or decreased operating time, decreased blood loss, decreased pain, decreased analgesic requirement, and decreased hospital stay with no increase in complications. It is not known whether these conclusions are similarly applicable to the laparoscopic management of a malignant adnexal mass.

Childers and coworkers (57) reported on a series of 138 patients who had a suspicious adnexal mass on the basis of abnormal ultrasonography findings or elevated CA 125 or both. In this series, 14% of the masses were subsequently found to be malignant. They reported a 1.4% rate of major intraoperative complications. There was one rectosigmoid enterotomy and one vena cava injury, both repaired laparoscopically and without sequelae, in addition to a port site bowel hernia that required laparotomy and bowel resection on postoperative day 2. Dottino and colleagues (58) reported on a series of 160 patients who were referred to a gynecologic oncology service with an adnexal mass; 9% of the masses were found to be malignant and 5% were LMP. They reported a 3% rate of intraoperative complications, with three trocar vascular injuries, one small bowel injury, and one case of persistent bleeding from pelvic adhesions requiring laparotomy. In neither series was it made clear whether the complications occurred in the malignant or the benign cases.

In the setting of traditional laparotomy, adnexectomy for the excision of a stage I ovarian malignancy is typically no more difficult than for a benign mass. In fact, the reverse is often true, with the most technically demanding cases often being those associated with benign conditions such as endometriosis, pelvic inflammatory disease, or dense postsurgical adhesions. These cases will continue to challenge the laparoscopic surgeon far more than the removal of an apparent stage I ovarian malignancy.

The size of a predominately solid adnexal mass may be a limiting factor in the use of laparoscopic surgery. Although laparoscopic adnexectomy may be performed fairly easily, the incision may need to be enlarged to allow removal of the mass intact. Morcellation of adnexal masses is always contraindicated. With larger solid masses there are diminishing returns for laparoscopy, because the size of the incision for removal of the mass approaches that which would have been required for a laparotomy at the outset. This issue may be less relevant for predominately cystic masses, which often can be decompressed within a bag or while applied to a transvaginal tube and removed via a laparoscopic port or colpotomy.

Does Rupture or Spill from a Malignant Ovarian Cyst Matter?

There is a theoretical concern that, in cases of early ovarian cancer confined to the ovary, intraoperative rupture of the capsule or spill of cyst contents may lead to intraperitoneal dissemination of malignant cells and ultimately to a poorer prognosis. This view was advocated by Webb and associates (63), who showed that a ruptured cyst was associated with a reduced 5-year survival rate in stage I epithelial ovarian cancer. This study failed to stratify for tumor adherence or high-grade lesions and did not include the routine use of peritoneal washings as part of the staging procedure and, so it probably underestimated the number of stage IC tumors. Subsequent studies have shown that intraoperative cyst rupture is not associated with reduced survival (64–67). Sjovall and associates (67) showed that there was a statistically significant reduction in survival in the group whose cyst ruptured before surgery, compared with those with intraoperative cyst rupture.

These studies all related to patients in whom any intraoperative rupture occurred during a primary laparotomy, and presumably in those cases copious peritoneal lavage was used. Caution must be used in applying conclusions derived from data obtained under one set of surgical conditions to a different set of surgical conditions. For example, it is unknown whether the high-pressure pneumoperitoneum, the carbon dioxide (CO_2) gas itself, or any other factors specific to laparoscopy might influence the outcome if rupture occurs during a laparoscopic procedure. It has been stated that laparoscopy is more likely than laparotomy to result in capsular rupture (57). Although this seems intuitively correct, no studies have addressed this issue.

Furthermore, the reason for the lack of supportive evidence to implicate intraoperative cyst rupture in poor survival may be that retrospective studies are not sensitive enough to detect small changes in mortality rates (44). An intact capsule may also be important to limit the inflammatory reaction and adhesion formation resulting from spill of a dermoid cyst and to reduce the risk of pseudomyxoma that might result from spill of a mucinous cyst (44). At the very least, intraoperative rupture will upstage some malignant cysts from stage IA to stage IC and therefore necessitate the use of adjuvant chemotherapy for patients who may not otherwise have required it (68).

It would be prudent in the surgical approach to take every care to maintain capsular integrity in order to minimize any possible risk of tumor dissemination. To minimize the likelihood of capsular rupture and tumor spill, several criteria have been suggested that may indicate that a mass should be managed by laparotomy rather than laparoscopy. These include a cystic mass larger than 10 cm diameter and a mass adherent to the pelvic sidewall requiring a difficult dissection (57). It is recommended that all cysts be removed from the abdomen either via a commercially available laparoscopic bag or via a colpotomy using a transvaginal tube (69). If a cyst is too large to be removed intact, it can be decompressed within the bag before exteriorization. Alternately, a large cystic mass can be fixed in the pelvis over a colpotomy and evacuated vaginally using suction. If cyst rupture does occur, the abdominal and pelvic contents should be thoroughly irrigated with copious fluid.

If a Malignancy Is Diagnosed at or after a Laparoscopic Procedure, Does It Matter If Definitive Surgical Staging Is Delayed until a Later Date?

There are two management options available on diagnosis of apparent stage I ovarian cancer at laparoscopy (usually after frozen section analysis of a specimen). One may either proceed to immediate surgical staging or stop the procedure and reschedule definitive surgical staging to a later date. Which of these options is most appropriate depends on individual circumstances and is influenced by the training and expertise of the surgeon (or the immediate availability of a suitably trained surgeon) and by the patient's preoperative counseling and expectations. What is not in doubt is that formal surgical staging is necessary, given that 28% of cases of apparent stage I ovarian cancer will be upgraded when a definitive staging procedure is carried out (70).

There have been no published studies regarding the effect of surgical delay on survival in ovarian cancer. Most of the available data involves surgical delay before laparotomy. The data is conflicting, with one study showing a correlation between surgical delay and increasing stage (71) and others showing no such correlation (72–74). Adding further uncertainty to this issue is the unknown effect of a laparoscopic procedure, which may include inspection only, cystectomy, or adnexectomy, before delayed definitive staging. A retrospective analysis of the influence of delayed staging laparotomy after laparoscopic removal of ovarian masses later found to be malignant reviewed 48 cases (75). In 24 of these, staging laparotomy was carried out within 17 days after laparoscopy, and in the other 24 cases there was a delay of more than 17 days. On univariate analysis there was seen to be a statistically significant increase in the proportion of advanced-stage tumors (both malignant and LMP) among patients in whom laparotomy was delayed for more than 17 days. However, on multivariate analysis this difference was statistically significant only for LMP tumors.

In a retrospective survey of 273 German departments of obstetrics and gynecology, the results of 192 cases of ovarian malignancy managed laparoscopically were reported (76). When the delay between laparoscopic biopsy and definitive surgery was longer than 8 days, port site metastases developed in 56% (5/9) of cases of apparent stage IC to II (but unstaged) ovarian cancer and in 47% (8/17) of cases of stage III ovarian cancer. Among 72 cases of apparent stage 1A (unstaged) ovarian cancer, there was rapid progression to stage III disease at laparotomy in 39% (28/72). Although the results of this survey are disturbing, it is not possible to isolate surgical delay as the main factor causing disease progression, given the careless surgical techniques employed. Even in apparent stage I tumors, only 7% of masses were removed intact via an endobag. In most of the cases, techniques such as capsule rupture, biopsy, and morcellation were utilized. Certainly these findings suggest that the combination of spill from the ovarian capsule and delay until definitive surgery can be associated with rapid progression of tumor stage.

Even with diligent preoperative triage of patients, the gynecologist may occasionally encounter unexpected malignancies when undertaking laparoscopic removal of an ovarian mass. In this situation it is probably better to terminate the surgery if a surgeon with the appropriate skills to perform a formal staging procedure is not immediately available. It is far more important that accurate staging be established, albeit at a later date. Undertreating of poorly staged or unstaged ovarian cancer is far more likely to compromise long-term survival than is delaying the surgical staging by a couple of weeks (77). Furthermore, in accurately staged low-grade tumors chemotherapy can be safely withheld (68).

The optimal timing of repeat surgery for staging purposes after a laparoscopic procedure has not been established, although Canis and associates (78) suggested that the staging surgery be considered an "oncologic emergency" and performed as soon as possible. The reality is that surgical delay is often longer than would be considered ideal. The mean time interval between the initial laparoscopic procedure and surgical staging was reported as 2.5 weeks in a Finnish study (79), 4.8 weeks in a U.S. study (80), 6.5 weeks in a study in the United Kingdom (81), and 12.5 weeks in an Austrian study (54).

Does Laparoscopy Cause Acceleration of the Spread of Malignant Cells?

There is speculation that factors specific to laparoscopy may encourage dissemination of malignant cells. Experimental evidence suggests that the CO_2 environment established during pneumoperitoneum may have a growth-stimulating effect on tumor cells (82). When tumor cells were instilled into the mouse peritoneal cavity with a CO_2 pneumoperitoneum and the results were compared with those of a control group in which tumor cells were instilled without a pneumoperitoneum, the pneumoperitoneum group displayed an increased seeding rate of tumor cells and a significant increase in the number and size of intraabdominal metastases compared with controls (83). This effect of the CO_2 pneumoperitoneum may be explained by diffuse damage to the peritoneum with exposure of the underlying basal lamina, which facilitates the attachment of tumor cells to the basal lamina (84). It is not known whether these experimental animal results are relevant to surgical practice in humans, but these findings nevertheless suggest caution in the application of laparoscopic surgery when there is likely to be rupture of a cyst or spill of malignant cells.

Several studies have compared tumor growth after laparotomy and after pneumoperitoneum in animal models. Although most found greater tumor growth after laparotomy (82,85–88), Volz and colleagues (89) found increased tumor growth associated with laparoscopy. Given the conflicting nature of these reports, it is not possible to draw firm conclusions.

How Does the Survival of Patients with Ovarian Cancer Managed Laparoscopically Compare with That of Patients Whose Disease Is Managed by the Traditional Approach of Laparotomy and Surgical Staging?

There are no currently available data from prospective trials comparing survival between patients with a malignant adnexal mass managed laparoscopically versus management by laparotomy and surgical staging. Table 11.2 (54–57,79–81,90–97) shows follow-up details of 689 cases of ovarian malignancy managed laparoscopically from 16 published reports since 1991. Most of

TABLE 11.2. *Studies of patients with ovarian cancer managed laparoscopically*

Source (ref. no.)	Ovarian cancers	Surgical staging		Follow-up period (months)		
		Laparotomy	Laparoscopy	No. Cases	Mean	Range
Reich et al., 1990 (95)	1	—	1	1	18	—
Maimen et al., 1991 (80)	42	37	—	?	"Significantly less than 1 year"	—
Nezhat et al., 1992 (94)	4	4	—	4	~23	12–36
Hulka et al., 1992 (55)	411	?	?	—	—	—
Canis et al., 1994 (59)	7	7	—	2	44	18–38
Pomel et al., 1995 (93)	10	—	10	?	?	?
Crawford et al., 1995 (81)	29	?	—	—	—	—
Chu et al., 1995 (91)	1	—	1	1	6	—
Childers et al., 1995 (92)	14	—	14	—	—	—
Spirtos et al., 1995 (97)	4	—	4	—	—	—
Wenzl et al., 1996 (54)	108	76	—	—	—	—
Childers et al., 1996 (57)	16	13	—	9	37	23–50
Canis et al., 1997 (56)	15	13	2	4	?	12–36
Possover et al., 1998 (96)	10	—	10	—	—	—
Dottino et al., 1999 (58)	9	5	2	—	—	—
Leminem and Lehtovirta, 1999 (79)	8	8	—	8	44	6–60

these patients underwent laparotomy and surgical staging after initial laparoscopic diagnosis/adnexectomy, although it is unclear what proportion had immediate laparotomy versus laparotomy delayed until a later date. In only 33 cases was the definitive surgical staging performed laparoscopically.

Follow-up data were reported for only 4% (30/689) of these cases, and in only one case did the follow-up period extend for 5 years. It is inappropriate to comment on short-term survival data in ovarian cancer, where recurrences can happen after more than 5 years even with early-stage disease (98). Therefore it is impossible to draw any valid conclusions regarding survival until the results of prospective trials with long-term follow-up are available.

Conclusion

Ten years ago, in a survey of members of The American Association of Gynecologic Laparoscopists, 12% of respondents stated that they performed laparoscopy on patients with an adnexal mass suspicious of malignancy (55). Today that rate is likely to be even higher. Published opinion regarding the role of laparoscopic surgery in the management of a mass at moderate/high risk for malignancy is divided between those advocating its use (58,92–94,99,100) and those advising laparotomy when malignancy is suspected (54,76,79,80,101,102). Others offer a compromise such as avoiding the use of laparoscopic management in all postmenopausal patients (103) or initiating laparoscopic assessment and proceeding to laparotomy and frozen section analysis if the mass appears suspicious (78).

Given the low risk of ovarian malignancy in an adnexal mass, it would seem reasonable to adopt a management policy based on a preoperative assessment of risk. The overall risk of malignancy depends on the patient population but may be expected to vary from less than 1% in low-risk populations to more than 10% in high-risk groups (Table 11.1). Depending on the exact criteria used, up to 94% of women with adnexal masses and "abnormal" ultrasound findings (56), and 86% of those with "abnormal" ultrasound findings or elevated CA 125 or both (57), who were managed laparoscopically, did not have ovarian cancer. These women should not be denied the advantages of laparoscopic management, nor should the women who do have a malignancy be compromised by inappropriate surgery. Achieving this balance requires careful preoperative evaluation and the application of cautious surgical judgment.

It is important that all women with a mass at moderate risk for malignancy be counseled preoperatively, so that they are aware of the possibility of malignancy and so that appropriate informed consent can be obtained to proceed to definitive surgery if the diagnosis is confirmed. Adnexal masses occurring in women with a past history of breast cancer or other nongynecologic malignancies are at high risk for both primary and secondary ovarian cancers and should be managed by a gynecologic oncologist (104).

The management algorithm shown in Figure 11.1 is intended as a guide to management for the competent gynecologic laparoscopist who is not trained in gynecologic oncology. The procedure should include careful inspection of all peritoneal surfaces, including the pelvis and pouch of Douglas, diaphragm, paracolic gutters, omentum, and bowel surfaces. It is recommended that peritoneal washings be obtained and that every care be taken to remove the cyst without rupture or spillage of cyst contents into the peritoneal cavity. Puncture, biopsy, and partial resection of suspicious masses are unacceptable practices. Morcellation of ovarian masses should not be performed. Frozen section analysis should be performed for all suspicious ovarian masses.

With the use of this schema it is likely that approximately 11% of all adnexal masses will be found to be "suspicious" at laparoscopy, of which 40% will be malignant or LMP and 60% will be benign (56). Laparoscopic excision of these "suspicious" masses cannot be recommended unless both frozen section analysis and the option to proceed to immediate surgical staging are available. If there is suspicion of ovarian cancer on laparoscopic evaluation, the ovarian capsule should not be violated and laparotomy should be initiated (80). The combination of spill and delay in definitive surgical management should be avoided at all costs (57).

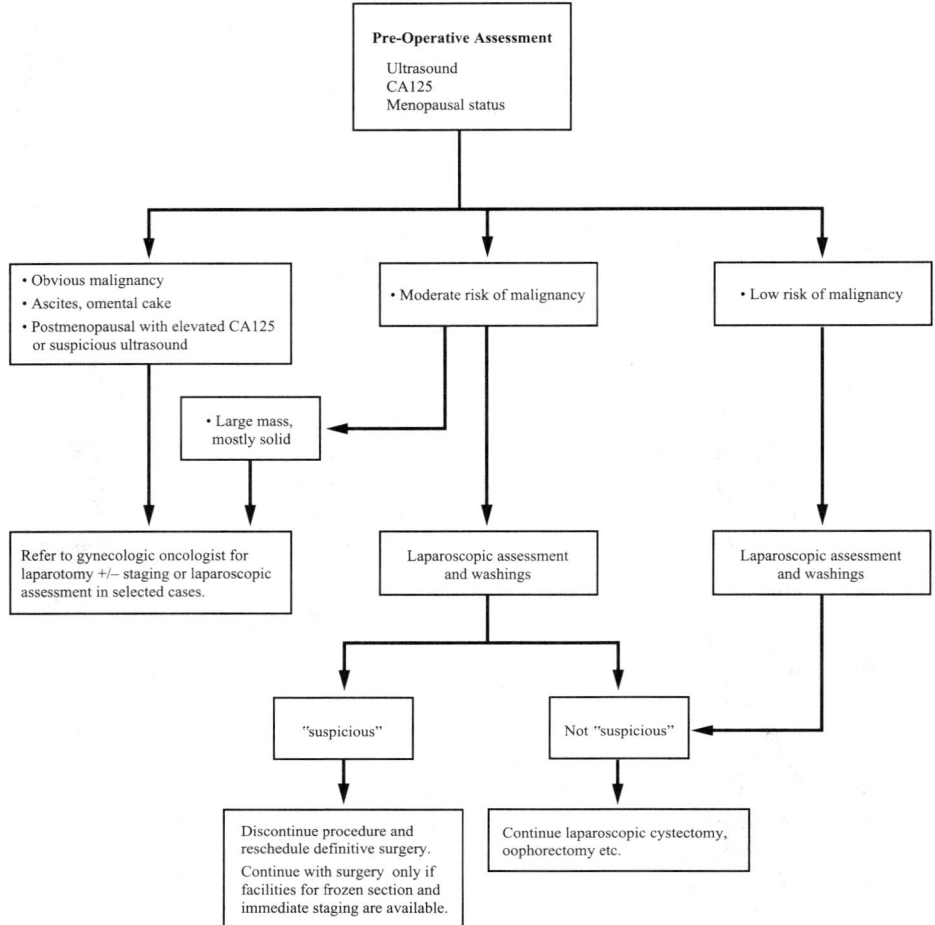

FIG. 11.1. Management guidelines for laparoscopic management of an adnexal mass.

Based on a series of 599 cases reported by Canis and associates (56), for every 100 adnexal masses seen by the general gynecologic laparoscopist who adopts this practice, 3 cases will be referred on to a gynecologic oncologist as obviously malignant or otherwise unsuitable for laparoscopic management on the basis of preoperative findings. Of the remaining 97 cases, 86 can be expected to be benign or nonsuspicious in appearance and can be managed entirely laparoscopically. In 11 cases the surgeon will discontinue the procedure based on the "suspicious" appearance of the mass at laparoscopy; if a gynecologic oncologist is not immediately available in these instances, rescheduling further surgery to a later date is appropriate. As a result, it is likely that a gynecologic oncologist will have operated on all the malignancies and LMP tumors (7 cases) in addition to 7 cases thought to be suspicious on laparoscopic appearance but subsequently found to be benign. The gynecologic laparoscopist will have entirely managed 86% of the original 100 cases. Using data from an updated series, it was estimated that if laparoscopy is used to assess all adnexal masses and an immediate laparotomy is performed for all masses found to be malignant or suspicious for malignancy, then 80% of all masses could be treated by laparoscopy with all malignancies treated by laparotomy (85). In practice, the figures will vary depending on age, menopausal status, and other risk factors of the patient population as well as the level of caution employed in interpretation of preoperative ultrasonography and CA 125 results and the laparoscopic skill of the individual surgeon.

There are numerous case reports of laparoscopic mismanagement of ovarian malignancies (75,76,79,80). In many of these, despite the preoperative suspicion of ovarian malignancy, malignant appearance of the ovarian tumor, and malignant frozen section report, immediate laparotomy was not performed (79). In one report, 93% of ovarian cysts subsequently found to be malignant were subjected to rupture, biopsy, or morcellation (76). Likewise at open surgery, inadequate and inappropriate procedures for ovarian cancer were reported in 48% of cases operated on by obstetricians/gynecologists in one series (105).

Errors in preoperative assessment and poor clinical and surgical judgment can occur with any type of surgery and may be reduced with education and training and by the development of guidelines for the appropriate use of laparoscopic surgery. Until there is more evidence available from prospective trials, it would be prudent to discontinue any laparoscopic procedure when a likely ovarian malignancy is encountered. In an ideal world, frozen section analysis and progression to immediate surgical staging would be universally available. Laparotomy through a vertical midline incision should still be regarded as the standard of care for patients with an ovarian malignancy.

LAPAROSCOPIC STAGING OF OVARIAN CANCER

The conventional management of ovarian cancer includes laparotomy and surgical staging through a midline vertical incision. Surgical staging requires exploration of the peritoneal surfaces in the pelvis and abdomen, peritoneal washings, omentectomy, biopsies of pelvic and paraaortic lymph nodes, and biopsies from the peritoneal surfaces and diaphragm. Many gynecologic oncologists advocate that the paraaortic lymph node dissection be continued up to the level of the juncture of the ovarian vein and the vena cava on the right side and the renal vein on the left side (106).

All of the surgical components that together constitute a comprehensive staging procedure can be performed laparoscopically. The techniques for laparoscopic pelvic and paraaortic lymphadenectomy and omentectomy have been well described (104,107,108). Laparoscopic assessment does have technical limitations with respect to staging of ovarian cancer. The surgeon is unable to palpate lymph nodes, manually examine the full extent of the bowel, or easily visualize the underside of the diaphragm. Compared with laparotomy, laparoscopy affords improved visualization of the diaphragm and the pelvic peritoneum.

The first laparoscopic staging procedure for ovarian cancer was reported by Reich and colleagues (95) in 1990 on a patient with apparent early stage ovarian cancer who had refused laparotomy. This procedure consisted of laparoscopic removal of both ovaries intact through a culdotomy incision, vaginal hysterectomy, laparoscopic omentectomy, and unilateral pelvic lymphadenectomy. The procedure did not include paraaortic lymphadenectomy and is therefore considered inadequate according staging guidelines of the International Federation of Gynecology and Obstetrics (FIGO). There have subsequently been at least 50 cases reported in the literature of laparoscopic staging of ovarian cancer (Table 11.3) (56,91–93,95–97,109,110). Most of these cases were previously diagnosed cancers subsequently referred for definitive management, and none include long-term follow-up.

Concerns regarding the adequacy of lymph node yields in laparoscopic surgery have been addressed in a number of studies in which laparoscopic pelvic lymphadenectomy was immediately followed by laparotomy. Querleu and associates (111) performed laparoscopic pelvic lymphadenectomy on 39 patients with cervical cancer and then evaluated the completeness of lymphadenectomy in 32 cases. They found that no positive nodes had been missed by the laparoscopic procedure; however, they did not state how many additional negative nodes were

TABLE 11.3. Laparoscopic staging of ovarian cancer[a]

Source (ref. no.)	Patients (n)	Operating time (min)	Pelvic lymph nodes (n)	PA lymph nodes (n)	Max. level of PA nodes	Blood loss (mL)	Hospital stay (d)	Complications
Reich et al., 1990 (95)	1	300	11 unilateral	Not done	Not done	200	1	Nil
Childers et al., 1993 (109)	6	NS	NS	6.3	To IMA	NS	1.3	Nil
Querleu and LeBlanc, 1994 (110)	8	227	NS	8.6	Infrarenal	<300	2.8	Nil
Childers et al., 1995 (92)	14	149 w/o hyst 196 with hyst	NS	NS	Infrarenal	NS	1.6	1 vena cava injury and 1 abdominal wall ecchymosis
Spirtos et al., 1995[b] (97)	4	193	11 right side 9.8 left side	7.9	? Infrarenal	<100	2.69	2 DVTs and 2 small bowel obstructions among 40 cases
Pomel et al., 1995 (93)	10	313	6 unilateral	8	Infrarenal	NS	4.75	1 pulmonary embolus and 1 hemorrhage requiring return to theater
Chu et al., 1995 (91)	1	260	NS	NS	Infrarenal	NS	2	Nil
Canis et al., 1997 (56)	1	NS	NS	NS	NS	NS	NS	NS
Possover et al., 1998[b] (96)	4	187	26.8	7.3	Infrarenal	NS	5.6	2 vascular injuries and 1 bowel perforation
Dottino et al., 1999[b] (90)	3	130	11.9	3.7	? Infrarenal	83.4	3.6	Vena cava laceration (2.50 mL blood loss)

PA, paraaortic; hyst, hysterectomy; w/o, without; DVT, deep venous thrombosis; IMA, inferior mesenteric artery; NS, not stated.
[a]Reports of staging in cases of low malignant potential tumors and second look surgery have been excluded.
[b]Data derived from studies that included staging procedures for other malignancies or indications; operating time, nodal counts, blood loss, hospital stay and complications specific to ovarian cancer could not be determined from these reports.

obtained at laparotomy. Childers and colleagues (112) reported on eight patients undergoing laparoscopic lymphadenectomy for cervical cancer. The average node count was 31, with positive nodes identified in three cases. The five remaining patients underwent laparotomy for radical hysterectomy, and on average three additional nodes per case were obtained. None of the additional nodes was positive. Fowler and coworkers (113) performed laparoscopic pelvic lymphadenectomy on 12 patients with cervical cancer along with paraaortic lymphadenectomy in 2 of these. The average lymph node count was 31, with two cases having positive nodes and an average of 7 additional nodes obtained at laparotomy, none of them positive.

Laparoscopic restaging of apparent stage I ovarian cancer is a potentially attractive surgical option. Gynecologic oncologists often encounter patients with previously diagnosed ovarian cancer who did not have surgical staging performed at the time of their primary surgery because the referring gynecologist performed oophorectomy without anticipating a malignancy. Currently, the standard management of these patients often incorporates a repeat laparotomy to facilitate definitive staging so that optimal adjuvant therapy can be assigned. A Gynecologic Oncology Group study has addressed the role of laparoscopy for restaging of ovarian cancers in this setting, with the results yet to be published.

It is possible laparoscopically to obtain adequate exposure, identify the pelvic anatomy, open the retroperitoneal spaces, completely dissect pelvic lymphatic tissue, and skeletonize the pelvic vessels, aorta, and vena cava. However, laparoscopic lymphadenectomy is not an easy technique to master and has a significant learning curve. It has been shown that the completeness of lymphatic tissue harvest increases with increasing surgical experience (113), whereas operative time decreases substantially (97). Laparoscopic pelvic and paraaortic lymphadenectomy is unlikely to be mastered by laparoscopic surgeons with no experience in the analogous open procedure, or by the experienced oncologic surgeon who does not also develops advanced laparoscopic skills (92). At present the safe use of this technique is limited to those few surgeons who have adequate training and experience in both gynecologic oncologic surgery and advanced laparoscopic procedures. Laparotomy is still the standard of care for the staging of ovarian cancer. The routine use of laparoscopy in this setting cannot be recommended until prospective trials with adequate follow-up have demonstrated its safety and reliability.

LAPAROSCOPIC MANAGEMENT OF OVARIAN TUMORS OF LOW MALIGNANT POTENTIAL

There are limited data available relevant to the laparoscopic management of ovarian tumors of LMP. Accurate preoperative diagnosis is impossible, because the cases are identified only on histologic analysis. The distinction between LMP and malignant ovarian tumors on frozen section analysis can be difficult, especially in the case of mucinous tumors. In their series of 48 patients with an intraoperative frozen section diagnosis of LMP tumor, Menzin and colleagues (114) found that the diagnosis was confirmed on permanent section in 67% of cases, upgraded to malignancy in 27%, and found to be benign in 6%.

Darai and associates (115) reported the largest series in the literature, with 25 patients with LMP ovarian tumors managed laparoscopically, representing 2.2% of 1,130 ovarian lesions managed laparoscopically over an 8-year period. Most (76%) were in premenopausal women and were asymptomatic (72%). The mean size of the tumors was 7.9 cm (range, 1.5 to 19 cm); 25% were "unilocular smooth sonolucent"; and the CA 125 was not elevated in 8 (70%) of the 12 cases in which it was measured. In 80% of cases the presumptive diagnosis based on preoperative evaluation and laparoscopic assessment was that of a benign ovarian tumor. There was a significantly higher rate of recurrence in patients treated with cystectomy compared with patients treated with complete salpingo-oophorectomy.

The diagnosis of LMP tumor is difficult to anticipate, and can be difficult to confirm intraoperatively. The laparoscopic management should follow the same principles as management at open surgery. Conservative surgery should be favored in women wishing to retain their fertility.

For confirmed LMP tumors at least ipsilateral salpingo-oophorectomy should be performed, with consideration of hysterectomy and bilateral salpingo-oophorectomy in postmenopausal women and appendectomy in the case of mucinous tumors. The role of surgical staging in LMP tumors is controversial (44).

LAPAROSCOPY IN THE MANAGEMENT OF ADVANCED OVARIAN CANCER

Even the most ardent proponents of laparoscopy would agree that "huge, fixed pelvic masses requiring extensive retroperitoneal dissection, often with bowel resection and retrograde hysterectomy cannot be removed laparoscopically" (99). There is growing evidence that, in patients with extensive disease, who have tumors unlikely to be optimally debulked even at laparotomy, neoadjuvant chemotherapy may be preferable to immediate surgery. Overall survival and progression-free survival rates in patients treated with neoadjuvant chemotherapy followed by interval debulking appear to be comparable to, or better than, those in women treated conventionally, whereas operative time, blood loss, and hospital stay may all be reduced (116–118). These findings are yet to be confirmed in a prospective randomized trial.

At this time, the standard of care for advanced ovarian cancer is still primary cytoreductive surgery via a midline laparotomy incision. Maximal surgical effort should be employed, with radical extirpation of tumor including bowel resection, urologic resection, liver resection, and splenectomy performed if necessary to achieve optimum cytoreduction and a state of minimum residual disease. The ability to assess the "resectability" of any given ovarian tumor and the ability to safely perform such radical surgery is influenced by the training and experience of the individual surgeon.

Identification of patients in whom optimal cytoreductive surgery is unlikely to be possible has usually been by clinical examination and CT scanning (116,117,119), although Vergote and coworkers (118) used laparoscopy as the basis for their decision to perform primary debulking surgery or give neoadjuvant chemotherapy in 77 cases from their series of 285 patients. They reported a mean operative time of 25 minutes, mean blood loss of 10 mL, and mean hospital stay of 2 days for the laparoscopy group and a mean time until laparotomy of 7 days in the group subsequently managed with primary cytoreductive surgery. They excised all trocar sites at the time of subsequent laparotomy and found 6 port site metastases. In all patients who received chemotherapy, the port site metastases disappeared during the course of their chemotherapy. It is difficult to reconcile the adequacy of laparoscopic assessment in this setting, given that it is usually the extent of disease in the upper abdomen or chest that limits the feasibility of cytoreductive surgery, rather than in the pelvis, where disease can almost always be resected with aggressive surgical techniques (116). In addition, it should be stressed that this approach is unorthodox and unproven.

Kadar (99) suggested that there is potential for definitive laparoscopic surgery to be performed as an interval procedure after neoadjuvant chemotherapy, but there is a lack of published evidence to support this concept.

SECOND-LOOK LAPAROSCOPY

Second-look surgery refers to the practice of reoperating on ovarian cancer patients after completion of the definitive surgery and first regimen of chemotherapy (typically six cycles) to determine whether a complete clinical response correlates with an absence of disease on surgical and pathologic assessment. The rationale for second-look laparotomy has been to provide information to aid in deciding whether to continue, alter, or discontinue a chemotherapy regimen and to provide an opportunity for secondary cytoreductive surgery if persistent or recurrent tumor is encountered (44). The role of second-look laparotomy in the management of ovarian cancer is controversial, and some authors suggest that the routine practice of second-look surgery, outside the confines of a clinical trial, is not appropriate in the modern management of the patient with ovarian cancer (120). Any assessment of the role of laparoscopy as an alternative to laparotomy in second-look surgery must be viewed in this context. In the evaluation of second-look laparoscopy, two specific criteria need to be addressed: laparoscopy should be as reliable as laparotomy in the diagnosis of complete remission, and there should be no increase in morbidity compared with laparotomy.

There is an improvement in visualization of the diaphragm and the superior surface of the liver with laparoscopy, and the magnification affords better identification of small lesions. However, laparoscopy may compromise assessment of the mesentery and small bowel and preclude the ability to palpate suspicious retroperitoneal lesions. Numerous studies from the 1970s and 1980s demonstrated that second-look laparoscopy was associated with a false-negative rate for the detection of persistent or recurrent disease of 18% to 50% (121–125). Taken in isolation, negative findings at second-look laparoscopy would be falsely reassuring, given that up to half of these patients will have undiagnosed recurrent or persistent tumor. It has been suggested that rather than replacing laparotomy, second-look laparoscopy could be a useful first step in second-look assessment, by identifying those patients with resectable, unresectable or diffuse disease after chemotherapy. Negative laparoscopies would be followed by laparotomy. If second-look laparoscopy were used in this way, one third of women would be spared laparotomy (122,123,126).

Given the advances in laparoscopic technologies during the last decade, the role of laparoscopy in second-look surgery has been reassessed. Clough and associates (127) undertook staging laparoscopy followed by immediate laparotomy in 20 cases of ovarian cancer. They reported a 14% false-negative rate for laparoscopy and found that the most common obstacle to reliable and safe laparoscopic assessment was the presence of dense adhesions. In this series, the presence of dense adhesions limited the number of cases that could be "completely explored" to 36%. Other series have reported "exhaustive" or "complete" laparoscopic assessments in 81% to 89% of cases (92,128). This wide range may reflect differences in the surgical effort employed and time taken to complete the procedure.

Bowel perforation is the most common major complication of second-look laparoscopy; it occurs with a frequency of 4% to 10% and usually requires laparotomy for repair (92,127–129). Other reported complications include major vessel injury, enterocutaneous fistula, and retroperitoneal hematoma (130). The overall major complication rate is 0% to 14%. The risk of major visceral or vascular injury is related to the complexity of the dissection (127). Comparing the morbidity at second-look laparoscopy to second-look laparotomy, Abu-Rustum and colleagues (130) reported a 27% complication rate for laparotomy and zero for laparoscopy, while Casey and associates (128) reported 8.6% for laparoscopy and 41% for laparotomy. Both these studies reported second-look laparoscopy to be associated with decreases in operating time, blood loss, hospital stay, and overall cost.

There have been no randomized, controlled trials of survival after negative second-look laparoscopy compared with negative second-look laparotomy. Similar risk of disease recurrence was reported in two series (128,130); however, a retrospective trial of 198 patients found a statistically significant increase in the relative risk for recurrence among patients who underwent second-look surgery by laparoscopy compared with laparotomy (131). It may be that this higher risk for recurrence reflects a lower accuracy in detecting subclinical persistent disease.

A new approach is the use of a 2.8-mm microlaparoscope for second-look surgery. A pilot study of eight cases concluded that this technique was feasible and was as accurate as conventional 10-mm laparoscopy (132). Microlaparoscopy can theoretically be performed under local anesthesia, but it is as yet unproven in the setting of second-look surgery.

PORT SITE METASTASES

The finding of tumor growth at the site of a previous laparoscopic trocar placement, commonly known as a port site metastasis, is one of the most feared complications of laparoscopic procedures in gynecologic cancer treatment. It is likely that there is underreporting of this complication in the literature, making an accurate estimate of incidence difficult to establish. However, retrospective series have reported an incidence ranging

TABLE 11.4. *Reported cases of port site recurrence in ovarian malignancy*

Source (ref. no.)	Diagnosis	Stage	Ascites	Procedure	Time to diagnosis (d)
Dobronte et al., 1978 (137)	CA	III	Yes	Diagnostic laparoscopy and biopsy	14
Stockdale and Pocock, 1985 (138)	CA	IV	Yes	Diagnostic laparoscopy and biopsy	8
Hsiu et al., 1986 (139)	LMP	III	?	Diagnostic laparoscopy and biopsy	21
	LMP	?III	?	Diagnostic laparoscopy and biopsy	21
Miralles et al., 1989 (140)	CA	?I	?	Laparoscopy after ?open adnexectomy	1 y
Gleeson et al., 1993 (144)	LMP	?IC	?	Oophorectomy and morcellation	14
	CA	III	Yes	Diagnostic laparoscopy and biopsy	14
	CA	III	Yes	Diagnostic laparoscopy and biopsy	14
Shepherd and Carter, 1994, (145)	LMP	?I	No	Laparoscopic cyst aspiration and excision	42
Childers et al., 1994 (142)	CA	IIA	No	Laparoscopic second-look procedure (positive for recurrence)	NS
Gungor et al., 1996 (141)	CA	IIIB	Yes	Laparoscopic third-look procedure	8 mo
Chu et al., 1996 (143)	CA	?IC, ?IIIC	Yes	Laparoscopic salping-oopherectomy	2 wk
Kruitwagen et al., 1996 (135)	7 CA	IIIC-IV	Yes	Diagnostic laparoscopy	9–35
Kindermann et al., 1996 (101)	8 CA	III	NS	Diagnostic laparoscopy and biopsy	8–60
	5 CA	IC-II	NS	Laparoscopic cystectomy/biopsy/morcellation	>8
	CA	?IA	NS	Laparoscopic removal with endobag	?
Van Dam et al., 1999 (134)	9 CA	IIIC–IV	NS	Laparoscopic assessment of primary and recurrent ovarian cancer to assess operability	14–90
Hopkins et al., 2000 (146)	LMP	?I	NS	Laparoscopic ovarian cystectomy, morcellation	28
	LMP	?I	NS	Laparoscopic partial excision	21
	LMP	?I	NS	Laparoscopic oophorectomy, bag rupture	14

NS, not stated; LMP, low malignant potential; CA, carcinoma.

from 1% to 16% of all laparoscopic procedures for ovarian cancer (133–135). There have been 44 cases reported in the English language literature, of which 37 have been in association with ovarian malignancies and 7 in association with LMP tumors (Table 11.4) (133,134,136–145).

There has been no well-documented case of stage I ovarian cancer associated with port site recurrence at primary surgery, although Kindermann and associates (101) reported a case of an apparent stage IA (unstaged) ovarian cancer removed laparoscopically with an endobag that subsequently developed a port site metastasis. A port site recurrence was found at laparotomy in association with large-volume stage IIIC disease, 2 weeks after laparoscopic removal of an apparent stage I (but unstaged) squamous cell carcinoma arising in a mature cystic teratoma with ascites (142). All other reported cases have been in association with stage II through IV ovarian malignancies or laparoscopic second-look procedures (Table 11.4). However, there have been at least five case reports of apparent stage I LMP tumors associated with port site metastases (143–145). In all of these it was not clear what, if any, staging procedures had been undertaken, and in at least four of the five cases laparoscopic techniques (morcellation or partial excision of ovarian mass) (143,145) or accidental rupture of a bag containing the ovarian specimen (145) may have accounted for iatrogenic spill of cells into the peritoneal cavity.

Two retrospective studies have analyzed the effect of port site metastases on survival in ovarian cancer (133,134). In both studies, all port site recurrences occurred in stage IIIC or stage IV disease, and in both there was no statistically significant difference in survival. The occurrence of a port site recurrence in a confirmed stage I ovarian malignancy could certainly have a negative impact on survival, although such a case has yet to be documented.

The exact etiology of port site metastases is unknown and may be multifactorial. Neuhaus and associates (146) reviewed a number of proposed mechanisms and physiologic factors that may be involved. Direct contamination of the port site with tumor cells may occur either during extraction of tumor through a small wound or indirectly from instruments contaminated with tumor cells. Tumor cells may exist in aerosol and be seeded into the wound, especially during desufflation of the pneumoperitoneum. It may be that seeding of tumor cells into the wound is no more likely at laparoscopy than at laparotomy, but metastases are more likely to occur because of locally acting immunologic or metabolic factors that are specific to laparoscopy. Hematogenous spread of malignant cells preferentially to the port site has also been proposed as a mechanism but seems unlikely (146). Factors specific to laparoscopy that may play a role in the development of port site metastases are the effect of increased intraperitoneal pressure, metabolic and immunologic effects of the CO_2 gas commonly used for insufflation, alterations in peritoneal humidity, stretching of the abdominal wall, electrostatic interactions with trocars, and pressure-flow effects related to the use of insufflating gas.

A number of strategies have been suggested to minimize the risk of port site recurrences. These are based on accepted surgical principles (in the absence of hard evidence), and most apply equally to the open or laparoscopic approach. First, one must attempt to prevent the spill of potentially malignant cells from any ovarian cyst. The possibility of malignancy should be considered in every case, so that care is taken to adopt surgical techniques to remove the tumor intact and without violating the capsule. Partial excision and morcellation should never be undertaken. Ovarian cystectomy or oophorectomy should be performed in preference to biopsy in most cases. Aspiration of any nonphysiologic ovarian cyst is not appropriate. The exposure of the anterior abdominal wall to tumor cells should be avoided by the use of a closed system such as a laparoscopic bag to remove ovarian tissue specimens. Cysts can be decompressed within the bag and the abdominal wound enlarged if necessary. Alternatively, specimens may be removed via a posterior colpotomy with the use of a transvaginal tube.

Irrigation of laparoscopic wounds may decrease the risk of tumor cell implantation and should be performed at the completion of surgery (135). Van Dam and colleagues (133) demonstrated that the rate of port site metastasis in 104 patients with primary or recurrent ovarian cancer undergoing laparoscopy to assess operability was 2% when all layers of the laparoscopic wounds were closed (peritoneum, rectus sheath, and skin) and 58% when only the skin layer was closed. This difference may be attributable to the fact that all patients in the series with port site metastases had advanced disease with ascites. Closing all layers separately may produce a more "watertight" seal and thus prevent chronic leakage of malignant ascites into the adipose layer. The same group also recommended that definitive treatment (either laparotomy with excision of the port sites or commencement of chemotherapy) should be undertaken within 1 week of laparoscopy to deal with any malignant cells that may be harbored in the port site wounds (133).

CONCLUSION

Advances in technology have broadened the indications for laparoscopic surgery, and it is now accepted practice in the routine management of benign adnexal masses. However, laparotomy remains the gold standard for the management of ovarian cancer. The role of laparoscopy in the diagnosis and management of the mass at moderate risk for malignancy varies depending on the skill and experience of the laparoscopic surgeon and on the availability of frozen section analysis and access to immediate surgical staging. The routine use of laparoscopy for surgical staging of early ovarian malignancies, second-look surgery, and assessment of suitability for cytoreductive surgery in advanced stage disease should all be considered still under evaluation. Prospective, randomized trials are needed to adequately evaluate the impact of laparoscopic surgery on ovarian cancer survival and the implications and true incidence of port site metastases.

Although laparoscopy is easy to apply, its use should not compromise the appropriate surgical management of ovarian cancer. The need for laparotomy to complete a difficult dissection or to facilitate adequate staging or cytoreductive surgery should not be seen as a laparoscopic failure. Laparotomy and laparoscopy should be regarded as complementary rather than mutually exclusive modalities. Finally, the proposed benefits of laparoscopic surgery, such as decreased cost, hospital stay, and complications as well as improved quality of life and productivity, have yet to be proven in prospective trials.

REFERENCES

1. Finkler NJ, Benacerraf B, Lavin PT, et al. Comparison of serum CA125, clinical impression and ultrasound in the preoperative evaluation of ovarian masses. *Obstet Gynecol* 1988;72: 659–664.
2. Roman LD, Muderspach LI, Stein SM, et al. Pelvic examination: tumor marker level and gray-scale and Doppler sonography in the prediction of pelvic cancer. *Obstet Gynecol* 1997;89:493–500.
3. Schutter EMJ, Kenemans P, Sohn C, et al. Diagnostic value of pelvic examination, ultrasound, and serum CA125 in postmenopausal women with a pelvic mass: an international multicenter study. *Cancer* 1994;74:1398–1406.
4. Van Nagell JR, Ueland FR. Ultrasound evaluation of pelvic masses: predictors of malignancy for the general gynecologist. *Curr Opin Obstet Gynecol* 1999;11: 45–49.
5. Kobayashi M. Use of diagnostic ultrasound in trophoblastic neoplasms and ovarian tumors. *Cancer* 1976;38:441–452.
6. Meire HB, Farrant P, Guha T. Distinction of benign from malignant ovarian cysts by ultrasound. *Br J Obstet Gynaecol* 1978;85:893–899.
7. Herrmann UJ, Locher GW, Goldhirsch A. Sonographic patterns of ovarian tumors: prediction of malignancy. *Obstet Gynecol* 1987;69:777–781.
8. Benacerraf BR, Finkler NJ, Wojciechowski C, Knapp RC. Sonographic accuracy in the diagnosis of ovarian masses. *J Reprod Med* 1990;35:491–495.
9. Granberg S, Norstrom A, Wikland M. Tumors in the lower pelvis as imaged by vaginal sonography. *Gynecol Oncol* 1990;37:224–229.
10. Sassone AM, Timor-Tritsch IE, Artner A, et al. Transvaginal sonographic characterization of ovarian disease: evaluation of a new scoring system to predict ovarian malignancy. *Obstet Gynecol* 1991;78:70–76.
11. Granberg S, Wikland M, Jansson I. Macroscopic characterization of ovarian tumors and the relation to histologic diagnosis: criteria to be used for ultrasound evaluation. *Gynecol Oncol* 1989;3:139–144.
12. Luxman D, Bergman A, Sagi J, David MP. The postmenopausal adnexal mass: correlation between ultrasonic and pathologic findings. *Obstet Gynecol* 1991;77:726–728.
13. Strigini FA, Gadducci A, DelBravo B, et al. Differential diagnosis of adnexal masses with transvaginal sonography, color flow imaging, and serum CA125 assay in pre- and postmenopausal women. *Gynecol Oncol* 1996;61:68–72.
14. Mangioni C, Bolis G, Molteni P, Belloni C. Indications, advantages and limits of laparoscopy in ovarian cancer. *Gynecol Oncol* 1979;7:47–55.
15. Jacobs I, Oram D, Fairbanks J, et al. A risk of malignancy index incorporating CA125, ultrasound and menopausal status for the accurate preoperative diagnosis of ovarian cancer. *Br J Obstet Gynaecol* 1990;97:922–929.
16. Davies AP, Jacobs I, Woolas R, et al. The adnexal mass: benign or malignant? Evaluation of a risk of malignancy index. *Br J Obstet Gynaecol* 1993;100:927–931.
17. Bourne T, Campbell S, Steer C, et al. Transvaginal color flow imaging: a possible new screening technique for ovarian cancer. *BMJ* 1989;299:1367–1370.
18. Kurjak A, Zalud I, Jurkovic Z, Miljan M. Transvaginal color flow Doppler for the assessment of pelvic circulation. *Acta Obstet Gynecol Scand* 1989;68:131–135.
19. Weiner Z, Thaler I, Beck D, et al. Differentiating malignant from benign ovarian tumors with transvaginal color flow imaging. *Obstet Gynecol* 1992;79:159–162.
20. Kawai M, Kano T, Kikkawa F, et al. Transvaginal Doppler ultrasound with color flow imaging in the diagnosis of ovarian cancer. *Obstet Gynecol* 1992;79:163–167.
21. Folkman J, Watson K, Ingber D, Hanahan D. Induction of angiogenesis during the transition from hyperplasia to neoplasia. *Nature* 1989;339:58–61.
22. Hamper U, Sheth S, Abbas FM, et al. Transvaginal color Doppler sonography of adnexal masses: differences in blood flow impedance in benign and malignant lesions. *AJR Am J Roentgenol* 1993;160:1225–1228.
23. Brown DL, Frates MC, Laing FC, et al. Ovarian masses: can benign and malignant lesions be differentiated with color and pulsed Doppler US? *Radiology* 1994;190:333–336.
24. Stein S, Laifer-Narin S, Johnson MB, et al. Differentiation of benign and malignant adnexal masses: relative value of gray scale, color Doppler, and spectral Doppler sonography. *AJR Am J Roentgenol* 1995;164:381–386.
25. Valentin L. Gray scale sonography, subjective evaluation of the color Doppler image and measurement of blood flow velocity for distinguishing benign and malignant tumors of suspected adnexal origin. *Eur J Obstet Gynecol* 1997;72:63–72.
26. Levine D, Feldstein VA, Babcook CJ, Filly RA. Sonography of ovarian masses: poor sensitivity of resistive index for identifying malignant lesions. *AJR Am J Roentgenol* 1994;162:1355–1359.
27. Bromley B, Goodman H, Benacerraf BR. Comparison between sonographic morphology and Doppler waveform for the diagnosis of ovarian malignancy. *Gynecol Oncol* 1994;83:434–437.

28. Schelling M, Braun M, Kuhn W, et al. Combined transvaginal B-mode and color Doppler sonography for differential diagnosis of ovarian tumors: results of a multivariate logistic regression analysis. *Gynecol Oncol* 2000;77:78–86.
29. Sengoku K, Satoh T, Saitoh S, et al. Evaluation of transvaginal color Doppler sonography, transvaginal sonography and CA125 for prediction of ovarian malignancy. *Int J Gynecol Obstet* 1994;46:39–43.
30. Chou CY, Chang CH, Yao BL, Kuo HC. Color Doppler ultrasonography and serum CA125 in the differentiation of benign and malignant ovarian tumors. *J Clin Ultrasound* 1994;22:491–496.
31. Antonic J, Rakar S. Color and pulsed Doppler US and tumor marker CA125 in differentiation between benign and malignant ovarian masses. *Anticancer Res* 1995;15:1527–1532.
32. Ferrier AJ, Picker RH, Sinosich M. A comparison of color flow Doppler and serum CA125 measurement in the preoperative evaluation of a complex pelvic mass. *Int J Gynecol Cancer* 1998;8:113–118.
33. Kusnetzoff D, Gnochi D, Damonte C, et al. Differential diagnosis of pelvic masses: usefulness of CA125, transvaginal sonography and echo-Doppler. *Int J Gynecol Cancer* 1998;8:315–321.
34. Schneider VL, Schneider A, Reed KL, Hatch KD. Comparison of Doppler with two-dimensional sonography and CA125 for prediction of malignancy of pelvic masses. *Obstet Gynecol* 1993;81:983–988.
35. Franchi M, Beretta P, Ghezzi F, et al. Diagnosis of pelvic masses with transabdominal color Doppler, CA125 and ultrasonography. *Acta Obstet Gynecol Scand* 1995;74:734–739.
36. Shy K, Dubinski T. Is color Doppler ultrasound useful in diagnosing ovarian cancer? *Clin Obstet Gynecol* 1999;42:902–915.
37. Yamashita Y, Torashima M, Hatanaka Y, et al. Adnexal masses: accuracy of characterization with transvaginal US and precontrast and postcontrast MR imaging. *Radiology* 1995;194:557–565.
38. Kurjak A, Kupesic S, Anic T, Kosuta D. Three-dimensional ultrasound and power Doppler improve the diagnosis of ovarian lesions. *Gynecol Oncol* 2000;76:28–32.
39. Kupesic S, Kurjak A. Contrast-enhanced, three dimensional power Doppler sonography for differentiation of adnexal masses. *Obstet Gynecol* 2000;96:452–458.
40. Grab D, Flock F, Stohr I, et al. Classification of asymptomatic adnexal masses by ultrasound, magnetic resonance imaging and positron emission tomography. *Gynecol Oncol* 2000;77:454–459.
41. Clayton RD, Snowden S, Weston MJ, et al. Neural networks in the diagnosis of malignant ovarian tumours. *Br J Obstet Gynaecol* 1999;106:1078–1082.
42. Biagiotti R, Desii C, Vanzi E, Gacci G. Predicting ovarian malignancy: application of artificial neural networks to transvaginal and color Doppler flow US. *Radiology* 1999;210:399–403.
43. Curtin JP. Management of the adnexal mass. *Gynecol Oncol* 1994;55:S42–S46.
44. Morrow CP, Curtin JP. Tumors of the ovary—classification: the adnexal mass. In: Morrow CP and Curtin JP, eds. *Synopsis of gynecologic oncology*, 5th ed. Philadelphia: Churchill Livingstone, 1998:215–232.
45. Nicklin JL, VanEijkeren M, Athanasatos P, et al. A comparison of ovarian cyst aspirate cytology and histology: the case against aspiration of cystic pelvic masses. *Aust N Z J Obstet Gynecol* 1994;34:546–549.
46. Trimbos JB, Hacker NF. The case against aspirating ovarian cysts. *Cancer* 1993;72:828–831.
47. Spanos WJ. Preoperative hormonal therapy of cystic adnexal masses. *Am J Obstet Gynecol* 1973;116:551–556
48. Ben-Ami M, Geslevich Y, Battino S, et al. Management of functional ovarian cysts after induction of ovulation: a randomized prospective study. *Acta Obstet Gynecol Scand* 1993;72:396–397.
49. Steinkampf MP, Hammond KR, Blackwell RE. Hormonal treatment of functional ovarian cysts: a randomized prospective study. *Fertil Steril* 1990;54:775–777.
50. Parker W, Berek J. Management of selected cystic adnexal masses in postmenopausal women by operative laparoscopy: a pilot study. *Am J Obstet Gynecol* 1990;163:1574–1577.
51. Mecke H, Lehmann-Willenbrock E, Ibrahim M, Semm K. Pelviscopic treatment of ovarian cysts in premenopausal women. *Gynecol Obstet Invest* 1992;34:36–42.
52. Nezhat C, Burrell M, Nezhat F. Laparoscopic radical hysterectomy with para aortic and pelvic node dissection. *Am J Obstet Gynecol* 1992;166:864–865.
53. Mage G, Canis M, Manes H, et al. Laparoscopic management of adnexal cystic masses. *J Gynecol Surg* 1990;6:71.
54. Wenzl R, Lehner F, Husslein P, Sevelda P. Laparoscopic surgery in cases of ovarian malignancies: an Austria wide survey. *Gynecol Oncol* 1996;63:57–61.
55. Hulka JF, Parker WH, Surrey MW, Phillips JM. Management of ovarian masses: AAGL 1990 survey. *J Reprod Med* 1992;37:599–602.
56. Canis M, Pouly JL, Wattiez A, et al. Laparoscopic management of adnexal masses suspicious at ultrasound. *Obstet Gynecol* 1997;89:679–683.
57. Childers JM, Nasseri A, Surwit EA. Laparoscopic management of suspicious adnexal masses. *Am J Obstet Gynecol* 1996;175:1451–1459.
58. Dottino PR, Levine DA, Ripley DL, Cohen CJ. Laparoscopic management of adnexal masses in premenopausal and postmenopausal women. *Obstet Gynecol* 1999;93:223–228.
59. Canis M, Mage G, Pouly JL, et al. Laparoscopic diagnosis of adnexal cystic masses: a 12 year experience with long term follow up. *Obstet Gynecol* 1994;83:707–712.
60. Hidlebaugh DA, Vulgaropulos S, Orr RK. Treating adnexal masses: operative laparoscopy vs laparotomy. *J Reprod Med* 1997;42:551–558.
61. Mais V, Ajossa S, Piras B, et al. Treatment of non endometriotic benign adnexal cysts: a randomized comparison of laparoscopy and laparotomy. *Obstet Gynecol* 1995;86:770–774.
62. Pittaway DE, Takacs P, Bauguess P. Laparoscopic adnexectomy: a comparison with laparotomy. *Am J Obstet Gynecol* 1994;171:385–391.
63. Webb MJ, Decker DG, Mussey E, Williams TJ. Factors influencing survival in stage I ovarian carcinoma. *Am J Obstet Gynecol* 1973;116:222–228.
64. Dembo AJ, Davy M, Stenwig AE, et al. Prognostic factors in patients with stage I epithelial ovarian cancers. *Obstet Gynecol* 1990;75:263–273.

65. Vergote IB, Kaern J, Abeler VM, et al. Analysis of prognostic factors in stage I epithelial ovarian carcinoma: importance of degree of differentiation and deoxyribonucleic acid ploidy in predicting relapse. *Am J Obstet Gynecol* 1993;169:40–52.
66. Sevelda P, Dittrich C, Salzer H. Prognostic value of the rupture of the capsule in stage I epithelial ovarian carcinoma. *Gynecol Oncol* 1989;35:321–322.
67. Sjovall K, Nilsson B, Einhorn N. Different types of rupture of the tumor capsule and the impact on survival in early ovarian carcinoma. *Int J Gynecol Cancer* 1994;4:333–336.
68. Berek JS. Epithelial ovarian cancer. In: Berek JS, Hacker NF, eds. *Practical gynecologic oncology*, 3rd ed. Philadelphia: Lippincott Williams & Wilkins, 2000:457–522.
69. McCartney AJ, Johnson N. Using a vaginal tube to exteriorize lymph nodes during a laparoscopic pelvic lymphadenectomy. *Gynecol Oncol* 1995;57:304–306.
70. Young RC, Decker DG, Wharton JT, et al. Staging laparotomy in early ovarian cancer. *JAMA* 1983;250:3072–3076.
71. Wikborn C, Pettersson F, Moberg PJ. Delay in diagnosis of epithelial ovarian cancer. *Int J Gynecol Obstet* 1996;52:263–267.
72. Fruchter RG, Boyce J. Delays in diagnosis and stage of disease in gynecologic cancer. *Cancer Detect Prev* 1981;4:481–486.
73. Smith E, Anderson B. The effect of symptoms and delay in seeking diagnosis among women with cancers of the ovary. *Cancer* 1985;56:2727–2732.
74. Flam F, Einhorn N, Sjoval K. Symptomatology of ovarian cancer. *Eur J Obstet Gynecol Reprod Biol* 1988;27:53–57.
75. Lehner K, Wenzl R, Heinzl H, et al. Influence of delayed staging laparotomy after laparoscopic removal of ovarian masses subsequently found to be malignant. *Obstet Gynecol* 1998;92:967–971.
76. Kindermann G, Massen V, Kuhn W. Laparoscopic management of ovarian tumors subsequently found to be malignant: a survey from 127 German departments of obstetrics and gynecology. *J Pelvic Surg* 1996;2:245–251.
77. Alvarez RD, Kilgore LC, Partridge EE, et al. Staging ovarian cancer diagnosed during laparoscopy: accuracy rather than immediacy. *South Med J* 1993;86:1256–1258.
78. Canis M, Botchorishvili R, Manhes H, et al. Management of adnexal masses: role and limitations of laparoscopy. *Semin Surg Oncol* 2000;19:28–35.
79. Leminem A, Lehtovirta P. Spread of ovarian cancer after laparoscopic surgery: report of eight cases. *Gynecol Oncol* 1999;75:387–390.
80. Maiman M, Seltzer V, Boyce J. Laparoscopic excision of ovarian neoplasms subsequently found to be malignant. *Obstet Gynecol* 1991;77:563–565.
81. Crawford RA, Gore ME, Shepherd JH. Ovarian cancers related to minimal access surgery. *Br J Obstet Gynaecol* 1995;102:726–730.
82. Jacobi CA, Sabbt R, Bohm B, et al. Pneumoperitoneum with carbon dioxide stimulates growth of malignant colonic cells. *Surgery* 1997;121:72–78.
83. Volz J, Koster S, Melchert F. The effects of pneumoperitoneum on intraperitoneal tumor implantation in nude mice. *Gynaecol Endosc* 1996;5:193–196.
84. Volz J, Koster S, Spacek Z, Paweletz N. The influence of pneumoperitoneum used in laparoscopic surgery on an intra abdominal tumor growth. *Cancer* 1999;86:770–774.
85. Canis M, Botchorishvili R, Wattiez A, et al. Tumor growth and dissemination after laparotomy and CO_2 pneumoperitoneum: a rat ovarian cancer model. *Obstet Gynecol* 1998;92:104–108.
86. Allendorf JD, Bessler M, Kayton ML, et al. Increased tumor establishment and growth after laparotomy vs laparoscopy in a murine model. *Arch Surg* 1995;130:649–653.
87. Mathew G, Watson DI, Rofe AM, et al. Wound metastases following laparoscopic and open surgery for abdominal cancer in a rat model. *Br J Surg* 1996;83:1087–1090.
88. Bouvy ND, Marquet RL, Jeekel J, Bonjer HJ. Laparoscopic surgery is associated with less tumor growth stimulation than conventional surgery: an experimental study. *Br J Surg* 1997;84:358–361.
89. Volz J, Koster S, Scaeff B. Laparoscopic management of gynecologic malignancies, time to hesitate. *Gynecol Endosc* 1997;6:145–146.
90. Dottino PR, Tobias DH, Beddoe AM, et al. Laparoscopic lymphadenectomy for gynecologic malignancies. *Gynecol Oncol* 1999;73:383–388.
91. Kiu-Kwong C, Fang-Ping C, Sheuenn-Dyh C. Laparoscopic surgical procedures for early ovarian cancer. *Acta Obstet Gynecol Scand* 1995;74:391–392.
92. Childers JM, Lang J, Surwitt EA, Hatch KD. Laparoscopic surgical staging of ovarian cancer. *Gynecol Oncol* 1995; 59:25–33.
93. Pomel C, Provencher D, Dauplat J, et al. Laparoscopic staging of early ovarian cancer. *Gynecol Oncol* 1995;58:301–306.
94. Nezhat F, Nezhat C, Welander CE, Benigno B. Four ovarian cancers diagnosed during laparoscopic management of 1011 women with adnexal masses. *Am J Obstet Gynecol* 1992;167:790–796.
95. Reich H, McGlynn F, Wilkie W. Laparoscopic management of stage I ovarian cancer: a case report. *J Reprod Med* 1990;35:601–605.
96. Possover M, Krause N, Plaul K, et al. Laparoscopic para-aortic and pelvic lymphadenectomy: experience with 150 patients and review of the literature. *Gynecol Oncol* 1998;71:19–28.
97. Spirtos NM, Schlaerth JB, Spirtos TW, et al. Laparoscopic bilateral pelvic and paraaortic lymph node sampling: an evolving technique. *Am J Obstet Gynecol* 1995;173:105–111.
98. Young RC, Walton LA, Ellenberg SS, et al. Adjuvant therapy in stage I and stage II epithelial ovarian cancer: results of two prospective randomized trials. *N Engl J Med* 1990;322:1021–1027.
99. Kadar N. Laparoscopic management of gynecological malignancies. *Curr Opin Obstet Gynecol* 1997;9:247–255.
100. Magrina J. Laparoscopic surgery for gynecologic cancers. *Clin Obstet Gynecol* 2000;43:619–640.
101. Chi DS, Curtin JP. Gynecologic cancer and laparoscopy. *Obstet Gynecol Clin North Am* 1999;26:201–215.
102. Parker WH. Management of adnexal masses by operative laparoscopy: selection criteria. *J Reprod Med* 1992;37:603–606.

103. Trimbos JB, Zola P. The present role of laparoscopy in gynaecological oncology: the EORTC point of view. *Eur J Cancer* 1995;31A: 803–805.
104. Chi DS, Curtin JP, Bakarat RR. Laparoscopic management of adnexal masses in women with a history of nongynecologic malignancy. *Obstet Gynecol* 1995;86:964–968.
105. McGowan L, Lesher LP, Norris HJ, Barnett M. Misstaging of ovarian cancer *Obstet Gynecol* 1985;65:568–572.
106. Morrow CP, Curtin JP. Surgery for ovarian neoplasia. In: *Gynecologic cancer surgery*. New York: Churchill-Livingstone, 1996:627–716.
107. Chen MD, Fowler JM. Laparoscopic pelvic lymphadenectomy. *Operative Techniques in Gynecologic Surgery* 1997;2:154–162.
108. Boike GM, Graham JE. Laparoscopic omentectomy in staging and treating gynecologic cancers. *J Am Assoc Gynecol Laparosc* 1995;2:S4.
109. Childers JM, Hatch KD, Tran AI, Surwit EA. Laparoscopic para-aortic lymphadenectomy in gynecologic malignancies. *Obstet Gynecol* 1993;82:741–747.
110. Querleu D, LeBlanc E. Laparoscopic infrarenal paraaortic lymph node dissection for restaging of carcinoma of the ovary or fallopian tube. *Cancer* 1994;73:1467–1471.
111. Querleu D, LeBlanc E, Castelain B. Laparoscopic lymphadenectomy in staging of early carcinoma of the cervix. *Am J Obstet Gynecol* 1991;164:579–581.
112. Childers J, Hatch K, Surwit E. The role of laparoscopic lymphadenectomy in the management of cervical carcinoma. *Gynecol Oncol* 1992;47:38–43.
113. Fowler J, Carter J, Carlson J. Lymph node yield from laparoscopic lymphadenectomy in cervical cancer: a comparative study. *Gynecol Oncol* 1993;51:187–192.
114. Menzin AW, Rubin SC, Noumoff JS, LiVolsi VA. The accuracy of frozen section diagnosis of borderline ovarian malignancy. *Gynecol Oncol* 1995;59: 183–185.
115. Darai E, Teboul J, Fauconnier A, et al. Management and outcome of borderline tumors incidentally discovered at or after laparoscopy. *Acta Obstet Gynecol Scand* 1998;77:451–457.
116. Schwartz PE, Rutherford TJ, Chambers JT, et al. Neoadjuvant chemotherapy for advanced ovarian cancer: long term survival. *Gynecol Oncol* 1999;72:93–99.
117. Surwit E, Childers J, Atlas I, et al. Neoadjuvant chemotherapy for advanced ovarian cancer. *Int J Gynecol Cancer* 1996;6:356–361.
118. Vergote I, DeWever I, Tjalma W, et al. Neoadjuvant chemotherapy or primary debulking surgery in advanced ovarian carcinoma: a retrospective analysis of 285 patients. *Gynecol Oncol* 1998;71:431–436.
119. Nelson BE, Rosenfeld AT, Schwartz PE. Preoperative abdominopelvic computed tomographic prediction of optimal cytoreduction in epithelial ovarian cancer. *J Clin Oncol* 1993;1:166–172.
120. Sijmons EA, Heintz PM. Second look surgery: second chance or second best? *Semin Surg Oncol* 2000;19: 54–61.
121. Xygakis AM, Politis GS, Michalas SP, Kaskarelis DB. Second look laparoscopy in ovarian cancer. *J Reprod Med* 1984;29:583–585.
122. Smith WG, Day TG, Smith JP. The use of laparoscopy to determine the results of chemotherapy for ovarian cancer. *J Reprod Med* 1977;18:257–260.
123. Piver MS, Shashikant BL, Barlow JJ, Gamarra M. Second look laparoscopy prior to proposed second look laparotomy. *Obstet Gynecol* 1980;55:571–573.
124. Quinn MA, Bishop GHJ, Campbell JJ, et al. Laparoscopic follow up of patients with ovarian carcinoma. *Br J Obstet Gynaecol* 1980;87:1132–1139.
125. Mangioni C, Bolis G, Molteni P, Belloni C. Indications, advantages and limits of laparoscopy in ovarian cancer. *Gynecol Oncol* 1979;7:47–55.
126. Rosenoff SH, DeVita VT, Hubbard S, Young RC. Peritoneoscopy in the staging and follow up of ovarian cancer. *Semin Oncol* 1975;2:223–228.
127. Clough K, Ladonre J, Nos C. Second look for ovarian cancer: laparoscopy or laparotomy? A Prospective Comparative Study. *Gynecol Oncol* 1999;72:411–417.
128. Casey AC, Farias-Eisner R, Pisani AL, et al. What is the role of reassessment laparoscopy in the management of gynecologic cancers in 1995? *Gynecol Oncol* 1996;60:454–461.
129. Berek JS, Griffiths CT, Leventhal JM. Laparoscopy for second look evaluation in ovarian cancer. *Obstet Gynecol* 1981;58:192–198.
130. Abu-Rustum NR, Barakat RR, Siegel PL, et al. Second look operation for epithelial ovarian cancer: laparoscopy or laparotomy? *Obstet Gynecol* 1996;88: 549–553.
131. Gadducci A, Sartori E, Maggino T. Analysis of failures after negative second-look in patients with advanced ovarian cancer: an Italian multicenter study. *Gynecol Oncol* 1998:150–155.
132. Franchi M, Ghezzi F, Beretta P, et al. Microlaparoscopy: a new approach to the reassessment of ovarian cancer patients. *Acta Obstet Gynecol Scand* 2000;79: 427–430.
133. Van Dam PA, DeCloedt J, Tjalma WA, et al. Trocar implantation metastasis after laparoscopy in patients with advanced ovarian cancer: can the risk be reduced. *Am J Obstet Gynecol* 1999;181:536–541.
134. Kruitwagen RF, Swinkels BM, Keyser KG, et al. Incidence and effect on survival of abdominal wall metastases at trocar or puncture sites following laparoscopy or paracentesis in women with ovarian cancer. *Gynecol Oncol* 1996;60:233–237.
135. Childers JM, Aqua KA, Surwit EA, et al. Abdominal wall tumor implantation after laparoscopy for malignant conditions. *Obstet Gynecol* 1994;84:765–769.
136. Dobronte Z, Wittmann T, Karacsony G. Rapid development of malignant metastases in the abdominal wall after laparoscopy. *Endoscopy* 1978;10:127–130.
137. Stockdale AD, Pocock TJ. Abdominal wall metastasis following laparoscopy: a case report. *Eur J Surg Oncol* 1985;11:373–375.
138. Hsiu JG, Given FT, Kemp GM. Tumor implantation after diagnostic biopsy of serous ovarian tumors of low malignant potential. *Obstet Gynecol* 1986;68: 90S–93S.
139. Miralles RM, Petit J, Gine L, Balaguero L. Metastatic cancer spread at the laparoscopic puncture site: report of a case in a patient with carcinoma of the ovary. *Eur J Gynecol Oncol* 1989;6:442–444.
140. Gungor M, Cengiz B, Turan YH, Ortac C. Implantation metastasis of ovarian cancer after third look laparoscopy. *J Pakistani Med Assoc* 1996;46:111–112.

141. Childers JM, Aqua KA, Surwit EA, et al. Abdominal wall tumor implantation after laparoscopy for malignant conditions. *Obstet Gynecol* 1994;84:765–769.
142. Chu HS, Jung NW, Kim JH, et al. Tumor implantation along abdominal trocar site after pelviscopic removal of malignant ovarian tumor. *J Korean Med Sci* 1996;11:440–443.
143. Gleeson NC, Nicosia SV, Mark JE, et al. Abdominal wall metastases from ovarian cancer after laparoscopy. *Am J Obstet Gynecol* 1993;169:522–523.
144. Shepherd JH, Carter PG. Wound recurrence by implantation of borderline ovarian tumour following laparoscopic removal. *Br J Obstet Gynaecol* 1994;101:265–266.
145. Hopkins MP, Von Gruenigen V, Gaich S. Laparoscopic port site implantation withy ovarian cancer. *Am J Obstet Gynecol* 2000;182:735–736.
146. Neuhaus SJ, Texler M, Hewett PJ, Watson DI. Port site metastases following laparoscopic surgery. *Br J Surg* 1998;85:735–741.

12

Primary Surgical Management of Advanced Epithelial Ovarian Cancer

Dennis S. Chi and William J. Hoskins

The American Cancer Society estimated that approximately 23,000 American women would be diagnosed with ovarian cancer in 2000, and more than 14,000 would die of the disease (1). Although modern therapy of ovarian cancer results in high cure rates for patients with early-stage disease, the majority of women are diagnosed when the cancer has progressed to an advanced stage and long-term survival rates are poor. Table 12.1 outlines the International Federation of Gynecology and Obstetrics (FIGO) staging classification for ovarian cancer (2). Table 12.2 summarizes the most recent report by FIGO regarding stage distribution and 5-year survival by stage for 2,854 patients with ovarian cancer (3). As can be seen from Table 12.2, more than 60% of patients were diagnosed with advanced stage III or IV disease, for which 5-year survival rates varied from 11% to 41% (3). Although the treatment of ovarian cancer generally requires a multimodality approach, surgery remains the cornerstone of therapy. The role that surgery plays in the treatment of ovarian cancer ranges from the establishment of diagnosis at initial laparotomy to the palliation of intestinal obstruction in cases of persistent disease. Table 12.3 outlines the many uses of surgery in the management of patients with advanced ovarian cancer.

The primary surgical management of ovarian carcinoma is essential to both diagnosis and treatment. In cases of apparently early-stage disease, proper surgical management involves comprehensive surgical staging based on the known patterns of spread, as described elsewhere in this book. Patients who present with advanced-stage disease frequently require aggressive surgical cytoreduction. The rationale and technique of primary cytoreductive surgery is the primary focus of this chapter.

DIAGNOSIS AND STAGING

The diagnosis of advanced ovarian cancer is rarely difficult. Unlike patients with early-stage disease, in whom the differential diagnosis of the adnexal mass must be considered, those who present with advanced-stage disease usually have symptoms, physical signs, or diagnostic study results demonstrating disease spread. The typical patient may complain of abdominal pain, increased abdominal girth, and/or disturbances of bowel or urinary tract function. Physical signs consist of palpable pelvic or pelvic/abdominal masses and ascites, which can usually be demonstrated by diagnostic studies such as ultrasound or computed tomography (CT) scans. Barium enema, when available, may demonstrate extrinsic compression of the large intestine. Invasion into the colonic lumen is infrequent. Chest radiographs often reveal pleural effusions.

The diagnostic or preoperative workup of patients with possible ovarian cancer focuses on proper preparation for surgery and the elimination of other primary cancers from the differential diagnosis. A diagnostic paracentesis or thoracentesis is rarely indicated. If pleural fluid collections are of sufficient quantity to cause significant impairment of pulmonary function, preoperative insertion of a chest tube should be considered. A pelvic and abdominal CT scan often provides useful information by ruling out pancreatic cancer, allowing evaluation of the liver and spleen, and providing evaluation of the urinary tract. A barium enema and colonoscopy can be used to

TABLE 12.1. *International federation of gynecology and obstetrics (FIGO) staging system for ovarian cancer*

Stage	Characteristics
I	Growth limited to the ovaries.
A	Growth limited to one ovary; no ascites; no tumor on the external surface; capsule intact.
B	Growth limited to both ovaries; no ascites; no tumor on the external surfaces; capsule intact.
C	Tumor either stage IA or IB, but with tumor on the surface of one or both ovaries; or with capsule ruptured; or with malignant cells in ascites or peritoneal washings.
II	Growth involving one or both ovaries with pelvic extension.
A	Extension and/or metastases to the uterus and/or tubes.
B	Extension to other pelvic tissues.
C	Tumor either stage IIA or IIB, but with tumor on the surface of one or both ovaries; or with capsule ruptured; or with malignant cells in ascites or peritoneal washings.
III	Tumor involving one or both ovaries with peritoneal implants outside the pelvis and/or positive retroperitoneal or inguinal lymp nodes. Superficial liver metastasis equals stage III. Tumor is limited to the true pelvis but with histologically verified malignant extension to small bowel or omentum.
A	Tumor grossly limited to the true pelvis but with histologically confirmed microscopic seeding of abdominal peritoneal surfaces.
B	Tumor involving one or both ovaries with histologically confirmed implants of abdominal peritoneal surfaces, none exceeding 2 cm in diameter. Nodes are negative.
C	Abdominal implants greater than 2 cm in diameter and/or positive retroperitoneal or inguinal nodes.
IV	Growth involving one or both ovaries with distant metastases. If pleural effusion is present, there must be positive cytology to allot a case to stage IV. Parenchymal liver metastasis equals stage IV.

From FIGO Cancer Committee. Staging announcement. *Gynecol Oncol* 1986;25:383–385, with permission.

rule out primary colon cancer and significant obstructive lesions of the colon. A chest radiograph and mammography are also advisable to rule out pulmonary disease and primary breast cancer, respectively. An intravenous pyelogram or cystoscopy is usually of little benefit unless symptoms indicate bladder involvement. A magnetic resonance imaging (MRI) study rarely provides additional useful information if a CT scan has already been performed.

In early ovarian cancer, comprehensive surgical staging is essential. In advanced disease, staging is usually obvious. Abdominal exploration frequently reveals gross evidence of widely metastatic ovarian cancer, and multiple biopsies to document occult disease are seldom necessary. In these cases, the aim of the procedure changes from establishing comprehensive surgical staging to attempting maximal tumor cytoreduction.

RATIONALE FOR PRIMARY SURGICAL CYTOREDUCTION

Frequently, at exploratory surgery, patients with advanced ovarian carcinoma are found to have large tumor masses in the abdomen and pelvis. Complete resection of all grossly visible tumor is

TABLE 12.2. *FIGO stage distribution and five-year survival rates*

Stage	No. patients	Percent of total	Five-year survival (%)
IA	342	12	87
IB	49	2	71
IC	352	12	79
IIA	64	2	67
IIB	92	3	55
IIC	136	5	57
IIIA	129	4	41
IIIB	137	5	25
IIIC	1,193	42	23
IV	360	13	11
Total	2,854	100	42

From Pecorelli S, Odicino F, Maisonnenve P, et al., Carcinoma of the ovary. In: Pecorelli S, Creasman WT, Pettersson F, et al., eds. *FIGO annual report on the results of treatment in gynaecological cancer, vol 23.* Oxford: Isis Medical Media Limited, 1998:75–102, with permission.

TABLE 12.3. *Roles of surgery in the management of advanced ovarian cancer*

Diagnosis
Staging
Primary cytoreduction
Surgical reassessment
Central venous access
Intraperitoneal access
Interval cytoreduction
Secondary cytoreduction
Palliation

usually impossible, and such patients cannot be cured by surgery alone. Primary surgical cytoreduction refers to the removal of as much tumor as possible at the initial operative procedure. For most human solid tumors, aggressive surgical resection is justified only if all visible tumor can be removed, rendering the operation potentially curative. For epithelial ovarian cancer, however, both theoretical and clinical benefits have been demonstrated for primary cytoreductive, or debulking, surgery even when all known tumor cannot be resected.

Theoretical Benefits of Primary Surgical Cytoreduction

The theoretical basis for cytoreductive surgery is derived from concepts about cancer growth kinetics. These concepts also provide insight into the mechanisms by which chemotherapy eradicates tumors. Successful therapy for ovarian cancer generally requires a combination of surgery and chemotherapy; therefore, growth kinetics must be considered in relation to both of these modalities.

Cells in any living tissue, including human cancers, are often categorized into either the growth fraction or the nonproliferating fraction based on their rate of growth. Tissues that constantly divide to replenish themselves have active growth fractions and are referred to as renewal tissues (e.g., hair, bone marrow, gastrointestinal mucosa). Tissues that are not constantly dividing and do not have active growth fractions are termed nonrenewal tissues (e.g., muscles, nerves). These terms are relative; the renewal tissues are not composed entirely of cells in the active growth fraction, and the nonrenewal tissues do have some portion of their cells in a growth fraction. Cancers behave like renewal tissues, with active growth fractions; however, as with other renewal tissues, only a portion of the cancer cells are in an active growth phase. The significant difference between cancers and renewal tissues is the lack of control exhibited by cancers. Cancers continue to grow without regulation and eventually kill their host through disruption of normal body functions. Cycling cells (Figure 12.1) (4) are in equilibrium with cells in the nonproliferating pool. Some cells are lost from each pool by cell death and are replaced by cells from the growth fraction. Cells that are in the G_1 (or G_0) phase of the cell cycle are said to be in the "resting phase." These cells are probably the source of nonproliferating cells. In some conditions, these nonproliferating cells can be recruited back into the cell cycle. This may be related to an improvement in cellular nutrition (4).

Within the cell cycle, the active phase consists of the S (synthesis) phase, the G_2 (premitotic) phase, and the M (mitotic) phase. Many chemotherapeutic agents are cell cycle–specific and act only during one of these phases. Other agents are non–cell cycle–specific and act during all phases of the cycle, including the resting phase. In general, cells that are actively dividing

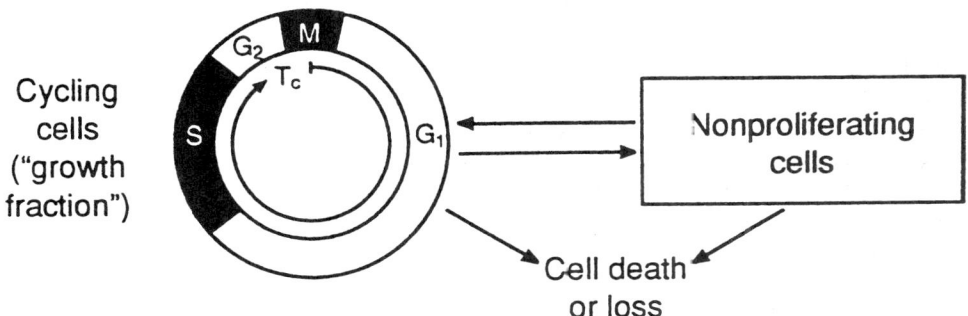

FIG. 12.1. Model of a tumor cell population. (From Tannock IF. Principles of cell proliferation: cell kinetics. In: DeVita VT, Hellman S, Rosenberg SA, eds. *Cancer: principles and practice of oncology.* Philadelphia: JB Lippincott, 1989:2–5, with permission.)

are more sensitive to chemotherapy than cells that are not actively dividing.

Initial tumor models suggested that cancers have exponential growth rates, which means that their growth follows a straight line when plotted on a logarithmic scale against time (4). The smallest tumor that can be detected is usually about 1 cm (1 g). This mass comprises 10^8 to 10^9 tumor cells and usually represents about 30 doublings of the tumor. If a tumor this small continued to grow, it would reach 1 kg in another 10 doublings. A tumor size of 1 kg is considered to be potentially lethal.

Studies have shown, however, that the actual growth of human solid tumors does not follow the ideal just described, but rather is marked by an increase in cancer doubling time as the tumor increases in size. This increase in doubling time results in a flattening of the growth curve that has been termed the "Gompertzian phenomenon" and is demonstrated mathematically by the Gompertz equation (4). The simulated growth curve of solid tumors is referred to as a Gompertzian growth curve and is shown in Figure 12.2 (4). One theoretical explanation for the flattening of the growth curve holds that tumors tend to outgrow their nutrients, with a resulting increase in doubling time. It has also been postulated that a high percentage of the cells in these large tumors are in a resting, or nondividing, phase of the cell cycle.

This information about the growth of human tumors provides the theoretical basis for cytoreductive surgery. These principles were summarized by Griffiths (5) and are listed in Table 12.4. The direct effect of cytoreduction involves improvement in the patient's nutritional status and overall sense of well-being. At the time of diagnosis, many patients with advanced ovarian cancer have a significant tumor burden, with involvement of the intestinal tract surfaces. Although the cancer usually does not invade deeply into the viscera, surface spread may involve much of the gastrointestinal tract, with devastating effects on bowel function. Consequently, these patients can have significant metabolic deficiencies (6). In such cases, the removal of large tumor masses can result in immediate improvement in gastrointestinal function and metabolic abnor-

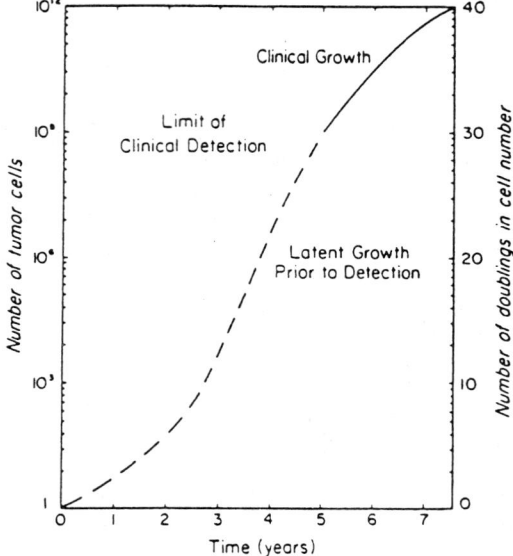

FIG. 12.2. Hypothetical growth curve for a human tumor. Note that the tumor grows for 5 years before attaining a size of approximately 1 g (approximately 10^9 cells), when it can first be clinically detected. Thereafter, despite some slowing of growth, it attains a lethal mass of approximately 1 kg (approximately 10^{12} cells) in a further 2.5 years. (From Tannock IF. Principles of cell proliferation: cell kinetics. In: DeVita VT, Hellman S, Rosenberg SA, eds. *Cancer: principles and practice of oncology.* Philadelphia: JB Lippincott, 1989:2–5, with permission.)

malities. Although these direct effects are unlikely to be of very significant benefit unless partial gastrointestinal or urinary obstruction were impairing nutrition or renal function, debulking surgery does appear to measurably improve the quality of life in these patients (7).

The concept of first-order kinetics states that removal of large tumor masses results in an exponential decrease in cancer cells, leaving fewer tumor cells to be eradicated by chemotherapy. Although the importance of this concept has been proposed by many authors, its significance probably exists only for patients with disease cytoreduced to microscopic size. Surgical reduction of tumor from 1 kg to 1 g represents a decrease in the total number of cancer cells from 10^{12} to 10^9 (a three-log decrease). This amount of cytoreduction is rarely attained. Even if it were, however,

TABLE 12.4. *Theoretical basis for cytoreductive surgery in epithelial ovarian cancer*

I. Direct effect
  A. Improved sense of well-being
  B. Improvement in metabolism
    1. Improved gastrointestinal function
    2. Removal of large necrotic tumor
II. First-order kinetics
    1. Removal of large volume of tumor results in an exponential reduction of tumor cells so that fewer cell kills are required to eradicate the tumor
    2. Fewer total number of cells results in less opportunity for the development of drug resistance
III. Excision of large tumor masses results in improved sensitivity to chemotherapy
    1. Removal of tumor with a poor blood supply
    2. Migration of increased numbers of cells into the active growth phase of the cell cycle with increased sensitivity to chemotherapy
    3. Residual small-volume tumor nodules are more likely to respond to chemotherapy

Modified from Griffiths CT. Surgery at the time of diagnosis in ovarian cancer. In: Blackledge G, Chanu KK, eds. *Management of ovarian cancer.* London: Butterworth, 1986:60, with permission.

considering tumor regrowth that occurs between chemotherapy cycles, an additional seven three-log kills would be required to eradicate the last cancer cell (5).

According to the mathematical model of Goldie and Coldman (8), the development of chemotherapy resistance is a function of the spontaneous mutation rate of tumor cells toward drug-resistant phenotypes. As tumor size and cell number increase, the probability of mutations and drug-resistant clones also increases. Therefore, primary cytoreductive surgery may remove existing resistant tumor clones while decreasing the spontaneous development of new resistant phenotypes (9).

The most important theoretical effect of primary cytoreductive surgery is thought to be the impact that the removal of large tumor masses has on the sensitivity to chemotherapy of the residual tumor nodules. Because most ovarian tumors are sensitive to a large number of chemotherapeutic agents, this effect is quite important. The resection of large bulky masses removes the portion of tumor with poor blood supply that would otherwise receive inadequate doses of chemotherapy. Furthermore, the Gompertzian model suggests that cytoreduction causes a high percentage of resting tumor cells to migrate into the pool of actively dividing cells, with a consequent increase in chemotherapy sensitivity. Small tumor implants (between 0.1 and 0.5 cm) have virtually 100% of their cells in the dividing pool (5).

Clinical Benefits of Primary Surgical Cytoreduction

All of the studies that support the clinical benefits of primary cytoreductive surgery are based on indirect analyses. To date, no prospective trial has ever been completed in which patients were randomly assigned to aggressive surgical cytoreduction versus less aggressive surgery. The Gynecologic Oncology Group (GOG) attempted such a trial but was unable to accrue enough patients reflecting the very strong indirect evidence for the benefits of cytoreductive surgery.

In 1968, Munnell (10) introduced the concept of "maximal surgical effort" for patients with ovarian cancer. He reported improved survival in patients who underwent "definitive surgery" compared with those who had "partial removal" or "biopsy only." Similar results were reported by Declos and Quinlan (11), who noted a 25% 4-year survival rate for patients with stage III ovarian cancer who had surgical cytoreduction to "nonpalpable" tumor, compared with 9% for those left with "palpable" residual tumor.

It was not until 1975, however, that residual tumor after primary cytoreduction was accurately quantified and correlated with survival. Griffiths (12) reported on 102 patients with stage II or III ovarian cancer who received single-agent melphalan after primary surgical cytoreduction. The patients were divided into four groups based on the diameter of the largest tumor nodule remaining after surgery. Median survival was 39 months for those patients with no gross residual tumor; 29 months for those with gross residual tumor less than 0.5 cm; 18 months for patients with 0.6 to 1.5 cm residual; and 11 months for those patients whose residual disease measured larger than 1.5 cm.

Other prognostic factors that have been studied are the total volume of residual disease and the number of residual lesions. In 1986,

Redman and associates (13) compared the effects according to total volume of residual disease (estimated in cubic centimeters) versus the volume of the largest residual mass (also estimated in cubic centimeters). Using the endpoints of overall median response rate to chemotherapy and median survival, they found essentially no difference between the volume of the single largest residual mass and the total residual tumor volume.

Gall and coworkers (14), in a GOG study of patients with less than 3 cm of residual disease, found improved survival in patients with one lesion compared with those who had more than one lesion. In a subsequent GOG report, Hoskins and colleagues (15) found a significant difference in progression-free interval and survival based on the number of residual lesions in 349 patients with stage III ovarian cancer cytoreduced to residual cancer of 1 cm or less. They found an increase in relative risk for patients with more than 20 residual lesions.

It appears that other factors, in addition to diameter of the largest residual mass, may influence prognosis. Nonetheless, since Griffith's seminal report, most authors have used the diameter of the maximal residual tumor nodule as the indicator of residual disease when reporting on the effects of cytoreductive surgery. Furthermore, although it may not be the only important factor, numerous studies in the literature have demonstrated that the diameter of residual disease strongly correlates with prognosis.

Most reports divide patients into "optimal" and "suboptimal" groups based on the residual disease diameter. Various cutoff points between 0.5 and 3.0 cm have been used for this division. The measurement of outcome has also varied, with some authors measuring response to chemotherapy, others measuring likelihood of achieving a negative second-look surgical assessment, and still others measuring rates of survival. The overall analysis of the results of primary cytoreductive surgery is, however, quite invariable. In all parameters, a clear prognostic benefit can be seen for patients who undergo "optimal" primary cytoreductive surgery compared with those who are "suboptimally" cytoreduced.

In 1978, Young and coauthors (16) reported the first randomized trial of multiagent nonplatinum-based chemotherapy versus single-agent alkylating therapy for advanced ovarian cancer. Patients with "optimal residual disease" had a significantly higher overall response rate than patients left with extensive residual disease (84% versus 53%, respectively). Table 12.5 lists several articles that have reported response rates to chemotherapy in relation to residual disease after primary cytoreductive surgery for advanced ovarian cancer (16–20). Consistent with the aforementioned theoretical benefits of cytoreduction, patients with less residual disease had a higher complete response rate and an improved overall response rate to postoperative chemotherapy, compared with those with more bulky residual tumor.

TABLE 12.5. *Effects of residual disease after primary cytoreductive surgery on response rate in advanced ovarian cancer*

Source (ref. no.)	Chemotherapy regimen	No. patients	Residual (cm)	Response (%) Complete	Total
Young et al., 1978 (16)	HexaCAF vs. L-PAM	19	<2	—	84
		58	>2	—	53
Ehrlich et al., 1979 (17)	PAC	14	<3	46	78
		25	>3	32	54
Wharton and Herson, 1981 (18)	L-PAM	45	<2	12	29
		59	>2	8	24
Conte et al., 1986 (19)	CAP vs. CP	37	<2	70	76
		38	>2	32	82
Total/Mean		115	Optimal	42.7	66.8
		180	Suboptimal	24.0	53.3

From Hoskins WJ: Primary cytoreduction. In: Markman M, Hoskins WJ, eds. *Cancer of the ovary.* New York: Raven Press, 1993:163–173, with permission.

TABLE 12.6. *Findings at second-look laparotomy by extent of residual disease after primary cytoreduction*

Residual[a]	Total patients	No. negative	Percent negative
None	460	331	72
Optimal	655	330	50
Suboptimal	682	158	23

[a] According to author's definition.
Modified from Barter JF, Barnes WA. Second-look laparotomy. In: Rubin SC, Sutton GP, eds. *Ovarian cancer.* New York: McGraw-Hill, 1993:269–300, with permission.

The most accurate method of evaluating the success of postoperative chemotherapy for patients with advanced ovarian cancer is the second-look surgical reassessment. The information it yields also provides a reliable prediction of survival. The amount of residual disease remaining after the initial surgical procedure for ovarian cancer has consistently proven to be a major determinant of the likelihood of disease being discovered at the time of the second-look procedure. Table 12.6 summarizes pooled data on 1,797 patients from 25 series, providing information on the relation of the extent of residual disease after primary surgery to the findings at second look (21). As can be seen from this review, a direct relation exists between the amount of residual disease at the conclusion of primary cytoreduction and the likelihood of a negative second-look surgical reassessment. These data are not corrected for stage and tumor grade, and therefore the "no residual" group includes patients with early-stage disease. Even considering this bias, however, there seems to be a strong correlation between extent of residual disease at primary surgery and the probability of discovering disease at second-look surgical assessment.

The ultimate test of any prognostic factor or therapy is its effect on survival. Before the routine use of postoperative platinum-based chemotherapy, two of the largest series that evaluated overall survival in relation to cytoreductive surgery were reported by Smith and Day (22) from the M.D. Anderson Cancer Center in Texas and Malkasian and colleagues (23) from the Mayo Clinic in Minnesota. In 1979, Smith and Day (22) reviewed the records of 2,115 patients with ovarian cancer treated during the 30-year period between 1944 and 1973. The 614 patients with stage III epithelial ovarian cancer were treated postoperatively with a variety of regimens including irradiation and chemotherapy with melphalan. Five-year survival rates based on residual tumor size were reported as follows: no residual tumor, 63%; 0 to 1 cm residual tumor, 41%; 1 to 2 cm, 15%; 3 to 6 cm, 8%; 7 to 9 cm, 0%; 10 cm or greater, 3%.

In 1984, Malkasian and colleagues (23) reported on the overall survival of 1,938 women with epithelial ovarian cancer who received their primary treatment at the Mayo Clinic in Minnesota. From 1950 to 1979, 730 patients with stage III disease were treated with a variety of postoperative regimens, as in the M.D. Anderson series. With 2 cm as the cutoff point for optimal versus suboptimal residual disease status, the estimated 5-year survival rates were 30% and 8%, respectively.

Two more recent GOG studies, reported by Hoskins and associates (15,24), have further clarified the role of primary cytoreductive surgery in patients with advanced ovarian cancer. In the first study the survival of patients with stage III disease who were found at surgery to have abdominal disease of 1 cm or less was compared with survival of those who had abdominal disease larger than 1 cm that was surgically cytoreduced to 1 cm or less (15). If surgery were the only important factor, then the survival rate should have been the same in the two groups. However, patients found to have small-volume disease survived longer than patients who were cytoreduced to small-volume disease. Further analysis showed that the age of the patient, the grade of the tumor, and the number of residual tumor nodules were independent prognostic factors. Although this study in no way showed a lack of effectiveness of primary cytoreductive surgery, it did show that other factors, including the biology of the tumor, are also important.

The second study demonstrated that surgical cytoreduction to 2 cm or less residual disease resulted in a significant survival benefit, but all residual diameters greater than 2 cm resulted in equivalent survival rates (Figure 12.3) (24). Unless the tumor could be cytoreduced to

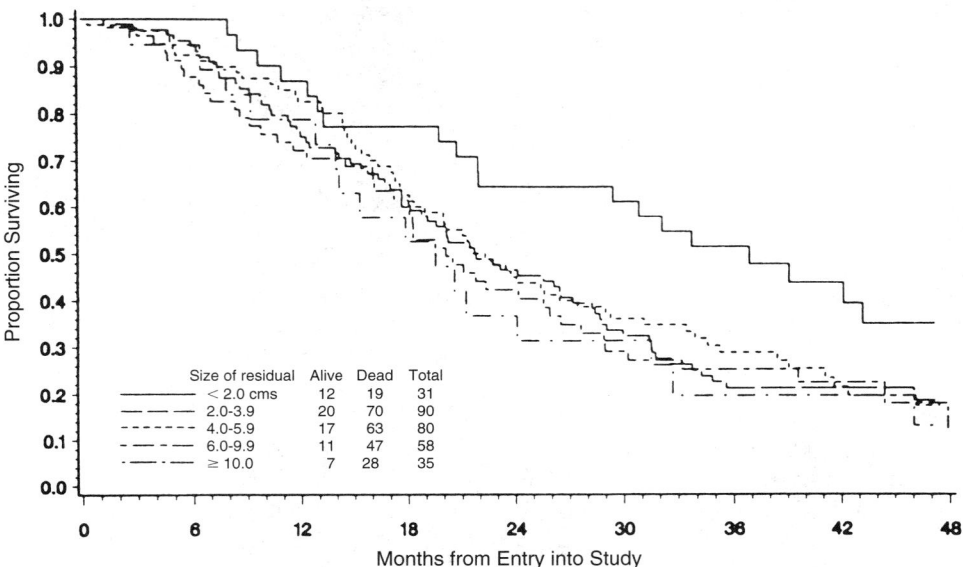

FIG. 12.3. Survival by maximum diameter of residual disease. (From Hoskins WJ, McGuire WP, Brady MF, et al. The effect of diameter of largest residual disease on survival after primary cytoreductive surgery in patients with suboptimal residual epithelial ovarian carcinoma: a Gynecologic Oncology Group study. *Am J Obstet Gynecol* 1994;170:974–980, with permission.)

a maximum residual tumor diameter of 2 cm or less, aggressive surgical cytoreduction did not affect survival.

Figure 12.4 is a composite graph of the survival curves for the two GOG studies reported by Hoskins and associates (24). Three distinct groups appear to emerge: (a) those with no grossly visible residual disease; (b) those with optimal residual disease (<2 cm); and (c) those with suboptimal disease (>2 cm in diameter). The 4-year survival rates were reported to be 60%, 35%, and less than 20%, respectively (24).

The results of the two GOG studies, along with other reports in the literature, were presented in 1994 at the National Institutes of Health (NIH) Consensus Development Conference on Ovarian Cancer. The consensus statement on the issue of the appropriate management of advanced epithelial ovarian cancer was that "aggressive efforts at maximal cytoreduction are important since minimal residual tumor is associated with improved survival" (25).

Although there is general consensus that optimal versus suboptimal surgical cytoreduction improves the prognosis for patients with advanced epithelial ovarian cancer, the most appropriate cutoff point remains somewhat controversial. In the 1970s, the most common definition of suboptimal disease was any residual disease measuring greater than 2 cm. In the early 1980s, the GOG defined suboptimal disease as any nodule 3 cm or greater in maximal diameter (26). Since 1986, however, despite the aforementioned GOG data published by Hoskins, the GOG has defined suboptimal disease as that measuring greater than 1 cm (24,27).

In the 1994 GOG study reported by Hoskins and associates (24), there were only 31 patients with residual disease measuring between 1 to 2 cm, which may account for their reluctance to change the definition of optimal cytoreduction from disease measuring 1 cm or less to that measuring 2 cm or less. In a recent analysis performed by Chi and coworkers (28) at the Memorial Sloan-Kettering Cancer Center (MSKCC), the 5-year survival rate for the 73 patients with advanced ovarian cancer cytoreduced to between 1 and 2 cm residual disease was not significantly different from that for patients with greater than 2 cm residual (28% versus 21%, respectively);

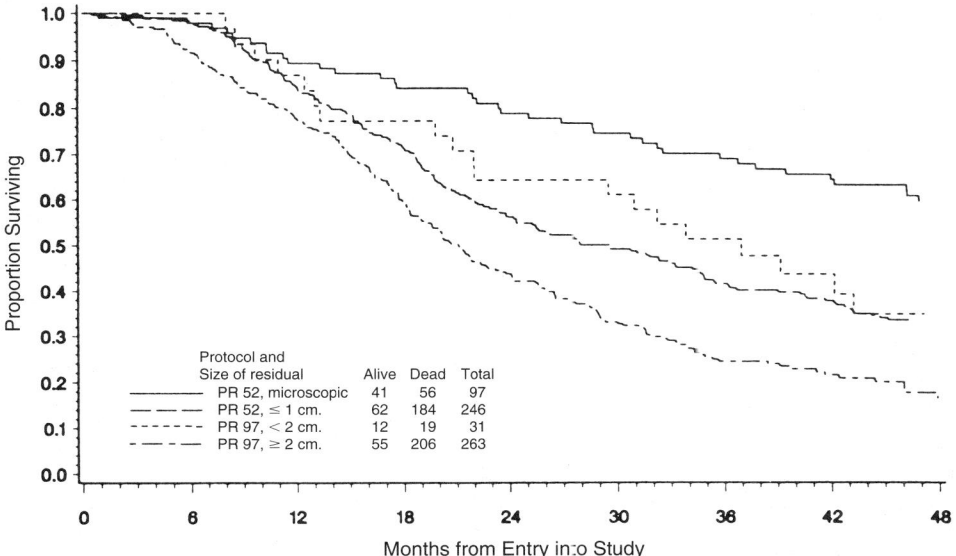

FIG. 12.4. Survival by residual disease, Gynecologic Oncology Group Protocols (PR) 52 and 97. (From Hoskins WJ, McGuire WP, Brady MF, et al. The effect of diameter of largest residual disease on survival after primary cytoreductive surgery in patients with suboptimal residual epithelial ovarian carcinoma: a Gynecologic Oncology Group study. *Am J Obstet Gynecol* 1994;170:974–980, with permission.)

however, both were significantly lower than the rate (50%) for patients whose residual disease was cytoreduced to 1 cm or less. These data appear to support the GOG's current definition of optimal cytoreduction. Table 12.7 demonstrates the survival data from the MSKCC study and summarizes the other recent large studies which have evaluated the effects of residual disease on survival for patients with stage III epithelial ovarian cancer treated with postoperative platinum-based chemotherapy (24,28–31). The data from Table 12.7 are remarkably consistent. For patients who undergo optimally debulking and treatment with platinum-based chemotherapy, the average median survival time is 55 months and the 5-year survival rate is approximately 50%. For patients with suboptimal disease, median survival decreases to 25 months, with the 5-year survival rate ranging from 15% to 29%.

Although the role of aggressive surgical cytoreduction in patients with stage III ovarian carcinoma appears to be well defined, its benefit in stage IV disease is less clear. Most of the studies supporting cytoreductive surgery have evaluated stage III patients alone or have analyzed stage III and stage IV patients collectively. Because patients with stage IV ovarian carcinoma have, by definition, extraperitoneal and/or intrahepatic metastases, some have questioned the benefit of intraperitoneal surgical cytoreduction in these cases (32,33). In a series of 35 women with stage IV ovarian cancer, Goodman and colleagues (34) found no significant survival benefit attributable to optimal versus suboptimal surgical cytoreduction.

In a more recent review, Curtin and colleagues (35) reported the survival data for 92 patients with stage IV ovarian carcinoma. All patients received platinum-based chemotherapy postoperatively. The median survival time was 40 months for the 41 patients who underwent optimal surgical cytoreduction (defined as maximal residual disease measuring 2 cm or less) and 18 months for the 51 patients who had suboptimal debulking. Other subsequent reports have confirmed the significant survival benefit associated with optimal surgical cytoreduction followed by platinum-based chemotherapy in patients with stage IV ovarian cancer; their results

TABLE 12.7. *Survival in stage III ovarian cancer by residual disease after primary cytoreductive surgery and postoperative platinum-based chemotherapy*

Source (ref. no.)	Residual (cm)	No. patients	Median survival (mo)	Five-year survival (%)
Neijt et al., 1987 (29)[a]	<1	62	40	—
	>1	129	21	—
Hoskins et al., 1994 (24)	0	97	—	60[b]
	<1	246	—	35[b]
	1–2	31	—	35[b]
	>2	263	—	<20[b]
Le et al., 1997 (30)	0	51	—	45
	Any	279	—	15
Eisenkop et al., 1998 (31)[c]	0	139	62	52
	Any	24	20	29
Chi et al., 2001 (28)	<1	56	56	50
	1–2	73	31	28
	>2	87	28	21
Total/Mean/Range	Optimal[d]	682	55	45–52[e]
	Suboptimal[d]	855	25	15–29[e]

[a] Includes 54 patients with stage IIB and IV disease.
[b] Four-year survival rates.
[c] Includes 27 patients with stage IV disease.
[d] According to authors' definition.
[e] Does not include 4-year survival data from study by Hoskins et al.

are summarized in Table 12.8 (34–38). Of the studies shown in Table 12.8, the series by Bristow and colleagues (38) was the only one to define suboptimal residual disease as that measuring greater than 1 cm and to separately analyze the effect of cytoreduction in patients with liver metastases. Their report of 84 patients included 37 with liver metastases. Six of these 37 patients underwent optimal resection of both extrahepatic and hepatic disease, and they had a median survival time of 50 months. Eleven patients had optimal extrahepatic cytoreduction but suboptimal residual hepatic tumor, and their median survival time was 27 months. Twenty patients were left with both suboptimal residual extrahepatic and hepatic disease, and they had a median survival time of 8 months. The authors concluded that even in patients with unresectable liver metastasis, optimal debulking of extrahepatic disease is associated with a significant survival advantage. This conclusion needs confirmation.

TABLE 12.8. *Median survival in stage IV ovarian cancer by residual disease after primary cytoreductive surgery and postoperative platinum-based chemotherapy*

Source (ref. no.)	Residual (cm)	No. patients	Median survival (mo)
Goodman et al., 1992 (34)	<2	23	28
	>2	12	22
Curtin et al., 1997 (35)	<2	41	40
	>2	51	18
Liu et al., 1997 (36)	<2	14	37
	>2	33	17
Munkarah et al., 1997 (37)	<2	31	25
	>2	61	15
Bristow et al., 1999 (38)	<1	25	38
	>1	69	10
Total/Mean	Optimal[a]	134	34
	Suboptimal[a]	226	15

[a] According to authors' definition.

TABLE 12.9. *Aggressive surgical procedures that may be considered to attain optimal tumor cytoreduction*

Multiple or extensive bowel resection
Rectosigmoid resection
Resection of ureteral/bladder segment
Extensive pelvic/aortic node dissection
Diaphragm stripping/resection
Splenectomy
Nephrectomy
Partial hepatectomy

Modified from Morrow CP, Curtin JP. Surgery for ovarian neoplasia. In: Morrow CP, Curtin JP, eds. *Gynecologic cancer surgery*. New York: Churchill Livingstone, 1996:627–716, with permission.

Overall, these recent series support the NIH consensus statement regarding the importance of aggressive surgical cytoreduction for advanced ovarian carcinoma, even in cases where the preoperative findings are compatible with stage IV disease. Table 12.9 lists aggressive surgical procedures that would be considered to remove metastatic disease in patients with advanced ovarian carcinoma, should such procedures help achieve optimal cytoreduction (39).

INTERVAL CYTOREDUCTION

The actual percentage of patients with advanced ovarian cancer whose disease can successfully be cytoreduced to optimal residual status at the initial surgical procedure ranges in the literature from 17% to 99%, with a mean of approximately 35% (31,40). However, most authorities believe that in major medical centers staffed with gynecologic oncologists the percentage of optimal cytoreduction is probably closer to 50%, which still leaves a substantial number of patients with advanced ovarian cancer suboptimally cytoreduced (41).

Because patients with suboptimal residual disease carry such a poor prognosis, further management in these cases is especially challenging. Some investigators have evaluated the benefit of a brief course of chemotherapy followed by a second attempt at "interval" cytoreduction before completion of a prescribed chemotherapy regimen (42–44). In 1984, Neijt and associates (42) reported that the survival of a small group of patients who were initially suboptimally cytoreduced was improved to a degree approaching that in optimally debulked patients when a second "intervention" debulking surgery was incorporated into the treatment program. Lawton and coworkers (43) subsequently attempted interval cytoreduction in 28 patients after three cycles of platinum-based chemotherapy and were successful in 21 patients in debulking to residual disease of less than 1 cm. Ng and colleagues (44) described 38 patients who underwent interval cytoreduction after two intense courses of platinum-based chemotherapy and reported that in 30 of these patients cytoreduction to less than 1 cm of residual disease was achieved. Therefore, it appears that interval cytoreduction can be quite successful in allowing patients a second opportunity for optimal cytoreduction.

These preliminary results led to the design of a randomized study of interval cytoreductive surgery by the European Organization for Research on Treatment of Cancer (EORTC). In the EORTC trial (45), patients with suboptimally cytoreduced advanced ovarian cancer (defined as residual disease of more than 1 cm) were given three cycles of cyclophosphamide and cisplatin chemotherapy. Patients without disease progression were then randomly assigned to undergo either interval debulking surgery or no surgery, with both arms subsequently receiving three more cycles of the same chemotherapy. Patients who underwent interval cytoreduction demonstrated a significant improvement in both progression-free survival (18 versus 13 months) and overall survival (26 versus 20 months) (Figures 12.5 and 12.6).

Based on the results of the EORTC trial, the GOG is currently performing another prospective, randomized trial to evaluate the benefit of interval cytoreduction. The schema of GOG Protocol 152 is similar to that of the EORTC trial except that patients will receive paclitaxel and cisplatin instead of cyclophosphamide and cisplatin. Although the benefits of aggressive primary surgical cytoreduction for advanced ovarian cancer are well accepted, the role of interval cytoreduction has yet to be established. Until the results of confirmatory studies such as GOG Protocol 152 become available, interval

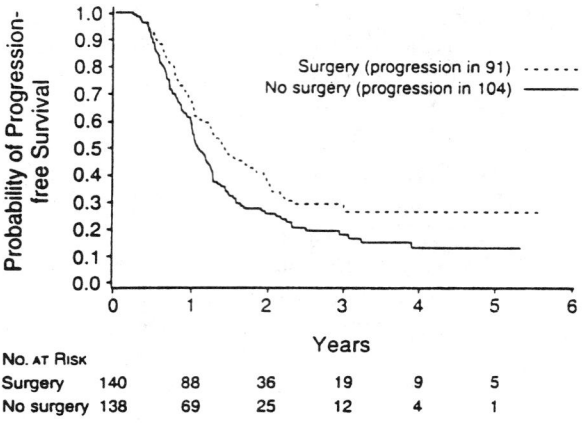

FIG. 12.5. Progression-free survival of patients with advanced epithelial ovarian cancer according to whether they underwent debulking surgery ($p = .013$ for the comparison between the groups by log-rank test). (From van der Burg MEL, van Lent M, Buyse M, et al. The effect of debulking surgery after induction chemotherapy on the prognosis in advanced epithelial ovarian cancer. N Engl J Med 1995;332:629–634, with permission.)

cytoreduction should be attempted only in a clinical trial setting.

TECHNIQUE OF CYTOREDUCTION

Few operations performed by the gynecologic surgeon are as demanding as the primary operation for ovarian cancer. Because of the intraabdominal spread patterns of the disease, the entire abdomen may be involved. The tumor tends to implant itself on any mesothelial surface, including abdominal gutters, pelvic peritoneum, surfaces of the intestine, and diaphragms. Pelvic disease can be especially difficult to remove because of the loss of normal surgical tissue planes. Fortunately, ovarian cancer often remains on the surface of organs, and full-thickness penetration of the intestine and urinary tract structures occurs late, if at all.

The approach to the pelvis should be via the retroperitoneum, with incisions that begin lateral to the infundibulopelvic ligament and, if necessary, lateral to the colon (Figure 12.7) (46). Using this approach, the surgeon can gain control of the infundibulopelvic ligament and uterine artery and can identify and preserve the iliac vessels, ureter, and obturator nerve (Figure 12.8) (46). With vital structures identified and protected, and with the blood supply under control, the surgeon proceeds by sweeping the tumor and pelvic viscera medially. If the anterior cul-de-sac is involved by tumor, it can be removed by stripping the peritoneum from the bladder muscularis. Opening the bladder to facilitate dissection and

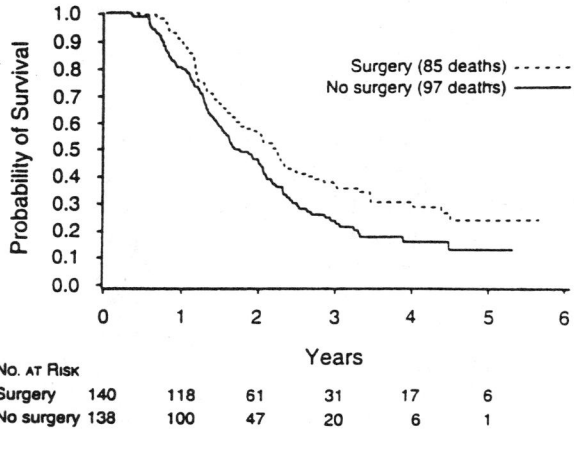

FIG. 12.6. Survival of patients with advanced epithelial ovarian cancer according to whether they underwent debulking surgery ($p = .012$ for the comparison between the groups by log-rank test). (From van der Burg MEL, van Lent M, Buyse M, et al. The effect of debulking surgery after induction chemotherapy on the prognosis in advanced epithelial ovarian cancer. N Engl J Med 1995;332:629–634, with permission.)

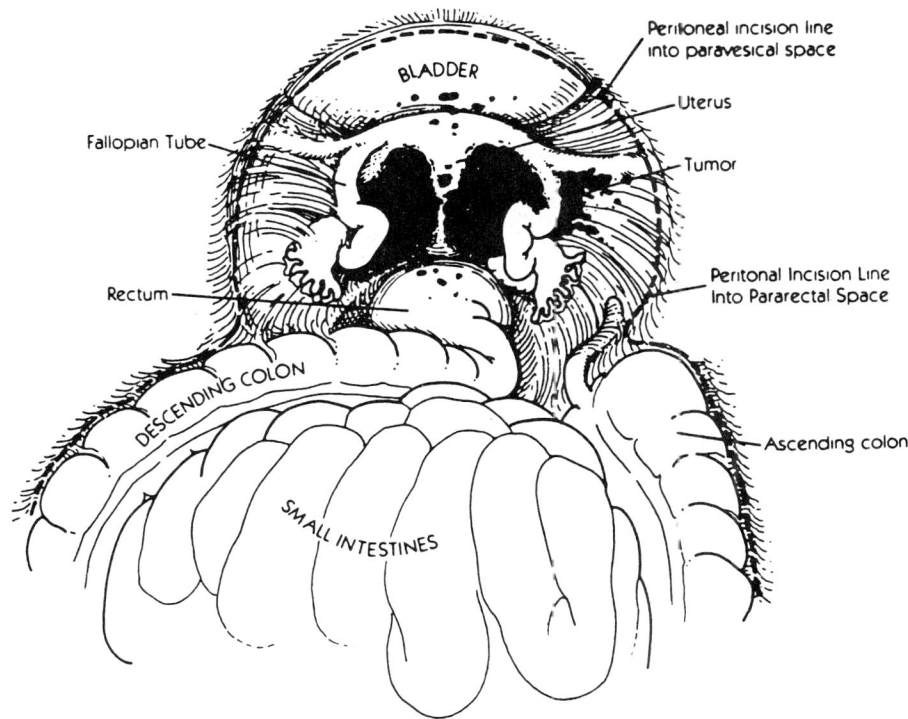

FIG. 12.7. Retroperitoneal approach for advanced ovarian cancer. (From PPO Updated 1(2), Feb 1987, with permission. Also see Markman M, Hoskins WJ, eds. *Cancer of the ovary.* New York, Raven Press, 1993:166–167.)

avoid injury to the base of the bladder is occasionally helpful. The management of the ureter depends on the degree to which the parametrium is involved by tumor. The ureter can usually be mobilized to the level of the parametrium and an extrafascial hysterectomy performed. Sometimes, however, the ureter must be dissected out of the parametrium to the level of the bladder so that involved parametrial tissue can be resected.

Complete removal of the pelvic peritoneum may be necessary and is usually not difficult, except over the rectosigmoid. If the posterior cul-de-sac is completely obliterated by tumor, a retrograde hysterectomy, as described by Hudson (47), may be required. In this procedure, the ureters are dissected out of the parametrium and the vagina is entered anteriorly. By circumscribing the vagina and severing the uterosacral ligaments without entering the posterior cul-de-sac, the surgeon can lift the entire tumor mass and uterus out of the pelvis. This mobilization of the pelvic viscera also facilitates removal of the cul-de-sac and dissection of the tumor from the surface of the rectum. The ureters must be dissected out of the parametrium early in this procedure so that they are not injured during the removal of the uterus and cul-de-sac. Occasionally, the tumor invades the rectal wall and resection of a segment is required as the tumor is removed. Transanal anastomosis with a stapling device is usually not difficult.

After the pelvis, the omentum is the second most frequently involved site. If only the infracolic omentum is involved, it can usually be separated at the edge of the transverse colon. An edematous plane usually exists, which facilitates this dissection. If the supracolic omentum is involved, the omentum should be separated from the transverse colon to expose the lesser sac. The entire omentum can then be resected along the greater curvature of the stomach. Care must be taken to ligate the gastroepiploic vessels on either

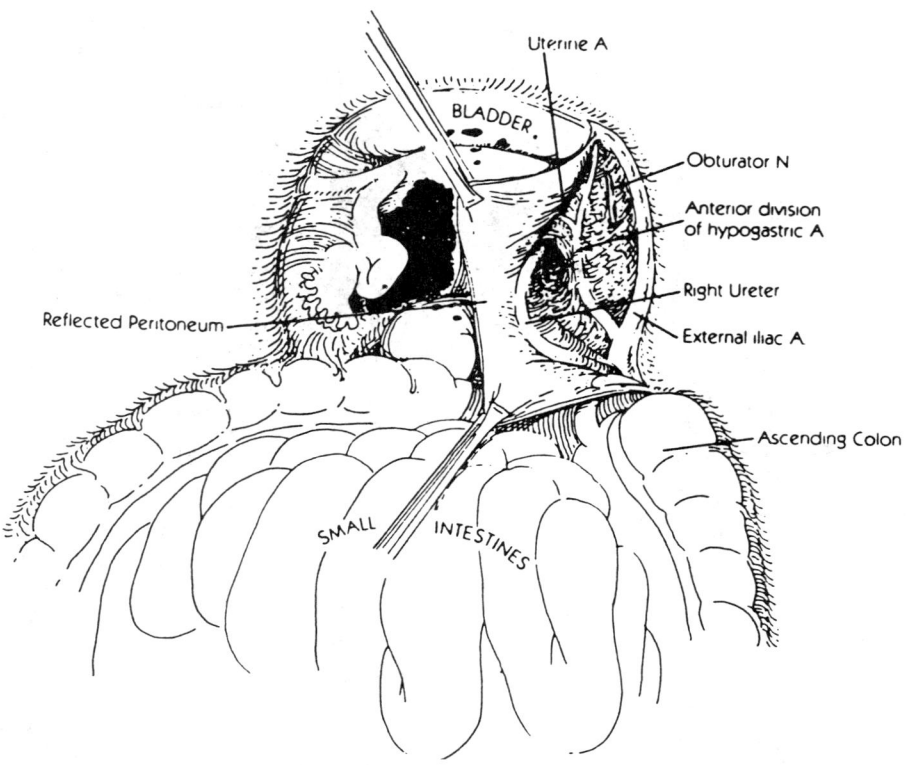

FIG. 12.8. Retroperitoneal approach for advanced ovarian cancer. (From PPO Updated 1(2), Feb 1987, with permission. Also see Markman M, Hoskins WJ, eds. *Cancer of the ovary*. New York, Raven Press, 1993:166–167.)

side, as well as the small gastric vessels from the gastroepiploic arcade. When the omentum is removed from the stomach, it is usually advisable to leave a nasogastric tube in place for a few days to prevent distension of the stomach and consequent disruption of the ligatures on these vessels. Dissection of the omentum from the splenic flexure, which requires care to avoid injury to the spleen, is facilitated by extending the abdominal incision to the xiphoid process.

Resection of other abdominal structures should be undertaken where feasible. Because of the surface growth pattern of ovarian cancer, tumor can often be removed from the surface of the intestine without the need for resection. On occasion, it is necessary to resect a portion of either the large or small intestine. The decision to perform one or more bowel resections for the purposes of cytoreduction requires mature judgment on the part of the surgeon. A good rule for intestinal resection is to determine whether resection will contribute to significant tumor reduction. It makes little sense to perform multiple intestinal resections if there is bulk disease elsewhere that is unresectable, unless bowel obstruction is present. Therefore, intestinal resection should be performed only if the procedure relieves an obstructive process and/or allows for optimal cytoreduction.

Isolated masses on the diaphragm can generally be excised with proper exposure, which may include partial mobilization of the liver. The ability to resect plaques of tumor on the diaphragm frequently depends on their size and location. Diaphragmatic stripping and tumor ablation using the argon beam coagulator (ABC, Conned Corp., Utica, New York) or the Cavitron Ultrasonic Aspirator (CUSA, Valley Lab, Boneder, Colorado) are the most frequently used methods to affect cytoreduction in this area (31,39).

Resection of other organs such as the spleen, a kidney, or a portion of the liver should be reserved for cases in which the resection would aid in leaving the patient with optimal residual disease. The same is true for lymphadenectomy. If a patient has enlarged pelvic and/or paraaortic lymph nodes, and if all or most of the intraabdominal disease is resectable, then therapeutic lymphadenectomy should be performed.

The decision as to how aggressively to pursue complete cytoreduction in the surgical treatment of ovarian cancer is one of the most difficult judgments that a gynecologic oncologist must make. Factors that influence this decision are the location and amount of disease, the medical condition of the patient, the skill of the surgeon, the surgeon's knowledge of the disease process, and the potential benefits of postoperative therapy. However, even an experienced surgeon is not always able to determine resectability without a significant amount of dissection. Several studies have analyzed the ability of various evaluations to predict optimal versus suboptimal cytoreduction before laparotomy. Preoperative CT scan, preoperative serum CA 125 levels, and operative laparoscopy have been reported to accurately predict optimal versus suboptimal cytoreduction in 66% to 87% of cases (48–52). These results, although encouraging, are still preliminary.

CONCLUSION

Although the diagnosis of advanced ovarian cancer is usually not difficult, other cancers such as those of the pancreas, colon, and breast can present a similar appearance. Careful diagnostic evaluation allows for correct diagnosis in most cases.

Staging of advanced disease is usually apparent at surgical exploration, and the major surgical issue is cytoreduction. A reasonable theoretical rationale exists for primary surgical cytoreduction, and clinical reviews provide good indirect evidence for its success. Despite the lack of prospective, randomized trials that clearly prove the efficacy of the procedure, there seems little doubt that patients who undergo optimal cytoreduction have higher complete and overall responses to chemotherapy, a greater likelihood of negative second-look surgical evaluations, and improved survival rates. Primary cytoreduction influences prognosis, and although it is not the only factor in a patient's chance of cure, it remains a very important part of therapy.

Other factors in addition to cytoreductive surgery can affect prognosis. The "biology of the disease" appears to have a significant role. To some extent, it is true that tumors in patients for whom optimal cytoreduction can be achieved are different from those in patients with suboptimal cytoreduction. Currently, however, there is no reliable way of determining this difference preoperatively.

In the new millennium, cytoreductive surgery will remain an integral component of the treatment of patients with advanced ovarian cancer. Technologic advances will facilitate the achievement of optimal primary cytoreduction while also refining the ability to predict which patients will not benefit from attempted primary debulking. For patients with suboptimal or recurrent disease, future studies will further define the roles of interval cytoreduction and secondary cytoreduction in relation to the numerous new chemotherapeutic agents currently being investigated.

REFERENCES

1. Greenlee RT, Murray T, Bolden S, et al. Cancer statistics, 1999. *CA Cancer J Clin* 2000;50:7–33.
2. FIGO Cancer Committee. Staging announcement. *Gynecol Oncol* 1986;25:383–385.
3. Pecorelli S, et al. Carcinoma of the ovary. In: Pecorelli S, Creasman WT, Pettersson F, et al., eds. *FIGO annual report on the results of treatment in gynaecological cancer*, vol 23. Oxford: Isis Medical Media Limited, 1998: 75–102.
4. Tannock IF. Principles of cell proliferation: cell kinetic. In: DeVita VT, Hellman S, Rosenberg SA, eds. *Cancer: principles and practice of oncology.* Philadelphia: JB Lippincott, 1989:2–5.
5. Griffiths CT. Surgery at the time of diagnosis in ovarian cancer. In: Blackledge G, Chan KK, eds. *Management of ovarian cancer.* London: Butterworth, 1986:60–75.
6. Fuller AF, Griffiths CT. Ovarian cancer cachexia-surgical interactions. *Gynecol Oncol* 1979;8:301–305.
7. Blythe JG, Wahl TF. Debulking surgery: does it increase the quality of survival? *Gynecol Oncol* 1982;14:396–400.
8. Goldie JH, Coldman JA. A mathematical model for relating the drug sensitivity of tumors to their spontaneous mutation rate. *Cancer Treat Rep* 1979;63:1727–1733.
9. Rubin SC, Hoskins WJ. Primary surgery for ovarian carcinoma. In: Sciarra JJ, Droegemueller W, eds.

Gynecology and obstetrics. Philadelphia: JB Lippincott, 1993:1–11.
10. Munnell EQ. The changing prognosis and treatment in cancer of the ovary: a report of 235 patients with primary ovarian carcinoma, 1952–1961. *Am J Obstet Gynecol* 1968;100:790–805.
11. Declos L, Quinlan EJ. Malignant tumors of the ovary managed with post operative megavolt irradiation. *Radiology* 1969;93:659–663.
12. Griffiths CT. Surgical resection of tumor bulk in the primary treatment of ovarian cancer. *Natl Cancer Inst Monogr* 1975;42:101–105.
13. Redman JR, Petroni GR, Saigo PE, et al. Prognostic factors in advanced ovarian carcinoma. *J Clin Oncol* 1986;4:515–523.
14. Gall S, Bundy B, et al. Therapy of stage III (optimal) epithelial carcinoma of the ovary with melphalan or melphalan plus *Corynebacterium parvum* (a Gynecologic Oncology Group study). *Gynecol Oncol* 1986;25:26–36.
15. Hoskins WJ, Bundy BN, Thigpen JT, Omura GA. The influence of cytoreductive surgery on recurrence-free interval and survival in small-volume stage III epithelial ovarian cancer: a Gynecologic Oncology Group study. *Gynecol Oncol* 1992;47:159–166.
16. Young RC, et al. Advanced ovarian adenocarcinoma: a prospective clinical trial of melphalan (L-PAM) versus combination chemotherapy. *N Engl J Med* 1978;299:1261–1266.
17. Ehrlich CE, Chabner BA, Mubbard SP, et al. Chemotherapy for stage II-IV epithelial ovarian cancer with cis-dichlorodiammineplatinum (II), Adriamycin and cyclophosphamide: a preliminary report. *Cancer Treat Rep* 1979;63:281–288.
18. Wharton JT, Herson J. Surgery for common epithelial tumors of the ovary. *Cancer* 1981;48:582–589.
19. Conte PF, Bruzzone M, Chiaro S, et al. A randomized trial comparing cisplatin plus cyclophosphamide versus cisplatin, doxorubicin and cyclophosphamide in advanced ovarian cancer. *J Clin Oncol* 1986;4:965–971.
20. Hoskins WJ. Primary cytoreduction. In: Markman M, Hoskins WJ, eds. *Cancer of the ovary.* New York: Raven Press, 1993:163–173.
21. Barter JF, Barnes WA. Second-look laparotomy. In: Rubin SC, Sutton GP, eds. *Ovarian cancer.* New York: McGraw-Hill, 1993:269–300.
22. Smith JP, Day TG. Review of ovarian cancer at the University of Texas Systems Cancer Center, M.D. Anderson Hospital and Tumor Institute. *Am J Obstet Gynecol* 1979;135:984–993.
23. Malkasian GD, Melton J, O'Brien PC, Greene MH. Prognostic significance of histologic classification and grading of epithelial malignancies of the ovary. *Am J Obstet Gynecol* 1984;149:274–284.
24. Hoskins WJ, et al. The effect of diameter of largest residual disease on survival after primary cytoreductive surgery in patients with suboptimal residual epithelial ovarian carcinoma: a Gynecologic Oncology Group study. *Am J Obstet Gynecol* 1994;170:974–980.
25. National Institutes of Health Consensus Development Conference Statement. Ovarian cancer: screening, treatment, and follow-up. April 5–7, 1994. *Gynecol Oncol* 1994;55:S4–S14.
26. Omura GA, et al. A randomized trial of cyclophosphamide and doxorubicin with or without cisplatin advanced ovarian carcinoma: a Gynecologic Oncology Group study. *Cancer* 1986;57:1725–1730.
27. McGuire WP, et al. Cyclophosphamide and cisplatin compared with paclitaxel and cisplatin in patients with stage III and stage IV ovarian cancer. *N Engl J Med* 1996;334:1–6.
28. Chi DS, Leon LF, Venkatraman ES, et al. Prognostic factors in advanced epithelial ovarian carcinoma. *(Submitted).*
29. Neijt JP, et al. Randomized trial comparing two combination chemotherapy regimens (CHAP-5 vs CP) in advanced ovarian carcinoma. *J Clin Oncol* 1987;5:1157–1168.
30. Le T, Krepart GV, Lotocki RJ, Heywood MS. Does debulking surgery improve survival in biologically aggressive ovarian carcinoma? *Gynecol Oncol* 1997;67:208–214.
31. Eisenkop SM, Friedman RL, Wang HJ. Complete cytoreductive surgery is feasible and maximizes survival in patients with advanced epithelial ovarian cancer: a prospective study. *Gynecol Oncol* 1998;69:103–108.
32. Schwartz PE. Cytoreductive surgery for the management of stage IV ovarian cancer [Editorial]. *Gynecol Oncol* 1997;64:1–3.
33. Bonnefoi H, et al. Natural history of stage IV epithelial ovarian cancer. *J Clin Oncol* 1999;17:767–775.
34. Goodman HM, et al. The role of cytoreductive surgery in the management of stage IV epithelial ovarian carcinoma. *Gynecol Oncol* 1992;46:367–371.
35. Curtin JP, et al. Stage IV ovarian cancer: impact of surgical debulking. *Gynecol Oncol* 1997;64:9–12.
36. Liu PC, et al. Effect of surgical debulking on survival in stage IV ovarian cancer. *Gynecol Oncol* 1997;64:4–8.
37. Munkarah AR, et al. Prognostic significance of residual disease in patients with stage IV epithelial ovarian cancer. *Gynecol Oncol* 1997;64:13–17.
38. Bristow RE, Montz FJ, Lagasse LD, et al. Survival impact of surgical cytoreduction in stage IV epithelial ovarian cancer. *Gynecol Oncol* 1999;72:278–287.
39. Morrow CP, Curtin JP. Surgery for ovarian neoplasia. In: Morrow CP, Curtin JP, eds. *Gynecologic cancer surgery.* New York: Churchill Livingstone, 1996:627–716.
40. Ozols RF, Rubin SC, Thomas G, Robboy S. Epithelial ovarian cancer. In: Hoskins WJ, Perez CA, Young RC, eds. *Principles and practice of gynecologic oncology,* 2nd ed. Philadelphia: Lippincott-Raven, 1997:919–986.
41. Hoskins WJ, Chi DS, Boente MP, Rubin SC. State of the art surgical management of ovarian cancer. *Cancer Res Ther Control* 1999;9:373–382.
42. Neijt JP, et al. Randomized trial comparing two combination chemotherapy regimens (HEXA-CAF vs CHAP-5) in advanced ovarian carcinoma. *Lancet* 1984;2:594–600.
43. Lawton FG, Reelman CW, Lueoley DM, et al. Neoadjuvant (cytoreductive) chemotherapy combined with intervention debulking surgery in advanced, unresected epithelial ovarian cancer. *Obstet Gynecol* 1989;73:61–65.
44. Ng LW, Rubin SC, Hoskins WJ. Aggressive chemosurgical debulking in patients with advanced ovarian cancer. *Gynecol Oncol* 1990;38:358–363.
45. van der Burg MEL, et al. The effect of debulking surgery after induction chemotherapy on the prognosis in advanced epithelial ovarian cancer. *N Engl J Med* 1995;332:629–634.

46. PPO Updated 1(2), Feb 1987. (Also see Markman M, Hoskins WJ (eds). *Cancer of the ovary.* New York, Raven Press, 1993:166–167.)
47. Hudson CN. Surgical treatment of ovarian cancer. *Gynecol Oncol* 1973;1:370–375.
48. Nelson BE, Rosenfeld AT, Schwartz PE. Preoperative abdominopelvic computed tomographic prediction of optimal cytoreduction in epithelial ovarian carcinoma. *J Clin Oncol* 1993;11:166–172.
49. Meyer JI, Kennedy AW, Friedman R, et al. Ovarian carcinoma: value of CT in predicting success of debulking surgery. *AJR Am J Roentgenol* 1995;165:875–878.
50. Vergote I, Dewever I, Tjalma W, et al. Neoadjuvant chemotherapy or primary debulking surgery in advanced ovarian carcinoma: a retrospective analysis of 285 patients. *Gynecol Oncol* 1998;71:431–436.
51. Surwit EA, Childers JM, Alberts DS. Survival and morbidity of neoadjuvant chemotherapy compared to primary cytoreductive surgery in advanced ovarian cancer [Abstract]. *Gynecol Oncol* 1998;68:122–123.
52. Chi DS, Venkatraman ES, Masson V, Hoskins WJ. The ability of preoperative serum CA-125 to predict optimal primary tumor cytoreduction in stage III epithelial ovarian carcinoma [Abstract]. *Gynecol Oncol* 1999;72:453.

13

Primary Chemotherapy for Epithelial Ovarian Cancer

William P. McGuire

The significant amount of research that epithelial ovarian cancer has generated over the past two decades is out of proportion to its incidence (14,500 deaths and 24,000 new cases in the United States annually) (1). This intense interest in ovarian cancer is probably the result of several factors: its occurrence in a population that is at the peak of productivity (women between 40 and 60 years of age); its general responsiveness to therapy, which suggests curability; and the realization that standard treatment for advanced ovarian cancer is still suboptimal in terms of long-term survival.

A minority of patients with ovarian cancer present with early disease (stage I and II). Most of these patients are offered some form of adjunctive therapy postoperatively, because approximately 30% to 40% of these cancers recur after surgery alone. The majority of patients, however, present with advanced disease (stage III and IV). These patients usually succumb after an initial gratifying response to cytotoxic chemotherapy followed by emergence of resistant clones and clinical progression. A small subgroup of patients fail primary therapy at the outset, and these patients with primary drug resistance present an even greater challenge.

This chapter reviews the current chemotherapeutic approaches to primary treatment of epithelial ovarian tumors of all stages. It is important to note that current chemotherapy regimens remain suboptimal treatment for ovarian cancer, and new approaches are clearly needed.

MANAGEMENT OF EARLY-STAGE DISEASE (I AND II)

Studies in the 1970s

Because only 20% to 25% of women with ovarian cancer present with early-stage disease, clinical research in this area has been limited by low patient numbers. Additionally, many of these patients present with premenopausal adnexal masses, are operated on by surgeons other than gynecologic oncologists who may incompletely stage the patient, and are never offered protocol therapy. A study initiated by the Gynecologic Oncology Group (GOG) in the early 1970s for stage I disease compared no postoperative therapy, postoperative pelvic radiation therapy, and 18 months of phenylalanine mustard (0.2 mg/kg/day × 5 days every 23 days) (2). Total accrual was fewer than 100 patients, and none were staged by current standards. Survival comparisons between any two groups were not statistically significant, although the group that received radiation therapy had the poorest outcome and the group that received chronic cytotoxic therapy did significantly better than the other two groups combined. The most important information generated by this study was a better understanding of differences in prognosis for subgroups of patients with early-stage disease. Patients with high-grade tumor or with extension of tumor through the capsule that caused adherence of the adnexal mass to peritoneal structures were found to have a high relapse rate (20% to 35%), while patients with low-grade tumor or tumor confined to the ovary displayed greater than 90% disease-free survival (DFS) at 5 years. Although this study did not help define optimal therapy for early-stage disease, it did help to delineate two groups of patients with early disease that have been handled separately in many subsequent treatment protocols.

Even in more modern studies, however, this separation of stage I patients into high-risk and low-risk categories has been suboptimal. In two studies of early ovarian cancer where prognostic variables were correlated with outcome, residual disease and high tumor grade were found to be powerful negative prognosticators in one study, with increasing age or stage and clear cell histology also prognostic to a lesser degree (3). In a second study of 252 patients with stage I disease by the same authors, high grade, dense adherence of the primary lesion, and large-volume ascites (in decreasing order) were predictive of adverse outcome (recurrence), after which a multivariate analysis showed that tumor bilaterality, cyst rupture, stage, capsular penetration, tumor size, histologic subtype, age, and type of postoperative therapy were not correlated with outcome (4).

Tumor grade has been shown in multiple other studies to be important to outcome (5), but reproducibility of histologic grade is only moderate (6). DNA ploidy has also been shown to be discriminatory for outcome in early disease (7), and it is a more reproducible parameter with automated flow cytometric techniques. Aneuploid tumors have a much worse prognosis than diploid tumors matched for other known prognostic factors. In a study from the Norwegian Radium Hospital there were no relapses among 77 patients with well differentiated and diploid tumors, in contrast to a 25% incidence of recurrence in 142 patients who had moderately to poorly differentiated tumors or well differentiated and nondiploid tumors. Another powerful predictor of outcome in both early and advanced disease is computerized morphometry, as popularized by Bruggle (8). In one study of 102 stage I patients, nuclear area and nuclear volume were strong predictors of outcome ($p = .0004$), those with higher values having a higher recurrence rate. In this same study, histologic grade was also predictive of outcome ($p = .008$) but interobserver correlation was poor (overall 34%). Morphometry has not been universally adopted and is not available at many hospitals.

There are additional risk factors that molecular biologic methodology has only recently allowed us to evaluate. This includes assessment of mutations in or overexpression of p53, p27, cyclin E, HER2/neu, platelet-derived growth factor (PDGF), transforming growth factor-β (TGF-β), vascular endothelial growth factor (VEGF), and Bcl-2. There are data suggesting that each may be important in determination of prognosis, but the data are conflicting, the sample sizes too small, or clinical outcomes not available to correlate with the parameter, precluding use of these factors routinely in risk assessment. An exhaustive review of this topic is beyond the scope of this review, but interested readers are referred to other publications (9). Several more years will be necessary to determine whether any of these factors is important enough in risk assessment to incorporate them into the staging system or use them to select candidates or noncandidates for adjuvant therapy.

Studies in the 1980s

The studies initiated in the 1980s included more detailed staging, which made the groups relatively more homogeneous and easier to compare. Two national trials in the United States were initiated and have reported mature data (10). The first, which included 81 patients, evaluated no postoperative therapy versus chronic oral phenylalanine mustard (0.2 mg/kg/day × 5 days every 4 to 6 weeks for 12 months) in patients with stage IA or IB tumors, grades 1 and 2. With a median follow-up period of more than 7 years, no discernable differences were seen in any outcome measure. DFS and survival were predicted to be in excess of 90% in both groups. Because of the risk of alkylating agent–induced leukemia in the treated group and the excellent survival demonstrated in both groups, this study recommended no postoperative therapy for low-grade stage I disease.

In the second trial, 141 patients with poorly differentiated stage IA, IB, IC, or stage II tumors of grades were randomly assigned to receive phenylalanine mustard (as in the earlier study) versus a single dose of intraperitoneal ^{32}P-chromic phosphate (15 mCi). Again, no significant differences were observed between the two groups for 5-year DFS or overall survival, both of which were predicted to be near 80%. Some 20% to 40% of patients from this study are expected to eventually have a recurrence, but review of prognostic factors does not allow the selection of favorable and nonfavorable groups for study.

Because ^{32}P was less toxic and easier to administer than melphalan, the standard of care for patients with early-stage disease was considered by many to be ^{32}P, although the authors made no recommendation for one therapy over the other. In these two trials, a significant number of patients with borderline ovarian tumors were included. These tumors have an indolent natural history (Chapter 22) and may have favorably skewed survival statistics. Additionally, no prospective trials have compared ^{32}P versus no therapy in high-risk, low-stage patients, and the acceptance of ^{32}P as the standard is therefore based on comparisons with historical controls showing 30% to 40% failure after surgery alone. However, these historical control patients often were not staged according to modern standards. Many may have been understaged, and they may have had significantly different pretreatment prognostic factors that make these comparisons less than optimal.

Incorporation of Cisplatin into Adjuvant Therapy

Cisplatin, the most active single agent in epithelial ovarian cancer, has only recently been incorporated into treatment regimens for early disease. Based on the previous GOG study, which concluded that high-risk patients benefited equally from intraperitoneal ^{32}P or chronic oral melphalan but that ^{32}P was less toxic, the next trial by the GOG compared ^{32}P versus three cycles of cyclophosphamide (1,000 mg/m^2 IV q 3 weeks) and cisplatin (100 mg/m^2 IV q 3 weeks) (11). A total of 204 evaluable patients were randomly assigned between September 1986 and March 1994. After a median follow-up period exceeding 5 years, 78% of the chemotherapy group and 66% of the ^{32}P group had recurrence; after adjusting for stage and histologic grade, the group receiving chemotherapy had a 31% decrement in estimated recurrence ($p = .08$, one-tail t test). The authors concluded that "although there were no statistically significant differences between the two treatment arms, the better progression-free interval for [chemotherapy] and the problems with adequate distribution and late toxicities associated with ^{32}P make platinum-based combinations the preferred standard treatment for patients with early high-risk ovarian cancer."

A Norwegian study mentioned previously regarding risk for recurrence as a function of DNA ploidy suggested that cisplatin alone was no better than ^{32}P in terms of outcome but had a better toxicity profile (12). In that study, 340 patients (stages I to IIIA) were randomly assigned to receive either cisplatin (50 mg/m^2 every 3 weeks × 6 cycles) or ^{32}P (7 to 10 mCi intraperitoneally), with some of the latter patients also receiving external beam radiation. After a median follow-up period of more than 5 years, no differences were apparent in either group, and the survival rate was 85% in both. The authors concluded that future studies in early ovarian cancer should have a control (no treatment) group.

In the two most recently completed GOG studies and the study from the Norwegian Radium Hospital there were no control (no treatment) arms. Because the two therapies compared in these three studies were equivalent in terms of outcome, it is difficult to assess the value of any form of therapy over simple observation after laparotomy. This issue was addressed in a study from a collaborative group in Italy (13). In that study patients underwent rigorous staging by modern criteria and 271 consecutive stage I patients were divided into two groups and treated on two separate protocols. Patients with stage IA or IB with grade 2 or 3 tumors were randomly allocated to observation or cisplatin (50 mg/m^2 IV q 28 days × 6 courses; $n = 83$). Patients with stage IC ($n = 152$) were randomly allocated to receive either the same cisplatin therapy or a single application of intraperitoneal ^{32}P (15 mCi). After a median observation time in excess of 6 years, the first trial showed a reduction in relapse among the patients treated with cisplatin (DFS 83%, versus 66% in the observation group; $p = .095$). Only grade of tumor and type of postoperative therapy were important in a multivariate analysis of risk of recurrence. Although these results do not reach statistical significance, there is a trend favoring therapy over observation and results after further follow-up may allow more sound conclusions. In this trial the differences in survival were less impressive than the recurrence data, in large part because of the rapid demise of those patients who had a recurrence after adjuvant cisplatin therapy; most of the chemonaive patients with recurrence were still alive and responding to and possibly cured by salvage therapy. In the second trial, for those patients with stage IC disease, the results were even more significant, with DFS of 85% for those treated with cisplatin versus 65% for those treated with ^{32}P ($p = .008$). Once again, survival differences were not significantly different, for the same reason as noted for the first trial. Two other observations about this study need mention. The tumors in the second group of patients, who were considered by the investigators to be at higher risk for failure, really did not behave any more aggressively than those in the supposedly lower-risk group, again highlighting the inadequacy of the current staging system. Additionally, the lack of a control arm in the second study begs the question of whether any therapy improves outcome. Only further maturity of these survival data may answer this question.

Conclusions

The only conclusion that can be made from these similar yet somewhat contradictory studies is that the need for any adjuvant therapy in early-stage ovarian cancer remains uncertain. If therapy is indicated, one without significant chronic toxicity should be chosen, because most of these patients live longer than 5 years after treatment and are at risk for chronic adverse effects. Although the Norwegian investigators may be correct in suggesting that future trials should include a control arm, such a trial is unlikely in the United States because of the significant bias in favor of adjuvant therapy of some form in a patient population in which the chance of recurrence is greater than 20%.

The reason why adjunctive therapy has not been shown to be more efficacious in ovarian cancer is unclear. Drugs with equivalent activity in advanced breast cancer have demonstrated a positive influence on survival in the postoperative adjuvant setting (high-risk node-negative and node-positive patients). However, high-risk breast cancer patients who are candidates for postoperative adjuvant therapies are 30 to 50 times more common than patients who are disease free after primary surgery for early ovarian cancer. Therefore, it is easier to complete studies and build on prior data. The greater number of eligible breast cancer patients also permits very large, randomized trials that allow detection of minor differences. The small number of patients with completely resected ovarian cancer makes accrual to trials slow (average trial length, more than 5 years) and total patient numbers in each trial so small as to make observations from those trials generally of low power.

It is generally agreed that patients with low-grade (1 or 2), stage IA or IB tumors have excellent survival after surgery alone, and adjuvant therapy is not required. All other patients with stage I or stage II tumors should be considered for entry into clinical trials, because data supporting the need for a specific adjuvant regimen remains to be defined.

MANAGEMENT OF ADVANCED-STAGE DISEASE (III AND IV)

Current trials in advanced ovarian cancer in the United States usually subdivide stage III patients by the amount of postoperative residual disease, because this factor has been shown to be prognostic for outcome in multiple studies and by multivariate analyses performed on large populations (14). Conversely, studies of advanced disease performed outside the United States frequently include patients with stage IIB to IV disease with stratification based on postoperative disease bulk. Additional factors found to be prognostic indicators for a positive outcome include low tumor grade, young age, good performance status, absence of ascites, cell type other than mucinous or clear cell, and treatment with cisplatin (15–18). Contemporary studies in the

United States use a residual mass size of 1 cm as the break point between optimal and suboptimal cytoreduction within stage III, whereas studies performed before 1985 usually used 2 to 3 cm as the breakpoint. This fact and its effect on outcome must be considered when studies from different time periods are compared.

By definition, patients with optimally debulked stage III disease rarely have measurable tumor at the completion of staging laparotomy. With the exception of the occasional patient who progresses during therapy, determination of response usually depends on findings at second-look laparotomy. However, the significance and value of this procedure outside a research setting remain controversial (19). Reassessment laparotomy has fallen into significant disfavor, and the surrogates of progression-free and overall survival have largely supplanted response in patients entered on clinical trials without measurable disease. However, these endpoints can be influenced by salvage therapies, when effective. Whether salvage therapy has an impact on survival or not, and what constitutes acceptable salvage therapy, are discussed in Chapters 15 and 16. The potential value of reassessment laparotomy consists in its allowing early identification of persistent or recurrent disease and rapid institution of effective salvage therapy. However, an 800-patient GOG trial was unable to demonstrate any difference in progression-free survival between patients who did or did not have this procedure performed (20). Nevertheless, it is the attainment of a complete pathologic response that may result in "cure" of advanced ovarian cancer. Patients with persistent disease after primary therapy are rarely alive 3 years later.

Drugs Active in Epithelial Ovarian Cancer

Single agents that are active in ovarian cancer include classic alkylating agents (most commonly cyclophosphamide, melphalan, and chlorambucil); platinum compounds (cisplatin and carboplatin); anthracyclines (doxorubicin, epirubicin, liposomally encapsulated doxorubicin, and mitoxantrone); taxanes (paclitaxel and docetaxel); chronic oral etoposide; topotecan; gemcitabine; hexamethylmelamine; methotrexate; and 5-fluorouracil. Tamoxifen and progestational agents have a low level of activity in patients with detectable cytoplasmic steroid receptors. This subject has been reviewed extensively (21).

Role of the Anthracyclines

Before the 1980s, the mainstay of therapy was alkylating agents, which produced clinical response rates of 40% to 50% and clinical complete response rates of 15% to 20%. Rare patients had surgical complete response, but those who did often remained disease-free for long periods. The use of anthracyclines were explored in the late 1970s and early 1980s, but there was little convincing evidence that they added significantly to efficacy of therapy, and they clearly added an extra dimension to toxicity (both hematologic and cardiac). Initially doxorubicin or other anthracyclines were added to an alkylating agent, but later, when the platinums were made part of primary therapy, these agents were once again explored. A metaanalysis of four trials in which patients were randomly assigned to receive a doxorubicin-based triplet or a doublet without doxorubicin found a 6% survival advantage for the triplet therapy (22). Other studies suggested some survival advantage by the addition of doxorubicin, but at the cost of increased toxicity (23,24). Nevertheless, anthracyclines were omitted from the primary treatment regimen in most U.S. studies of ovarian cancer in 1986 due to unclear advantage and concern over the additional toxicity associated with their use. Studies from Europe continued to explore their use, with epirubicin used more commonly than doxorubicin. Today, where a new doublet has become the standard of care, further exploration of the role of anthracyclines is underway.

Incorporation of the Platinums

Cisplatin was developed in the late 1970s and carboplatin in the early 1980s. After both were shown to be active in a series of phase II trials in recurrent and persistent ovarian cancer, they were rapidly incorporated into primary therapy. With the addition of the platinums to primary therapy, clinical response rates rose to 80%

and clinical complete response to 40% to 50%. Depending on disease bulk, 20% (suboptimal disease) to 50% (optimal disease) of clinical complete responders could be expected to have negative second-look operations. However, the durations of these responses appeared to be briefer than with alkylating therapy. This probably was related to the length of drug exposure. With the then-current platinum-based regimens, only six courses of therapy were typically administered (due to development of cumulative toxicities), and usually treatment was completed within 5 months. With alkylating agents the treatment was typically 12 cycles, often spanning 15 months, and the patients who were candidates for second-look operations at that point (i.e., those with no early progression after response) were self-selected to have long disease-free intervals. By the mid 1980s platinum-based therapy had become the "gold standard" worldwide.

Some believed that platinum monotherapy was adequate, although in the United States the doublet of platinum and cyclophosphamide was more commonly used. A metaanalysis of some 1,200 patients across many trials suggested that platinum-based combinations were superior to single-agent platinum in terms of response and progression-free interval but not overall survival (25). This metaanalysis was performed before the change to paclitaxel-based therapy (discussed later). The data also clearly supported the significant role of platinum in the primary therapy of advanced ovarian cancer, demonstrating that incorporation of platinum into the primary treatment regimen improved outcome in comparison to regimens that did not contain a platinum compound. Further, this study suggested equivalent efficacy for cisplatin and carboplatin, with less toxicity and better patient acceptance of the latter. From the mid-1980s onward, then, combination therapy with a platinum compound and cyclophosphamide became the standard of care in the United States. Single-agent carboplatin was more commonly used in the United Kingdom, and an anthracycline-based three-drug regimen remained a common practice in Western Europe. Nevertheless, it remained a point of controversy as to whether single-agent platinum or some platinum-based combination was preferable.

Combination Therapy versus Single Agents

The past two decades of research have established that cisplatin-based combination therapy is more effective in the initial treatment of ovarian cancer than therapy with single alkylating agents (26) or combinations without cisplatin (27,28), although the relative merits of single-agent platinum and platinum-based combinations are debated even today. This improvement in efficacy with the platinums, however, applies only to response rates and possibly to DFS. No large impact on long-term survival has been noted, particularly in patients with bulky disease postoperatively. This is most probably a result of the frequent use of platinum compounds as salvage therapy in patients for whom nonplatinum regimens have failed, which blurs the primary effect of platinum on survival. However, one retrospective study that compared survival before the platinum era and after the introduction of these agents strongly suggested that the platinums have had some impact, as well, on survival. In that study from the Netherlands (29), patients diagnosed with ovarian cancer diagnosed between 1981 and 1985 had a better survival than a similar group of patients diagnosed between 1975 and 1980. The two reasons proposed for this improvement were the more routine use of aggressive surgical cytoreduction and the use of cisplatin-based therapy. Thus, incorporation of cisplatin into primary therapy may have improved survival, although no single study has demonstrated this convincingly.

Although the metaanalysis cited previously (25) suggested very strongly that platinum-containing combinations are statistically superior to single-agent cisplatin, some investigators argued that single-agent cisplatin or carboplatin used in a more intensive manner (made more feasible when it is not combined with other agents) is just as effective as platinum-based combinations, has less toxicity, and is less likely to lead to secondary tumors. Some support for this approach was generated when a very large multinational collaborative trial was reported (30). In that study, carboplatin and the three-drug regimen of cyclophosphamide, doxorubicin, and cisplatin led to similar outcomes in a diverse group of patients, and the carboplatin monotherapy was significantly less toxic. To the contrary, however, are multiple studies over the past two decades that have explored dose intensity of the platinums and have not been able to demonstrate any outcome advantage for clinically achievable platinum dose intensity (see later discussion).

Substitution of Carboplatin for Cisplatin

Many studies suggest that carboplatin may be substituted for cisplatin in combination regimens with equivalent end results (31,32), and that the two drugs are equivalently active as single agents (33). Carboplatin is much easier to administer (outpatient administration without hydration) and has less gastrointestinal, renal, and peripheral neurologic toxicity. It does cause dose-limiting myelosuppression, especially thrombocytopenia, but this has been easily managed by using doses based on calculated creatinine clearance. This topic has been reviewed extensively (34).

Role of Paclitaxel

Paclitaxel, the first of a new class of compounds, the taxanes, causes excessive polymerization of tubulin and prolonged stability of the polymers. Although it was originally identified in 1966, clinical development was thwarted until the mid-1980s owing to problems with supply as well as insolubility of the agent. Early activity of paclitaxel was noted during phase I trials, and soon thereafter limited phase II studies were initiated (limited because of problems with drug supply). This topic has been reviewed elsewhere (35,36). In multiple phase II studies in ovarian cancer, activity was noted most uniquely in a population of patients whose disease was refractory to cisplatin (37,38). It was this activity in platinum-resistant recurrent disease, as defined by Markman and colleagues (39), that piqued the interest for further investigation and rapid movement of this compound into front-line therapy.

After the completion of these phase II studies, paclitaxel was combined with cisplatin in a phase I study design. This study revealed that each drug could be given in clinically relevant doses, particularly when the cisplatin followed paclitaxel given as a 24-hour continuous infusion (40). Sequences in which cisplatin preceded paclitaxel were more toxic to granulocytes. Further, the combination using this schedule did not appear to enhance neurotoxicity, which had been a concern since each single agent was known to be neurotoxic (total dose–related for cisplatin and dose- and infusion rate–related for paclitaxel). With this new agent that appeared to be non-cross-resistant with cisplatin, phase III trials were initiated; the results have firmly established that the combination of paclitaxel and a platinum analog constitutes the new standard of care for treatment of advanced ovarian cancer (41,42).

Although these two studies were similar, they did differ in two regards. The study from the United States (GOG Protocol 111) comprised a patient population with suboptimal disease (bulky), and the paclitaxel was administered at a dose of 135 mg/m^2 over 24 hours; in contrast, the multinational study had 35% optimal patients, and the paclitaxel was administered at a dose of 175 mg/m^2 as a 3-hour infusion. In both studies the control was identical, with cisplatin at 75 mg/m^2 administered as a short infusion over 2 hours and cyclophosphamide administered at 750 mg/m^2 as a bolus. Results from both studies showed a significant improvement in clinical response rate, median progression-free interval, and median survival all favoring the paclitaxel arm. A trend in favor of complete pathologic response was also noted in the study from the United States, where reassessment laparotomy was performed in most patients who had a clinical complete response. In the multinational study, subset analysis showed that the effect of paclitaxel was equivalent in patients with either bulky or optimal disease. With follow-up in the GOG study in excess of 60 months, there remained a significant reduction in risk of progression and a reduction in risk of death among those patients treated with cisplatin/paclitaxel compared with cisplatin/cyclophosphamide. The hazard ratio for the benefit decreased with further follow-up, but at 60 months there were 27% of patients alive in the paclitaxel group, compared with 18% in the cyclophosphamide group (W.P. McGuire, personal communication, 2000).

Some lessons can be learned by comparing outcomes in these two trials. Neurotoxicity was very significant on the paclitaxel arm in the multinational study, with 19% of patients on the experiencing grade 3 toxicity, compared with only 1% in the cyclophosphamide arm. Only 4% of patients on the GOG study who received cisplatin and paclitaxel over 24 hours experienced similar levels of neurotoxicity. Similar levels of neurotoxicity had been reported by investigators from Cleveland (43) and were unanticipated at the time of that report. Neurotoxicity with paclitaxel appears to be both dose and schedule dependent, with higher does and shorter infusion schedules leading to more neurotoxicity. The only differences between the multinational study and the GOG study were dose and schedule of paclitaxel and the fact that some patients in the multinational study were treated with a total of nine cycles of therapy, whereas few patients in the GOG study received more than six cycles. A further comparison between the multinational and GOG studies seems appropriate also. The outcomes in the two trials were remarkably similar even with the inclusion of 35% optimally debulked cases in the multinational study and supposedly none in the GOG study. As mentioned previously, stage III patients with optimal debulking enjoy much better progression-free and overall survival compared with those patients who have bulky disease. The reasons for the similar outcomes rather than better outcomes in the multinational study are not entirely clear but may relate to inclusion of some patients in the GOG study with cryptic optimal disease. The protocol that was sponsored by the GOG for optimal disease in the same period that GOG 111 was accruing patients compared intravenous and intraperitoneal therapies, and many investigators were biased against that trial.

The GOG has also produced results of a large study in bulky ovarian cancer which, on the surface, make the data just described somewhat difficult to interpret (44). In that study 615 evaluable patients with suboptimal stage III or stage IV disease were randomly assigned to the combination of cisplatin and paclitaxel in the same dose and schedule as in GOG 111, paclitaxel as a single agent at 200 mg/m^2 over 24 hours, or cisplatin as a single agent at 100 mg/m^2. The results showed that paclitaxel as a single agent is inferior to either the combination regimen or cisplatin used alone in terms of response rate and progression-free survival. However, survival rates in all three arms of the study were similar. In this study reassessment laparotomy was required for patients with clinical complete response at the conclusion of six cycles of therapy. Among patients receiving paclitaxel alone as primary therapy, 71% received cisplatin as salvage therapy; and, 52% of patients receiving primary monotherapy with cisplatin received paclitaxel as salvage therapy. Approximately half of these patients were given second-line therapy before clinical progression based on either persistent disease radiographically or findings of persistent disease at reassessment laparotomy. So what this study actually addressed was the use of cisplatin and paclitaxel either concurrently or sequentially. Toxicity appeared to be more severe in patients treated with cisplatin monotherapy; 12% of these patients had early discontinuation of therapy for toxicity (primarily neurotoxicity), compared with 1% for paclitaxel and 4% for the combination. Further, 21% of patients treated with cisplatin monotherapy refused second-look surgery, compared with 8% for paclitaxel and 9% for the combination. This was presumably a result of persistent toxicity and/or reduced quality of life, although this parameter was not specifically measured.

One could question how it is that crossover in this trail blurred survival differences while survival differences were maintained in the multinational trial described previously. In the multinational trial, crossover occurred primarily at the time of clinical progression, whereas in this study significant preemptive crossover occurred. Therefore, it must be concluded from these results that paclitaxel and a platinum compound remain the treatment of choice for advanced ovarian cancer. The better therapeutic index seems occur with application of both agents simultaneously. When outcomes of this study and the multinational study are compared, it must also be concluded that, if the platinum and taxane are to be administered sequentially, they should be given in rapid sequence rather than at clinical progression. Finally the median survival times in all arms of this trial (30, 26, and 27 months for cisplatin, paclitaxel, and combination therapy, respectively) were inferior to those seen in the cisplatin and paclitaxel arms of the GOG and multinational studies (37 and 35 months, respectively). This once again supports the suggestion that there may have been cryptic optimal patients in the GOG original trial.

The final trial to explore the incorporation of paclitaxel into primary therapy is the large ICON 3 study, in which more than 2,000 patients were randomly assigned to a nonpaclitaxel regimen (either carboplatin monotherapy or cyclophosphamide, doxorubicin, and cisplatin) or to the carboplatin/paclitaxel doublet (45). The early results of that trial showed no outcome advantage for the paclitaxel regimen; however, those results were very immature (median follow-up, less than 18 months). In addition, the conclusion of lack of efficacy of paclitaxel was based on the entire study population (30% with stage I/II disease or microscopic disease), whereas analysis of outcome in patients with residual disease after surgery showed a positive outcome effect for paclitaxel (W.P. McGuire, personal communication, 1999).

It is fair to state that the standard of care for treatment of advanced ovarian cancer is now paclitaxel (dose and schedule unknown; see later discussion) in conjunction with a platinum coordination complex (see later discussion of compounds used) for six cycles. Two recent consensus statements have opined that the platinum and paclitaxel doublet is the standard of care (46,47).

Controversies Surrounding the Paclitaxel and Platinum Doublet

Since it has been established that a platinum compound and paclitaxel in some dose and schedule is now the standard of care for primary therapy of advanced ovarian cancer, the major controversies surrounding this treatment relate to (a) the dose of paclitaxel, (b) the duration of the paclitaxel infusion, and (c) which platinum compound to use.

There is little evidence to support an improved outcome with increasing doses of paclitaxel beyond those currently recommended, 135 to 175 mg/m^2. Although most studies of more dose-intense paclitaxel as monotherapy have been performed in a salvage setting and a different outcome could occur in a primary disease setting, the randomized study performed by the GOG is rather convincing that dose increments of 1.5-fold are unlikely to generate significantly improved clinical outcomes (48). In that study patients with both platinum-sensitive and platinum-resistant recurrent ovarian cancer were randomly assigned to receive either 175 mg/m^2 or 250 mg/m^2 paclitaxel, both administered over 24 hours. Only a small difference in response rate (35% versus 28%) was observed, with no improvement in progression-free survival or overall survival related to dose. Further, significantly more thrombocytopenia, anemia, gastrointestinal toxicity, neurotoxicity, and myalgia were associated with the higher-dose regimen, in addition to the need for cytokine support with its attendant cost and toxicity. Rowinsky (49) also showed in a retrospective analysis that doses in excess of 175 mg/m^2 actually caused a survival decrement. Therefore, the currently recommended starting dose of paclitaxel is 135 mg/m^2 for the 24-hour schedule and 175 mg/m^2 for the 3-hour infusion, the two schedules with which there is the largest experience.

Regarding the duration of paclitaxel infusion, controversy still exists. The original studies used a continuous 24-hour infusion (37,40,41), based on the assumption that a long infusion would abrogate severe allergic reactions seen in the phase I trials. Early phase I studies using infusions of 1 to 3 hours had noted a 5% to 10% incidence of severe anaphylactic reactions. Concomitant with increasing infusion duration, corticosteroids and antagonists of both H$_1$ and H$_2$ histamine receptors were employed. This reduced the incidence of allergic reaction to 1% to 3%, but it was unclear which of these measures led to the reduction. As investigators became more comfortable with paclitaxel, shorter infusions were again explored. In a large, randomized trial which compared 3-hour versus 24-hour infusion of paclitaxel in the salvage treatment of ovarian cancer (50), no increase in allergic reactions was noted with the shorter infusion time (all patients were given medications to abrogate allergic reactions). Further, it was noted that myelosuppression was much more common with the 24-hour than the 3-hour schedule. The investigators concluded that, with reduced hematologic toxicity and no evidence of a difference in response or survival endpoints, the 3-hour infusion was the preferred schedule. At the same time, however, data from *in vitro* studies suggested that the ability of paclitaxel to kill cells was strongly correlated with exposure duration and not dose (51). Thus, the possibility existed that the differential toxicity noted in this trial was related to exposure duration of the bone marrow stem cell and that a similar effect could occur in the tumor stem cell. Although infusion duration made no difference in efficacy endpoints in a salvage setting, the same might not be true in a primary treatment setting.

The recently reported results of another GOG study help to address this question. During the conduct of the GOG 111 trial, a phase I study was initiated exploring the feasibility of combining carboplatin with paclitaxel. The rationale for this combination was the better therapeutic index of the carboplatin/cyclophosphamide doublet as compared with the cisplatin/cyclophosphamide doublet when they were compared in the 1980s. Much to the surprise of most, the carboplatin/paclitaxel doublet was well tolerated and could be administered at full doses of both agents without unacceptable hematologic toxicity (52). The regimen of carboplatin (AUC [area under curve] 5-7) with paclitaxel at 175 mg/m^2 was rapidly adopted by most clinicians in the United States as a substitute for the superior regimen in the GOG trial, which used the more inconvenient 24-hour paclitaxel with cisplatin regimen. Therefore, not only was infusion duration of the paclitaxel altered with the possible implications already noted, but the platinum analog was changed simultaneously and without a randomized trial to support its equivalency. For these reasons, the GOG began a trial to compare these two platinum/paclitaxel doublets in a cohort of patients with optimally debulked ovarian cancer. The results of that trial, although preliminary, make it very unlikely that the more convenient carboplatin and short-infusion paclitaxel regimen will be inferior to the more cumbersome cisplatin/paclitaxel doublet (53). Although this was a single trial to address this issue, it was large ($n = 800$) and it is unlikely that the issue will be tested in any subsequent trial. Carboplatin and short-infusion paclitaxel has become the new standard of care by default. Nevertheless, an ongoing GOG study is comparing the 24-hour infusion of paclitaxel and cisplatin with a continuous 96-hour infusion (30 mg/m^2/day × 4 days) paclitaxel and cisplatin. This study was initiated before the results of the above study were known, and unless the even more cumbersome continuous infusion is better, there is little reason to further explore paclitaxel infusion duration.

The study described previously addresses both the choice of platinum analog and the infusion duration of paclitaxel. Two additional studies have explored the single question of which platinum analog is better. One study of 182 patients with various stages of disease randomly assigned patients to receive paclitaxel at 175 mg/m^2 given over 3 hours with either cisplatin at 75 mg/m^2 or carboplatin to an AUC of 5 as primary postoperative therapy (54). There were no apparent differences in efficacy between the two doublets, and the paclitaxel/carboplatin regimen was better tolerated; neutropenia and thrombocytopenia were somewhat more common in the carboplatin arm, whereas gastrointestinal toxicity and neurotoxicity were more common in the cisplatin arm. However, the study is probably too small to answer with any significant power the question of equivalency, which would require 200 to 250 patients per arm. A larger study from Germany (55) randomly assigned 798 patients to paclitaxel, 185 mg/m^2 over 3 hours, combined with either carboplatin (AUC = 6) or cisplatin (75 mg/m^2). The results once again demonstrated no significant differences in efficacy in outcome measures with the two doublets, and the carboplatin arm had better patient acceptance based on a quality-of-life measurement conducted in conjunction with the study. In both of the investigations, the use of cisplatin with short- infusion paclitaxel was associated with high levels of serious peripheral neurotoxicity, confirming the statement made earlier that this particular doublet should be avoided. In patients who are intolerant of carboplatin because of severe hematologic toxicity, an alternate regimen that is acceptable is cisplatin with long-infusion paclitaxel, which is associated with less neurotoxicity. In the rare patient who develops early neurotoxicity with the carboplatin and short-infusion paclitaxel doublet, carboplatin may be administered at an AUC of 5 to 7 with paclitaxel at 135 mg/m^2 over 24 hours, with the anticipation that this will reduce the degree of neurotoxicity. This regimen was also found to be safe and well tolerated in the phase I study combining paclitaxel and carboplatin (52).

It has not yet been proved that the doublet of a taxane and platinum will improve outcome in patients with optimally debulked disease; however, when platinum was incorporated into primary therapy almost two decades ago the greatest impact was seen in this population, and there is some evidence to suggest a survival advantage at least in some groups of patients since the introduction of platinum. It is hoped that the same will be observed with the introduction of paclitaxel into primary therapy. Although most physicians in the United States have already adopted the platinum/paclitaxel doublet for all stages of advanced disease, there is not and likely will never be a randomized trial in optimal stage III disease to prove that paclitaxel improves outcome in this subset of patients. Only with further use of paclitaxel-containing regimens and a subsequent metaanalysis will information be available concerning the value of adding paclitaxel to the treatment in earlier ovarian cancer.

Dose Intensity

Manipulation of dose intensity (milligrams of drug administered per square meter of body surface area per unit of time) was suggested more than a decade ago to be one way to overcome drug resistance (55). To date, that anticipation has not been met. There are now studies comparing standard doses to moderately increased (two-fold) doses of cisplatin or carboplatin without a clear indication of outcome benefit and with a significant increase in toxicity. This topic has been reviewed elsewhere (56,57). More aggressive attempts to increase dose intensity have used very high doses of chemotherapy followed by autologous stem cell transfusion. The largest U.S. experience was with cyclophosphamide, carboplatin, and mitoxantrone (58). This therapy used in patients with low-volume and platinum-sensitive recurrent disease achieved high response rates but very poor long-term survival rates. An attempt to move high-dose chemotherapy and stem cell transplantation into the primary treatment of ovarian cancer by the GOG was not possible owing to very poor accrual and premature closure of the study. The reasons for this failure included both patient and physician bias and lack of support by insurance companies. In Europe two randomized trials are comparing standard and high-dose therapies, and the results are anxiously awaited. Certainly until those studies are completed and results are available, high-dose chemotherapy and stem cell transplantation must be considered experimental.

FUTURE THERAPIES

The current therapy of advanced epithelial ovarian cancer remains inadequate. Even with incorporation of paclitaxel into the primary treatment regimen, the long-term (5-year) survival rate is only 27% in the study with the longest reported follow-up (41). Although this represents a 50% increase in survival over cyclophosphamide-based regimens, there are multiple agents now available with documented activity in the salvage treatment of platinum-resistant ovarian cancer. These "new" agents include pegylated liposomal doxorubicin, oral etoposide, gemcitabine, and topotecan. Soon international trials will be initiated to move these candidate agents into primary therapy. It is hoped that one or more of them will further improve the therapeutic envelope for advanced ovarian cancer. Additionally a large number of new cytostatic agents are now poised for clinical trial. These include angiogenesis inhibitors, metalloproteinase inhibitors, farnesyltransferase inhibitors, and tyrosine kinase inhibitors. These agents are best studied in patients with very low tumor burdens. The tumor burden in most patients with ovarian cancer can be reduced several logs with currently available cytotoxic therapies, but recurrence remains the rule rather than the exception. Evaluation of these agents for use in consolidation or maintenance after cytotoxic therapy offers another avenue of exploration that may improve the long-term outlook for these patients.

REFERENCES

1. Parker SL, Tong T, Bolden S, et al. Cancer statistics, 1997. *CA Cancer J Clin* 1997;47:5–27.
2. Hreschshyshyn MM, Park RC, Blessing JA, et al. The role of adjuvant therapy in stage I ovarian cancer. *Am J Obstet Gynecol* 1980;138:139–145.
3. Dembo AJ, Bush RS. Choice of postoperative therapy based on prognostic factors. *Int J Rad Oncol Biol Phys* 1982;8:893–897.
4. Dembo AJ, Davy M, Stenwig AE, et al. Prognostic factors in patients with stage I epithelial ovarian cancer. *Obstet Gynecol* 1990;75:263–273.
5. Bertelsen K, Hølund B, Andersen JE, et al. Prognostic factors and adjuvant treatment in early epithelial ovarian cancer. *Int J Gynecol Cancer* 1993;3:211–218.
6. Bertelsen K, Hølund B, Andersen E. Reproducibility and prognostic value of histologic type and grade in early ovarian cancer. *Int J Gynecol Cancer* 1993;3:72–79.
7. Vergote IB, Kaern J, Abeler VM, et al. Analysis of prognostic factors in stage I epithelial ovarian cancer: importance of degree of differentiation and deoxyribonucleic acid ploidy in predicting relapse. *Am J Obstet Gynecol* 1993;169:40–52.
8. Brugghe J, Baak JP, Wiltshaw E, et al. Quantitative prognostic features in FIGO I ovarian cancer patients without postoperative treatment. *Gynecol Oncol* 1998;68:47053.
9. Boente MP, Hamilton TC, Godwin AK, et al. Early ovarian cancer: a review of its genetic and biologic factors, detection and treatment. *Curr Probl Cancer* 1996;20:83–137.
10. Young RC, Walton LA, Ellenberg SS, et al. Adjuvant therapy in stage I and stage II epithelial ovarian cancer. *N Engl J Med* 1990;322:1021–1027, 1990.
11. Young RC, Brady MF, Nieberg RM, et al. Randomized clinical trial of adjuvant treatment on women with early (FIGO I–IIA high risk) ovarian cancer–GOG #95. *Proc Am Soc Clin Oncol* 1999;18:A1376.
12. Vergote IB, Vergote-De Vos LN, Abeler VM, et al. Randomized trial comparing cisplatin and radioactive phosphorus or whole-abdomen irradiation as adjuvant treatment of ovarian cancer. *Cancer* 1992;69:741–749.
13. Bolis G, et al. Multicenter controlled trial in patients with stage I epithelial ovarian cancer. *Proc Int Gynecol Cancer Soc* 1991; 3:16.
14. Hoskins WJ, Rubin SC. Surgery in the treatment of patients with advanced ovarian cancer. *Semin Oncol* 1991;18:213–221.
15. Neijt JP, ten Bokkel Huinink WW, van der Burg ME, et al. Long-term survival in ovarian cancer: mature data from the Netherlands Joint Study Group for Ovarian Cancer. *Eur J Cancer* 1991;27:1367–1372.
16. Omura GA, et al. Long-term follow-up and prognostic factor analysis in advanced ovarian carcinoma: the Gynecologic Oncology Group experience. *J Clin Oncol* 1991;9:1138–1150.
17. Marsoni S, et al. Prognostic factors in advanced epithelial ovarian cancer. *Br J Cancer* 1990;62:444–450.
18. van Houwelingen JC, et al. Predictability of the survival of patients with advanced ovarian cancer. *J Clin Oncol* 1989;7:769–773.
19. Luesley D, et al. Failure of second-look laparotomy to influence survival in epithelial ovarian cancer. *Lancet* 1988;2:599–603.
20. Ozols RF, Bundy BF, Fowler J, et al. Randomized phase III trial of cisplatin (CIS)/paclitaxel (PAC) versus carboplatin (CARBO)/PAC in optimal stage III epithelial ovarian cancer: a Gynecologic Oncology Group trial (GOG 158). *Proc Am Soc Clin Oncol* 1999;18: A1376.
21. McGuire WP, Harris WL. Chemotherapy of epithelial ovarian cancer. In: Deppe G, Baker VV, eds. *Gynecologic oncology*. New York: Oxford University Press, 1999:212–240.
22. Ovarian Cancer Meta-Analysis Group. Cyclophosphamide plus cisplatin versus cyclophosphamide, doxorubicin, and cisplatin chemotherapy of ovarian carcinoma: a meta-analysis. *J Clin Oncol* 1991;9:1669–1674.
23. Ahern RP, Gore ME. Impact of doxorubicin on survival in advanced ovarian cancer. *J Clin Oncol* 1995;13: 726–732.
24. Fanning J, Bennett TZ, Hilgers RD. Meta-analysis of cisplatin, doxorubicin, and cyclophosphamide chemotherapy of ovarian carcinoma. *Obstet Gynecol* 1993;80: 954–960.
25. Advanced Ovarian Trials Group. Chemotherapy in advanced ovarian cancer: an overview of randomized clinical trials. *Br Med J* 1991;303:884–893.
26. Williams CJ, Mend GM, Macbeth FR, et al. Cisplatin combination chemotherapy versus chlorambucil in advanced ovarian carcinoma: mature results of a randomized trial. *J Clin Oncol* 1985;3:1455–1462.
27. Neijt JP, et al. Randomised trial comparing two combination chemotherapy regimens (HEXACAF vs CHAP-5) in advanced ovarian cancer. *Lancet* 1984;2: 594–600.
28. Omura GA, et al. A randomized trial of cyclophosphamide and doxorubicin with or without cisplatin in advanced ovarian cancer. *Cancer* 1986;57:1725–1730.
29. Balvert-Locht HR, et al. Improved prognosis of ovarian cancer in the Netherlands during the period 1975–1985: a registry-based study. *Gynecol Oncol* 1991;42:3–8.
30. ICON2 Collaborators. ICON2: randomized trial of single-agent carboplatin against three-drug combination of CAP (cyclophosphamide, doxorubicin, and cisplatin) in women with ovarian cancer. *Lancet* 1998;352: 1571–1577.
31. Swenerton KD. Cisplatin/cyclophosphamide vs carboplatin/ cyclophosphamide in advanced ovarian cancer. *Proc Int Gynecol Cancer Soc* 1991;3:44.
32. Alberts DS, Green S, Hannigan EV, et al. Improved therapeutic index of carboplatin plus cyclophosphamide versus cisplatin plus cyclophosphamide: final report by the Southwest Oncology Group of a phase III randomized trial in stages III and IV ovarian cancer. *J Clin Oncol* 1992;10:683–685.
33. Mangioni C, Bolis G, Pecorelli S, et al. Randomized trial in advanced ovarian cancer comparing cisplatin and carboplatin. *J Natl Cancer Inst* 1989;81:1464–1471.
34. Alberts DS, Canetta R, Mason-Liddil N. Carboplatin in the first-line chemotherapy of advanced ovarian cancer. *Semin Oncol* 1990;17:54–60.

35. Rowinsky EK, Donehower RC. Paclitaxel. *N Engl J Med* 1995;332:1004–1014.
36. McGuire WP. Taxol: a new drug with significant activity as a salvage therapy in advanced epithelial ovarian carcinoma. *Gynecol Oncol* 1993;51:78–85.
37. McGuire WP, Rowinsky EK, Rosenshein NB, et al. Taxol: a unique antineoplastic agent with significant activity in advanced ovarian epithelial neoplasms. *Ann Intern Med* 1989;111:273–279.
38. Thigpen JT, Blessing JA, Ball H, et al. Phase II trial of paclitaxel in patients with progressive ovarian carcinoma after platinum-based chemotherapy; a Gynecologic Oncology Group study. *J Clin Oncol* 1994;12:1748–1753.
39. Markman M, Rothman R, Hakes T, et al. Second-line platinum therapy in patients with ovarian cancer previously treated with cisplatin. *J Clin Oncol* 1991;9:1692–1703.
40. Rowinsky EK, Gilbert MR, McGuire WP, et al. Sequences of taxol and cisplatin: phase I and pharmacologic study. *J Clin Oncol* 1991;9:1692–1703.
41. McGuire WP, Hoskins WJ, Brady MF, et al. Cyclophosphamide and cisplatin compared with paclitaxel and cisplatin in patients with stage III and stage IV ovarian cancer. *N Engl J Med* 1996;334:1–6, 1996.
42. Stuart G, Bertelsen K, Mangioni C, et al. Updated analysis shows a highly significant improved overall survival (OS) for cisplatin-paclitaxel as first line treatment of advanced ovarian cancer: mature results of the EORTC-GCCG, NOCOVA, NCIC-CTG, and Scottish Intergroup Trial. *Proc Am Soc Clin Oncol* 1998;17:A1394.
43. Connelly E, Markman M, Kennedy A, et al. Paclitaxel delivered as a 3-hr infusion with cisplatin in patients with gynecologic cancers: unexpected incidence of neurotoxicity. *Gynecol Oncol* 1996;62:166–168.
44. Muggia FM, Braly PS, Brady MF, et al. Phase III randomized study of cisplatin versus paclitaxel versus cisplatin and paclitaxel in patients with suboptimal stage III or IV ovarian cancer: a Gynecologic Oncology Group study. *J Clin Oncol* 2000;18:106–115.
45. Harper P. A randomized comparison of paclitaxel and carboplatin versus a control arm of single agent carboplatin or CAP (cyclophosphamide, doxorubicin and cisplatin): 2075 patients randomized into the 3rd International Collaborative Ovarian Neoplasms Study (ICON-3). *Proc Am Soc Clin Oncol* 1999;18:A1375.
46. Berek JS, Bertelsen K, du Bois A, et al. Advanced epithelial ovarian cancer: 1998 consensus statements. *Ann Oncol* 1999;10 [Suppl 1]:87–92.
47. Piccart MJ, du Bois A, Gore ME, et al. A new standard of care for treatment of ovarian cancer. *Eur J Cancer* 2000;36:10–12.
48. Omura GA, Brady MF, Delmore JE, et al. A randomized trial of paclitaxel at 2 dose levels and filgrastim at 2 dose levels in platinum pretreated epithelial ovarian cancer: Gynecologic Oncology Group, SWOG, NCCTG and ECOG study. *Proc Am Soc Clin Oncol* 1996;15:A755.
49. Rowinsky EK. The taxanes: dosing and scheduling considerations. *Oncology* 1997;11[3 Suppl 2]:7–19.
50. Eisenhauer EA, ten Bokkel Huinink WW, Swenerton KD, et al. European-Canadian randomized trail of paclitaxel in relapsed ovarian cancer: high-dose versus low-dose and long versus short infusion. *J Clin Oncol* 1994;12:2654–2666.
51. Liebman JE, Cook JA, Lipschultz C, et al. Cytotoxic studies of paclitaxel in human tumour cell lines. *Br J Cancer* 1993;68:1104–1109.
52. Bookman MA, McGuire WP, Kilpatrick D, et al. Carboplatin and paclitaxel in ovarian carcinoma: a phase I study of the Gynecologic Oncology Group. *J Clin Oncol* 1996;14:1895–1902.
53. Ozols RF, Bundy BN, Fowler J, et al. Randomized phase III study of cisplatin/paclitaxel vs. carboplatin/paclitaxel in optimal stage III ovarian cancer: a Gynecologic Oncology Group trial. *Proc Am Soc Clin Oncol* 1999;18:A1373.
54. Neijt JP, Engelholm SA, Witteveen PO, et al. Paclitaxel (175 mg/m^2 over 3 hours) with cisplatin or carboplatin in previously untreated ovarian cancer. *Semin Oncol* 1997;24[5 Suppl 15]:36–39.
55. Levin L, Hryniuk WM. Dose intensity analyses of chemotherapy regimens in ovarian cancer. *J Clin Oncol* 1987;5:756–767.
56. McGuire WP. How many more nails to seal the coffin of dose intensity. *Ann Oncol* 1997;8:311–313.
57. Thigpen JT. Dose intensity in ovarian carcinoma: hold, enough? *J Clin Oncol* 1997;15:1291–1293.

14
Second-Look Laparotomy

Thomas C. Randall and Stephen C. Rubin

The term second-look laparotomy (SLL) is used to indicate a systematic surgical reexploration performed in asymptomatic patients who have no clinical evidence of persistent tumor after initial surgery and a planned program of chemotherapy for ovarian cancer. The procedure remains both an important surrogate for overall survival in the evaluation of clinical trials and the only reliable indicator of disease status in ovarian cancer patients after initial therapy (1).

Despite this precise and widely accepted definition, there is often confusion in the literature of SLL with other secondary operations for ovarian cancer. Some of these secondary operations for ovarian cancer are the following.

- *Surgical staging*—The patient was found to have ovarian cancer on a previous surgery, but has not undergone indicated systematic surgical staging.
- *Debulking*—The patient had only diagnostic surgery or otherwise had residual disease after surgery under less than ideal circumstances and is taken to the operating room in the interest of achieving optimal surgical cytoreduction before chemotherapy is initiated.
- *Interval surgical cytoreduction*—At initial surgery, the patient is found to have unresectable disease; she is taken back to the operating room after several cycles of chemotherapy with the intention of removing tumor that has now been rendered resectable.
- *Reassessment laparotomy*—The patient is known to have persistent disease after initial surgery and chemotherapy, but she is taken to the operating room to more accurately evaluate the extent of response to therapy or to facilitate some form of salvage therapy.
- *Palliative operations*—The patient has known persistent or progressive disease and undergoes surgery for bowel obstruction, fistula, or some other complication of her disease.

Over the past 50 years, SLL has emerged from an obscure, reportable technique to become an integral component of ovarian cancer management. In the 1970s and 1980s, performance of SLL became the expected standard of care, and at many centers the majority of women who were eligible underwent SLL. Greater understanding of the implications and utility of SLL findings and a greater interest in patient autonomy and quality of life have inspired many surgeons to individualize the use of SLL (2), whereas others have simply abandoned it (3).

Proponents of SLL cite its accuracy, its low morbidity, and the potential therapeutic value of consolidation therapy and secondary cytoreduction at the time of SLL. Detractors of the procedure note the potential negative influence on the patient's quality of life, significant recurrence rate despite negative SLL, lack of effective salvage therapy for women shown to have persistent disease, and lack of proven consolidation therapy for women shown to be free of detectable disease. A further criticism is that only a small proportion of women traditionally undergoing SLL are likely to benefit from secondary cytoreduction in this setting.

An unfortunate corollary of this ongoing controversy is that the performance of SLL has become somewhat variable, and practice patterns often seem related more to the preference of the individual surgeon than to the indications and preferences of the particular patient. It is important, therefore, for each physician caring for women with ovarian cancer to become sufficiently versed in the history, indications, implications, and execution of the procedure so as to enable the patient to make an informed personal decision about this potentially valuable component of ovarian cancer care.

HISTORY OF SECOND-LOOK SURGERY

In 1951, Wangensteen coined the term "second-look" operation to describe his findings in a series patients who underwent surgical exploration to assess the results of treatment of their gastrointestinal malignancies (4). These patients were selected for their high risk of recurrence based on the finding of involved regional lymph nodes at the initial operation, and reexplorations were subsequently carried out at specific intervals even though the patients were asymptomatic and without clinical evidence of carcinoma. The purpose was to identify residual or recurrent disease as early as possible, when the chances for further effective treatment were best. Wangensteen showed that about half of these patients had persistent disease, the morbidity of the surgery was low, and a small number of patients with residual carcinoma could be salvaged by further therapy.

With regard to ovarian cancer, the term "second-look" was initially used with a variety of meanings. In 1941, Marchetti described a series of patients with "inoperable" ovarian cancer who underwent exploratory laparotomy, biopsy, and then radiation therapy, making possible a second operation for cancer removal (5). In 1945, Parks reported a similar experience (6).

The contemporary understanding and definition of SLL for ovarian cancer has evolved from investigations at the M.D. Anderson Cancer Center in Houston. In 1966, Rutledge and Burns reported on 288 patients with advanced ovarian cancer who had been treated with melphalan and asked the question, "Should laparotomy be used more often when a patient has an unusually good response to determine if the drug should be discontinued?" (7). In their series, 28 patients underwent exploration for this indication, and 12 had presented after 4 to 35 months of chemotherapy. Two of these patients had a recurrence during the follow-up of the study. The authors concluded that "a good response to the drug is reason for laparotomy" and further pointed out that the absence of cancer at reexploration does not guarantee cure.

In 1970, reports of chemotherapy-induced leukemia provided further motivation to discontinue chemotherapy after true remission is attained. To this end, in 1976, Smith and colleagues at M.D. Anderson reported long-term follow-up results on 103 patients who had undergone SLL (8). They stipulated the absence of clinical disease as a precondition for the surgery and stressed the importance of the procedure in allowing discontinuation of therapy for those women who were surgically disease free. By the late 1970s SLL began to become a part of the routine management of most patients with ovarian cancer.

Initial series of SLLs were performed in the setting of prolonged treatments with alkylating agents, and overall response rates for patients with advanced ovarian cancer were reported to be 30% to 50%. With the advent of multiagent regimens (9), single-agent cisplatinum, and, ultimately, multiagent platinum-containing regimens, overall response rates in excess of 70% became achievable. Interestingly, the proportion of patients found to be disease free at the time of SLL remained somewhat consistent across series using different chemotherapy regimens across a wide range of efficacy. Presumably this was related to the fact that the prolonged use of less effective agents allowed many patients to experience recurrence before SLL. Since patients tend to respond more rapidly to platinum-based chemotherapy, patients so treated became eligible for SLL sooner in their clinical course, and therefore no such elimination of women with early relapses occurred. Unfortunately, it has now been shown that relapse rates are higher for patients with negative SLL after treatment with platinum-based chemotherapy (10). For some surgeons, this has led to disenchantment with the procedure. However, as reviewed later in this chapter, a negative SLL after platinum-based therapy, although not synonymous with cure, provides considerable prognostic information and may help to better direct further management.

In 1993, Williams and colleagues reported the experience of the Gynecologic Oncology Group (GOG) with SLL in the management of malignant ovarian germ cell tumors (11). Among 45 women in their series who underwent SLL after complete surgical cytoreduction and chemotherapy, 43 had surgically documented complete responses to initial therapy. One of these women had a recurrence and died despite aggressive salvage therapy. Of the women found to have disease at SLL, both were alive and disease free on follow-up. Among patients with incomplete cytoreduction at initial surgery, it was found that the presence of teratoma elements determined the utility of SLL. Of 48 patients with suboptimal debulking who had no teratoma elements in their primary tumors, 45 had negative SLL and three had persistent endodermal sinus tumor or embryonal cell carcinoma. All of these latter 3 patients died despite aggressive salvage therapy. Among the 22 women who had teratoma elements in their primary tumors, 16 had mature teratoma at SLL, which in 7 women was bulky or progressive. Fourteen of these 16 women and 6 of the 7 with bulky or progressive disease were disease free at follow-up after surgical resection. Therefore, it appears that, among patients with malignant germ cell tumors of the ovary, SLL should be restricted to those women who have teratoma elements in their primary tumors and who have incomplete cytoreduction at initial surgery.

Similarly, in 1993, Rubin and colleagues published their experience at Memorial Sloan-Kettering Cancer Center with SLL in women with stage I epithelial ovarian cancer (12). In this group of 54 women who had undergone thorough surgical staging, only 3 (5.5%) had a positive SLL. At 48 months of follow-up, more than half of the women with grade 3 tumors and none of those with grade 1 or 2 tumors, had experienced a recurrence. Therefore, SLL does not appear to contribute to the management of properly surgically staged patients with stage I epithelial ovarian cancer. Concordant with this finding is the trend over time for surgeons to restrict SLL to those women who present with advanced-stage disease.

DETERMINATION OF DISEASE STATUS BEFORE SECOND-LOOK LAPAROTOMY

The evaluation of any ovarian cancer patient after her planned course of chemotherapy should begin with a careful physical examination, with particular attention paid to the pelvic examination. An individual with an extensive understanding of the postoperative pelvic anatomy, ideally the person who performed the initial surgery, should perform this examination. Any abnormal mass or nodularity found in this clinical setting can be assumed to signify recurrent or persistent disease. If there is any reason to doubt this, it is usually straightforward to perform a fine-needle aspiration or core biopsy of the affected area.

Many authors have reported the relationship of the serum marker CA 125 to SLL findings. As shown in Table 14.1, an elevated CA 125 value at the conclusion of primary chemotherapy is almost invariably associated with persistent disease at SLL. A normal result in this setting is less meaningful, because about half of such patients will be found to have persistent disease at SLL. It is unclear why patients can have normalization of an increased CA 125 level after surgery and chemotherapy in the setting of persistent disease. Although it has been speculated that this phenomenon might be caused by the elimination of CA 125+ cell clones (13), immunohistochemical studies have shown that the residual tumor frequently has rich expression of the antigen (14). Therefore, the absence of detectable CA 125 in serum may be caused by poor perfusion of the

TABLE 14.1. *CA 125 Value before second-look laparotomy (SLL) (data from 15 series, 686 patients)*

CA 125	Positive SLL/ total surgeries	Percent positive
Normal	229/497	46
Elevated	179/189	95

From references 13, 42, 45, 92, 94–102, and 104, with permission.

TABLE 14.2. *Correlation of computed tomography scan results with second-look laparotomy (SLL) (data from 10 series, 397 patients)*

Scan result	Positive SLL/ total surgeries	Percent positive
Positive	73/92	79
Negative	111/216	49

From references 16, 45, 91, 92, and 106–111, with permission.

tumor or some other isolation of the tumor from the circulation.

Computed tomography (CT) also has been extensively used in the diagnosis and monitoring of ovarian cancer. Although improvements in this technology have been frequently made, its sensitivity in practice remains too low to reasonably replace SLL. As shown in Table 14.2, the sensitivity of CT to detect disease in patients at high risk for persistence at a variety of academic centers is less than 50%. In many series, masses 2 cm in diameter or larger were found after negative CT (15). The specificity of CT in this setting is generally quite good. If there is reason to doubt that a mass represents persistent or recurrent disease, confirmation can usually be obtained by fine-needle aspiration.

A number of other techniques have been investigated to determine disease status in ovarian cancer patients who are in clinical remission after primary surgery and chemotherapy. Although some of these techniques have appeared promising in their ability to identify a proportion of patients with persistent disease, none has proved as accurate as SLL.

Ultrasonography has been investigated as a means to determine disease in ovarian cancer patients and appears to offer little advantage over CT (16). Sonography is somewhat less suited in its imaging characteristics for detecting small-volume persistent disease. Documented limitations of ultrasound studies include their inability to detect retroperitoneal adenopathy smaller than 3 cm in diameter, omental plaques less than 1.5 cm in thickness, mesenteric masses smaller than 5 cm, and peritoneal masses of 2 cm or less (17–20).

Magnetic resonance imaging (MRI) has also been used to monitor ovarian cancer and is increasingly used to evaluate ovarian masses. MRI usually provides excellent views of retroperitoneal or other extraperitoneal pathology. Perhaps because this technology is sensitive to motion artifact, MRI shows no improvement over CT scanning in the detection of 1- to 5-mm implants within the peritoneal cavity.

In 1976, McGowan and Bunnag described the use of culdocentesis to obtain cytologic specimens from the peritoneal cavity in women being monitored for ovarian cancer and were able to demonstrate that the presence of malignant cells was a poor prognostic indicator (21). In 1985, Goldberg and colleagues performed postchemotherapy culdocentesis in 44 women with advanced-stage ovarian cancer (22). Among 12 patients with negative cytology on culdocentesis, 11 were found to have a histologically negative SLL. Although these authors concluded that culdocentesis might therefore be performed in place of SLL, their finding is inconsistent with a number of larger trials, in which patients were frequently found to have a pathologically positive SLL in the absence of positive washings. In a study of 96 women reexplored for ovarian cancer, for example, Rubin and colleagues found that only 28% of patients with microscopic disease and 34% of those with grossly visible disease had positive washings (23). Because culdocentesis appears to be significantly less accurate than SLL and does not allow assessment of the location and extent of tumor or removal of tumor, it is rarely used today.

TECHNIQUE OF SECOND-LOOK LAPAROTOMY

SLL is intended to be a thorough surgical reassessment of the entire peritoneal cavity and retroperitoneal lymph nodes. Before performing the procedure, the surgeon should review the findings of the patient's initial surgery with particular attention the extent of the original disease, the surgical procedures performed, and the size and location of any residual tumor masses. The patient should have a thorough bowel preparation, because it is not uncommon to encounter significant adhesions intraoperatively. The operation should begin with a careful examination under anesthesia. Cystoscopy and proctoscopy may be performed to further exclude persistent disease, although in most patients in complete clinical remission the yield of these procedures is very low. If there is evidence of disease on the examination under anesthesia, an exploration may be carried out to better define the extent and resectability of disease, but the operation should not be recorded as an SLL.

The abdomen is entered through a generous midline incision that allows adequate exposure of the upper abdominal structures. Washings should be obtained from the pelvis, from the right and left paracolic gutters, and from under the right and left hemidiaphragms. Detectable adhesions should be lysed. Because adhesions often form at the site of tumor nodules, a portion of any adhesion should be submitted for pathologic analysis. A complete and systematic exploration of the upper abdomen is then performed, and any suspicious areas should be biopsied. Any residual momentum or paraaortic nodal tissue should be inspected and resected. The bowel must be freed and examined in its entirety. A thorough exploration of the pelvis is performed, with particular attention paid to any sites of residual tumor at the time of the initial surgery; as observed by Phibbs and colleagues (24), these sites are frequently found to have persistent disease at SLL.

If tumor is found, the most common site of disease is the pelvis. Podczaski and colleagues reported that among 27 patients with grossly positive SLL, disease was found at the primary site in 25 (93%) (25). In the same series, patients who had only microscopic residual tumor were found to have disease at the site of their primary tumor 67% of the time. If tumor is identified or suspected, the tissue should be sent for frozen section. The location and extent of all tumor masses should be carefully documented. Once disease is identified, the goal becomes the removal of as much tumor as is possible and reasonable. The procedure may be concluded after no gross disease remains.

If tumor is not identified, the surgeon should undertake to biopsy or remove areas that frequently harbor residual disease. The pedicles of the ovarian vessels should be identified and biopsied. Hysterectomy should be performed if it was not done at the initial operation. Multiple peritoneal biopsies should be performed, particularly from the pelvic cul-de-sac, the pelvic sidewalls, both paracolic gutters, and both hemidiaphragms. The retroperitoneal spaces should be explored and biopsies taken from the paraaortic and pelvic lymph nodes. If no disease is found, most surgeons will take 20 to 30 biopsies. Friedman and associates reported that the yield and significance of SLL is improved when more than 100 specimens are obtained (26). The search for tumor at SLL must be meticulous and exhaustive. Frequently, only tiny areas of tumor are identified that could easily be overlooked.

TIMING OF SECOND-LOOK LAPAROTOMY

The optimal time for the performance of SLL has been a source of considerable controversy. The question actually encompasses two separate issues: the optimal duration of the chemotherapy itself and the optimal interval from the conclusion of chemotherapy to the surgery. As mentioned earlier, early series of SLL involved patients who had been treated with single alkylating agent therapy for 18 to 24 months or longer. It is now clear that platinum-containing regimens are superior to those previously used. Two large trials have attempted to determine the optimal duration of platinum-based chemotherapy regimens (27,28). In comparisons of 12 versus 6 and 10 versus 5 cycles of platinum, Adriamycin, and cyclophosphamide, neither trial demonstrated a superiority of prolonged treatment in either initial response or long-term survival.

The issue of the optimal interval from the conclusion of chemotherapy to SLL has not been thoroughly investigated. It has been common practice to perform the surgery as soon as the patient's blood counts show satisfactory recovery. This has generally been done so that treatment may be reinstituted for those women with persistent disease as quickly as possible. In the absence of clear evidence that this very early second-line therapy confers a survival advantage, however, it seems quite reasonable to leave the timing of the surgery up to the patient's preference and convenience.

COMPLICATIONS OF SECOND-LOOK LAPAROTOMY

Given that SLL is a major abdominal operation undertaken in patients with cancer and recent chemotherapy who have had prior extensive abdominal surgeries, the rate of complications might be expected to be high. In 18 series of SLLs involving 1,292 patients, there was 1 death (0.08%) related to severe adhesions and bowel obstruction. The overall rate of other complications was low, with wound infection (5.7%), urinary tract infection (4.2%), and paralytic ileus (3.3%) being the most common (25,29–45). Despite the fact that it is frequently necessary to perform an extensive lysis of intestinal adhesions to complete the procedure, the rates of intestinal injury and obstruction are low.

FINDINGS AT SECOND-LOOK LAPAROTOMY

The primary purpose of SLL is the identification of persistent disease. In 74 reported series of SLLs including 5,518 patients, 2,905 (53%) were found to have persistent disease (Table 14.3). Remarkably, this proportion of positive SLL is found consistently even in recent series. Despite constant reports of promising approaches and technologies, the ability to nonsurgically determine disease status remains poor.

Many authors have related clinical and pathologic factors to the probability of finding disease at SLL. The most consistent predictors of persistent disease at the time of SLL are stage and the volume of tumor remaining at the completion of initial surgery. Patients found to have stage III or IV disease at initial surgery have a much higher likelihood of positive SLL (67%) than do women with stage I or II disease (20% to 30%).

TABLE 14.3. Findings at second-look laparotomy from 74 combined series

Finding	Number	Percent
No tumor found	2,613	47
Tumor found	2,905	53
Total	5,518	100

From references 13, 15, 18, 20, 29–48, 54, 57, 58, 61, 64, 65, 80, and 6, with permission.

TABLE 14.4. Findings at second-look laparotomy by extent of residual disease after primary cytoreduction

Residual[a]	No. negative	Total patients	Percent negative
None	331	460	72
Optimal	369	706	52
Suboptimal	187	746	25

[a] According to authors' definition.
From references 25, 29, 30, 32, 33, 35–38, 41, 45, 46, 50, 54, 85, 87, 90, 112, 115, 117, 120, 122, 124, and 128, with permission.

The volume of tumor remaining at the close of the initial surgery is also highly predictive of the outcome of SLL. As shown in Table 14.4, patients with no residual tumor at the close of initial surgery had only a 28% chance of having a positive SLL, compared with 48% for women with visible but optimally debulked tumor after initial surgery and 75% for women with suboptimally debulked tumor. Although many older series included stage I patients among those with no residual tumor, it appears clear that there is an independent effect of residual tumor volume at initial surgery on the outcome of SLL.

In many series it appears that tumor grade is also a predictor of SLL outcome, and pooling the data to include patients with stage I to IV disease, who were treated with a variety of chemotherapy regimens, supports this observation. Therefore, it appears that women with poorly differentiated tumors have a somewhat higher risk of positive SLL. These data are not adjusted for stage and amount of residual tumor at initial surgery, and grade may simply be a covariate with these other predictors. In addition, this trend is less apparent in series of patients with advanced-stage tumors treated with platinum-based chemotherapy regimens.

Although a negative SLL is not indicative of cure, the information gained is clearly of prognostic value. Lippman and associates (46) showed a significantly increased survival rate for patients with negative versus positive SLL (0.013). Podczaski and colleagues (47) demonstrated a 5-year survival rate of 80% after negative SLL, compared with 47% for microscopically positive SLL, 30% for gross disease up to 2 cm in diameter at SLL, and 10% if tumor greater than 2 cm in diameter were found. DeGramont and associates (48) had similar findings and additionally observed that patients whose tumor was larger than 2 cm at SLL appeared to live longer if the disease was partially removed. In a recent series, Katsoulis and coworkers (50) found that, among patients with stages III and IV ovarian cancer, the presence of residual disease at initial surgery and the outcome of SLL were the strongest predictors of survival. When stepwise logistic regression was performed, only the result of SLL remained a significant predictor of survival in their material.

NEGATIVE SECOND-LOOK LAPAROTOMY

The development of current chemotherapy regimens for ovarian cancer, using platinum and paclitaxel, has resulted in very high initial response rates; however, many of these women ultimately have recurrence and die from their disease. It is now of mainly historical significance that early series of SLL found rates of recurrence after negative SLL in the range of 20% to 30% (21). In an analysis of patients with negative SLL after platinum-based chemotherapy, however, Rubin and colleagues documented a recurrence rate of 50% (51). It is likely that earlier series observed a lower rate of recurrence after negative SLL because the longer treatments required with alkylating agents had the effect of screening out patients who had early recurrences before they became candidates for SLL. In subsequent analyses, Rubin and colleagues found disease-free survival rates of 75% at 2 years, 55% at 5 years, and 52% at 10 years after negative SLL (10,52). Bolis and coworkers found disease-free survival rates of 57% at 3 years, 50% at 5 years, and 43% at 8 years after negative SLL (53). It appears from these long-term follow-up studies that the majority of patients who have a recurrence after negative SLL do so in the first 2 to 3 years after the procedure, while those who are disease free at 5 years have an excellent survival outlook.

Clinical and pathologic factors that predict disease recurrence after a negative SLL have been evaluated in a number of series. In the majority of series the presence of residual tumor at the conclusion of initial surgery, increasing tumor grade, and advanced-stage disease are associated with an increased risk of recurrence (48,51,54–57). As reported by Rubin and colleagues, the long-term survival rate for patients with less than 2 cm residual tumor after initial surgery was almost 70%, while that of patients with more than 2 cm of tumor at the end of initial surgery was less than 30%. Other factors that have been less consistently reported as predictive of recurrence after negative SLL include age, unfavorable histology (e.g., clear cell, undifferentiated), and number of biopsies performed during the SLL.

Although the finding has not been supported by all series, both Rome and Fortune (44) and Gershenson and coworkers (58) showed a trend toward decreased recurrence with a greater number of biopsies that in the latter study reached significance. Friedman and colleagues (26) reported on a series of patients who had surgical cytoreduction to less than 1 cm residual tumor, followed by platinum-based chemotherapy and SLL. At an average follow-up of 3 years, 28% of these patients had experienced a recurrence. The authors noted that this rate is lower than in other series and suggested that they may have had a lower rate of false-negative SLL because all of their patients who underwent SLL had at least 100 peritoneal biopsies performed as well as lymph node sampling. It is also possible, however, that the low recurrence rate reported is more a tribute to the initial surgical effort than to the SLL technique employed.

Known risk factors for recurrence can provide the oncologist and the patient with a fairly clear idea of the stratum of risk that is faced. This in turn can suggest which patients would be best served by further therapy. One frustration of SLL has been the absence of suitable consolidation regimens for those patients who are without documented disease on reexploration. Some recent results, however, begin to offer hope that reasonably effective consolidation regimens may soon become available.

Barakat and colleagues (59) reported the results of a phase II trial performed at the Memorial Sloan-Kettering Cancer Center in which 36 patients were treated with intraperitoneal cisplatin and etoposide after negative SLL. They found that the toxicity of the regimen was acceptable and, on comparison to a contemporaneous group of 46 women who underwent observation alone after SLL, there was a significant increase in disease-free survival. In a small trial, Pickel and associates (60) found that disease-free survival of 15 patients who received intermittent cisplatin after negative SLL was superior to that of a control group who underwent observation alone.

Another possible application of intraperitoneal therapy in this setting is the administration of the radiocolloid ^{32}P chromic phosphate. Varia (61) and Spencer (62) and their colleagues have shown that the intraperitoneal administration of ^{32}P appears to improve disease-free survival after negative SLL, and the GOG has completed accrual for a randomized clinical trial (GOG Protocol 93) to better answer this question.

POSITIVE SECOND-LOOK LAPAROTOMY

Patients found to have persistent disease at SLL represent a heterogeneous clinical group. Many patients in this group, for instance those with bulky residual tumor after initial surgery who now have only microscopic persistent disease at SLL, have had a significant partial response to platinum-based chemotherapy. Others may have simply progressive tumor that demonstrates little or no sensitivity to platinum. This disparity is most easily expressed by the volume of tumor that is found at the time of SLL. As stated earlier, the 5-year survival rates for women with microscopic disease, gross disease smaller than 2 cm, and gross disease larger than 2 cm at SLL are 47%, 30%, and 10%, respectively. The published experience with salvage therapy is concordant with these figures in that some activity has been observed in salvage treatment of low-volume persistent disease, but only minimal activity has been found with any modality in patients who have a significant volume of tumor remaining after first-line therapy.

Secondary Cytoreduction at Second-Look Laparotomy

About 75% of patients with persistent disease at SLL have gross tumor. The observation that the volume of disease remaining after SLL is highly correlated with survival, as well as a wealth of data supporting the therapeutic value of cytoreduction at initial surgery (63), has prompted the majority of surgeons to attempt to resect tumor at the time of SLL. This has not been found to be associated with undue morbidity. Although series have been reported that both support (64,65) and refute (42,44) the value of surgical cytoreduction at the time of SLL, the data reported from larger, more rigorously defined series of patients treated with platinum-based chemotherapy favor a significant beneficial effect.

Hoskins and colleagues (65) reported that the 5-year survival rate for those patients, disease reduced to microscopic volume at SLL was as good as that for patients found to have microscopic disease on SLL (51% versus 62%, $p = .55$). In contrast, the rate for patients with gross disease remaining after SLL was 10%. Most of these women had stage III or IV disease and were treated with platinum-based chemotherapy. Podratz and colleagues (64) found that women with secondary cytoreduction to microscopic disease at SLL had a 5-year survival rate of 55%, compared with 14% for women with tumor residual greater than 5 mm diameter after SLL. Similarly, Lippman and coworkers (46) found that patients who underwent resection at SLL to less than 2 cm tumor masses had a 5-year survival rate of 40%, whereas no patients with residual tumor of 2 cm diameter or larger lived 3 years after SLL.

Using data prospectively acquired by the GOG, Williams and colleagues (66) evaluated the utility of secondary debulking at the time SLL. All of these patients had suboptimally cytoreduced advanced-stage disease and were treated with platinum-based chemotherapy under the scrutiny of the cooperative group. Although the ultimate survival of all patients was poor, they found that the survival of patients with gross disease "redebulked" to microscopic disease was as good as that of patients who were found to have microscopic disease on SLL. They further found that in each category of tumor volume the risk of death was decreased by cytoreduction to a lower level. Consistent with previous data, fewer than 5% of patients experienced any bowel or urinary injury, and fewer than 10% received a transfusion.

As with primary cytoreduction, it is not clear whether the improved survival that is associated with debulking at the time of SLL is a result of removal of tumor or simply a surrogate marker for a more favorable tumor biology. Although it has been correctly observed that this question cannot be answered until a randomized, controlled trial is performed, given the number of outcomes and variables involved such a trial would be difficult to design and execute. Many patients will be treated before such a trial is completed. From the available data it is clear that "redebulking" at the time of SLL is feasible, is associated with limited morbidity, and is strongly associated with an improvement in survival. Certainly cytoreduction should be performed in women who are undergoing SLL. Whether there is sufficient benefit to justify SLL as a therapeutic intervention for a subset of patients remains to be determined.

Salvage Chemotherapy after Positive Second look Laparotomy

Consistent with the apparent survival benefit of tumor reduction at SLL, clinical response to salvage chemotherapy varies significantly according to the volume of tumor remaining at the end of SLL. As stated earlier, much of this variation is a reflection of the patient's response to initial therapy; bulky disease is generally resistant to platinum-based therapy, and the response of such disease to salvage regimens is unusual. There are numerous reports in the literature of trials of various salvage regimens for platinum-resistant ovarian cancer. Perhaps most indicative of the poor results achieved in this setting is the fact that, although several generations of primary chemotherapy for ovarian cancer have been developed, no regimen aimed at platinum-resistant disease has been tested in a phase III trial in the cooperative group setting. Despite the activity of platinum-based regimens in other settings, and others Podratz (64) have noted the futility of continuing platinum-based therapy for women with apparent progression on initial therapy.

Although cure is uncommon for patients with persistent disease at SLL, some improvement in palliation or duration of survival has been achieved inpatients with low-volume disease. One approach for patients with low-volume disease has been the use of intraperitoneal chemotherapy. The theoretical advantage of intraperitoneal administration of chemotherapy is that higher concentrations of the agent may be achieved within the peritoneal cavity, where most if not all of the persistent disease is found. Preclinical and phase I studies led by Markman (67) showed that the concentrations achieved with intraperitoneal administration of cisplatinum are two to three logs higher than those achieved with intravenous administration. A significant minority of patients with persistent disease at SLL have extraperitoneal disease (51). One possible disadvantage of such treatment is that exposure of extraperitoneal tumor is not improved, so toxicity might be increased without improving cure.

The GOG studied the effect of intraperitoneal cisplatinum and thiotepa in patients with 0.5 cm or less of surgically documented residual tumor and demonstrated partial platinum sensitivity. They demonstrated a total response rate of 21%, comparable to the response rates seen with a variety of second-line chemotherapy agents in patients with platinum-resistant tumor (68). Therefore, it does not appear that intraperitoneal administration of platinum allows one to "overcome partial-platinum resistance" as has been suggested (67).

Markman and associates reported a trial in which patients were treated with intraperitoneal paclitaxel after SLL findings positive for 0.5 cm or less residual tumor volume (49). Of 28 patients with microscopic disease at the start of intraperitoneal therapy, 17 (61%) had a surgically defined complete response, but of 31 patients with residual macroscopic disease at the start of intraperitoneal therapy, only 1 (4%) had a complete response.

Another possible improvement suggested in therapy after positive SLL has been the addition of immunotherapy to chemotherapy. Bruzzone and colleagues reported the results of a trial of intraperitoneal carboplatin with and without interferon-$\alpha 2$ for patients found to have small-volume residual disease at SLL (69). They found that the median progression-free survival time was the same for both groups (11 months for chemotherapy alone, 10 months for chemotherapy plus interferon) while the toxicity of the combined regimen was higher.

The absence of a clearly effective salvage regimen for patients found to have disease at SLL is pertinent to a recent analysis published by Ozols and colleagues (70). They evaluated the influence of SLL on the survival of patients enrolled in a prospective, randomized trial of Taxol and either cisplatin or carboplatin for women who had minimal residual tumor after initial surgery for ovarian cancer (GOG Protocol 158). At the time of enrollment patients were asked to decide whether to undergo a second-look procedure after the planned chemotherapy. Ozols and colleagues observe that the patients who had SLL performed had no appreciable improvement in survival over those not undergoing SLL and argued that SLL should no longer be a part of the management of ovarian cancer. Such a proscription of the procedure based on these data may not be appropriate, however, for several reasons. First, one should not underestimate the value that patients place on the prognostic information gained from the procedure. Second, because all patients in this trial had optimal residual tumor volume after their initial surgery, those who were found to have disease at SLL in this setting had disease that was progressive on platinum-based chemotherapy. Therefore, in these women there is no opportunity to evaluate the effect of secondary cytoreduction in patients with partially chemosensitive disease. Third, because patients were treated with second-line chemotherapy after recurrence, these data demonstrate that the early institution of second-line chemotherapy based on a positive SLL provides no benefit over waiting for clinical signs of recurrence. Therefore, it may be more appropriate to recognize these data as an indictment of our currently available second-line chemotherapy rather than a condemnation of SLL in all settings.

RADIATION THERAPY AFTER SECOND-LOOK LAPAROTOMY

Although the idea of using a different treatment modality for consolidation or salvage therapy is conceptually attractive, because of the theoretical and practical limitations of radiation therapy it is no longer in widespread use for the secondary treatment of ovarian cancer. Possible advantages of radiation therapy for ovarian cancer include use of a different antitumor modality and treatment of the entire abdominal cavity, to which ovarian cancer is limited for most of its natural history. Disadvantages of radiation therapy include (a) lack of convincing data to demonstrate its efficacy, (b) lack of therapeutic effect outside of the abdominal cavity, (c) significant short- and long-term side-effects, and (d) limit of doses to the upper abdomen due to the relatively low radiotolerance of the liver and kidneys.

Both preclinical studies (71) and clinical experience (72) show that ovarian cancer radiosensitivity is decreased in platinum-resistant tumors. In reviewing the experience of ovarian cancer treatment using whole-abdomen radiotherapy, Thomas observed that "overall, the balance of evidence is against a significant curative effect for radiotherapy as salvage or consolidation therapy, at least in the situations where it has been used" (73). She also observed that, if morbidity is to be limited, abdominal radiotherapy should be limited to 25 Gy or less, initial chemotherapy should be limited to six cycles, and surgery should be limited to initial debulking and SLL. Such patients have certainly not exhausted their options for chemotherapy treatment, and therefore whole-abdomen radiation therapy seems ill advised unless it is given in the setting of a clinical trial or unless stronger evidence of its efficacy emerges.

SECOND-LOOK LAPAROSCOPY

Cost and postoperative morbidity and recovery are significant disadvantages of SLL. Since 1973 it has been established that it is feasible to perform laparoscopy to assess disease status after initial surgery and chemotherapy for ovarian cancer. Ozols and coworkers reported on 66 "restaging" laparoscopies performed at the NCI (74). In their experience, no patient had intestinal injury or other complications requiring exploration; however, 55% of those patients who had negative laparoscopies were found to have persistent disease on laparotomy. Similarly, in 1981, Berek and associates reported 119 laparoscopies performed on 57 ovarian cancer patients (75). In

14% of their cases, there were major complications requiring laparotomy. Most of these cases involved bowel injury caused by adhesions.

In the interim, however, the safety and utilization of laparoscopy have increased dramatically. Given the advances in technology and facility with laparoscopy, it may be appropriate to reconsider the value of the technique. Several reports suggest that second-look laparoscopy may be a reasonable alternative to SLL assuming that the proper equipment, training, and skills have been obtained.

Childers and colleagues reported on 44 "restaging" laparoscopies, of which 24 (55%) were positive (76). The mean operative time was 75 minutes, and significant complications occurred in 14% of patients, including injuries to the vena cava, the colon, and the ileum (one each). At a mean follow-up of 28 months, 8 (40%) of 20 patients had recurrence after negative laparoscopy, consistent with data from series of SLLs in platinum-treated patients.

Abu-Rustum and colleagues presented a series of second-look surgeries in advanced stage patients treated with platinum-based chemotherapy at the Memorial Sloan-Kettering Cancer Center (77). Thirty-one patients underwent laparoscopy, 70 had laparotomy, and 8 underwent both procedures in the same operation. They found persistent disease in the same proportion of patients in each group (54.8%, 61.4%, and 62.5% respectively). Four of the patients who underwent both procedures had initially negative laparoscopies in the setting of persistent disease. All of these patients had positive washings, and only one had a positive biopsy on laparotomy. Over a median follow-up period of 22 months, patients experienced the same rate of recurrence regardless of the second-look surgery performed. The laparoscopy group was found to have significantly lower mean operative time, lower estimated blood loss, shorter mean hospital stay, and lower total hospital charges. All of the complications observed in this series occurred in the group undergoing laparotomy, and no patients were reported as having dense adhesions that obviated laparoscopic assessment. This suggests that excellent preoperative judgment may have been executed to select those patients with fewer adhesions for laparoscopy; the success of laparoscopy might be less if laparoscopy were employed indiscriminately in this setting.

Casey and colleagues at the Cedars-Sinai Medical Center in Los Angeles reported their experience with 154 patients who underwent reassessment procedures, including 57 second-look laparoscopies and 69 SLLs (78). Eleven of 104 laparoscopies were converted to laparotomy because of the presence of extensive dense adhesions. These troublesome cases were evaluated in the laparotomy group, which possibly skewed the analysis in favor of laparoscopy. These researchers found the same proportion of patients with persistent disease in both laparoscopy and laparotomy groups (52.6% and 53.6%, respectively) and the same rate of recurrence after negative surgical reassessment (14.6% and 17.9%), despite the fact that 50% fewer biopsies were taken in the laparoscopy group. Because most of the patients with advanced ovarian cancer undergo lymph node sampling at primary surgery at the authors' center, none of the laparoscopy patients and only seven of the laparotomy patients underwent nodal sampling at second look-surgery. Consistent with Abu-Rustum's report, these authors found shorter operative time, lower estimated blood loss, shorter hospitalization, and lower total costs in the laparoscopy group.

All of these reports come from centers that treat many cases of ovarian cancer and where laparoscopy is extensively utilized in a variety of complex surgeries. Therefore, although their results are encouraging and admirable, they are not necessarily generalizable to practice in facilities where lower volumes of ovarian cancer surgery or complex laparoscopic surgeries are performed. Clough and colleagues, for example, reported their experience at the Institute Curie in Paris (79). They performed second-look laparoscopies immediately followed by laparotomy in 20 women with advanced-stage ovarian cancer. Using laparotomy as their "gold standard," they found that laparoscopy had a specificity of 100% but a sensitivity of only 86%. Extensive, dense adhesions prevented the performance of a complete surgical assessment in 59% of their patients.

It appears that laparoscopy may be an effective means of performing reassessment surgery in selected patients. Laparoscopy has the potential advantages of decreasing the cost, recovery time, and morbidity of the procedure. Each surgeon must assess himself or herself, or one's facilities, and the individual patient carefully before determining that these goals can be reached with laparoscopy without compromising the intent of the procedure.

CONCLUSIONS

Over the past two decades the initial treatment of ovarian cancer has changed significantly. The importance of surgical staging for apparent early ovarian cancer and the importance of maximal surgical cytoreduction for advanced-stage ovarian cancer have been established by extensive retrospective and prospective cooperative group studies. Because the ability to nonsurgically assess disease status is quite poor in ovarian cancer, SLL is often a vital component of clinical trials. The role of SLL outside of this setting, on the other hand, has become controversial. With the advent of platinum-based chemotherapy there was a dramatic increase in the proportion of patients who experienced a complete clinical response after initial therapy for ovarian cancer. There was also a significant increase in the number of patients who had recurrence of disease after a surgically documented complete response to initial therapy. This decreased the prognostic power of a negative SLL. In contrast to the experience with alkylating agent therapy, there is little evidence that additional courses of platinum-based chemotherapy improve response rates. Therefore, another indication for SLL, early discontinuation of therapy, became less relevant. For patients who do not respond to platinum-based chemotherapy, response to second-line therapy is frequently so poor that many oncologists question the value of early initiation of therapy. Largely for these reasons, SLL is no longer a reflexive component of ovarian cancer therapy, and for some patients, such as women with documented early-stage ovarian cancer, SLL is no longer recommended.

For selected patients however, SLL remains an important component of ovarian cancer therapy. For women who are at high risk for recurrent or persistent disease, SLL may offer some benefit. Recent investigations of consolidation therapy have been encouraging, and additional findings, such as those from the trial of intraperitoneal ^{32}P, may offer further hope in this setting. Results from several studies published in the last decade have established a clear apparent benefit of secondary cytoreduction at the time of SLL. Evidence for an effective salvage regimen for women who have bulky disease at the conclusion of SLL is lacking. The patient should understand the issues and controversy surrounding this intervention, and the surgeon should remain open-minded about developments in ovarian cancer therapy that might render SLL more or less valuable. For women who have a high risk for recurrence, who are medically fit, and who desire more accurate prognostication and/or aggressive treatment of their cancer, we believe that SLL remains a beneficial procedure.

REFERENCES

1. Rubin SC, Lewis J Jr. Second-look surgery in ovarian carcinoma. *CRC 8* 1988;75:91.
2. Podratz K, Cliby W. Second-look surgery in the management of epithelial ovarian carcinoma. *Gynecol Oncol* 1994;55:S128–S133.
3. Creasman W. Second look laparotomy in ovarian cancer. *Gynecol Oncol* 1994;55:S122–S127.
4. Wangensteen OH. Cancer of the colon and rectum. *Wisc Med J* 1949;48:591–597.
5. Marchetti AA. Ovarian cancer: clinicopathologic evaluation. *NY State J Med* 1941;41:24.
6. Parks TJ. Carcinoma of the ovary treated preoperatively with deep x-ray: report of three cases. *Am J Obstet Gynecol* 1945;49:676.
7. Rutledge F, Burns BC. Chemotherapy for advanced ovarian cancer. *Am J Obstet Gynecol* 1966;96:761.
8. Smith JP, Delgado G, Rutledge F. Second-look operation in ovarian carcinoma: post-chemotherapy. *Cancer* 1976;38:1438.
9. Young RC, et al. Advanced ovarian adenocarcinoma: a prospective clinical trial of melphalan (L-PAM) versus combination chemotherapy. *N Engl J Med* 1978;299:161.
10. Rubin SC, Hoskins WJ, Saigo PE, et al. Prognostic factors for recurrence following negative second-look laparotomy in ovarian cancer patients treated with platinum-based chemotherapy. *Gynecol Oncol* 1991;42:137–141.
11. Williams SD, et al. Second-look laparotomy in ovarian germ cell tumors: the Gynecologic Oncology Group experience. *Gynecol Oncol* 1994;52:287–291.
12. Rubin SC, et al. Second-look laparotomy in stage 1 ovarian cancer following comprehensive surgical staging. *Obstet Gynecol* 1993;82:139–142.
13. Vergote I, Bormer O, Abeler V. Evaluation of serum CA 125 levels in the monitoring of ovarian cancer *Am J Obstet Gynecol* 1987;157:88.

14. Maughan T, et al. CA 125 in ovarian tumour tissue at second-look laparotomy. *Br J Cancer* 1989;59:259–260.
15. Brenner DE, et al. Abdominopelvic computed tomography: evaluation in patients undergoing second-look laparotomy for ovarian carcinoma. *Obstet Gynecol* 1985;65:715.
16. Sanders RC, McNeil BJ, Finberg NJ, et al. A prospective study of computed tomography and ultrasound in the detection and staging of pelvic masses. *Radiology* 1983;146–439.
17. Wicks J, et al. Correlation of ultrasound and pathologic findings in patients with epithelial carcinoma of the ovary. *J Clin Ultrasound* 1984;12:397.
18. Murolo C, Constantini S, Foglia G, et al. Ultrasound examination in ovarian cancer patients. *J Ultrasound Med* 1989;8:441.
19. Sonnendecker E, Butterworth A. Comparison between ultrasound and histopathological evaluation in ovarian cancer patients with complete clinical remission. *J Clin Ultrasound* 1985;13:5.
20. Rubinstein E, Knudsen J. Clinical aspects of second-look laparotomy in ovarian cancer. *Ann Chir Gynaecol* 1986;75:177.
21. McGowan L, Bunnag B. The evaluation of therapy for ovarian cancer. *Gynecol Oncol* 1976;4:375.
22. Goldberg G, Learmonth G, Blodi B, et al. Role of cul-de-sac aspiration cytology in the management and follow-up of patients with ovarian carcinoma. *J Reprod Med* 1985;30:867.
23. Rubin SC, Dulaney ED, Markman M, et al. Peritoneal cytology as an indicator of disease in patients with residual ovarian carcinoma. *Obstet Gynecol* 1988;3:851.
24. Phibbs GD, Smith JP, Stanhope CR. Analysis of sites of persistent cancer at "second-look" laparotomy in patients with ovarian cancer. *Am J Obstet Gynecol* 1983;147–611.
25. Podczaski E, et al. Use of second-look laparotomy in the management of patients with ovarian epithelial malignancies. *Gynecol Oncol* 1987;28:205.
26. Friedman RL, Eisenkop SM, Wang HJ. second-look laparotomy for ovarian cancer provides reliable prognostic information and improves survival. *Gynecol Oncol* 1997;88–94.
27. Hakes T, et al. Randomized prospective trial of 5 versus 10 cycles of cyclophosphamide, doxorubicin and cisplatin (CAP) in stage III and IV ovarian cancer. *Proc ASCO* 1990;9:156.
28. Bertelsen K, et al. A prospective randomized comparison of 6 and 12 cycles of cyclophosphamide, Adriamycin, and cisplatin in advanced epithelial ovarian cancer: a Danish Ovarian Study Group trial (DACOVA). *Gynecol Oncol* 1993;49:30.
29. Schwartz P, Smith J. Second lookoperations in ovarian cancer. *Am J Obstet Gynecol* 1980;138:112.
30. Curry SL, Zumbo MM, Nahhas WA, et al. second-look laparotomy for ovarian cancer. *Gynecol Oncol* 1981;11:114.
31. Jones Soo IS, Khoo K, Whitaker S. Evaluation of ovarian cancer by second-look laparotomy after treatment. *Aust N Z J Surg* 1981;51:30.
32. Roberts W, Hrdel K, Rich WM, et al. second-look laparotomy in the management of gynecologic malignancy. *Gynecol Oncol* 1982;13:345.
33. Webb M, et al. second-look laparotomy in ovarian cancer. *Gynecol Oncol* 1982;14:285.
34. Phibbs S, Smith J, Stanhope R. Analysis of sites of persistent cancer at second-look laparotomy in patients with ovarian cancer. *Am J Obstet Gynecol* 1983;147:61.
35. Berek JS, et al. second-look laparotomy in stage III epithelial ovarian cancer: clinical variables associated with disease status *Obstet Gynecol* 1984;64:207.
36. Smirz L, et al. second-look laparotomy after chemotherapy in the management of ovarian malignancy. *Am J Obstet Gynecol* 1935;152:661.
37. Podratz K, et al. second-look laparotomy in ovarian cancer: evaluation of pathologic variables. *Am J Obstet Gynecol* 1985;152:230.
38. Dauplat J, et al. second-look laparotomy in managing epithelial ovarian carcinoma. *Cancer* 1986;57:1626.
39. Miller D, et al. A critical reassessment of second-look laparotomy in epithelial ovarian carcinoma. *Cancer* 1986;57:530.
40. McCusker M, Hoffman JS, Curry SL, et al. The role of second-look laparotomy in treatment of epithelial ovarian cancer. *Gynecol Oncol* 1987;28:83.
41. Gallup DG, Tollendo OE, Dndzinski MR, et al. Another look at the second assessment procedure for ovarian epithelial carcinoma. *Am J Obstet Gynecol* 1987;157:590.
42. Chambers SK, et al. Evaluation of the role of second looksurgery in ovarian cancer. *Obstet Gynecol* 1988;72:404.
43. Lucas J, et al. Restaging laparotomy and ovarian cancer. *South Med J* 1988;81:584.
44. Rome R, Fortune DW. The role of second-look laparotomy in the management of patients with ovarian carcinoma. *Aust N Z J Obstet Gynaecol* 1988;28:318.
45. Torretta L, et al. Diagnostic alternatives to second-look in ovarian cancer. *Eur J Gynaecol Oncol* 1990;2:145.
46. Lippman S, et al. second-look laparotomy in epithelial ovarian carcinoma prognostic factors associated with survival duration. *Cancer* 1988;61:2571.
47. Podczaski E, et al. Survival of patients with ovarian epithelial carcinomas after second-look laparotomy. *Gynecol Oncol* 1990;36:43.
48. DeGramont A, et al. Survival after second-look laparotomy in advanced ovarian epithelial cancer: study of 86 patients. *Eur J Cancer Clin Oncol* 1989;25:3.
49. Markman M, Brady MF, Spirton NM, et al. Phase II trial of intraperitoneal paclitaxel in carcinoma of the ovary, tube, and peritoneum: a Gynecologic Oncology Group study. *J Clin Oncol* 1998;16:2620–2624.
50. Katsoulis M, et al. The prognostic significance of second-look laparotomy in advanced ovarian cancer. *Eur J Gynaecol Oncol* 1997;18:200–202.
51. Rubin S, Hoskins WJ, Hakes TB, et al. Recurrence after negative second-look laparotomy for ovarian cancer: analysis of risk factors. *Am J Obstet Gynecol* 1988;159:1094.
52. Rubin SC, et al. Ten-year follow-up of ovarian cancer patients after second-look laparotomy with negative findings. *Obstet Gynecol* 1999;93:21–24.
53. Bolis G, Villa A, Guarnino P, et al. Survival of women with advanced ovarian cancer and complete pathologic response at second-look laparotomy. *Am Cancer Soc* 1996;128–131.

54. Carmichael JA, et al. A predictive index of cure versus no cure in advanced ovarian carcinoma patients: replacement of second-look laparotomy as a diagnostic test. *Gynecol Oncol* 1987;27:269.
55. Podczaski E, et al. Recurrent disease after negative second-look laparotomy in stages III and IV ovarian carcinoma. *Gynecol Oncol* 1988;29:274.
56. Podratz K, et al. Survival of patients with ovarian epithelial carcinomas after second-look laparotomy. *Gynecol Oncol* 1990;36:43.
57. Ghtage P, Krepact GV, Lotocki R, et al. Factor analysis of false-negative second-look laparotomy. *Gynecol Oncol* 1990;36:172.
58. Gershenson DM, et al. Prognosis of surgically determined complete responders in advanced ovarian cancer. *Cancer* 1985;5:1129.
59. Barakat R, Almadrones L, Venkatraman ES, et al. A phase II trial of intraperitoneal cisplatin and etoposide as consolidation therapy in patients with stage II–IV epithelial ovarian cancer following negative surgical assessment. *Gynecol Oncol* 1998;69:17–22.
60. Pickel H, Lahousen M, Petru E, et al. Consolidation radiotherapy after carboplatin-based chemotherapy in radically operated advanced ovarian cancer. *Gynecol Oncol* 1999;72:215–219.
61. Varia M, et al. Intraperitoneal chromic phosphate therapy after second-look laparotomy for ovarian cancer. *Cancer* 1988;61:919.
62. Spencer T, et al. Intraperitoneal P-32 after negative second-look laparotomy in ovarian carcinoma. *Cancer* 1989;63:2434.
63. Randall T, Rubin S. Surgical management of ovarian cancer. *Semin Surg Oncol* 1999;17:173–180.
64. Podratz K, Schray MF, Wieland HS, et al. Evaluation of treatment and survival after positive second-look laparotomy. *Gynecol Oncol* 1988;31:9.
65. Hoskins WJ, et al. Influence of secondary cytoreduction at the time of second-look laparotomy on the survival of patients with epithelial ovarian carcinoma. *Gynecol Oncol* 1989;34:365.
66. Williams L, et al. Secondary cytoreductive surgery at second-look laparotomy in advanced ovarian cancer: a gynecologic oncology group study. *Gynecol Oncol* 1997;66:171–178.
67. Markman J. Intraperitoneal chemotherapy. *Semin Oncol* 1991;18:248.
68. Feun L, Blessing JA, Major FJ, et al. A phase II study of intraperitoneal cisplatin and thiotepa in residual ovarian carcinoma: a gynecologic oncology group study. *Gynecol Oncol* 1999;71:410–415.
69. Bruzzone M, et al. Intraperitoneal carboplatin with or without interferon-α advanced ovarian cancer patients with minimal residual disease at second look: a prospective randomized trial of 111 patients. *Gynecol Oncol* 1997;65:499–505.
70. Ozols RF, et al. Randomized phase III study of cisplatin (CIS)/paclitaxel (PAC) versus carboplatin (CARBO)/PAC in optimal stage III epithelial ovarian cancer (OC): a gynecologic oncology group trial (GOG 158). *Proc ASCO* 2000.
71. Schwartz J, et al. X-ray and cisplatin cross-resistance in human tumor cell lines. *Cancer Res* 1988;48:5133.
72. Peters W, Blasko JC, Bagley CM, et al. Salvage therapy with whole-abdominal irradiation in patients with advanced carcinoma of the ovary previously treated by combination chemotherapy. *Cancer* 1996;58:880.
73. Thomas G. Is there a role for consolidation or salvage radiotherapy after chemotherapy in advanced epithelial ovarian cancer? *Gynecol Oncol* 1993;51:97–103.
74. Ozols R, et al. Peritoneoscopy in the management of ovarian cancer. *Am J Obstet Gynecol* 1981;140:611.
75. Berek JS, et al. Laparoscopy for second-lookevaluation in ovarian cancer. *Obstet Gynecol* 1981;58:192.
76. Childers J, Lang J, Surwit EA, et al. Laparoscopic surgical staging of ovarian cancer. *Gynecol Oncol* 1995;59:25–33.
77. Abu-Rustum N, et al. Second lookoperation for epithelial ovarian cancer: laparoscopy or laparotomy? *Obstet Gynecol* 1996;88:549–553.
78. Casey AC, et al. What is the role of reassessment laparoscopy in the management of gynecologic cancers in 1995? *Gynecol Oncol* 1996;60:454–461.
79. Clough K, Ladonne JM, Nos C, et al. Second-look for ovarian cancer: laparoscopy or laparotomy? A prospective comparative study. *Gynecol Oncol* 1999;72:411–417.
80. Stuart G, Jeffries M, Stuart JL, et al. The changing role of second-look laparotomy in the management of epithelial carcinoma of the ovary. *Am J Obstet Gynecol* 1982;142:612.
81. Creasman WT, Gall S, Bundy BN, et al. second-look laparotomy in the patient with minimal residual stage III ovarian cancer (a Gynecologic Oncology Group study). *Gynecol Oncol* 1989;35:378.
82. Omura G, Blessing JA, Ehrlich CE, et al. A randomized trial of cyclophosphamide and doxorubicin with or without cisplatin in advanced ovarian carcinoma. *Cancer* 1986;57:1725.
83. Kirwan PH, Naftalin NJ, Khanna S, et al. The role of second-look laparotomy in the management of patients with stage II, III and IV ovarian cancers following chemotherapy with cisplatin, Adriamycin and cyclophosphamide. *Br J Obstet Gynaecol* 1986;93:629.
84. Menczer J, et al. second-look laparotomy in ovarian carcinoma patients after 8 and after 12 courses of cisplatin based chemotherapy. *Gynecol Obstet Invest* 1989;27:102.
85. Cohen CJ, Goldberg JD, Nolland JF, et al. Improved therapy with cisplatin regimens for patients with ovarian carcinoma (FIGO stages III and IV) as measured by surgical end-staging (second-look operation). *Am J Obstet Gynecol* 1983;145:955.
86. Shelley W, et al. Adriamycin and cisplatin in the treatment of stage III and IV epithelial ovarian carcinoma. *Gynecol Oncol* 1988;29:208.
87. Bertelsen K, Hansen MK, Pedersen PH, et al. The prognostic and therapeutic value of second-look laparotomy in advanced ovarian cancer. *Br J Obstet Gynaecol* 1988;95:1231.
88. Schneider J, et al. Cisplatin-containing versus cisplatin-free adjuvant chemotherapy in ovarian carcinoma. *Oncology* 1990;47:109.
89. Watring W, et al. Second lookprocedures in ovarian cancer patients receiving six vs nine courses of platinum, Adriamycin, Cytoxan (PAC) chemotherapy: the SCPMG experience 1982–1985. *Gynecol Oncol* 1989;32:245.

90. Cain JM, Saigo PE, Pierce VK, et al. A review of second-look laparotomy for ovarian cancer. *Gynecol Oncol* 1986;23:14.
91. Megibow A, et al. Accuracy of CT in detection of persistent or recurrent ovarian carcinoma: correlation with second-look laparotomy. *Radiology* 1988;166:341.
92. Kamura T, et al. Efficacy of second-look laparotomy for patients with epithelial ovarian carcinoma. *Int J Gynecol Obstet* 1990;33:141.
93. Stehman F, Calkins AR, Wass JL, et al. A comparison of findings at second-look laparotomy with preoperative computed tomography in patients with ovarian cancer. *Gynecol Oncol* 1988;29:37.
94. Niloff J, et al. Predictive value of CA 125 antigen levels in second lookprocedures for ovarian cancer. *Am J Obstet Gynecol* 1985;151:981.
95. Atack D, et al. CA 125 surveillance and second-look laparotomy in ovarian carcinoma. *Am J Obstet Gynecol* 1986;154:287.
96. Berek J, Knapp RC, Malkasian GD, et al. CA 125 serum levels correlated with second lookoperations among ovarian cancer patients. *Obstet Gynecol* 1985;67:685.
97. Facchini V, et al. second-look laparotomy in the management of malignant epithelial ovarian neoplasias. *Eur J Gynaecol Oncol* 1986;2:152.
98. Rome R, Koh H, Fortune D, et al. CA 125 serum levels and secondary laparotomy in epithelial ovarian tumours. *Aust N Z J Obstet Gynaecol* 1987;27:142.
99. Alvarez R, et al. CA 125 as a serum marker for poor prognosis in ovarian malignancies. *Gynaecol Oncol* 1987;26:284.
100. Rubin S, Hoskins WJ, Hakes TB, et al. Serum CA 125 levels and surgical findings in patients undergoing secondary operations for epithelial ovarian cancer. *Am J Obstet Gynecol* 1989;160–166.
101. Potter M, et al. Value of serum CA 125 levels: does the result preclude second look? *Gynaecol Oncol* 1989;33:201.
102. Panich P, et al. Predictive value of multiple tumor marker assays in second lookprocedures for ovarian cancer. *Gynecol Oncol* 1989;36:286.
103. Podczaski E, Whitney C, Manetta A, et al. Use of CA 125 to monitor patients with ovarian epithelial carcinomas. *Gynecol Oncol* 1989;33:193.
104. Patsner B, et al. Does serum CA 125 level prior to second-look laparotomy for invasive ovarian adenocarcinoma predict size of residual disease? *Gynecol Oncol* 1990;37:319.
105. Ho AG, Beller U, Speyer JL, et al. A reassessment of the role of second-look laparotomy in advanced ovarian cancer. *J Clin Oncol* 1987;5:1316.
106. Stern J, Buacama, et al. Can computed tomography substitute for second-look operation in ovarian carcinoma? *Gynaecol Oncol* 1981;11:82.
107. Goldhirsch A, et al. Computed tomography prior to second-look operation in advanced ovarian cancer. *Obstet Gynaecol* 1983;62:630.
108. Clarke-Pearson D, Bandy LC, Dndzinski M, et al. Computed tomography in evaluation of patients with ovarian carcinoma in complete clinical remission. *JAMA* 1986;255:62.
109. Calkins A, Stehman FB, Wass JL, et al. Pitfalls in interpretation of computed tomography prior to second-look laparotomy in patients with ovarian cancer. *Br J Radiol* 1987;60:975.
110. Silverman P, Osborne M, Dunnick NR, et al. CT prior to second lookoperation in ovarian cancer. *AJR Am J Roentgenol* 1988;150:829.
111. Reuter K, et al. Comparison of abdominopelvic computed tomography results and findings at second-look laparotomy in ovarian carcinoma patients. *Cancer* 1989;63:1123.
112. Sonnendecker E. Is routine second-look laparotomy for ovarian cancer justified? *Gynecol Oncol* 1988;31:249.
113. Rocereto T, Morgan CE, Guintoli RL, et al. The second lookceliotomy in ovarian cancer. *Gynaecol Oncol* 1984;19:34.
114. Ballon SC, et al. second-look laparotomy in epithelial ovarian carcinoma: precise definition, sensitivity, and specificity of the operative procedure. *Gynaecol Oncol* 1984;17:154.
115. Free KE, Webb MJ. second-look laparotomy: clinical correlations. *Gynecol Oncol* 1987;26:290.
116. Webster KD, Ballard LA. Ovarian carcinoma: second-look laparotomy post chemotherapy. *Cleve Clin Q* 1981;48:365.
117. Barnhill DR, Hoskins WJ, Herler PB, et al. The second looksurgical reassessment for epithelial ovarian carcinoma. *Gynaecol Oncol* 1984;19:148.
118. Milstead R, Milsted R, Sangster G, et al. Treatment of advanced ovarian cancer with combination chemotherapy using cyclophosphamide, Adriamycin and cisplatinum. *Br J Obstet Gynaecol* 1984;91:927.
119. Phillips B, Buchsbaum HJ, Lifshitz S, et al. Reexploration after treatment for ovarian carcinoma. *Gynecol Oncol* 1979;8:339.
120. Ayhan A, Yarali H, Develioglu O, et al. Prognosticaters of second-look laparotomy findings in patients with epithelial ovarian cancer. *J Surg Oncol* 1991;46:222
121. Kudo R, Takashina T, Ito E, et al. Peritoneal washing cytology at second-look laparotomy in cisplatin treated ovarian cancer patients. *Acta Cytol* 1990;34:545.
122. Davidson NGP, et al. Advanced ovarian cancer: long-term results following chemotherapy and second-look laparotomy. *Gynaecol Oncol* 1990;39:295.
123. Jager W, Adam R, Wildt L, et al. Serum CA 125 as a guideline for the timing of a second-look operation and second line treatment in ovarian cancer. *Arch Gynecol Obstet* 1988;243:91.
124. Lund B, Williamson P. Prognostic factors for outcome of and survival after second-look laparotomy in patients with advanced ovarian carcinoma. *Obstet Gynecol* 1990;76:617.
125. Ngan H, Wong LC, Ma HK, et al. Place of second-look laparotomy after 18 courses of chemotherapy in epithelial ovarian cancer. *Aust N Z J Obstet Gynaecol* 1989;29:52.
126. Mead G, Williams CJ, MacBeth FR, et al. second-look laparotomy in the management of epithelial cell carcinoma of the ovary. *Br J Cancer* 1984;50:185.
127. Yakushiji M, Kato T. Evaluation of the second-look laparotomy in the management of carcinoma of the ovary. *Semin Surg Oncol* 1986;2:72.
128. Vardi J, Rafla SD, Malhotra C, et al. The feasibility of early administration of combination chemotherapy following cytoreductive surgery and second lookoperation in patients with stage III ovarian carcinoma: a pilot study. *Gynecol Oncol* 1989;34:12.

15
Secondary Cytoreductive Operations

Thomas W. Burke and Mitchell Morris

CYTOREDUCTIVE SURGERY

The prognostic importance of small-volume residual disease in women with advanced epithelial ovarian carcinoma was proposed by Griffiths in the late 1970s (1,2). His reviews demonstrated that patients with residual tumor diameters of less than 1.5 cm after initial exploration and resection had significantly better long-term and disease-free survival rates than patients with residual disease of greater than 1.5 cm. This finding has been confirmed by almost every other large clinical review of patients with advanced ovarian cancer. Primary cytoreductive surgery has been firmly established as the initial therapy in the management of these tumors.

Various target tumor sizes have been suggested as "optimal." Residual tumor diameters of less than 1.0, 1.5, or 2.0 cm are usually advocated. Residual disease diameters of greater than 2.0 cm convey a poorer prognosis, and these tumor sizes are consistently termed "suboptimal." A review of published residual disease data and patient outcome suggests that optimal primary cytoreduction represents a continuum: the smaller the residual disease volume, the better the outcome.

The use of more aggressive approaches to tumor resections and the application of innovative surgical techniques allow more patients to be left with minimal tumor volume after the initial operation for ovarian cancer. Most surgeons routinely perform bowel or urinary tract resections in order to remove a significant volume of disease. The argon beam coagulator, ultrasonic surgical aspirator, and other techniques that are useful in the removal of plaque disease from the pelvic peritoneum and diaphragm are additional tools for optimal resection. The benefits achieved by these aggressive primary cytoreduction techniques depend on the sensitivity of any remaining tumor to followup treatment with systemic chemotherapy and must be balanced against the potential for greater perioperative morbidity.

CLINICAL SETTINGS FOR SECONDARY CYTOREDUCTION

Because optimal primary cytoreductive operations appear to have a significant impact on survival, several groups have proposed the use of secondary cytoreduction in women with persistent or recurrent ovarian cancer. Series that describe these surgical efforts employ a variety of definitions of secondary cytoreduction. Many include heterogeneous groups of patients with a wide range of tumor sizes and volumes. Nevertheless, several general clinical scenarios can be delineated as follows: (a) patients undergoing second-look laparotomy who are found to have macroscopic disease; (b) patients who develop clinically evident recurrent disease at some point after completing primary surgery and chemotherapy; (c) patients who do not respond to initial surgery and chemotherapy; and (d) patients whose tumors are considered unresectable at initial operation and who undergo a second operation to attempt tumor reduction after an abbreviated course of chemotherapy.

This last situation has commonly been referred to as "interval debulking surgery." In many cases, the initial exploration was by nononcologic surgeons, and it can be difficult to determine whether these patients would have had a successful primary cytoreduction if a more experienced surgeon had been present. Studies that report on patients in this category undoubtedly include some patients whose disease is truly unresectable, as well as those who had an inadequate primary cytoreductive effort. The interval debulking operation can be considered an initial attempt at cytoreduction for some women previously treated by nononcologic surgeons.

LIMITATIONS OF AVAILABLE INFORMATION

Evaluation of the published data regarding secondary cytoreduction is complicated by several factors. Most studies that review secondary cytoreduction are retrospective and cover a relatively long time interval. Because current concepts regarding cytoreduction and secondary surgery were still evolving during the time the data were accumulated, the criteria for surgery and types of operations performed vary significantly. Most studies include a mixed group of patients who have been subjected to different criteria throughout the review period. Multiple selection criteria have often been employed to define and examine a homogeneous subset of patients. However, this approach can result in substantial selection bias.

Cytoreductive efforts, both primary and secondary, are most applicable to patients with advanced epithelial tumors. Reviews that evaluate only stage III and IV patients should provide the most useful information. Unfortunately, some studies include patients with early-stage tumors, inadequate staging, or nonepithelial cancers. Patients with germ cell, metastatic, or stromal tumors should be discussed separately, because the biology of these cancers may not be identical to that of epithelial tumors.

Because of the lengthy time intervals, patients reported in many retrospective series were treated with significantly different chemotherapeutic regimens, ranging from single alkylating agents to platinum combinations. The general trend in ovarian cancer treatment over the past 10 years is toward more aggressive primary surgery and platinum-paclitaxel chemotherapy. The precise impact of secondary cytoreduction in this complex setting is difficult to define.

FEASIBILITY AND MORBIDITY

Reported success rates for optimal cytoreduction vary considerably, mainly because they depend on the criteria used to select patients for secondary surgery. Success rates are also affected by the definition of "ideal" resection used in individual studies. The clinical aspects of most of the published reports are compiled in Table 15.1. Complete cytoreduction to microscopic disease (no gross residual) was achievable in 110 (42%) of 262 cases. The achievement of complete cytoreduction seems to be related to both the persistence and skill of the surgeon and the biologic behavior of the tumor. The series that describe complete cytoreduction usually involved groups of patients who underwent second-look laparotomy (3–8). Because most candidates for second-look laparotomy have no clinically detectable disease, most represent chemotherapy responders. Excision of all gross tumor may be more feasible in this subset of patients.

Optimal cytoreduction, variably defined as residual disease with diameters between 1.0 and 2.0 cm, was accomplished in 498 (58%) of 864 patients who underwent second surgical procedures. Included in this group were patients who met current criteria for second-look laparotomy, patients with persistent disease after primary surgery and chemotherapy, and some patients with progressive disease (9–24). Despite the heterogeneity of the clinical setting, optimal secondary cytoreduction is technically possible in a substantial percentage of patients.

As described previously, interval debulking surgery is a recent concept developed to avoid immediate reexploration in patients with extensive abdominal disease at initial exploration. Optimal resection after abbreviated chemotherapy was possible in 185 (70%) of 266 patients from six published series (15–19,21). This success rate seems impressive because most of these patients were initially deemed unresectable. However, patients selected for interval debulking have often demonstrated clinical responses to initial chemotherapy, whereas nonresponders do not usually undergo a second operation.

The morbidity of secondary cytoreductive operations represents a cross-section of the usual

TABLE 15.1. Clinical features, feasibility, and morbidity of secondary cytoreduction

Study	Clinical situation	No. patients	FIGO stage	Definition of "optimal" (cm)	Optimal resection No.	Optimal resection %	Morbidity (%)	Mortality (No.)
Schwartz (1980)	SLL + PD	112	I–IV	<2.0	75	67	33%	0
Berek (1983)	SLL + RD	32	III–IV	<1.5	12	38	34%	0
Vogl (1984)	SLL	12	III–IV	<2.0	9	75	NS	0
Wesley (1984)	SLL	26	I–IV	NGR	15	58	70%	0
Wils (1986)	IDS	24	III–IV	<1.5	18	75	NS	0
Dauplat (1986)	SLL	27	I–IV	NGR	13	48	NS	0
Neijt (1987)	IDS	47	II–IV	<1.0	30	63	NS	NS
Podratz (1988)	SLL	43	I–IV	NGR	9	21	35%	0
Lippman (1988)	SLL	27	I–IV	<2.0	14	52	NS	0
Morris (1988)	RD	30	I–IV	<2.0	17	57	37%	0
Morris (1989)	PRD	33	I–IV	<2.0	18	55	24%	0
Hoskins (1989)	SLL	43	I–IV	NGR	16	37	NS	NS
Michel (1989)	SLL + PD	109	I–IV	<2.0	57	52	NS	NS
Lawton (1989)	IDS	28	III–IV	<2.0	25	89	50%	0
Ng (1990)	IDS	18	III–IV	<1.0	12	67	33%	1
Jacob (1991)	IDS	22	III–IV	<2.0	17	77	23%	0
Segna (1993)	RD + PRD	100	I–IV	<2.0	61	61	13%	1
Van der Burg (1995)	IDS	130	II–IV	<1.0	81	64	15%	0
Eisenkop (1995)	RD	36	I–IV	NGR	30	83	30%	1
Vaccarello (1995)	RD	38	I–IV	<0.5	14	37	24%	0
Williams (1997)	SLL	124	III–IV	NGR	57	46	7%	0
Lichtenegger (1998)	RD	81	III–IV	<2.0	53	65	26%	0

SLL, second-look laparotomy; PD, persistent disease; RD, recurrent disease NS, not stated; NGR, no gross residual; IDS, interval debulking surgery; PRD, progressive disease.

complications associated with major abdominal surgery. Although the definitions of morbidity vary, total rates of about 30% are commonly reported (Table 15.1). Some operative complications may be more commonly seen in secondary cytoreduction patients. Blood loss that requires transfusion is frequent. In Morris and colleagues' series of patients with recurrent disease, median blood loss was 890 mL, with a median replacement of 2.4 units (13). A median loss of 1,650 mL and median intraoperative replacement of 3 units was noted in patients with progressive disease (12). Thirty-one percent of patients undergoing interval debulking surgery at our institution had an operative blood loss of more than 2,000 mL (19). Undoubtedly, surgical blood loss is a function of the extent of the resection; many secondary cytoreductive operations are complex and extensive procedures. Eisenkop and coworkers noted a clear correlation between operative time, blood loss, and perioperative morbidity (23).

Prolonged adynamic ileus is another relatively common complication (3,9,12,13). The long anesthetic and operative times, complicated abdominal procedures, frequent need for bowel resection, and a history of previous laparotomy all predispose patients to the development of postoperative ileus. The natural spread pattern of epithelial ovarian cancer, which results in multiple serosal tumor implants, hinders normal bowel function and enhances the potential for prolonged ileus. Sequelae of this complication include the frequent need for parenteral alimentation and longer hospitalization.

In the review by Morris and coworkers (12), perioperative morbidity was more common in patients who underwent bowel resection as part of a cytoreductive effort (31%) than in those who did not require bowel resection (9%). However, patients with and without bowel resection had similar complication rates (31% and 38%, respectively) in the series reported by Berek and colleagues (9). The perioperative mortality described by Ng and coworkers occurred after breakdown of a colonic reanastomosis that was performed as part of an interval debulking operation (18).

The observed morbidity of secondary cytoreduction appears to be acceptable in view of the scope and complexity of the cases. Invasive cardiovascular monitoring, blood component replacement, perioperative parenteral nutrition, and appropriate antibiotic therapy should be employed as indicated. Careful attention to perioperative care permits an aggressive operative approach while minimizing patient risk.

SURVIVAL IMPACT

Although optimal secondary cytoreduction is possible in many ovarian cancer patients, the most important clinical issues are whether such procedures will result in tangible quality-of-life benefits, increased cure rates, or prolonged survival. As noted previously, interpretation and comparison of the available data are hampered by two major limitations. First, secondary cytoreduction has been attempted in clinically dissimilar patient subsets; and second, many patients who undergo secondary resections are subjected to some selection criteria before cytoreduction is attempted. The subgroups with the poorest prognosis, particularly those who do not respond to primary chemotherapy, often do not become candidates for cytoreduction. Patients who ultimately undergo second-look or interval debulking operations may therefore represent a more favorable population.

The survival impact of secondary cytoreduction in patients who have received primary surgery and chemotherapy is summarized in Table 15.2. Schwartz and Smith described the experience with cytoreduction at second-look operations in 112 patients from our institution (7). The concept of second-look surgery was evolving during the period of this study, so the population includes both patients who were clinically disease free and some patients with responsive, but clinically detectable, persistent disease. Two-year survival rates of 47.5%, 29.5%, and 9% were observed for patients with microscopic, less than 2.0 cm, and greater than 2.0 cm residual disease, respectively. As reported by Raju and colleagues (25), survival after second-look cytoreduction to microscopic residual disease was 20% in a similar mixed group of complete and partial clinical responders. No 3-year survival was seen in patients with macroscopic residual disease. Berek and associates found a median survival time of 20 months in patients who had residual tumors of 1.5 cm or less, compared with 5 months in those with residual tumors of more than 1.5 cm (9). Patients in this study also represented a mixture of clinical situations; 9 had persistent disease, and 12 had clinically evident tumor with bowel obstruction. Segna and coworkers (20) also found a significant survival advantage in women with optimal resection who had recurrent disease (Figure 15.1). In a similar study that mixed patients with complete clinical response and those with persistent or progressive disease, Michel and colleagues (14) calculated 2-year survival rates of 31% (optimal) and 21% (suboptimal); these differences were not significant. The investigators concluded that the quality-of-life advantages for optimally resected patients with bulky disease was a short-term benefit that did not translate into prolonged survival. Luesley and coworkers found no survival advantage for patients who underwent complete cytoreduction compared with those who were left with macroscopic residual disease (3). Of 15 patients with complete resection of macroscopic disease, only 2 were alive without disease at the time of analysis. However, patients with maximally resected disease did have a survival advantage in the series reported by Dauplat and associates (4) and by Potter and colleagues (26). In the former review, 7 of 13 patients with completely resected tumors had disease-free survival, compared with only 3 of 17 patients with partial resections.

Morris and coworkers stratified candidates for secondary cytoreduction into three categories: (a) those who had stable or progressive disease while receiving first-line chemotherapy after primary cytoreduction (i.e., chemotherapy nonresponders); (b) those who responded to primary therapy and experienced a disease-free interval, but who later developed a delayed recurrence; and (c) those who completed primary therapy without clinical evidence of disease but

TABLE 15.2. Survival impact of "optimal" secondary cytoreduction

Study	Clinical situation	Residual disease (cm)	Survival	Survival measure	Significance (p)
Schwartz (1980)	SLL	Micro ≤2.0 >2.0	47.5% 29.5% 9.0%	2 y	NS
Raju (1982)	SLL	Micro Macro	20% 0%	3 y	NS
Berek (1983)	SLL + RD	≤1.5 >1.5	20 mo 5 mo	Median	<.01
Luesley (1984)	SLL	Micro ≤2.0 >2.0	50% 23% 0%	20 mo	>.05
Dauplat (1986)	SLL	Micro Macro	NS	2 y	<.05
Lippman (1988)	SLL	≤2.0 >2.0	42% 0%	4 y	.001
Morris (1988)	RD	≤2.0 >2.0	18.8 mo 13.3 mo	Median	>.05
Podratz (1988)	SLL	Micro ≤0.5 >0.5	55% 21% 14%	4 y	<.01
Hoskins (1989)	SLL	Micro Macro	51% <10%	5 y	.013
Michel (1989)	SLL + PD	≤2.0 >2.0	18 mo 13 mo	Median	>.05
Morris (1989)	PRD	>2.0 <2.0	12 mo 8 mo	Median	<.03
Segna (1993)	RD + PRD	≤2.0 >2.0	27 mo 9 mo	Median	.0001
Eisenkop (1995)	RD	Micro Macro	43 mo 5 mo	Median	.03
Vacarello (1995)	RD	≤0.5 >0.5	4+ mo 23 mo	Median	<.0001
Williams (1997)	SLL	Micro ≤1.0 >1.0	23 mo 14 mo 8 mo	Median	.0001

SLL, second-look laparotomy; Micro, microscopic residual disease; NS, not stated; Macro, macroscopic residual disease; RD, recurrent disease; PD, persistent disease; PRD, progressive disease.

were found to have persistent disease at planned second-look laparotomy (12). Examination of the survival impact of secondary cytoreduction within these defined subsets reduces the bias that can be seen when patients with tumors of different biologic behavior are compared. The investigators initially evaluated 33 chemotherapy nonresponders and found a statistically significant survival advantage for patients whose disease had been optimally resected (12). The median survival time was 12 months for patients with less than 2.0 cm of residual disease and 7.8 months for those with more than 2.0 cm. Median survival times were 19.5 months (optimal) and 8.3 months (suboptimal) when 1.0 cm of residual disease was used as the definition of an optimal resection. Despite these survival differences, response to second-line therapy was universally poor. Survival curves for optimal and suboptimal groups overlapped by 20 months. Overall median survival from diagnosis was 21.5 months, which led to the conclusion that any benefit from optimal secondary cytoreduction in chemotherapy nonresponders is short-lived.

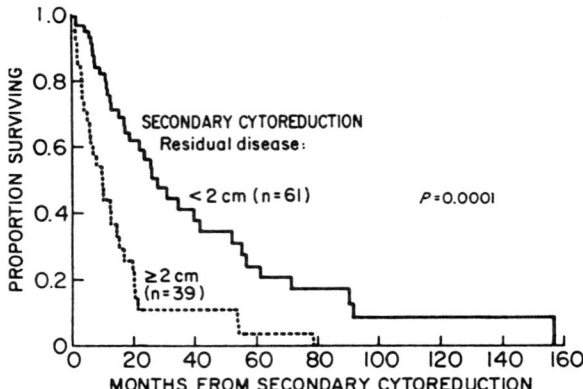

FIG. 15.1. Survival was significantly influenced by diameter of residual disease in this group of 100 women who underwent secondary cytoreduction for recurrent disease. (From Segna RA, Dottino PR, Mandelil JP, et al. Secondary cytoreduction for ovarian cancer following cisplatin therapy. *J Clin Oncol* 1993;11:435, with permission.)

In a second study from our center, Morris and colleagues reviewed 30 patients with recurrent disease who had secondary cytoreduction after a period of clinical remission (more than 6 months) (13). Presumably these patients had less biologically aggressive tumors than those who failed to respond to primary therapy. With 2.0 cm of residual disease as the definition of optimal resection, survival times of 18 and 13.3 months were observed for optimal and suboptimal groups, respectively. Response to subsequent therapy was poor, with only 3 patients remaining disease free at the time of analysis. The obvious conclusion from both studies is that any potential benefit of optimal secondary cytoreduction is dependent on effective second-line treatment. This conclusion is further supported by Vogl and coworkers, who attempted secondary cytoreduction after six cycles of chemotherapy in 18 patients who had been judged "unresectable" at primary laparotomy (10). Only 1 patient with completely resected residual tumor had a significant duration of disease-free survival.

Lippman and associates examined prognostic factors for survival in 70 consecutive patients undergoing second-look laparotomy (11). Most of these patients had advanced-stage and high-grade tumors, most had received primary cisplatin-based chemotherapy, and all were without clinical evidence of disease at the time of surgery. Secondary cytoreduction was attempted in 27 patients who had macroscopic tumor greater than 2.0 cm. Survival for patients whose tumors were reduced to less than 2.0 cm was significantly better than for those whose tumors could not be cytoreduced to this level. The authors concluded that optimal secondary resection may be beneficial in the subgroup of patients with bulky residual disease that is discovered at second look.

Podratz and coauthors reported their experience with 116 patients who had positive findings at second-look laparotomy (5). These patients had completed primary therapy (surgery and chemotherapy) and were clinically tumor free. Secondary cytoreduction was routinely attempted when feasible. The residual disease categories were defined as microscopic only, less than 0.5 cm, and more than 0.5 cm. Estimated 4-year survival times were 55%, 21%, and 14%, respectively (Figure 15.2). The difference between the results with disease of less than versus more than 0.5 cm was not significant. Overall median survival time was 22.5 months. Hoskins and coworkers published their findings in a similar group of 67 patients with positive second-look operations in whom secondary cytoreduction was routinely attempted (6). The median survival time for the entire group was 28 months. Patients with microscopic disease and those whose disease was reduced to microscopic levels had similar survival times, whereas those with macroscopic residual of any size had extremely poor outcomes. The excellent report of Williams and colleagues on 124 women with macroscopic tumor detected at second-look laparotomy clearly demonstrated a survival advantage for those who undergo successful cytoreduction (8). Women

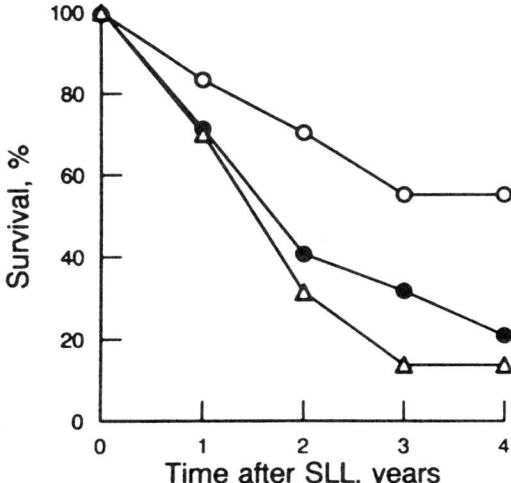

FIG. 15.2. Patients with microscopic residual disease (open circles) following second-look laparotomy fared better than those with residual disease <5 mm (closed circles) or >5 mm (triangles). (From Podratz KC, Schray MF, Wieand HS, et al. Evaluation of treatment and survival after positive second-look laparotomy. *Gynecol Oncol* 1988;31:9, with permission.)

with microscopic residual survived a median of 23 months, compared with only 8 months for those with more than 1.0 cm residual tumor (Figure 15.3). These three reviews suggest that a significant survival advantage for patients with positive second-look laparotomy can be demonstrated only when disease is reducible to microscopic levels.

INTERVAL DEBULKING OPERATIONS

Many patients with advanced epithelial ovarian tumors undergo initial exploratory surgery and diagnosis in small community hospitals. Typically, these patients are then referred to subspecialists or cancer centers for further therapy. A proportion of these patients have suboptimal primary resections and significant residual disease at the time of referral. Interval debulking surgery provides a management scheme that does not compromise outcome but avoids immediate reexploration in these usually debilitated patients. Published information on the long-term results of this approach is limited (Table 15.3). Reviews by Lawton and coworkers (17) and Ng and associates (18) address the treatment details, feasibility, and morbidity of the concept, but survival impact was not assessed in these reports because of short follow-up.

Wils and others described their results in 50 of 88 patients with stages III and IV ovarian cancer who had suboptimal (more than 1.5 cm residual disease) primary operations (15). After the primary operation, all patients were treated with cisplatin, doxorubicin, and cyclophosphamide chemotherapy. Twenty-four patients with responsive tumors were explored for interval debulking, and 18 tumors were optimally resected to less than 1.5 cm. Three-year survival in the optimal interval resection group was comparable to that for patients who had optimal primary resection, which suggests that delayed cytoreduction may result in an equivalent outcome for patients whose tumors are sensitive to first-line chemotherapy. Neijt and associates summarized their experience with 47 patients who had interval cytoreductions while receiving primary platinum-based combination chemotherapy (16). All of these patients had clinically evident tumor and had undergone exploratory surgery, with their tumors being deemed primarily unresectable by experienced surgeons. No survival advantage was detected for patients whose tumors were cytoreduced to less than 1.0 cm. The authors concluded that interval debulking is of no benefit when an initial aggressive attempt at cytoreduction has failed.

In a retrospective matched-control study from our service, Jacob and coworkers examined a group of 22 patients referred after exploration and biopsy only (19). The patients were treated with platinum-based chemotherapy and then had interval debulking operations. The survival rates for this group were compared with those for patients with suboptimal primary cytoreduction who received chemotherapy and second-look laparotomy, and with those for a second control group who underwent immediate reexploration and an attempt at primary cytoreduction before starting chemotherapy. Each group was limited to patients with advanced-stage, high-grade tumors. All patients in the control groups received platinum-based chemotherapy. No significant

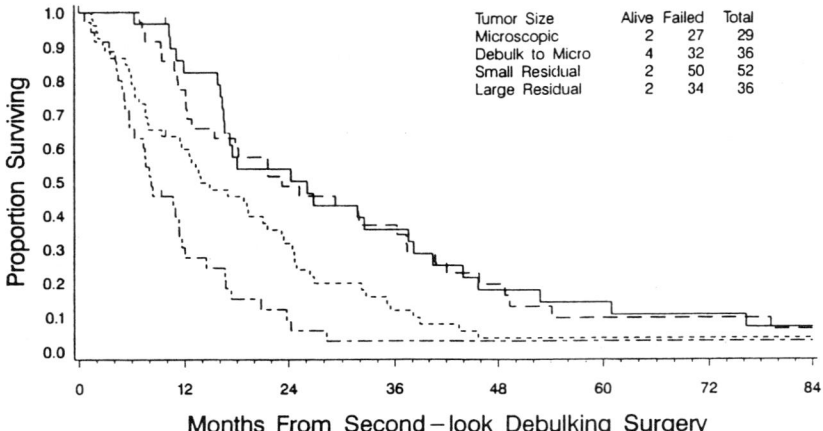

FIG. 15.3. Survival was clearly related to the residual disease volume at the completion of second-look laparotomy in this analysis by Williams and others. Patients whose tumors were reduced to microscopic disease at the completion of the operation had an outcome identical to those whose tumors were already at microscopic levels at the beginning of the operation. (From Williams L, Brunetto VL, Yordan E, et al. Secondary cytoreductive surgery at secondary-look laparotomy in advanced ovarian cancer: a Gynecologic Oncology Group study. *Gynecol Oncol* 1997;66:174, with permission.)

survival differences were seen between the group that underwent interval debulking and either of the control groups. Within the interval resection group, a survival advantage for optimal residual disease (less than 2.0 cm) was noted (18 versus 7.5 months). Because of the comparable survival results in these three groups, the authors concluded that patients with bulky disease after primary operation have a poor prognosis, regardless of the type or timing of additional attempts at surgical resection.

Van der Berg and colleagues performed the only reported randomized trial of interval debulking surgery from the EORTC (21). All eligible patients had disease volumes greater than 1.0 cm. After three courses of cisplatin and cyclophosphamide chemotherapy, study participants were randomly assigned to surgery or no surgery arms. Patients receiving an interval debulking operation had longer progression-free and overall survival times and a lower risk for death from disease (Figure 15.4).

TABLE 15.3. *Survival impact of residual disease in interval debulking operations*

Study	Neoadjuvant chemotherapy	Residual disease (cm)	Survival	Survival measure	Significance (*p*)
Wils (1986)	PAC	≤1.5 >1.5	50%	3 y	<.05
Neijt (1987)	CHAP/CP	≤1.0 >1.0	28% 30%	3 y	.70
Jacob (1991)	PAC/CP[a]	≤2.0 >2.0	18 mo 7.5 mo	Median	.02
Van der Burg (1995)	PC	No surgery ≤1.0 >1.0	20 mo 26.6 mo 19.4 mo	Median	>.04

[a] Most patients were treated with PAC or CP regimen.
PAC, cisplatin, doxorubicin, and cyclophosphamide; CHAP, cyclophosphamide, hexamethamelamine, doxorubicin, and cisplatin; CP, cyclophosphamide and cisplatin.

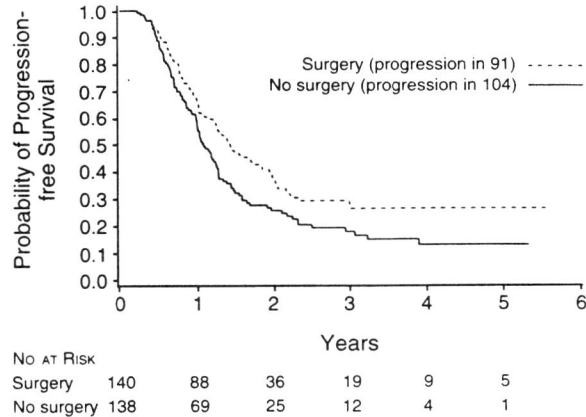

FIG. 15.4. Patients randomized to receive an interval debulking operation had a significant improvement in survival when compared to those who received no interval operation. (From Van der Burg MEL, van Lent M, Buyse M, et al. The effect of debulking surgery after induction chemotherapy on the prognosis in advanced epithelial ovarian cancer. *N Engl J Med* 1995;332:633, with permission.)

CONCLUSIONS

Despite the difficulties in comparing and assessing the available information about secondary cytoreductive surgery, some general conclusions can be drawn. Secondary resection is technically possible in a significant proportion of patients whose tumors are not eradicated by primary surgery and first-line chemotherapy. With currently available surgical techniques, secondary cytoreduction can be accomplished with significant but acceptable morbidity. The mortality risk is negligible. Because patients with suboptimal resections have 5-year survival rates of less than 10%, aggressive secondary surgical procedures should be limited to cases in which optimal resection is thought to be achievable. Complex operations that leave residual disease of more than 2.0 cm should be avoided unless they provide a clear palliative benefit.

Routine categorization of the clinical situation is helpful in determining whether a given patient is likely to derive a survival advantage from secondary cytoreduction. Patients with progressive disease during primary therapy; those with clinically evident, persistent disease at the conclusion of primary therapy; and those whose disease recurs soon after the completion of primary treatment have a limited life expectancy. In the absence of proven second-line treatment, secondary cytoreduction should not be attempted in these settings.

Patients who have complete clinical responses to primary therapy may benefit from cytoreduction at the time of second-look laparotomy, but it should be attempted only when an optimal result is possible. The greatest impact is seen in the subset of patients who undergo removal of all gross residual tumor, which suggests that survival, even in the optimal group, is strongly related to the volume of disease that remains at completion of the operation. Patients with complete clinical responses whose tumors recur after very long disease-free intervals (longer than 1 year) may also derive a survival benefit from a repeat cytoreductive effort. Our clinical impression is that patients with tumors that recur after long intervals are more likely to respond to repeat treatment with platinum-taxol chemotherapy (Figure 15.5). The ability to resect all gross disease at second-look laparotomy may be an inherent reflection of tumor biology and chemotherapeutic sensitivity rather than surgical technique or skill.

The limited experience with interval debulking surgery suggests that patients who respond to an abbreviated course of chemotherapy and then undergo optimal resection have outcomes that are equivalent to those of patients with optimal initial resection and subsequent chemotherapy. The major advantage of this approach is the elimination of an immediate reexploration in patients with advanced disease. Further investigations of this concept need to stratify patients into two groups:

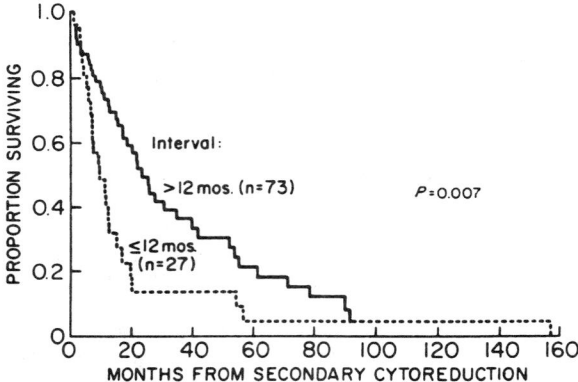

FIG. 15.5. Enhanced survival was noted when the disease-free interval after primary treatment exceeded 1 year in this series of patients. (From Segna RA, Dottino PR, Mandelil JP, et al. Secondary cytoreduction for ovarian cancer following cisplatin therapy. *J Clin Oncol* 1993;11:435, with permission.)

(a) those who have had an inadequate attempt at primary cytoreduction, and (b) those whose tumors are truly unresectable. Patients in these subpopulations probably have tumors of differing biologic aggressiveness and should not be analyzed as a single group.

The single greatest factor in the failure of secondary cytoreduction is the lack of effective second-line therapy. Virtually all patients who undergo secondary cytoreduction are left with some residual tumor, and their long-term survival depends on additional postoperative treatment. Epithelial ovarian tumors that have not responded to platinum-taxol regimens are notoriously resistant to other currently available second-line systemic chemotherapy agents. Alternative second-line options now under investigation include intraperitoneal isotopes, whole-abdomen irradiation, intraperitoneal chemotherapy, monoclonal antibody-directed agents, intraperitoneal immune-modulating molecules, and p53 gene therapy. However, these therapies are generally thought to be ineffective against significant gross disease. Experimental therapies may enhance survival only in those patients with optimally resected tumors.

More information about the impact of secondary cytoreductive surgery is needed. Further refinement of our current approach to secondary cytoreduction is likely, and a survival advantage may be demonstrated for additional patient subsets. If successful second-line treatment becomes available, the survival impact of secondary resection will need to be reexamined in this context.

REFERENCES

1. Griffiths CT. Surgical resection of tumor bulk in the primary treatment of ovarian carcinoma. *Natl Cancer Inst Monogr* 1975;42: 101.
2. Griffiths CT, Parker LM, Fuller Jr, AF. Role of cytoreductive surgical treatment in the management of advanced ovarian cancer. *Cancer Treat Rep* 1979;63:235.
3. Luesley DM, Chan KK, Fielding JWL, et al. Second-look laparotomy in the management of epithelial ovarian carcinoma: an evaluation of fifty cases. *Obstet Gynecol* 1984;64:421.
4. Dauplat J, Ferriere JP, Gorbinet M, et al. Second-look laparotomy in managing epithelial ovarian carcinoma. *Cancer* 1986;57:1627.
5. Podratz KC, Schray MF, Wieand HS, et al. Evaluation of treatment and survival after positive second-look laparotomy. *Gynecol Oncol* 1988;31:9, 1988.
6. Hoskins WJ, Rubin SC, Dulaney E, et al. Influence of cytoreduction at the time of second-look laparotomy on the survival of patients with epithelial ovarian carcinoma. *Gynecol Oncol* 1989;34:365.
7. Schwartz PE, Smith JP. Second-look operations in ovarian cancer. *Am J Obstet Gynecol* 1980;138:1124.
8. Williams L, Brunetto VL, Yordan E, et al. Secondary cytoreductive surgery at secondary-look laparotomy in advanced ovarian cancer: a Gynecologic Oncology Group study. *Gynecol Oncol* 1997;66:171.
9. Berek JS, Hacker NF, Lagasse LD, et al. Survival of patients following secondary cytoreductive surgery in ovarian cancer. *Obstet Gynecol* 1983;61:189.
10. Vogl SE, Seltzer V, Calanog A, et al. "Second-effort" surgical resection for bulky ovarian cancer. *Cancer* 1984;54:2220.
11. Lippman SM, Alberts DS, Slymen DJ, et al. Second-look laparotomy in epithelial ovarian carcinoma: prognostic factors associated with survival duration. *Cancer* 1988;61:2571.
12. Morris M, Gershenson DM, Wharton JT. Secondary cytoreductive surgery in epithelial ovarian cancer: nonresponders to first-line therapy. *Gynecol Oncol* 1988; 33:1.
13. Morris M, Gershenson DM, Wharton JT, et al. Secondary cytoreductive surgery for recurrent epithelial ovarian cancer. *Gynecol Oncol* 1989;34:334.

14. Michel G, Zarca D, Castaigne D, Prade M. Secondary cytoreductive surgery in ovarian cancer. *Eur J Surg Oncol* 1989;15:201.
15. Wils J, Blijham G, Naus A, Belder C, et al. Primary of delayed debulking surgery and chemotherapy consisting of cisplatin, doxorubicin, and cyclophosphamide in stage III-IV epithelial ovarian carcinoma. *J Clin Oncol* 1986;4:1068.
16. Neijt JP, ten Bokkel Huinink WW, van der Burg MEL, et al. Randomized trial comparing two combination chemotherapy regimens (CHAP-5 v CP) in advanced ovarian carcinoma. *J Clin Oncol* 1987;5:1157.
17. Lawton FG, Redman CW, Luesley DM, et al. Neoadjuvant (cytoreductive) chemotherapy combined with intervention debulking surgery in advanced, unresected epithelial ovarian cancer. *Obstet Gynecol* 1989; 73:61.
18. Ng LW, Rubin SC, Hoskins WJ, et al. Aggressive chemosurgical debulking in patients with advanced ovarian cancer. *Gynecol Oncol* 1990;38:358.
19. Jacob JH, Gershenson DM, Morris M, et al. Neoadjuvant chemotherapy and interval debulking for advanced epithelial ovarian cancer. *Gynecol Oncol* 1991; 42:146.
20. Segna RA, Dottino PR, Mandelil JP, et al. Secondary cytoreduction for ovarian cancer following cisplatin therapy. *J Clin Oncol* 1993;11:434.
21. Van der Burg MEL, van Lent M, Buyse M, et al. The effect of debulking surgery after induction chemotherapy on the prognosis in advanced epithelial ovarian cancer. *N Engl J Med* 1995;332:629.
22. Vaccarello L, Rubin SC, Vlamis V, et al. Cytoreductive surgery in ovarian carcinoma patients with a documented previously complete surgical response. *Gynecol Oncol* 1995;57:61.
23. Eisenkop SM, Friedman RL, Wang H-J. Secondary cytoreductive surgery for recurrent ovarian cancer: a prospective study. *Cancer* 1995;76:1606.
24. Lichtenegger W, Sehouli J, Buchmann E, et al. Operative results after primary and secondary debulking-operations in advanced ovarian cancer (AOC). *J Obstet Gynaecol Res* 1998;24:447.
25. Raju KS, McKinna JA, Barker GH, et al. Second-look operations in the planned management of advanced ovarian carcinoma. *Am J Obstet Gynecol* 1982;144:650.
26. Potter ME, Hatch KD, Soong S-J, et al. Second-look laparotomy and salvage therapy: a research modality only? *Gynecol Oncol* 1992;44:3.

16

Recent Developments in the Treatment of Recurrent Ovarian Carcinoma

James T. Thigpen and Vincent E. Herrin

INTRODUCTION

Celomic epithelial carcinoma of the ovary accounts for more deaths than any other gynecologic malignancy. In the United States alone, approximately 28,200 women were diagnosed with celomic epithelial ovarian cancer in 1999; and an estimated 14,500 women died from their disease (1). These figures result from the lack of an effective screening test and the resultant diagnosis of ovarian cancer at an advanced stage in the majority of patients.

The management of newly diagnosed patients depends on the extent of disease at the time of diagnosis, as reflected in the International Federation of Gynecology and Obstetrics (FIGO) staging system (Chapter 10). The initial step in management is an accurate staging; in the vast majority of patients, this requires an exploratory laparotomy. Using this system, the physician can divide patients into two major categories: the majority who present with advanced disease (stages III and IV) and those who present with limited disease (stages I and II). For patients with advanced disease, optimal first-line management takes advantage of the advances that have been made in chemotherapy over the last 20 years, first with platinum drugs and then with taxanes, to improve response rates and outcomes for women with ovarian cancer (2–6). Women with bulky disease, representing 60% of patients with advanced disease, have a 10-year relapse rate of 80% to 85%. Among women with small-volume disease, defined as tumors smaller than 2 cm in diameter, 60% to 70% eventually relapse.

Those with limited disease (stage I disease confined to the ovary or stage II disease with tumor beyond the ovary but confined to the pelvis) are managed initially with surgical resection (7,8). Those with favorable features (grade 1, no tumor on the surface of the ovary, no extraovarian disease, no ascites, and negative peritoneal cytology) receive no further therapy, and fewer than 10% experience relapse. All other patients with stage I disease and those with stage II disease are at high risk for relapse and receive adjuvant platinum-based chemotherapy. After adjuvant therapy, the relapse rate is 20%. Those with low-risk disease have a better than 90% rate of survival at 5 years survival with surgical resection only (total abdominal hysterectomy, bilateral salpingo-oophorectomy, careful surgical exploration, and removal of all gross disease). Those with high-risk disease have a 5-year survival rate of only 60% with surgical resection and appear to benefit from platinum-based adjuvant chemotherapy, with a reduction in recurrence rate from 40% to 20% (7,8).

These outcome figures represent significant progress in the last two decades. Long-term survival is now possible even for those with bulky advanced disease. Nevertheless, by taking into account the frequency of each stage and its projected relapse rate, the overall likelihood of relapse after initial therapy is 62% (Table 16.1). This 62% is the patient population that is the focus of efforts to develop successful second-line therapy (6–8). The discussion in this chapter focuses on the nature of the patient population requiring second-line therapy, those factors that should influence therapeutic

TABLE 16.1. *Source of patients eligible for second-line therapy*

Initial disease	Frequency (%)	Recurrence rate (%)
Stage I–II low risk	10	10
Stage I–II high risk	15	20
Stage III small volume	30	60–70
Stage III–IV large volume	45	80–85
Overall	100	62

TABLE 16.2. *Patients eligible for second-line therapy based on type of initial therapy and response*

Group	Definition
A	Patients who have a recurrence after initial complete surgical resection of low-risk stage I disease (chemonaive)
B	Patients who complete front-line chemotherapy with no evidence of residual disease and experience a treatment-free interval before recurrence longer than 12 months (chemosensitive)
C	Patients who achieve a complete response to front-line chemotherapy and experience a treatment-free interval longer than a specified minimum duration but no longer than 12 months (chemosensitive)
D	Patients who achieve a complete response to front-line chemotherapy but experience a treatment-free interval of less than a specified minimum duration (chemoresistant)
E	Patients who achieve only a partial response or who have at best stable disease (chemoresistant)
F	Patients who experience progression of disease while receiving front-line therapy (chemoresistant)

choices, and specific recommendations for systemic therapy.

THE PATIENT POPULATION

The most important step in deciding appropriate second-line or salvage therapy for patients with recurrent or persistent ovarian carcinoma is to understand the nature of the patient population eligible for such treatment. Long-term follow-up of women treated for ovarian carcinoma has identified a number of characteristics associated with increased likelihood of persistence or recurrence: clear cell or mucinous histology, nonplatinum-based treatment, poor performance status, older age, higher stage, clinically measurable disease, larger residual tumor volume, ascites, and histologic grade. None of these factors, however, helps in the selection of appropriate salvage therapy.

One factor that does provide a basis for choosing salvage therapy is the outcome of first-line therapy (9). Patients eligible for second-line therapy are a heterogeneous mix of six distinct groups (Table 16.2). These groups are defined by the type of initial therapy, the response to initial therapy, and the interval between completion of initial therapy and subsequent requirement for further treatment of persistent or recurrent disease. The first group of patients (group A) are those who have a recurrence after initial complete surgical resection of low-risk stage I disease. These patients comprise at most 10% of those who initially present with low-risk limited disease. Based on the current standard of care, they will have undergone surgical resection only and will have received no prior systemic therapy; hence, they are classified as chemonaive (and thus chemosensitive).

The second group of patients (group B) includes those who completed front-line chemotherapy with no evidence of residual disease, whether the chemotherapy was adjuvant therapy for high-risk stage I–II disease or treatment for advanced disease, and experienced recurrence more than 12 months after completion of that therapy. Such patients are chemosensitive on the basis of their initial response and have a high probability of responding again to the same systemic therapy.

The third group of patients (group C) consists of those who achieved a complete response to front-line chemotherapy and then experienced recurrence after a treatment-free interval of a specified minimum duration but less than a maximum duration of 12 months. The minimum that the treatment-free interval should last for patients to be included in this group is not clear. The most common definition of minimum duration of the treatment-free interval, 6 months, is now thought to be too long, and an emerging consensus favoring 3 months as the minimum period seems likely. Such patients are chemosensitive on the basis of their initial response but have a probability of responding again to the same systemic therapy that is lower than that of the group with the treatment-free intervals longer than 12 months.

The fourth group of patients (group D) includes those who achieved a complete response to initial therapy but experienced only a brief interval before disease progression. The definition of what constitutes a brief interval has been discussed. Patients in this group are unlikely to respond to retreatment with the same drugs and hence should be considered chemoresistant (at least to the initial drugs).

The fifth group of patients (group E) consists of those patients who achieved only a partial response or who had at best stable disease. Because it is unlikely that the remaining disease will respond further to the initial regimen, these patients should also be considered chemoresistant.

The sixth and final group of patients (group F) includes those patients whose disease progressed during initial therapy. The tumors in these patients are clearly chemoresistant and represent the greatest challenge for second-line treatment.

These six categories define six distinct groups of patients based primarily on the nature of response to front-line therapy. For practical purposes, these six categories have been further reduced to two: those with chemosensitive disease (groups A through C) and those with chemoresistant disease (groups D through F) (Table 16.3). Studies performed before 1990 rarely drew a distinction between those patients with chemosensitive versus chemoresistant disease. Because those with chemosensitive disease are far more likely to respond to treatment and to survive longer, it is difficult to assess the meaning of response rates and rates of progression-free and overall survival without knowing the proportion of patients who had chemosensitive disease. More recent studies have defined the populations at least in terms of the two categories, chemosensitive and chemoresistant. These trials with reasonable descriptions of the patient population in terms of response to front-line therapy are emphasized as a basis for patient management.

PATIENT MANAGEMENT

Decisions on patient management should be based on an examination of the literature and a clear understanding of the goals of second-line chemotherapy.

Role of Second-Line Chemotherapy

It should be noted at the outset that the role, if any, of second-line therapy is debated. The decision to start second-line therapy should be based on a clear understanding with the patient that, although occasional long-term remissions are possible, cure is not the goal.

One of the most difficult decisions is whether to start second-line therapy at the first discovery of recurrence of disease. First evidence of disease may take the form of symptomatic recurrence, in which case immediate start of second-line therapy is reasonable, with the goal of palliation of symptoms. If, on the other hand, recurrence is manifested by a rising value for the serum marker CA 125, visualization of a mass on computed tomographic scan of the abdomen, or discovery of a mass on pelvic examination in the absence of symptoms, the role of immediate second-line therapy is less clear. Those who take a less aggressive view of such a situation argue that therapy should await the onset of symptoms, particularly in those patients with only a rise in CA 125. They claim evidence that shows low response rates and little gain in survival. On the other hand, those who argue for immediate second-line therapy in such patients contend that smaller-volume masses respond better and that responders almost always do better thant nonresponders.

Although the real answer is not known, a rational approach would take into account whether the

TABLE 16.3. *Common definitions of platinum-sensitive and platinum-resistant patients*

Platinum sensitive (groups A–C)	Initial complete response to platinum
	Treatment-free interval >6 mo
Platinum resistant (groups D–F)	Progression on platinum
	Best response stable to platinum
	Relapse <6 mo after prior platinum

TABLE 16.4. *Phase II randomized trial of cap versus paclitaxel in platinum-sensitive disease*

Parameter	CAP	Paclitaxel
Response	54%	49%
Clinical complete response	32%	20%
Response duration	18.9 mo	7.3 mo
Median survival	24.3 mo	20.3 mo

CAP, cyclophosphamide, doxorubicin, and cisplatin.
From Colombo N, Marzola M, Parma G, et al. Paclitaxel vs CAP in recurrent platinum-sensitive ovarian cancer: a randomized phase II study [Abstract]. *Proc ASCO* 1996;15:279, with permission.

disease responded to front-line therapy. In those with chemosensitive disease, response rates (RR) as high as 60% and median survival times as long as 2 years have been reported (see later discussion) (Table 16.4) (10–12). These patients arguably should have immediate therapy on discovery of recurrence. In those with chemoresistant disease, response rates are relatively low and survival times short (see later discussion). A reasonable approach would argue for immediate treatment only when actual masses are observed or symptoms occur. Rising CA-125 values would serve only as an indicator that further evaluation is needed. With this as background, a discussion of platinum-sensitive and platinum-resistant disease follows.

Management of Platinum-Sensitive Disease

Patients who fit into groups A through C (Table 16.3) have disease that exhibits a high propensity to respond to therapy with paclitaxel plus a platinum compound. Most will have received these agents as front-line therapy and, by definition, will have responded to the treatment. Many reports provide examples of the successful use of second-line platinum-based salvage therapy in such platinum-sensitive cases but not in those with platinum-resistant disease. For example, a randomized phase II study of either paclitaxel or PAC (cisplatin, doxorubicin, cyclophosphamide) in patients with platinum-sensitive disease reported high response rates and clinical complete response rates (CR) and median survival times approaching 2 years with both regimens (Table 16.4) (10).

As another example, intravenous cisplatin-based therapy was evaluated retrospectively in 72 patients with measurable disease who had received at least two cisplatin-based or carboplatin-based regimens and had demonstrated a platinum-free interval of at least 4 months between completion of the first regimen and initiation of the second (11). The overall RR was 43%. Among the 31 responsive patients were 10 with surgically defined, or pathologically confirmed, complete responses. The response rate increased as the platinum-free interval lengthened. Among those with an interval between 5 and 12 months, the RR was 27%, with a surgical CR of 5%. Among those with a platinum-free interval of 13 to 24 months, the RR was 33% and the surgical CR was 11%. With a platinum-free interval of longer than 24 months, the RR was 59% and the surgical CR was 22% (11).

A third example is a study of 40 consecutive patients who had responded to initial platinum-based therapy. A second-line regimen of weekly cisplatin combined with either epirubicin or etoposide yielded a 60% RR, a 25% CR, a median duration of response of 7 months, and a median survival of 13.5 months (12). The longer the disease-free interval before relapse, the greater was the likelihood of response.

In a fourth example, a study of 28 patients who had relapses after initial cisplatin combination chemotherapy, the combination of carboplatin (300 mg/m^2 on day 8) preceded by cyclophosphamide (100 mg/m^2/day on days 1 through 7) produced 9 objective responses (5 complete and 4 partial responses) (13). Six of these responses (46%) occurred among 13 patients whose disease responded to the initial platinum-based therapy and was therefore defined as platinum-sensitive. Only 3 responses (20%) were observed among the 15 platinum-resistant patients. The relatively high response rate among the platinum-resistant group may be explained by the definitions of response used in this study, because the platinum-resistant group included patients with platinum-free intervals as long as 12 months.

A fifth study evaluated the platinum analog iproplatin, given at an initial dose of 270 mg/m^2 to patients with recurrent ovarian carcinoma after cisplatin or carboplatin therapy (14). Among

78 patients whose disease was resistant to either cisplatin or carboplatin, there were 9 responses (12%); 3 were complete, and 6 were partial responses. Among 19 patients with platinum-sensitive disease, 5 responses (26%) were observed; 2 were complete, and 3 were partial.

These five representative trials (10–14) demonstrate that patients who respond to platinum-based therapy initially and then experience relapse after a significant platinum-free interval have a high likelihood of responding again to intravenous platinum-based treatment. The correct definition of a significant platinum-free interval is not clear. The data suggest that the longer the interval, the more likely it is that the response will be favorable. A significant number of responses were observed in patients with treatment-free intervals as short as 4 months (11).

In addition to the length of the treatment-free interval that is appropriate as a cutoff point between sensitive and resistant patients, other important questions remain to be answered. First, what constitutes the optimal regimen for retreatment in these patients with platinum-sensitive disease? Secondly, should the second-line therapy be a single-agent regimen or a combination of active agents? The cited studies (10–14) show clearly that repeat therapy with a platinum-based regimen is active. Although other agents exhibit significant activity in platinum-sensitive patients, platinum-based regimens yield overall response rates that tend to be higher.

Whether combining a platinum compound with a nonplatinum agent improves outcome is not clear. At least some evidence suggests that a combination similar to that used for front-line therapy (a paclitaxel/platinum regimen) may be advantageous. For example, one study showed that, among patients who received paclitaxel and platinum in combination initially and who then experienced relapse after 6 months, retreatment with the same combination produced an RR as high as 91% (15). The activity of alternative second-line agents in a population with chemotherapy-sensitive disease must be interpreted with these results in mind.

Three reasonable recommendations for the management of platinum-sensitive disease can be proposed on the basis of current evidence

TABLE 16.5. *Recommendation for second-line chemotherapy for patients with platinum-sensitive disease*

1. General recommendations
   a. Patients should be retreated with the same or a similar regimen to which they responded as a part of front-line therapy.
   b. The optimal regimen is not known, but alternatives include paclitaxel plus a platinum compound, a platinum compound alone, and paclitaxel alone.
2. Special circumstances
   a. Allergic reactions to carboplatin may prevent further use of this compound.
   b. Cumulative toxicity, such as cumulative myelosuppression or neurotoxicity, may limit further utility of paclitaxel and the platinum compounds.

(Table 16.5). First, the patient should be administered a platinum-based regimen. This is based on much higher response rates reported with the use of platinum-based regimens. Secondly, a combination of a platinum compound plus paclitaxel is reasonable for retreatment. The bases for this choice are the combination's superiority in front-line therapy (2–5) and the high response rates reported for this combination in the second-line setting in platinum/paclitaxel-sensitive disease (15). Third, the expected frequency of response to second-line therapy varies directly with the length of the treatment-free interval (11).

The foregoing discussion has focused on patients with platinum-sensitive disease. What about the patient who has demonstrated taxane sensitivity? This population should respond well to repeat treatment with a taxane/platinum combination. There is only one study that at least indirectly addresses this situation. The Gynecologic Oncology Group (GOG) conducted a randomized phase III trial in which one of the arms called for the use of paclitaxel alone at 200 mg/m^2 every 3 weeks. Thirty-eight patients whose disease progressed on paclitaxel received therapy with cisplatin 100 mg/m^2 (16). The RR in these patients was 61% (25% CR), with a median progression-free survival time (PFS) of 11 months and a median overall survival time (OS) of 14.3 months. These data, together with the marked response rate to paclitaxel in platinum-sensitive patients (RR 49%, CR 20%, PFS 7.3 months, OS 20.3 months) (10), provide strong support for the previous conclusion that a paclitaxel/platinum combination is a reasonable and probably preferred choice in chemosensitive disease, whether the initial regimen included a platinum compound, paclitaxel, or both.

Management of Platinum-Resistant Disease

Successful management in patients who have demonstrated clinical resistance to platinum-based therapy requires the use of agents that are not cross-resistant with the platinum compounds. Until approximately 10 years ago, essentially no such agents had been identified. Now at least nine agents have been shown to produce objective responses in patients who have failed to respond to platinum-based initial therapy: paclitaxel, oral etoposide, Doxil, topotecan, gemcitabine, tamoxifen, Navelbine, ifosfamide, and 5-fluorouracil (5-FU)/leucovorin. Although each of these agents appears to be more active in platinum-sensitive patients, major interest has been generated primarily by their activity in patients with resistant disease (Table 16.6).

Taxanes

Initial interest in paclitaxel in ovarian carcinoma developed from reports of phase II trials involving patients with platinum-resistant disease. Paclitaxel achieved responses in 24% to 30% of these patients (17–20). Because of the extensive documentation of paclitaxel activity in this setting, this agent is clearly the treatment of choice when an objective response has not been achieved with an initial platinum-based regimen not containing a taxane.

The schedule and dosing for paclitaxel in second-line chemotherapy are still being evaluated, but administration every 3 weeks as either a 3-hour or a 24-hour infusion seems to be most appropriate. These two schedules yield similar efficacy but different toxicity profiles (21). The 24-hour infusion produces little nonhematologic toxicity but significant myelosuppression. The 3-hour infusion results in much less myelosuppression but more neurotoxicity and other nonhematologic adverse effects. Both schedules are well tolerated despite earlier concerns about hypersensitivity reactions and cardiotoxicity.

Longer infusions of paclitaxel have been reported to produce a significant number of responses in breast cancer patients in whom shorter infusions have failed. In a report of paclitaxel given as a 96-hour infusion to patients with ovarian carcinoma who had failed shorter infusions of paclitaxel, only 1 response was observed among 17 patients (22). It should be noted, however, that these 17 patients had been heavily pretreated with up to seven prior regimens and may well represent an unfair test of this approach. At least one study reported that weekly paclitaxel for salvage of ovarian carcinoma may allow more intense dosing because the safety profile for weekly paclitaxel appeared to be better than that associated with administration every 3 weeks (23). The value of such increased dose-intensity is, however, debatable (21–24).

Docetaxel, another taxane, is also active as second-line therapy in ovarian carcinoma, although reports to date have consisted of small phase II trials. Of potentially great interest is a recent report suggesting that docetaxel may be

TABLE 16.6. *Drugs with activity in platinum-resistant disease (data from best series)*

Drug (ref. no.)	Response rate		Progression-free survival (mo)
	No./total patients	%	
Paclitaxel (19)	9/27	33	4.0
Oral etoposide (27)	11/41	27	5.7
Doxil (29)	15/63	24	6.6
Topotecan (5-day schedule) (31)	14/113	12	3.0
Gemcitabine (39)	7/40	18	2.8
Vinorelbine (42)	4/24	17	4.0
Ifosfamide (46)	5/41	12	N/A
5-Fluorouracil/leucovorin (48)	5/29	17	N/A
Tamoxifen (50)	10/77	13	N/A

N/A, not applicable.

active when paclitaxel fails (25). This study documented a partial RR of 25% (3 of 12 patients) for docetaxel in patients whose disease was unresponsive to paclitaxel. Before applying this observation to general oncologic practice, the activity of docetaxel in this setting will have to be confirmed and the adequacy of the prior paclitaxel therapy will have to be evaluated.

Because paclitaxel is now a part of standard front-line therapy, attention is currently focused on agents with activity in patients who have disease resistant to both the platinum compounds and paclitaxel: oral etoposide, Doxil, topotecan, and gemcitabine.

Oral Etoposide

Among eight other agents with demonstrated activity in platinum-resistant disease, etoposide is the most interesting. Earlier studies of intravenous etoposide given for 3 to 5 days every 3 weeks produced variable response rates. The largest of these studies, conducted by the GOG (26), reported an RR of only 8.3% among 24 patients—a rate so low that no further studies were planned.

The subsequent availability of oral etoposide permitted a more prolonged course of 50 mg/m^2 daily for 21 days every 4 weeks. The GOG reported an RR of 27% among 41 patients with platinum-resistant disease (27). Three of these responses were durable complete responses. Although there are other reports of the activity of oral etoposide as second-line therapy, none has provided clear definitions of the population as either platinum sensitive or platinum resistant. More importantly, among 25 patients with disease resistant to both the platinum compounds and paclitaxel, 8 responses (32%) were observed. This is the highest reported response rate in patients with disease resistant to both of the front-line agents.

Oral etoposide produces toxicity that is centered primarily on myelosuppression and nausea and vomiting. In the GOG trial, 41% of patients who received 50 mg/m^2/day for 21 days experienced grade 3 or 4 myelosuppression; but this is less than that reported with topotecan. The second most common side effect was gastrointestinal; 10 of the 82 patients in the study experienced severe nausea and vomiting. On balance, the drug is better tolerated than two other prominent agents in the second-line setting, Doxil and topotecan. It produces numerically higher response rates, although such comparisons should be interpreted with caution. It can be given orally. For all these reasons, oral etoposide should probably be considered as the first agent to be employed in patients whose disease is resistant to paclitaxel and platinum.

Doxil

In a report from 1997, liposomal-encapsulated doxorubicin (Doxil) produced nine responses among 35 patients described as having refractory ovarian cancer (28). Among the 26 patients with resistant disease (defined as a treatment-free interval of less than 6 months), there were 7 responses (27%). None of these responders had experienced progression while receiving front-line therapy but rather exhibited treatment-free intervals of 1 to 3 months. Among the 9 patients with sensitive disease, there were 2 responses (22%), with treatment-free intervals of 12 and 15 months, respectively. These data certainly suggest that Doxil has activity in both platinum-sensitive and platinum-resistant patients.

A further report supports the 1997 study (29). Among 89 patients with platinum-resistant disease, 82 of whom also had disease resistant to paclitaxel, the RR to 50 mg/m^2 every 3 weeks was 23.8% in the 63 patients who could be evaluated for response. This is the second highest response rate reported among patients with disease resistant to both the platinum compounds and the taxanes and identifies Doxil as an excellent choice for management of such multiple-resistant ovarian cancers.

The most significant toxicity associated with Doxil is plantar-palmar erythrodysesthesia (hand-foot syndrome) which was observed in 20% of patients treated at 50 mg/m^2 every 3 weeks (29). Lower doses, in the range of 40 mg/m^2 every 3 weeks, are associated with significantly less hand-foot syndrome. Myelosuppression, primarily in the form of neutropenia, was seen in only 16% and is therefore less a problem than is the case with oral etoposide or topotecan.

Topotecan

Topotecan, a topoisomerase I inhibitor, has significant activity against ovarian cancer. In several reports, it appears to be active as second-line therapy in patients with either platinum-sensitive or platinum-resistant disease (30–38). Results appear to depend significantly on schedule; regimens involving courses of 5 or more days yield higher response rates (33–35,37).

The largest study of topotecan as second-line therapy was a randomized comparison of topotecan versus paclitaxel (30). There were no differences with regard to response rate, response duration, time to progression, or survival in a mixed population of patients with platinum-sensitive and platinum-resistant disease. The preliminary report actually suggested that topotecan had a superior time to progression, but the final analysis, as yet unpublished, showed no difference.

Results of several, smaller studies support the conclusion that topotecan is active and emphasize the importance of dose and schedule. In a study using a 5-day infusion schedule and a dosage of 1.5 mg/m^2, 4 responses (14%) were achieved among 28 evaluable patients with platinum-resistant disease (32–37). A Canadian trial evaluated a 5-day schedule versus a weekly 24-hour infusion in a randomized phase II trial involving patients who were not platinum resistant (33). The important observations were a 23% RR with the 5-day schedule and a 3% RR with the weekly 24-hour infusion. Yet another phase II trial evaluated a 24-hour infusion of 8.5 mg/m^2 every 3 weeks; only 2 partial responses among 29 patients were observed (37).

Another phase II trial assessed a 21-day infusion of topotecan in 24 patients and reported responses in 8 (35%) of 23 patients (36). A 3-day dosing schedule is being evaluated in another phase II trial; preliminary results from 29 patients indicate reduced toxicity and a reduced objective response rate (2 partial responses among the 29 patients) (35). These results do not prove the superiority of prolonged schedules, but such a conclusion is certainly suggested.

An alternative approach to lengthening the duration of the topotecan course is the use of an oral formulation of the drug. A phase II study of oral topotecan given on a 5-day schedule to 116 women who had failed one prior platinum-based regimen reported an overall RR of 18% with responses confirmed by independent review. This response rate appears to be similar to that of intravenous topotecan with somewhat less hematologic toxicity. Although this appears to be a promising approach, it should be noted that the percentage of patients with platinum-resistant disease was not reported in this study and that these patients had had only one prior chemotherapy regimen.

The major toxicity associated with topotecan was hematologic toxicity manifested primarily as neutropenia. With the 5-day dosing schedule at 1.5 mg/m^2/day in the largest of the topotecan groups, 82% of the patients experienced grade 4 neutropenia. Febrile neutropenia with suspected or actual infection occurred in 27%. No deaths from myelosuppression-related complications occurred.

In summary, topotecan appears to be active as second-line therapy in patients with platinum-resistant ovarian cancer. Results appear to be particularly sensitive to schedule; regimens employing courses of 5 or more days in duration produce higher response rates.

Gemcitabine

In a phase II study of patients with recurrent disease after initial platinum-based chemotherapy, gemcitabine at 800 mg/m^2 weekly for 3 weeks followed by a week of rest demonstrated significant activity (8 partial responses among 42 evaluable patients or 19%) (39). In the platinum-resistant subset, 7 responses were observed among 35 patients (20%). This established that gemcitabine is clearly active in platinum-resistant disease. Two other studies support this conclusion. A phase II trial of gemcitabine in a similar schedule at 1,200 mg/m^2 weekly in 38 patients with platinum-resistant disease reported an overall RR of 13.9% (40). More recently, another phase II trial of gemcitabine in a similar schedule at 2,000 mg/m^2

weekly reported 3 partial responses among 16 patients for an RR of 19% (41). In this last trial, all three responses occurred in patients who were both platinum and taxane resistant.

Toxicity consisted primarily of neutropenia in the first two studies and was characterized as mild. In the high dose trial, thrombocytopenia was the dose-limiting toxicity. There appeared to be no advantage to either of the higher-dose schedules.

Vinorelbine

Vinorelbine (Navelbine) has activity in platinum-resistant disease. In the largest phase II study, vinorelbine 25 mg/m^2 was given weekly; activity was reported in 33 patients, 24 of whom had platinum-resistant disease (42). Five responses—1 complete and 4 partial—occurred in the 24 patients with platinum-resistant disease (21%). In a subsequent report (43), investigators used a dose of 30 mg/m^2 weekly in 38 patients, 12 of whom had platinum-resistant disease. The overall RR was 29%, with 4 complete and 7 partial responses among the 38 patients. Among the 12 patients with platinum-resistant disease, the RR was 33%, with 1 complete and 3 partial responses.

A phase I study of vinorelbine for refractory disease evaluated 23 women with platinum-resistant disease who received vinorelbine for 3 days every 3 weeks (44). The overall RR among 20 evaluable patients was 30%. Because this phase I study was designed to test a potentially more convenient administration schedule for the drug, the very high incidence of nonhematologic manifestations of toxicity (especially bone pain) led the authors to recommend that this schedule not be pursued further despite the fact that the response rate was slightly higher that those reported in previous studies of vinorelbine given weekly.

On the negative side, the Southwest Oncology Group reported that the objective RR was only 3% among 81 patients with disease that was both paclitaxel- and platinum-resistant (45).

In all of these studies, vinorelbine was well tolerated, with major toxicities related to myelosuppression. However, none of the studies addressed disease resistant to both platinums and taxanes

Ifosfamide

Activity of ifosfamide in platinum-resistant ovarian cancer has been observed in two studies. The earlier study included 41 patients, who received between 1.0 and 1.2 gm/m^2/day for 5 days every 3 weeks (46). Five responses—1 complete and 4 partial—were observed. The more recent study, involving 21 patients, confirmed the suggested activity (47).

Of even greater interest, however, is the fact that the investigators in the more recent trial sought to confirm the hypothesis that the response rate to ifosfamide would be higher in patients who were naive to alkylating agent therapy. All of the patients had been treated with first-line paclitaxel and platinum and had not been exposed to any alkylating agents, unlike patients in the earlier study, who had received cyclophosphamide before the ifosfamide. The objective RR was 10% in the later study, similar to that reported in the earlier study. Although the hypothesis regarding efficacy in alkylating agent–naive patients was not confirmed, it is important to note that refractoriness to taxanes may not diminish the activity of ifosfamide and that ifosfamide has definite, albeit modest, activity in the patient population with disease resistant to the platinums and taxanes.

Major toxicity of ifosfamide includes myelosuppression and central nervous system toxicity. Myelosuppression is manifested primarily as neutropenia, which occurs at a grade 3 or 4 level in only 20% of patients at the dose of 1 to 1.2 g/m^2 daily for 5 days every 3 weeks. Central nervous system toxicity occurs in 12% of the patients and is characterized by disorientation, hallucinations, somnolence, and agitation. The frequency of central nervous system toxicity increases with low albumin, renal impairment, and shorter schedules of administration.

5-Fluorouracil plus Leucovorin

The combination of 5-FU plus leucovorin given daily for 5 days every 4 weeks produced 5 responses (1 complete and 4 partial) among 29 patients in a phase II trial of the GOG (48). This suggests that the combination is active. The only caveat is the fact that, among 15 patients with platinum-sensitive disease, only 1 responded (7%). The activity of this regimen needs to be confirmed.

Tamoxifen

The GOG studied the effectiveness of tamoxifen 20 mg orally twice daily in patients with recurrent or persistent ovarian cancer (49). Among 105 patients, there were 19 responses (18%). In a subsequent report, this study was reanalyzed according to whether the patients had platinum-sensitive or platinum-resistant disease (50). In the platinum-resistant population, there were 10 responses among 77 patients (13%). Of note is the analysis of estrogen receptor status in patients who achieved a complete response. Eight of nine were estrogen receptor–positive. However, 59% of those with stable or progressive disease also were positive for estrogen receptors.

Other Agents

Among other agents tested, mitoxantrone has demonstrated potential activity in patients with disease resistant to the platinums and the taxanes. In a phase II study, mitoxantrone 28 mg/m^2 every 3 to 4 weeks produced 5 responses among 33 patients (15%) (51). Because four of the responses were defined only by a decline in the serum CA-125 level, further study is needed to determine whether mitoxantrone has activity as second-line therapy for ovarian carcinoma.

Another agent approved for second-line therapy is hexamethylmelamine. There are three key studies addressing the role of hexamethylmelamine. Vergote and colleagues treated 57 patients with platinum-resistant disease with 260 mg/m^2 daily for 14 days every 4 weeks. Three complete and 4 partial responses were observed among 50 patients evaluable for response (RR, 14%) (52). The GOG observed with hexamethylmelamine at the same dose and schedule 1 complete and 2 partial responses among 36 patients, 30 of whom were evaluable for response (RR, 10%) (53). In a much earlier study, Manetta and colleagues saw no responses among 11 patients with platinum-resistant disease (54). These data provide a somewhat mixed picture, but the response rate to hexamethylmelamine is at best modest in patients with resistant disease. In exchange for this modest response rate, the drug induces significant gastrointestinal toxicity, manifested primarily by nausea and vomiting.

A number of other agents have been tested with little or no success in the platinum-resistant disease population, including melphalan, cyclophosphamide, doxorubicin, and hydroxyurea. Two of these agents (melphalan and hydroxyurea) are approved for use as second-line therapy for ovarian carcinoma. Although both have some activity in platinum-sensitive disease (as do the other two), use of a platinum compound or paclitaxel is better in such a population. In resistant disease, the agents discussed earlier are better choices.

Significant Questions Regarding Second-Line Therapy

Although a rational approach to second-line therapy can be based on the response to initial chemotherapy, a number of questions remain unanswered. These concern the selection of a regimen and the roles of high-dose and intraperitoneal (IP) chemotherapy.

Selection of Regimen

The choice of specific regimen in the second-line setting is to some extent a matter of personal bias. There are, however, some considerations that should be taken into account (2–5). In the front-line setting, randomized trials show a clear advantage for paclitaxel-platinum combinations over single agents. Extrapolation from these studies to the management of chemosensitive patients in the setting of second-line therapy has led to the generally accepted recommendation that a paclitaxel-platinum combination be used. Dose and schedule should reflect what is known about front-line therapy.

TABLE 16.7. *Recommendations for second-line chemotherapy for patients with platinum-resistant disease*

1. General recommendations
   a. Patients should be treated with a drug or regimen that achieves responses in disease resistant to the regimen used as part of front-line therapy.
   b. Assuming that front-line therapy consisted of paclitaxel plus a platinum compound, alternatives include oral etoposide, Doxil, topotecan, gemcitabine, tamoxifen, navelbine, ifosfamide, and 5-fluorouracil plus leucovorin.
2. Selection of drug (in order of recommended priority)
   a. Oral etoposide
   b. Doxil
   c. Topotecan

TABLE 16.8. *Randomized trial of doxil versus topotecan in second-line therapy for ovarian carcinoma*

Parameter	Doxil	Topotecan
Patients	239	235
Response (%)		
Overall	20	17
Sensitive	28	29
Resistant	12	7
Survival (wk)		
Overall	53	51
Sensitive[a]	86	64
Resistant	33	37

[a] $p = .012$.

From Gordon A, Fleagle J, Guthrie D, et al. Interim analysis of a phase III randomized trial of Doxil/Caelyx versus topotecan in the treatment of patients with relapsed ovarian cancer [Abstract]. *Proc ASCO* 2000;19:3802, with permission.

In the management of chemoresistant patients (Table 16.7), virtually no studies of combination chemotherapy have been conducted. Single-agent therapy is usually chosen. Choice of the specific agent should be based on reported response rates and other factors. The agent with the highest RR in paclitaxel-platinum resistant patients (32%) is oral etoposide; hence, etoposide should be considered as the first salvage therapy (27).

The second highest RR reported in an abstract in the 1999 *Proceedings of ASCO* was that produced by Doxil (23%) (29). This agent has just been approved for use in the second-line setting and is a logical second choice. The most intensively studied of the salvage agents is topotecan, which has clear activity (13% RR in platinum-resistant patients) as well as approval of the U.S. Food and Drug Administration in the setting of second-line therapy. This drug would be a logical third choice.

In particular, the choice between Doxil and topotecan has been evaluated in a randomized trial (Table 16.8) (55). A total of 474 patients who had received prior front-line chemotherapy with a platinum-based combination were randomly assigned at recurrence or progression to either Doxil 50 mg/m^2 every 3 weeks or topotecan 1.5 mg/m^2/day for 5 days every 3 weeks. Patients were stratified according to whether they had platinum-sensitive or platinum-resistant disease and also according to whether or not they had bulky (more than 5 cm) disease. In the overall analysis and in the platinum-resistant group, there were no significant differences in response rate, time to progression, or overall survival. In the platinum-sensitive subset, Doxil produced superior survival results. In terms of toxicity, topotecan produced significantly more myelosuppression; whereas Doxil caused plantar-palmar erythrodysesthesia in 23% of patients. Doxil appeared to offer advantages over topotecan in terms of greater ease of administration (1 day versus 5 days) and less overall toxicity. This would support the recommendation to choose Doxil as the second agent in the second-line setting and topotecan as the third.

Situations will arise in which the use of one of these three agents is inappropriate or not feasible. In other instances, patients who have failed these three second-line drugs will have sufficient performance status and desire to be treated further that other agents might be considered. Because of its relative lack of toxicity and its reported 13% RR in platinum-resistant patients, tamoxifen would make a reasonable choice in situations in which toxicity was a major concern. Gemcitabine, Navelbine, 5-FU/leucovorin, and ifosfamide all have similar response rates in platinum-resistant patients and can be considered. The one other drug often used as second-line therapy is hexamethylmelamine, but studies in platinum-resistant patients each produced RRs of less than 10%.

High-Dose Chemotherapy

Although the role of high-dose chemotherapy supported by stem cell transplantation as initial therapy for ovarian cancer or as consolidation therapy in remission remains unclear and requires further evaluation, this approach does not have a defined place in the salvage setting. A review article from February 1999 found that, almost uniformly, high-dose chemotherapy for bulky and/or heavily pretreated disease gave high initial response rates but no significant survival advantage (56). Because palliation is the primary goal in the salvage setting, the excessive toxicity from high-dose chemotherapeutic regimens is undesirable.

Intraperitoneal Chemotherapy

The role of IP therapy in front-line treatment of ovarian carcinoma awaits refinement by an ongoing phase III trial by the GOG. The role of IP therapy in the salvage setting, however, is in serious question. A study of IP platinum-based therapy in 1991 reported that, among those with platinum-sensitive disease, a 42% CR was observed; whereas the CR among platinum-resistant patients was only 7% (57). Because these response rates are similar to those achieved with intravenous platinum-based therapy in the second-line setting, the advantage of IP therapy as compared to intravenous therapy is not clear at all.

In a review article on salvage therapy for ovarian cancer, IP therapy with platinum was recommended as the second-line therapy for patients with platinum-sensitive disease (58), but the basis for the preference was not clear. At present, there seems to be little role for IP chemotherapy in the management of patients with platinum-resistant disease or patients with residual tumor of any size (especially larger than 2 cm).

CONCLUSIONS

The current management of ovarian carcinoma in patients with recurrence after initial platinum-based chemotherapy depends on consideration of the results of initial chemotherapy. Patients who respond to initial platinum-based therapy and relapse after a reasonable platinum-free interval should be considered to be clinically sensitive to further platinum-based treatment. Such therapy will yield RRs as high as 60%, with up to 25% of patients achieving a complete response. There is no evidence that more dose-intense approaches yield better results in these patients than standard intravenous schedules.

Patients with failure to respond to initial platinum-based therapy or relapse shortly after completion of initial therapy should be regarded as clinically resistant to further platinum-based treatment. Such patients should be treated with drugs which have been shown to have activity against resistant disease. These include taxol, oral etoposide, Doxil, topotecan, tamoxifen, gemcitabine, Navelbine, 5-FU/leucovorin, and ifosfamide. There is no evidence that combinations of these drugs are more effective than single-agent therapy.

REFERENCES

1. Landis SH, Murray T, Bolden S, Wingo PA. Cancer statistics, 1999. *CA Cancer J Clin* 1999;49:8–31.
2. McGuire WP, Hoskins WJ, Brady MF, et al. Cyclophosphamide and cisplatin compared with paclitaxel in patients with stage III and stage IV ovarian cancer. *N Engl J Med* 1996;334:1–6.
3. Piccart MJ, Bertelsen K, Stuart G, et al. Is cisplatin-paclitaxel the standard in first-line treatment of advanced ovarian cancer? The EORTC-GCCG, NOCOVA, NCI-C and Scottish intergroup experience [Abstract]. *Proc Am Soc Clin Oncol* 1997;16:352a.
4. Muggia FM, Braly PS, Brady MF, et al. Phase III trial of cisplatin or paclitaxel versus their combination in suboptimal stage III and IV epithelial ovarian cancer: Gynecologic Oncology Group study #132 [Abstract]. *Proc Am Soc Clin Oncol* 1997;16:352a.
5. Harper P. A randomised comparison of paclitaxel (T) and carboplatin (J) versus a control arm of single agent carboplatin (J) or CAP (cyclophosphamide, doxorubicin, and cisplatin): 2075 patients randomised into the 3rd International Collaborative Ovarian Neoplasm study (ICON3) [Abstract]. *Proc Am Soc Clin Oncol* 1999; 18:356a.
6. Thigpen T: Second-line therapy for ovarian carcinoma: general concepts. In Perry M, ed, *American society of clinical oncology 1999 educational book,* ASCO, Alexandria, Virginia, 1999, 564–566.
7. Bolis G, Colombo N, Pecorelli S, et al. Adjuvant treatment for early epithelial ovarian cancer: results of two randomised clinical trials comparing cisplatin to no further treatment or chromic phosphate. *Ann Oncol* 1995; 6:887–893.

8. Young R, Walton L, Ellenberg S, et al. Adjuvant therapy in stage I and stage II epithelial ovarian cancer. *N Engl J Med* 1990;322:1021–1027.
9. Thigpen T, Vance R, Khansur T. Second-line chemotherapy for recurrent carcinoma of the ovary. *Cancer* 1993; 71:1559–1564.
10. Colombo N, Marzola M, Parma G, et al. Paclitaxel vs CAP in recurrent platinum-sensitive ovarian cancer: a randomized phase II study [Abstract]. *Proc ASCO* 1996; 15:279.
11. Markman M, Rothman R, Hakes T, et al. Second line platinum therapy in patients with ovarian cancer previously treated with cisplatin. *J Clin Oncol* 1991;9:389–393.
12. Zanaboni R, Scarfone G, Presti M, et al. Salvage chemotherapy for ovarian cancer recurrence: weekly cisplatin in combination with epirubicin or etoposide. *Gynecol Oncol* 1991;43:24–28.
13. Van der Burg M, Hoff A, van Lent M, et al. Carboplatin and cyclophosphamide salvage therapy for ovarian cancer patients relapsing after cisplatin combination chemotherapy. *Eur J Cancer* 1991;27:248–250.
14. Weiss G, Green S, Alberts D, et al. Second-line treatment of advanced measurable ovarian cancer with iproplatin: a Southwest Oncology Group study. *Eur J Cancer* 1991;27:135–138.
15. Rose PG, Fusco N, Fluellen L, Rodriguez M. Second-line therapy with paclitaxel and carboplatin for recurrent disease following first-line therapy with paclitaxel and platinum in ovarian or peritoneal carcinoma. *J Clin Oncol* 1998;16:1494–1497.
16. Thigpen T, Blessing J, Homesley H, et al. Cisplatin as salvage therapy in ovarian carcinoma treated initially with single agent paclitaxel: a Gynecologic Oncology Group study [Abstract]. *Proc Am Soc Clin Oncol* 1996;15:286.
17. McGuire WP, Rowinsky EK, Rosenshein NB, et al. Taxol: a unique antineoplastic agent with significant activity in advanced ovarian epithelial neoplasms. *Ann Intern Med* 1989;111:273–279.
18. Einzig AI, Wiernik PH, Sasloff J, et al. Phase II study and long-term follow-up of patients treated with taxol for advanced ovarian adenocarcinoma. *J Clin Oncol* 1992;10:1748–1753.
19. Thigpen JT, Blessing JA, Ball H, et al. Phase II trial of paclitaxel in patients with progressive ovarian carcinoma after platinum-based chemotherapy: a Gynecologic Oncology Group study. *J Clin Oncol* 1994;12:1748–1753.
20. Kohn EC, Sarosy G, Bicher A, et al. Dose-intense taxol: high response rate in patients with platinum-resistant recurrent ovarian cancer. *J Natl Cancer Inst* 1994;86: 18–24.
21. Eisenhauer E, ten Bokkel Huinink W, Swenerton K, et al. European-Canadian randomized trial of paclitaxel in relapsed ovarian cancer: high-dose versus low-dose and long versus short infusion. *J Clin Oncol* 1994;12:2654.
22. Markman M, Rose PG, Jones E, et al. Ninety-six hour infusional paclitaxel as salvage therapy of ovarian cancer patients previously failing treatment with 3-hour or 24-hour paclitaxel infusion regimens. *J Clin Oncol* 1998;16:1849–1851.
23. Rosenberg P, Andersson H, Boman K, et al. A randomized multicenter study of single agent paclitaxel (TAXOL) given weekly versus every three weeks to patients (PTS) with ovarian cancer (OC) previously treated with platinum therapy [Abstract]. *Proc Am Soc Clin Oncol* 1999;18:368a.
24. Omura G, Brady M, Delmore J, et al. A randomized trial of paclitaxel at 2 dose levels and filgastrim at 2 dose levels in platinum pretreated epithelial ovarian cancer: a GOG, SWOG, NCCTTG, and ECOG study. *Proc Am Soc Clin Oncol* 1996;15:280.
25. Kavanagh JJ, Winn R, Steger M, et al. Docetaxel for patients with ovarian cancer refractory to paclitaxel, an update [Abstract]. *Proc Am Soc Clin Oncol* 1999;18:368a.
26. Slayton R, Creasman W, Petty W, et al. A phase II trial of VF-16-213 in the treatment of advanced squamous cell carcinoma of the cervix and adenocarcinoma of the ovary: a Gynecologic Oncology Group study. *Cancer Treat Rep* 1982;66:1569–1671.
27. Rose P, Blessing J, Mayer A, et al. Prolonged oral etoposide as second-line therapy for platinum-resistant and platinum-sensitive ovarian carcinoma: a Gynecologic Oncology Group study. *J Clin Oncol* 1998;16:405–410.
28. Muggia F, Hainsworth J, Jeffers S, et al. Phase II study of liposomal doxorubicin in refractory ovarian cancer: antitumor activity and toxicity modification by liposomal encapsulation. *J Clin Oncol* 1997;15:987–993.
29. Rose P, Gordon AN, Granai CO, et al. Interim analysis of a non-comparative, multicenter study of DOXIL/CAELYX in the treatment of patients with refractory ovarian cancer [Abstract]. *Proc Am Soc Clin Oncol* 1999;18:360a.
30. ten Bokkel Huinink W, Gore M, Carmichael J, et al. Topotecan versus paclitaxel for the treatment of recurrent epithelial ovarian cancer. *J Clin Oncol* 1997;15:2183–2193.
31. Bookman MA, Malmstrom H, Bolis G, et al. Topotecan for the treatment of advanced epithelial ovarian cancer: an open-label phase II study in patients treated after prior chemotherapy that contained cisplatin or carboplatin and paclitaxel. *J Clin Oncol* 1998;16:3345–3352.
32. Kudelka A, Tresukosol D, Edwards C, et al. Phase II study of intravenous topotecan as a 5-day infusion for refractory epithelial ovarian cancer. *J Clin Oncol* 1996;14:1552–1557.
33. Hoskins P, Eisenhauer E, Beare S, et al. Randomized phase II study of two schedules of topotecan in previously treated patients with ovarian cancer: a National Cancer Institute of Canada Clinical Trials Group study. *J Clin Oncol* 1998;16:2233–2237.
34. Hochster H, Wadler S, Runowicz C, et al. Activity and pharmacodynamics of 21-day topotecan infusion in patients with ovarian cancer previously treated with platinum-based chemotherapy. *J Clin Oncol* 1999;17:2553–2561.
35. Belinson J, Kennedy A, Webster K, et al. Preliminary results of a Cleveland Clinic Cancer Center Gynecologic Oncology Program phase 2 trial of topotecan (TOPO) administered on a 3-day schedule as salvage therapy of platinum and paclitaxel refractory ovarian cancer (ROC) [Abstract]. *Proc Am Soc Clin Oncol* 1999;18:369a.
36. Clarke-Pearson DL, Van Le L, Iveson T, et al. A phase II study of oral topotecan as a single agent, second-line therapy, administered for five days in patients with advanced ovarian cancer [Abstract]. *Proc Am Soc Clin Oncol* 1999;18:368a.
37. Markman M, Blessing J, Alvarez R, et al. Phase II evaluation of 24-h continuous infusion topotecan in recurrent, potentially platinum-sensitive ovarian cancer: a Gynecologic Oncology Group study. *Gynecol Oncol* 2000;77:112–115.

38. McGuire W, Blessing J, Bookman M, et al. Topotecan has substantial antitumor activity as first-line salvage therapy in platinum-sensitive epithelial ovarian carcinoma: a Gynecologic Oncology Group study. *J Clin Oncol* 2000;18:1062–1067.
39. Lund B, Hansen O, Theilade K, et al. Phase II study of gemcitabine in previously treated ovarian cancer patients. *J Natl Cancer Inst* 1994;86:1530–1533.
40. Friedlander M, Millward MJ, Bell D, et al. A phase II study of gemcitabine in platinum pre-treated patients with advanced epithelial ovarian cancer. *Ann Oncol* 1998;9:1343–1345.
41. Kudelka AP, Verschraegen CF, Edwards CL, et al. A preliminary report of a phase 2 study of gemcitabine in women with platinum refractory mullerian (ovarian, fallopian tube and primary peritoneal) carcinomas [Abstract]. *Proc Am Soc Clin Oncol* 1999;18:377a.
42. Bajetta E, Di Leo A, Biganzoli L, et al. Phase II study of vinorelbine in patients with pretreated advanced ovarian cancer: activity in platinum-resistant disease. *J Clin Oncol* 1996;14:2546–2551.
43. Burger RA, DiSaia PJ, Roberts JA, et al. Phase II trial of vinorelbine in recurrent and progressive epithelial ovarian cancer. *Gynecol Oncol* 1999;72:148–153.
44. Gershenson DM, Burke TW, Morris M, et al. A phase I study of a daily ×3 schedule of intravenous vinorelbine for refractory epithelial ovarian cancer. *Gynecol Oncol* 1998;70:404–409.
45. Rothenberg ML, Liu PY, Nahhas WA, et al. A phase II trial of vinorelbine in relapsed and refractory ovarian cancer: a Southwest Oncology Group study (SWOG-9324) [Abstract]. *Proc Am Soc Clin Oncol* 1999;18:383a.
46. Markman M, Hakes T, Reichman B, et al. Ifosfamide and mesna in previously treated advanced epithelial ovarian cancer: activity in platinum-resistant disease. *J Clin Oncol* 1992;10:243–248.
47. Markman M, Kennedy A, Sutton G, et al. Phase 2 trial of single agents ifosfamide/mesna in patients with platinum/paclitaxel refractory ovarian cancer who have not previously been treated with an alkylating agent. *Gynecol Oncol* 1998;70:272–274.
48. Look K, Muss H, Blessing J, Morris M. A phase II trial of 5-fluorouracil and high-dose leucovorin in recurrent epithelial ovarian carcinoma: a gynecologic Oncology Group study. *Am J Clin Oncol* 1995;18:19–22.
49. Hatch K, Beecham J, Blessing J, Creasman W. Responsiveness of patients with advanced ovarian carcinoma to tamoxifen. *Cancer* 1991;68:269–271.
50. Markman M, Iseminger K, Hatch K, et al. Tamoxifen in platinum-refractory ovarian cancer: a Gynecologic Oncology Group ancillary report. *Gynecol Oncol* 1996;62:4–6.
51. Markman M, Lichtman S, Homesley H, et al. Phase 2 trial of moderately high dose single agent mitoxantrone in platinum and paclitaxel-refractory ovarian cancer. *Gynecol Oncol* 1998;70:123–126.
52. Vergote I, Himmelmann A, Frankendal B, et al. Hexamethylmelamine as second-line therapy in platin-resistant ovarian cancer. *Gynecol Oncol* 1992;47:282–286.
53. Markman M, Blessing J, Moore D, et al. Altretamine (hexamethylmelamine) in platinum-resistant and platinum-refractory ovarian cancer: a Gynecologic Oncology Group phase II trial. *Gynecol Oncol* 1998;69:226–229.
54. Manetta A, Tewari K, Podczaski E. Hexamethylmelamine as a single second-line agent in ovarian cancer: follow-up report and review of the literature. *Gynecol Oncol* 1997;66:20–26.
55. Gordon A, Fleagle J, Guthrie D, et al. Interim analysis of a phase III randomized trial of Doxil/Caelyx versus Topotecan in the treatment of patients with relapsed ovarian cancer [Abstract]. *Proc Am Soc Clin Oncol* 2000;19:380a.
56. Herrin VE, Thipgen JT. High-dose chemotherapy in ovarian carcinoma. *Semin Oncol* 1999;26:99–105.
57. Markman M, Reichman B, Hakes T, et al. Responses to second-line cisplatin-based intraperitoneal therapy in ovarian cancer: influence of a prior response to intravenous cisplatin. *J Clin Oncol* 1991;9:1801–1805.
58. Alberts DS. Treatment of refractory and recurrent ovarian cancer. *Semin Oncol* 1999;26[Suppl 1]:8–14.

17
Intraperitoneal Chemotherapy

Maurie Markman

INTRACAVITARY CHEMOTHERAPY OF MALIGNANT DISEASE: HISTORICAL PERSPECTIVE

The earliest experience with the intraperitoneal administration of cytotoxic agents in the management of the patient with cancer was reported in the 1950s and 1960s and included the use of nitrogen mustard, hemisulfur mustard, 5-fluorouracil (5-FU), and thiotepa (1). Although these studies were limited in patient number and the response criteria were generally not well defined, individual patients were reported to experience objective and subjective improvement in cancer-related symptoms, particularly the control of malignant ascites reaccumulation.

Unfortunately, the *local side effects* of this therapeutic approach (e.g., abdominal pain, adhesion formation, bowel obstruction) were frequently quite severe, especially when agents were employed that were known to cause direct toxicity to tissue when extravasation occurred after *intravenous* administration. In addition, actual shrinkage of tumor masses was rarely observed after intracavitary cytotoxic drug delivery. Finally, with the demonstrated ability of systemically administered cytotoxic agents to control ascites formation, particularly in ovarian cancer, there appeared to be little reason to instill the drugs directly into the abdominal cavity.

Therefore, not surprisingly, there was little enthusiasm generated for this therapeutic strategy based on the early experience. However, investigators at a number of centers continued to report success with the use of intracavitary cytotoxic drug delivery for the control of malignant fluid reaccumulation, particularly pleural effusions (2). Bleomycin is the cytotoxic agent most commonly used for this purpose (3).

However, this drug, as well as other cytotoxic agents, has enjoyed only limited success when administered intraperitoneally to control ascites reaccumulation.

BASIC PRINCIPLES OF INTRAPERITONEAL THERAPY IN THE MANAGEMENT OF OVARIAN CANCER

Interest in the intraperitoneal administration of chemotherapeutic agents for their *cytotoxic* rather than sclerosing properties was renewed in the late 1970s after the publication of a now classic paper by Dedrick and his colleagues at the National Cancer Institute (NCI), in which the authors presented a sound pharmacokinetic rationale for this therapeutic approach in the management of ovarian cancer (4).

The mathematical model put forth by the NCI investigators suggested that, depending on the unique characteristics of individual antineoplastic agents, tumor present within the peritoneal cavity could be exposed to 10 to 1,000 times higher concentrations of the drug, compared with the systemic circulation, after direct intraperitoneal administration. The *slower* a drug exits the cavity and the more *rapidly* it is removed from the systemic compartment (renal or biliary excretion, metabolism), the greater the pharmacokinetic advantage associated with the intraperitoneal instillation of the agent.

Properties known to *increase* the pharmacokinetic advantage associated with intraperitoneal delivery include larger drug size and limited lipid solubility (1). In addition, drugs that are rapidly and extensively metabolized into nontoxic metabolites during their first passage through the liver have been shown to possess

TABLE 17.1. *Pharmacokinetic advantage associated with the intraperitoneal administration of selected agents with activity in ovarian cancer*

Agent	Peak peritoneal cavity/plasma concentration ratio
Cisplatin	20
Carboplatin	18
Melphalan	93
Mitoxantrone	620
Doxorubicin	474
5-Fluorouracil	298
Paclitaxel	1,000

the greatest pharmacokinetic advantage after intraperitoneal delivery, because the major route of drug exit from the peritoneal cavity is by way of the portal circulation, rather than by direct uptake into the systemic compartment (1). Therefore, it is not surprising that the agents that have demonstrated the greatest pharmacokinetic advantage after intraperitoneal delivery are the antineoplastic drugs, such as 5-FU, doxorubicin, and paclitaxel, which are metabolized in the liver (Table 17.1).

A second important principle of intraperitoneal therapy is the need for instilled drug to come in *direct* contract with the tumor. When antineoplastic agents are delivered systemically, they reach tumor by capillary flow. However, with intraperitoneal administration there is no vascular compartment to ensure that the drug-containing fluid actually reaches the site of the malignant cells. This problem is compounded by the fact that patients considered for intraperitoneal chemotherapy may have previously undergone one or more laparotomies, with subsequent adhesion formation secondary to the surgical injury, which may interfere with the adequacy of drug distribution throughout the peritoneal cavity.

Both preclinical evaluation and the results of limited human trials have demonstrated that distribution of the drug-containing treatment fluid can be enhanced by instilling the agent in a large volume (5,6). In most clinical trials the treatment volume used has been approximately 2 L, but it can certainly be argued that in many patients an even larger volume might further improve the distribution of the cytotoxic agent or agents. Patients who are unable to tolerate a treatment volume of 2 L, due to abdominal pain or extremely slow instillation times, are not good candidates for intraperitoneal therapy because it is almost certain that only a limited portion of the peritoneal cavity will be bathed with the drug-containing fluid. If the adequacy of distribution is questioned in an individual patient, either a radionuclide scan or a computed tomographic scan with intraperitoneal contrast can be employed to evaluate the cavity after drug administration (7,8).

Perhaps the major limiting factor in defining the patient population in whom intraperitoneal therapy is a reasonable therapeutic option is the known limited depth of penetration of chemotherapeutic agents directly into tissue by *free surface diffusion*. Both *in vitro* and *in vivo* experimental systems have confirmed that, depending on the specific therapeutic agent employed, the depth of penetration of antineoplastic agents is limited to several cell layers, with a maximum of 1 to 3 mm from the surface of the peritoneal lining (9–11). However, if is not just the depth of penetration after intraperitoneal therapy that is at issue, but rather the actual concentration of drug within the tissue observed after the regional approach, compared with tissue levels achieved with systemic drug administration. For example, if levels of the cytotoxic drug obtained within tumor tissue after intravenous therapy essentially equaled those achieved through the regional approach, it would be difficult to justify the added time, expense, and morbidity associated with intraperitoneal therapy.

A direct comparison of platinum tissue levels attained after intraperitoneal cisplatin administration compared with intravenous delivery of the agent was reported in an experimental system, with higher tissue concentrations of cisplatin being demonstrated only to a depth of 0.1 to 1 mm from the peritoneal surface (11). Patients usually undergo more than a single course of therapy. Therefore, subsequent treatment cycles may be associated with a cytotoxic effect to tumor cells that were initially deeper than 1 mm from the peritoneal surface, as malignant cells killed from previous treatment courses are removed from the cavity. However, on the basis of this experimental model, it would be predicted that any clinically relevant advantage of intraperitoneal cisplatin administration, compared with systemic drug delivery, would be limited to those patients with ovarian cancer who have tumor nodules of very small volume (0.5 cm or less in maximal diameter) or only microscopic disease at the initiation of the regional treatment program. As discussed later in this chapter, this hypothesis has been shown to be remarkably accurate in predicting the clinical activity of intraperitoneal cisplatin-based therapy when it is used as a second-line treatment strategy in patients with ovarian cancer.

Finally, there is the important issue of the relative importance of cytotoxic drug delivery to tumor by *capillary flow* versus *free surface diffusion*. It is appropriate to question the potential negative consequences associated with achieving high local tumor drug interactions on the surface of the peritoneal lining if an additional feature of regional drug administration is a *decrease* in the concentration of the cytotoxic agent reaching the tumor through the vascular system. It is theoretically possible that the overall effectiveness of this therapeutic strategy may be inferior to systemic drug administration, despite the levels of the cytotoxic agent demonstrated in the peritoneal cavity after regional delivery.

If the agent or agents selected for intraperitoneal administration are not limited by their local side effects, the dose-limiting toxicity will be systemic (e.g., bone marrow suppression, mucositis). Therefore, it is reasonable to suggest that under these circumstances (antineoplastic drug delivered at its maximally tolerated dose) the same amount of cytotoxic agent is entering the systemic compartment and reaching the tumor by capillary flow after intraperitoneal instillation as would be observed if the drug were administered systemically. Therefore, at least in theory, there should be no compromise in efficacy associated with the regional administration of the cytotoxic agent. Conversely, if the amount of an antineoplastic agent that can be administered into the peritoneal cavity is limited by its local rather than its systemic side effects, the exposure of the tumor to drug by capillary flow will be reduced, compared with systemic delivery. As discussed later, the intraperitoneal administration of paclitaxel produces extremely high cavity but minimal systemic levels of the agent (12,13). Therefore, *optimal* use of this agent in ovarian cancer might be to deliver it by both the intraperitoneal and systemic routes.

UNIQUE TOXICITIES ASSOCIATED WITH INTRAPERITONEAL THERAPY

Before embarking on a discussion of the specific drugs and drug combinations examined for clinical activity in patients with ovarian cancer, it is important to address two unique potential toxicities associated with this therapeutic strategy.

The first issue is the need to establish a safe and convenient access to the peritoneal cavity for administration of the antineoplastic agent. Although it is possible to place a percutaneous catheter into the peritoneal cavity at the time of each treatment course, this approach is very time-consuming, runs a high risk of causing a bowel perforation in a patient with adhesions from prior surgeries, and may be associated with poor treatment volume distribution if the catheter is inserted into a region of the cavity that is separated from other parts of the compartment by adhesions. Most investigators have employed semipermanent indwelling catheters, which are surgically placed, to administer the intraperitoneal therapy (14,15). This strategy has been associated with excellent patient acceptance and acceptable rates of catheter failure and infection (15–18).

Of greater concern are the potential complications associated with the drugs administered into the peritoneal cavity. Drugs that are irritants may cause minor, moderate, or severe pain. Although symptoms usually subside within several days, the inflammation associated with irritation of the peritoneal lining may lead to adhesion formation and interference with future treatment courses or subsequent bowel obstruction (19). Not surprisingly, cytotoxic agents that are known *vesicants*, such as doxorubicin, are associated with the most serious local toxicity (20,21). However, even drugs that have not been associated with serious local reactions when they extravasate into the subcutaneous tissues may be associated with significant peritoneal irritation because of the extremely high concentrations of the agents that come in direct contact with the peritoneal lining after regional drug instillation (12,13,22,23).

Perhaps of greatest concern for the toxicity of intraperitoneal therapy is the potential for the development of acute or late bowel obstruction, secondary to extensive adhesion formation. Although bowel obstruction does occur, the extensive data currently available for single-agent intraperitoneal cisplatin therapy demonstrates that such events are uncommon (19,24). With other agents, such as mitoxantrone, the incidence of serious local toxic events may be considerably higher (22). Clinicians employing either single agents or combination regimens for intraperitoneal therapy must be aware of the relative potential of the specific program to induce peritoneal irritation, adhesion formation, and subsequent bowel obstruction.

SECOND-LINE INTRAPERITONEAL CHEMOTHERAPY TRIALS IN OVARIAN CANCER

A number of chemotherapeutic agents have been examined for their safety, pharmacokinetic advantage (Table 17.1), and potential efficacy when administered by the intraperitoneal route as therapy for ovarian cancer.

Cisplatin

Because of its central role in the management of ovarian cancer, cisplatin is the single agent that has undergone the most extensive evaluation for intraperitoneal delivery (25). Several phase I trials demonstrated a 10- to 20-fold increased exposure of the peritoneal cavity to cisplatin, compared with the systemic compartment, after regional delivery (6,26–28). As noted previously, there are minimal local effects observed when cisplatin is administered into the peritoneal cavity as a single agent, and the dose-limiting toxicities for intraperitoneal instillation of cisplatin are the systemic effects of the drug (e.g., emesis, nephrotoxicity, neurotoxicity).

Phase II trials of single-agent intraperitoneal cisplatin (29–31) and cisplatin-based combination regimens (32–37) have been conducted in patients with ovarian cancer previously treated with intravenous cisplatin. In the absence of randomized clinical trials comparing single-agent intraperitoneal cisplatin to any of the cisplatin-based intraperitoneal combination regimens, it cannot be concluded that any of the drug combinations are superior to cisplatin administered alone. Overall, approximately 20% to 30% of ovarian cancer patients have been reported to achieve a surgically defined complete response if "small-volume disease" was present at initiation of the second-line cisplatin-based intraperitoneal regimen.

In an effort to define ovarian cancer patient populations who might be considered reasonable candidates for second-line platinum-based intraperitoneal therapy, investigators have attempted to more critically evaluate the specific subgroups among individuals with "small-volume residual disease." In several trials, approximately 30% to 40% of patients whose largest tumor nodule measured 0.5 cm or less (including patients with only microscopic disease) were found to achieve surgically defined complete responses (32,33,36,38). In sharp contrast, fewer than 10% of patients with any mass greater than 1 cm in diameter achieved a complete response.

In addition, prior response to systemically administered cisplatin appears to significantly affect an individual's chances of achieving a response to second-line intraperitoneal cisplatin. In one report, patients who failed to respond to intravenous cisplatin achieved a low surgically defined complete response rate (less than 10%), despite the presence of very-small-volume residual disease (microscopic, or tumor masses less than 0.5 cm in diameter) (38). In contrast, patients who had previously responded to systemic cisplatin and who had very-small-volume residual disease when cisplatin-based intraperitoneal therapy was initiated experienced a 45% surgically defined complete response rate (Table 17.2).

On the basis of these data is it reasonable to suggest that a second-line cisplatin-based intraperitoneal chemotherapy program is an appropriate regimen for patients with surgically documented very-small-volume residual disease

TABLE 17.2. *Influence of a prior response to intravenous cisplatin on the secondary surgically-documented complete response rate to intraperitoneal cisplatin in patients with small-volume residual disease (maximum tumor diameter, ≤ 1 cm)*

Prior response status	No. patients	Complete response rate (%)
Prior response to cisplatin	36	42
No response to cisplatin	14	7

From Markman M, Reichman B, Hakes T, et al. Responses to second-line cisplatin-based intraperitoneal therapy in ovarian cancer: influence of a prior response to intravenous cisplatin. *J Clin Oncol* 1991;9:1801–1805, with permission.

(microscopic only, or macroscopic cancer no more than 0.5 cm in maximum diameter) who have demonstrated a major response to front-line cisplatin or carboplatin-based systemic therapy.

Two different approaches to the use of intraperitoneal cisplatin-based chemotherapy in ovarian cancer have been reported. The first is a standard cisplatin dosing program, approximately 75 to 100 mg/m^2. Pharmacokinetic data have demonstrated that approximately 70% to 90% of the cisplatin administered into the peritoneal cavity reaches the systemic compartment (6,26–28). Therefore, it is argued that a reasonable dose of cisplatin will also reach the tumor by capillary flow after regional drug delivery with this intraperitoneally administered dose of cisplatin.

The alternative approach, pioneered by investigators at the University of California, San Diego Medical Center, uses a significantly escalated dose of intraperitoneal cisplatin (200 mg/m^2 or more) (6,34,37,39–41). This strategy requires the simultaneous systemic administration of sodium thiosulphate to protect the kidneys from the nephrotoxic effects of the cisplatin (42,43). Pharmacokinetic studies have demonstrated that there is little inactivation of cisplatin in the systemic circulation or peritoneal cavity when this strategy is employed (6), but it remains to be determined whether doubling the dose of cisplatin in this manner results in a higher objective response rate and improved survival compared with a lower intraperitoneal dose of cisplatin without the neutralizing agent. At the present time, because of the potential for increased toxicity secondary to the high concentration of cisplatin used, this strategy should not be employed outside the clinical trial setting.

In the absence of data from randomized, controlled clinical trials, it is currently not possible to make a definitive statement regarding the ultimate impact on survival of a surgically documented response to second-line cisplatin-based intraperitoneal therapy in ovarian cancer. Even survival for 4 to 5 years after a second-line treatment regimen in individuals with small-volume residual ovarian cancer documented at second-look laparotomy may simply represent the natural history of disease in a subset of such patients (44–46). This point is relevant to all second-line treatment approaches administered to patients with small-volume residual ovarian cancer, including intensive chemotherapy with autologous bone marrow support. However, the fact that several groups have now reported prolonged survival for a subset of patients treated with second-line intraperitoneal cisplatin-based chemotherapy in this malignancy of interest (47–49), and their findings may lead to the conduct of randomized trials in this clinical setting.

Investigators at the Memorial Sloan-Kettering Cancer Center reported a provocative experience employing an intraperitoneal cisplatin/etoposide regimen in patients with advanced ovarian cancer who had achieved a surgically defined complete response to platinum-based systemic chemotherapy, where it is known that the ultimate relapse rate is greater than 50% (50). The relapse rate of patients treated with this "consolidation strategy" was compared with that of a nonrandomized institutional "control population" who were treated at Memorial during the same period as the conduct of the phase II intraperitoneal trial (51). Although patients in the control group had more favorable clinical characteristics (i.e., more stage II disease, less bulky residual disease at the initiation of initial systemic chemotherapy), they experienced a statistically significantly higher relapse rate. This observation needs to be confirmed through the conduct of a randomized trial.

Carboplatin

Compared with cisplatin, there has been considerably less experience with the use of carboplatin for intraperitoneal administration in the management of ovarian cancer. However, several phase I trials have both confirmed the safety of this route of drug delivery for carboplatin and established that the pharmacokinetic advantage associated with the intraperitoneal administration of this cytotoxic drug is similar to that of cisplatin (approximately 20-fold increased exposure of the peritoneal cavity compared with the systemic circulation) (52,53).

As might have been anticipated, the dose-limiting toxicity observed in these trials has been bone marrow suppression, particularly thrombocytopenia. This is a concern with the use of carboplatin as a second-line treatment strategy in patients with ovarian cancer. Because the drug is associated with considerable marrow toxicity, its use may be limited as a second-line intraperitoneal agent, particularly in patients treated with a systemic carboplatin-paclitaxel regimen, currently the "standard of care" for initial systemic chemotherapy of ovarian cancer (54,55).

In the several phase I clinical trials, the local toxicity of intraperitoneal carboplatin was observed to be particularly mild. In fact, surgical reassessment after intraperitoneal carboplatin therapy has been notable for minimal adhesion formation. In this regard, the local toxicity of carboplatin may be superior to that of cisplatin, although both cytotoxic agents are tolerated extremely well after intraperitoneal administration.

In addition, phase II trials of single-agent intraperitoneal carboplatin administered as a second-line therapy in patients with persistent or recurrent ovarian cancer have confirmed that objective antitumor responses, including surgically documented complete remissions, can be observed after the use of this agent (56,57). The surgical complete response rate in these trials (25%) was approximately equivalent to that achieved with either single-agent or combination cisplatin-based intraperitoneal chemotherapy programs for persistent or recurrent ovarian cancer.

However, a note of caution must be introduced before it is concluded that carboplatin and cisplatin are *equivalent* drugs for intraperitoneal administration in patients with ovarian cancer. Investigators in the Netherlands examined the intraperitoneal administration of carboplatin in the same rat model previously used to evaluate the depth of penetration of cisplatin in the peritoneal cavity after either intraperitoneal or systemic drug delivery (11,58). Despite the persistence of higher concentrations of carboplatin within the peritoneal cavity for longer periods than noted with intraperitoneal cisplatin, the levels of carboplatin within the tissue itself were significantly lower than those observed with an equitoxic dose of cisplatin. One likely explanation for these findings is that carboplatin is less able than cisplatin to penetrate into the normal tissue.

Although the clinical implications of these experimental findings are uncertain, one comparison of results of a nonrandomized trial experience suggested that the surgically documented complete response rate when intraperitoneal carboplatin is employed as a second-line strategy in small-volume macroscopic residual ovarian cancer is lower than that observed with intraperitoneal cisplatin (59). In this report, the surgically documented complete response rate in *microscopic* residual ovarian cancer was similar when either intraperitoneal cisplatin or carboplatin was used. This experience supports (but does not prove) the hypothesis that cisplatin is superior to the newer agent in regard to its ability to directly penetrate into small macroscopic tumor nodules.

For the present, based on these preclinical and clinical observations as well as the greater experience with intraperitoneal cisplatin, a second-line regional chemotherapy program in ovarian cancer employing cisplatin should be preferred over one using carboplatin outside a study setting, unless there is a contraindication to the use of the older platinum agent (e.g., nephrotoxicity, neurotoxicity from previous cisplatin).

Doxorubicin

Based on preclinical data demonstrating that intravenous treatment of a murine ovarian cancer was ineffective but intraperitoneal delivery of the agent produced long-term disease free survival (60), doxorubicin was one of the first agents to be examined for intraperitoneal use in patients with persistent ovarian cancer after front-line therapy. However, although a major pharmacokinetic advantage for this route of drug delivery was observed and objective antitumor responses were documented, the local toxicity of the agent was found to be excessive (21,34).

This should not have been surprising in view of the known vesicant properties of doxorubicin and experimental data demonstrating local toxicity after intraperitoneal delivery (20). However, it had been hoped that dilution of the drug in a treatment volume of several liters would minimize the toxic effects of the agent. It was shown in one trial that the toxicity of a combination regimen of cisplatin, cytarabine, and doxorubicin could be minimized if the dose of doxorubicin were markedly reduced (2 mg versus 20 to 30 mg used in single-agent trials), but the pharmacokinetic advantage associated with the regional administration of the agent was also greatly diminished with this approach (34). Therefore, most investigators have abandoned the use of intraperitoneal doxorubicin for trials in ovarian cancer.

It should be noted that the local toxicity associated with intraperitoneal administration of doxorubicin appears to be substantially reduced if the agent is delivered in liposomes (61). With the demonstrated activity of a systemically delivered liposomal doxorubicin preparation in platinum-resistant ovarian cancer (62), there may be interest in exploring this novel agent administered by the intraperitoneal route.

Mitoxantrone

In contrast to doxorubicin, mitoxantrone, a cytotoxic agent closely related to doxorubicin in toxicity and antitumor efficacy (63), is not considered a vesicant (64). In preclinical evaluation, mitoxantrone was demonstrated to be remarkably cytotoxic to most human ovarian cancers at concentrations of the agent achievable within the peritoneal cavity after intraperitoneal delivery, but not with systemic drug administration (65). The pharmacokinetic advantage of intraperitoneal mitoxantrone was demonstrated in several phase I trials, with cavity exposure exceeding systemic exposure by approximately 1,000-fold after regional drug delivery (66). However, the dose-limiting toxicity of the agent administered regionally is local toxicity, including abdominal pain, adhesion formation, and subsequent bowel obstruction. Although surgically documented responses and prolonged survival have been noted in several trials of second-line intraperitoneal mitoxantrone in ovarian cancer, the local toxicity of the agent severely limits the potential of the drug for regional delivery (22,67,68).

Alkylating Agents

Alkylating agents had been considered of interest for intraperitoneal administration in patients with ovarian cancer because of their known activity in the disease (25). For an agent to have the potential for exhibiting clinical utility after intraperitoneal administration, it is essential that the drug be active in its natural state and *not* require activation in the liver to become a cytotoxic drug. Thus, cyclophosphamide, which requires activation in the liver, could not be considered for intraperitoneal administration despite its antineoplastic activity in ovarian cancer.

In contrast, melphalan does not require activation in the liver. Several phase I clinical trials have demonstrated a pharmacokinetic advantage (approximately 100-fold), as well as tolerability, associated with the intraperitoneal administration of melphalan (69,70). The dose-limiting toxicity observed with its intraperitoneal delivery is bone marrow suppression.

A second alkylating agent, thiotepa, has also been examined for intraperitoneal administration (71). In contrast to experience with melphalan, the pharmacokinetic advantage associated with this alkylating agent was very modest (four-fold).

Although these data are of some interest, with the demonstration of the superiority of a platinum/paclitaxel regimen compared with a cisplatin/cyclophosphamide program in advanced ovarian cancer, there is currently limited enthusiasm for further investigation of the use of alkylating agents in ovarian cancer, for either systemic or regional delivery (72,73).

Etoposide

Interest in the administration of etoposide by the intraperitoneal route in patients with ovarian cancer comes from a large body of both preclinical evaluation and clinical trials which have demonstrated synergy between the agent and cisplatin (1). Single-agent etoposide has shown activity with prolonged oral administration in platinum-resistant ovarian cancer (74).

In several small phase I trials, single-agent intraperitoneal etoposide was demonstrated to be associated with acceptable local toxicity. The pharmacokinetic advantage observed with intraperitoneal administration was found to be modest (approximately 16-fold) (75). However, etoposide is a highly protein-bound drug. After intraperitoneal delivery, the pharmacokinetic advantage for cavity exposure associated with the "active" (nonprotein bound) drug was found to be 64-fold greater than that of the systemic circulation.

Etoposide has been combined with cisplatin in a number of phase II intraperitoneal trials of second-line therapy of ovarian cancer (36,37,76). Although surgically documented responses were observed, it remains unknown whether this combination regional chemotherapy strategy is superior to single-agent cisplatin in this clinical setting. There is particular concern for the potential for increased local toxicity associated with the two-drug intraperitoneal regimen. Therefore, outside the study setting, there appears little justification to employ a regional cisplatin/etoposide regimen rather than single-agent cisplatin or carboplatin.

5-Fluorouracil and 5-Floxuridine

Before the introduction of cisplatin into clinical practice, 5-FU was frequently used in several combination chemotherapy regimens in advanced ovarian cancer (77). Because the agent is rapidly and extensively metabolized into a nontoxic metabolite during its first passage through the liver, 5-FU is an ideal drug to consider for intraperitoneal delivery. It was one of the first drugs to be examined for its potential utility for intraperitoneal administration in patients with ovarian cancer.

Studies demonstrated that 5-FU was reasonably well tolerated after delivery into the peritoneal cavity, with both local pain and systemic toxicity (mucositis, marrow suppression) being dose-limiting (23,78). In addition, a major pharmacokinetic advantage (300-fold) for cavity exposure was demonstrated. However, minimal activity was shown in a phase II trial of intraperitoneal 5-FU in previously treated patients with ovarian cancer (79).

Limited data on delivery of the related fluoropyrimidine, FUDR (floxuridine), by the intraperitoneal route in ovarian cancer are more promising (80). Single-agent activity was observed, and the results of a randomized phase II trial in ovarian cancer suggested the potential superiority of intraperitoneal FUDR compared with intraperitoneal mitoxantrone (81).

Paclitaxel

Paclitaxel was an important cytotoxic agent to examine for regional delivery in ovarian cancer. First, the drug is active in platinum-resistant disease (82). Second, paclitaxel's large size and known hepatic metabolism would predict a significant pharmacokinetic advantage associated with intraperitoneal administration (83,84).

Phase I evaluation of the agent delivered by the intraperitoneal route demonstrated a greater than 1,000-fold pharmacokinetic advantage associated with exposure to the peritoneal cavity compared with the systemic compartment (12,13). In addition to high peak concentration and high AUC (area under the concentration-versus-time curve) associated with regional delivery of paclitaxel, significant cytotoxic concentrations of the drug persist within the peritoneal cavity for longer than 5 to 7 days after a single administration. Therefore, at least in theory, weekly intraperitoneal delivery of paclitaxel might be capable of producing a continuous exposure of at least the surface of the peritoneal lining to this potent cycle-specific antineoplastic agent.

As previously noted, the dose-limiting toxicity of intraperitoneal paclitaxel is local (abdominal pain) (12). There is only mild bone marrow suppression associated with intraperitoneal administration despite the extremely high concentrations of the agent achieved within the peritoneal cavity.

A phase II trial of second-line single-agent intraperitoneal paclitaxel demonstrated considerable activity for this route of administration in microscopic residual disease (85). In the presence of macroscopic residual tumor, however, intraperitoneal paclitaxel was essentially inactive, supporting the minimal penetration of the agent directly into tumor tissue and the limited delivery of the drug to cancer by capillary flow after regional treatment. As noted previously, the optimal use of this agent in small-volume ovarian cancer might be delivery by both the intravenous and intraperitoneal routes.

INTRAPERITONEAL ADMINISTRATION OF BIOLOGIC AGENTS

Over the past decade there has been increasing interest in the use of biologic agents in the treatment of malignant disease. Interest in this strategy for the treatment of cancer has been heightened with the availability of large quantities of these agents made through recombinant DNA techniques. As with cytotoxic chemotherapeutic agents, there is a strong rationale to consider the intraperitoneal use of biologic agents in ovarian cancer (86). Two major points can be made to support this therapeutic strategy. First, after intraperitoneal administration, tumor present in the cavity can be exposed to significantly higher concentrations of the drugs compared to those achieved with systemic delivery (86). To the extent that the activity of the biologic agents against ovarian cancer is concentration dependent, this may increase the effectiveness of therapy. Second, the direct intraperitoneal administration of biologic agents may lead to the stimulation and activation of local effector cells (e.g., lymphocytes, natural killer cells) that are cytotoxic to tumor.

A number of clinical trials have examined a variety of biologic agents for intraperitoneal delivery, including *Corynebacterium parvum* (87), recombinant α- and γ-interferon (88–91), recombinant interleukin-2 (92,93), and recombinant tumor necrosis factor (94). Objective antitumor activity was observed in a number of these trials. At the current time it remains unknown whether any of these agents will prove superior to intraperitoneal cisplatin or whether different patient populations will respond to cytotoxic virsus biologic agents. Randomized controlled trials are required to address these clinically important issues.

INTRAPERITONEAL THERAPY AS INITIAL TREATMENT OF OVARIAN CANCER

With the demonstrated activity of second-line cisplatinbased intraperitoneal therapy in the treatment of ovarian cancer, it was natural that this therapeutic strategy would be examined as a front-line approach. However, several points must be addressed before considering a possible role for intraperitoneal therapy in this clinical setting.

First, as previously discussed, any advantage of intraperitoneal drug delivery over that achieved with systemic administration of the same (or similar) agents will be limited to those situations in which very small residual tumor volumes are present at the initiation of therapy. Despite the general acceptance of surgical tumor debulking as a standard management strategy in the treatment of ovarian cancer, most patients with advanced disease (stage III/IV) have considerable tumor bulk present (tumor masses greater than 0.5 cm in diameter) before the initiation of chemotherapy. Therefore, the patient population with the greatest potential to benefit from this approach (i.e., those with very-small-volume residual disease) is limited in number.

Second, because cisplatin is an active drug in ovarian cancer and reaches the systemic compartment in considerable concentrations after intraperitoneal delivery, it will be difficult to know what role, if any, the intraperitoneal route has played in determining an individual patient's response to treatment.

Therefore, randomized controlled clinical trials are required to determine whether the higher local concentrations associated with the intraperitoneal administration of cisplatin (or carboplatin) can be translated into an improved response rate and longer survival time for patients with ovarian cancer treated in this manner.

Publication of the results of a landmark randomized trial in 1996 that compared intraperitoneal with intravenous cisplatin as initial treatment of small-volume residual advanced ovarian cancer did much to address the question of the clinical relevance of the pharmacokinetic advantage associated with regional drug delivery (24). All patients in this trial also received intravenous cyclophosphamide. In this study, conducted by the Southwest Oncology Group (SWOG) and the GOG, patients receiving treatment by the intraperitoneal route were found to have a survival advantage and experienced less toxicity (neutropenia, tinnitus) compared with those given intravenous cisplatin. However, because this study was initiated before the introduction of paclitaxel into standard oncologic practice (72,73), it might reasonably be asked what role intraperitoneal cisplatin would play in individuals receiving systemic paclitaxel.

A second randomized trial conducted by the GOG and SWOG partially addressed this question. In this study, patients received either intravenous or intraperitoneal cisplatin along with intravenous paclitaxel (95). In the experimental arm of the study, patients initially received two courses of moderately high-dose carboplatin (AUC 9), designed to "chemically debulk" tumor before the administration of the regional treatment program (96). In a preliminary report of this study, patients treated with the intraperitoneal cisplatin regimen had a statistically significant improvement in progression-free survival and a borderline improvement in overall survival, compared with the all-intravenous regimen (95). However, this specific regimen resulted in an excessive degree of thrombocytopenia due to the initial intravenous carboplatin, and it cannot be recommended for further investigation.

A recent GOG trial may provide a definitive answer in regard to the use of intraperitoneal chemotherapy as initial treatment of ovarian cancer. In this study, patients with small-volume residual stage III ovarian cancer were randomly assigned to receive either a regimen of intraperitoneal cisplatin, intraperitoneal paclitaxel, and intravenous paclitaxel or a "standard program" of intravenous cisplatin and paclitaxel. The results of this study are awaited with interest.

TABLE 17.3. *Clinical situations in which it is appropriate to consider intraperitoneal therapy in the management of ovarian cancer*

1. Small-volume residual disease (microscopic, tumor nodules ≤ 0.5 cm in maximum diameter) after initial platinum-based systemic therapy (REASONABLE STANDARD MANAGEMENT STRATEGY).
2. Negative second-look laparotomy in patients with stage III/IV disease and high-grade tumor (ultimate relapse rate approaches 50%–60%) (INVESTIGATIVE APPROACH).
3. Initial therapy for stage I/II disease with high-grade tumor (INVESTIGATIVE APPROACH).
4. Initial therapy for stage III disease with all or certain drugs administered by the intraperitoneal route (INVESTIGATIVE APPROACH).

CONCLUSION

The use of intraperitoneal therapy in the management of ovarian cancer is based on a sound experimental and pharmacological rationale. The safety and activity of a number of antineoplastic agents when administered by the intraperitoneal route to patients with ovarian cancer has been established. The results of randomized, controlled clinical trials have confirmed the potential clinical efficacy of this approach in specific patient populations. In appropriately selected individuals with ovarian cancer, intraperitoneal therapy is a reasonable therapeutic approach, both in the investigative setting and in the standard management of this malignancy (Table 17.3).

REFERENCES

1. Markman M. Intraperitoneal anti-neoplastic agents for tumors principally confined to the peritoneal cavity. *Cancer Treat Rev* 1986;13:219–242.
2. Austin EH, et al. The treatment of malignant pleural effusions. *Ann Thorac Surg* 1979;28:190.
3. Ostowski MJ. An assessment of the long-term results of controlling the reaccumulation of malignant effusions using intracavitary bleomycin. *Cancer* 1986;57:721.
4. Dedrick RL, Myers CE, Bungay PM, et al. Pharmacokinetic rationale for peritoneal drug administration in the treatment of ovarian cancer. *Cancer Treat Rep* 1978;62:1.
5. Rosenshein N, et al. The effect of volume on the distribution of substances instilled into the peritoneal cavity. *Gynecol Oncol* 1978;6:106.

6. Howell SB, Pfeifle CL, Wung WE, et al. Intraperitoneal cisplatin with systemic thiosulphate protection. *Ann Intern Med* 1982;97:845.
7. Dunick NR, et al. Intraperitoneal contrast infusion for assessment of intraperitoneal fluid dynamics. *AJR Am J Roentgenol* 1979;133:221.
8. Van Weelde BJ, et al. Scintigraphic peritoneography in advanced ovarian malignancies: its value for chemotherapeutic distribution studies. *Clin Radiol* 1984;35:465.
9. Ozols RF, Louar GY, Doroshow JH, et al. Pharmacokinetics of Adriamycin and tissue penetration in murine ovarian cancer. *Cancer Res* 1979;39:3209.
10. Nederman T, et al. Penetration and binding of vinblastine and 5-fluorouracil in cellular spheroids. *Cancer Chemother Pharmacol* 1984;13:131.
11. Los G, et al. Direct diffusion of cis-diamminedichloroplatinum(II) in intraperitoneal rat tumors after intraperitoneal chemotherapy: a comparison with systemic chemotherapy. *Cancer Res* 1989;49:3380.
12. Markman M, Rovoinsky M, Hakes T, et al. Phase 1 trial of intraperitoneal Taxol: a Gynecologic Oncology Group study. *J Clin Oncol* 1992;10:1485.
13. Francis P, et al. Phase 1 feasibility and pharmacologic study of weekly intraperitoneal paclitaxel: a Gynecologic Oncology Group pilot study. *J Clin Oncol* 1995;13:2961.
14. Pfeifle CE, et al. Totally implantable system for peritoneal access. *J Clin Oncol* 1984;2:1277.
15. Piccart MJ, et al. Intraperitoneal chemotherapy: technical experience at five institutions. *Semin Oncol* 1985;12[3 Suppl 4]:90.
16. Kaplan RA, Markman M, Lucas WE et al. Infectious peritonitis in patients receiving intraperitoneal chemotherapy. *Am J Med* 1985;78:49.
17. Rubin SC, et al. Long term access to the peritoneal cavity in ovarian cancer patients. *Gynecol Oncol* 1988;33:46.
18. Davidson S, et al. Intraperitoneal chemotherapy: analysis of complications with an implantable subcutaneous port and catheter system. *Gynecol Oncol* 1991;41:101–106.
19. Markman M, et al. Complications of extensive adhesion formation following intraperitoneal chemotherapy. *Surg Gynecol Oncol* 1986;112:445.
20. Litterst CL, Collins JM, Lowe ML, et al. Local and systemic toxicity resulting from large-volume Ip administration of doxorubicin in the rat. *Cancer Treat Rep* 1982;66:157.
21. Ozols RF, et al. Phase 1 and pharmacological studies of Adriamycin administered intraperitoneally to patients with ovarian cancer. *Cancer Res* 1982;42:4265.
22. Markman M, et al. Phase 2 trial of intraperitoneal mitoxantrone in the management of refractory ovarian carcinoma. *J Clin Oncol* 1990;8:146.
23. Speyer JL, et al. Phase 1 pharmacological studies of 5-fluorouracil administered intraperitoneally. *Cancer Res* 1980;40:567.
24. Alberts DS, et al. Intraperitoneal cisplatin plus intravenous cyclophosphamide versus intravenous cisplatin plus intravenous cyclophosphamide for stage III ovarian cancer. *N Engl J Med* 1996;335:1950.
25. Cannistra SA. Cancer of the ovary. *N Engl J Med* 1993;329:1550.
26. Casper ES, et al. Ip cisplatin in patients with malignant ascites: pharmacokinetic evaluation and comparison with the iv route. *Cancer Treat Rep* 1983;67:235–238.
27. Pretorius RG, et al. Pharmacokinetics of Ip cisplatin in refractory ovarian carcinoma. *Cancer Treat Rep* 1983;67:1035.
28. Lopez JA, Krikorian JH, Reich SD, et al. Clinical pharmacology of intraperitoneal cisplatin. *Gynecol Oncol* 1985;20:1.
29. Cohen AM, et al. Surgical considerations in ovarian cancer. *Semin Oncol* 1985;12[3 Suppl 4]:53.
30. Hacker NF, et al. Intraperitoneal cis-platinum as salvage therapy for refractory epithelial ovarian cancer. *Obstet Gynecol* 1987;70:759.
31. Ten Bokkel Huinink WE, et al. Experimental and clinical results with intraperitoneal cisplatin. *Semin Oncol* 1985;12[3 Suppl 4]:43.
32. Markman M, et al. Intraperitoneal cisplatin and cytarabine in the treatment of refractory or recurrent ovarian carcinoma. *J Clin Oncol* 1991;9:204–210.
33. Piver MS, et al. Surgically documented response to intraperitoneal cisplatin, cytarabine, and bleomycin after intravenous cisplatin-based chemotherapy in advanced ovarian adenocarcinoma. *J Clin Oncol* 1988;6:1679.
34. Markman M, Howell SB, Lucas WE, et al. Combination intraperitoneal chemotherapy with cisplatin, cytarabine, and doxorubicin for refractory ovarian carcinoma and other malignancies principally confined to the peritoneal cavity. *J Clin Oncol* 1984;2:1321.
35. Piccart MJ, et al. Intraperitoneal chemotherapy with cisplatin and melphalan. *J Natl Cancer Inst* 1988;80:1118.
36. Reichman B, et al. Intraperitoneal cisplatin and etoposide in the treatment of refractory/recurrent ovarian carcinoma. *J Clin Oncol* 1989;7:1327.
37. Kirmani S, et al. A phase II trial of intraperitoneal cisplatin and etoposide as salvage treatment for minimal residual ovarian carcinoma. *J Clin Oncol* 1991;9:649–657.
38. Markman M, et al. Responses to second-line cisplatin-based intraperitoneal therapy in ovarian cancer: influence of a prior response to intravenous cisplatin. *J Clin Oncol* 1991;9:1801–1805.
39. Markman M, et al. Intraperitoneal chemotherapy employing a regimen of cisplatin, cytarabine and bleomycin. *Cancer Treat Rep* 1986;70:755.
40. Markman M, et al. Intraperitoneal chemotherapy with high dose cisplatin and cytarabine for refractory ovarian carcinoma and other malignancies principally involving the peritoneal cavity. *J Clin Oncol* 1985;3:925.
41. Howell SB, et al. A phase II trial of intraperitoneal cisplatin and etoposide for primary treatment of ovarian epithelial cancer. *J Clin Oncol* 1990;8:137.
42. Howell SB, Tae He R. Effect of sodium thiosulphate on cis-diamminedichloroplatinum(II) toxicity and antitumor activity in L1210 leukemia. *Cancer Treat Rep* 1980;64:611.
43. Shea M, et al. Kinetics of sodium thiosulphate, a cisplatin neutralizer. *Clin Pharmacol Ther* 1984;35:419.
44. Hoskins WJ, et al. Influence of secondary cytoreduction at the time of second-look laparotomy on the survival of patients with epithelial ovarian carcinoma. *Gynecol Oncol* 1989;34:365.
45. Wharton JT, et al. Long-term survival after chemotherapy for advanced epithelial ovarian carcinoma. *Am J Obstet Gynecol* 1984;148:997.
46. Podratz KC, et al. Evaluation of treatment and survival after positive second-look laparotomy. *Gynecol Oncol* 1988;31:9.

47. Howell SB, Zimm S, Markman M, et al. Long term survival of advanced refractory ovarian carcinoma patients with small-volume disease treated with intraperitoneal chemotherapy. *J Clin Oncol* 1987;5:1607.
48. Markman M, Reichman B, Hakes T, et al. Impact on survival of surgically-defined favorable responses to salvage intraperitoneal chemotherapy in small volume residual ovarian cancer. *J Clin Oncol* 1992;10:1479.
49. Piver MS, et al. Evaluation of survival after second-line intraperitoneal cisplatin-based chemotherapy for advanced ovarian cancer. *Cancer* 1994;73:1693.
50. Rubin SC, Hoskins WJ, Saigo PE, et al. Recurrence following negative second-look laparotomy for ovarian cancer: analysis of risk factors. *Am J Obstet Gynecol* 1988;159:1094.
51. Barakat RR, et al. A phase II trial of intraperitoneal cisplatin and etoposide as consolidation therapy in patients with stage II–IV epithelial ovarian cancer following negative surgical assessment. *Gynecol Oncol* 1998;69:17.
52. Deregorio MW, et al. Preliminary observations of intraperitoneal carboplatin pharmacokinetics during a phase I study of the Northern California Oncology Group. *Cancer Chemother Pharmacol* 1986;18:235.
53. Elferink F, et al. Pharmacokinetics of carboplatin after intraperitoneal administration. *Cancer Chemother Pharmacol* 1988;21:57.
54. Bookman MA, et al. Carboplatin and paclitaxel in ovarian carcinoma: a phase I study of the Gynecologic Oncology Group. *J Clin Oncol* 1996;14:1895.
55. Ozols RF, Bundy BN, Fowler J, et al. Randomized phase III study of cisplatin/paclitaxel versus carboplatin/paclitaxel in optimal stage III epithelial ovarian cancer: a Gynecologic Oncology Group trial (GOG 158). *Proc Am Soc Clin Oncol* 1999;18:356a.
56. Speyer JL, et al. Intraperitoneal carboplatin: favorable results in women with minimal residual ovarian cancer after cisplatin therapy. *J Clin Oncol* 1990;8:1335.
57. Pfeiffer P, et al. Intraperitoneal carboplatin in the treatment of minimal residual ovarian cancer. *Gynecol Oncol* 1990;36:306.
58. Los G, et al. Penetration of carboplatin and cisplatin into rat peritoneal tumor nodules after intraperitoneal chemotherapy. *Cancer Chemother Pharmacol* 1991;28:159–165.
59. Markman M, Reichman B, Hakes T, et al. Evidence supporting the superiority of intraperitoneal cisplatin compared to intraperitoneal carboplatin for salvage therapy of small volume residual ovarian cancer. *Gynecol Oncol* 1993;50:100.
60. Ozols RF, et al. Kinetic characterization and response to chemotherapy in a transplantable murine ovarian cancer. *Cancer Res* 1979;39:3202.
61. Delgado G, et al. A phase I/II study of intraperitoneally administered doxorubicin entrapped in cardiolipin liposomes in patients with ovarian cancer. *Am J Obstet Gynecol* 1989;160:812.
62. Muggia FM, et al. Phase II study of liposomal doxorubicin in refractory ovarian cancer: antitumor activity and toxicity modification by liposomal encapsulation. *J Clin Oncol* 1997;15:987.
63. Shenkenberg TD, et al. Mitoxantrone: a new anticancer drug with significant activity. *Ann Intern Med* 1986;105:67.
64. Dorr RT, et al. Lack of experimental vesicant activity for the anticancer agents cisplatin, melphalan and mitoxantrone. *Cancer Chemother Pharmacol* 1986;16:91.
65. Alberts DS, Young L, Mason N, et al. In vitro evaluation of anticancer drugs against ovarian cancer at concentrations achievable by intraperitoneal administration. *Semin Oncol* 1985;12[3 Suppl 4]:38.
66. Alberts DS, et al. Phase 1 clinical and pharmacokinetic study of mitoxantrone given to patients by intraperitoneal administration. *Cancer Res* 1988;48:5874.
67. Markman M, Herkis T, Reichman B, et al. Phase 2 trial of weekly or biweekly intraperitoneal mitoxantrone in epithelial ovarian cancer. *J Clin Oncol* 1991;9:978–982.
68. Husain A, et al. Phase II trial of intraperitoneal cisplatin and mitoxantrone in patients with persistent ovarian cancer. *Gynecol Oncol* 1999;73:96.
69. Howell SB, et al. Intraperitoneal chemotherapy with melphalan. *Ann Intern Med* 1984;101:14.
70. Holcenberg J, et al. Intraperitoneal chemotherapy with melphalan plus glutaminase. *Cancer Res* 1983;43:1381.
71. Wadler S, Egorin MJ, Zuhowski EG, et al. Phase 1 clinical and pharmacokinetic study of thiotepa administered intraperitoneally in patients with advanced malignancies. *J Clin Oncol* 1989;7:132.
72. McGuire WP, et al. Cyclophosphamide and cisplatin compared with paclitaxel and cisplatin in patients with stage III and stage IV ovarian cancer. *N Engl J Med* 1996;334:1.
73. Stuart G, et al. Updated analysis shows a highly significant improved overall survival for cisplatin-paclitaxel as first line treatment of advanced ovarian cancer: mature results of the EORTC-GCCG, NOCOVA, NCIC CTG and Scottish Intergroup trial. *Proc Am Soc Clin Oncol* 1998;17:361a.
74. Rose PG, et al. Prolonged oral etoposide as second-line therapy for platinum-resistant and platinum-sensitive ovarian carcinoma: a Gynecologic Oncology Group Study. *J Clin Oncol* 1998;16:405.
75. Zimm S, Cleary S, Lucas W, et al. Phase I/pharmacokinetic study of intraperitoneal cisplatin and etoposide. *J Clin Oncol* 1987;47:1712.
76. Markman M, Blessing JA, Major F, et al. Salvage intraperitoneal therapy of ovarian cancer employing cisplatin and etoposide: a Gynecologic Oncology Group study. *Gynecol Oncol* 1993;50:191.
77. Thigpen T, Vanu R, Lamburth B, et al. Chemotherapy for advanced or recurrent gynecologic cancer. *Cancer* 1987;60:2104
78. Demicheli R, Jirillo A, Bonćiarelli G, et al. Pharmacological data and technical feasibility of intraperitoneal 5-fluorouracil administration. *Tumori* 1982;68:437.
79. Ozols RF, Speyer JL, Jankins J, et al. Phase II trial of 5-FU administered Ip to patients with refractory ovarian cancer. *Cancer Treat Rep* 1984;68:1229.
80. Muggia FM, Chan KK, Russell C, et al. Phase I and pharmacologic evaluation of intraperitoneal 5-fluoro-2'-deoxyuridine. *Cancer Chemother Pharmacol* 1991;28:241.
81. Muggia FM, Liu PY, Alberts DS, et al. Intraperitoneal mitoxantrone or floxuridine: effects on time-to-failure and survival in patients with minimal residual ovarian cancer after second-look laparotomy. A randomized phase II study by the Southwest Oncology Group. *Gynecol Oncol* 1996;61:395.

82. McGuire W, Rowinsky EK, Rosenskeiu NB, et al. Taxol: a unique antineoplastic agent with significant activity in advanced ovarian epithelial neoplasms. *Ann Intern Med* 1989;111:273.
83. Rowinsky EK, Cazenave LA, Donehower RC, et al. Taxol: a novel investigational antimicrotubule agent. *J Natl Cancer Inst* 1990;82:1247.
84. Monsarrat B, Mariel E, Gois S, et al. Taxol metabolism: isolation and identification of three major metabolites in rat bile. *Drug Metab Dispose* 1990;18:895.
85. Markman M, Bandy MF, Spirtos NM, et al. Phase II trial of intraperitoneal paclitaxel in carcinoma of the ovary, tube, and peritoneum: a Gynecologic Oncology Group study. *J Clin Oncol* 1998;16:2620.
86. Markman M. The intracavitary administration of biological agents. *J Biol Response Mod* 1987;6:404.
87. Bast RC, Berek JS, Obrist R, et al. Intraperitoneal immunotherapy of human ovarian carcinoma with *Corynebacterium parvum*. *Cancer Res* 1983;43:1395.
88. Berek JS, Hacker NF, Lichtenstein A, et al. Intraperitoneal recombinant alpha-interferon for "salvage" immunotherapy in stage III epithelial ovarian cancer: a Gynecologic Oncology Group study. *Cancer Res* 1985;45:4447.
89. Nicoletto MO, et al. Experience with intraperitoneal alpha-2a interferon. *Oncology* 1992;49:467.
90. D'Acquisto R, Markman M, Hakes T, et al. A phase 1 trial of intraperitoneal recombinant-gamma interferon in advanced ovarian carcinoma. *J Clin Oncol* 1988;6:689–695.
91. Pujade-Lauraine E, Guastalla JP, Colombo W, et al. Intraperitoneal recombinant interferon gamma in ovarian cancer patients with residual disease at second-look laparotomy. *J Clin Oncol* 1996;14:343.
92. Chapman PB, Kolitz JE, Hakes TB, et al. A phase 1 pilot study of intraperitoneal recombinant interleukin 2 in patients with ovarian carcinoma. *Invest New Drugs* 1988;5:179.
93. Edwards RP, Gooding W, Lembersky BC, et al. Comparison of toxicity and survival following intraperitoneal recombinant interleukin-2 for persistent ovarian cancer after platinum: twenty-four-hour versus 7-day infusion. *J Clin Oncol* 1997;15:3399.
94. Markman M, Reichman B, Ianotti N, et al. Phase 1 trial of recombinant tumor necrosis factor administered by the intraperitoneal route. *Reg Cancer Treat* 1989;2:174.
95. Markman M, Bundy B, Benda J, et al. Randomized phase 3 study of intravenous cisplatin/paclitaxel versus moderately high dose IV carboplatin followed by IV paclitaxel and intraperitoneal cisplatin in optimal residual ovarian cancer: an Intergroup Trial (GOG, SWOG, ECOG) [Abstract 1392]. *Proc Am Soc Clin Oncol* 1998;17:361.
96. Shapiro F, Schneider J, Markman J, et al. High-intensity intravenous cyclophosphamide and cisplatin, interim surgical debulking, and intraperitoneal cisplatin in advanced ovarian carcinoma: a pilot trial with ten-year follow-up. *Gynecol Oncol* 1997;67:39.

18

Palliative Surgery for Epithelial Ovarian Cancer

Daniel L. Clarke-Pearson, Gustavo C. Rodriguez, and Matthew Boente

INTRODUCTION

Ovarian carcinoma patients who have failed to respond to surgery and platin-based chemotherapy can rarely be salvaged by second- or third-line therapies. The great majority of such patients experience continued, unrelenting disease progression ultimately resulting in death. Progressive ovarian cancer usually results in symptoms associated with intraperitoneal tumor spread: abdominal distention and pressure, anorexia, nausea, vomiting, and shortness of breath. Because most ovarian cancer patients are not in severe pain and retain their mental faculties, the successful palliation of intestinal obstruction, ascites, pleural effusions, and urinary tract obstruction may allow additional weeks or months of useful life outside of the hospital.

The surgical approach to these particular problems is discussed in this chapter. Some problems may be easily palliated by relatively minor surgery, such as paracentesis or placement of a thoracostomy tube. On the other hand, major surgical interventions intended to provide palliation may actually result in serious complications and decreased quality and duration of remaining life. In considering surgical palliation, therefore, the surgeon must strive to improve quality of life by relieving symptoms and at the same time must limit surgery to situations in which palliative goals may be accomplished in the majority of patients. Although some data now exist that can aid in identifying prognostic factors portending a better or worse surgical outcome, most information is based on retrospective single-institution series collected over several decades. Much of this information is likely biased by personal or institutional philosophy of management and may not be entirely applicable to a particular patient. Because it is unlikely that prospective, randomized trials will ever be conducted, the physician must rely on currently available information combined with individualization of patient care and good surgical judgment. We believe that the best patient management decisions will be made by an experienced gynecologic oncologist who has the capability of providing the full range of medical and surgical options for palliation. These therapeutic options must be used on an individual patient basis after considering the patient's overall medical status, prognosis, and desires. We agree with Rubin, who believes that the "issues revolve around the questions of the advisability of surgical interventions–what are the chances that surgery can relieve the obstruction, what is the morbidity of the operation, what are the chances of reobstruction, and importantly, what is the cost?" (1).

INTESTINAL OBSTRUCTION

Although intestinal obstruction may be a presenting symptom of undiagnosed ovarian cancer, there is no doubt, in our opinion, that the patient will benefit from surgery to relieve the obstruction as well as to allow proper diagnosis, staging, and cytoreductive surgery. After initial therapy, because of the peculiar spread patterns of ovarian cancer throughout the peritoneal cavity, intestinal obstructions are a common problem for patients with progressive ovarian cancer. Krebs and Goplerud (2) found that of 208 patients who died of ovarian cancer, 96 (46%)

had 165 episodes of small bowel obstruction requiring hospitalization, surgery, or both. In a review of 310 patients treated in a single institution, Lund and associates (3) found that the estimated incidence of intestinal obstruction requiring hospitalization and surgery was 26% at 5 years. In another series of 150 patients with epithelial ovarian carcinoma treated in a 4-year period, Solomon and colleagues (4) found that 22 women (15%) developed intestinal obstruction requiring surgical intervention. These latter two reports probably underestimate the problem of intestinal obstruction, because short duration of follow-up failed to capture the majority of patients who develop symptoms of progressive terminal disease. In addition to these clinically obvious events of small bowel obstruction, it has been our experience that an even larger proportion of the population of women with ovarian carcinoma suffer more subtle gastrointestinal (GI) symptoms of poor appetite, abdominal fullness, nausea, and pelvic pressure, all caused by progressive intraperitoneal carcinomatosis and ultimately resulting in death from malnutrition.

The cause of intestinal obstruction is most commonly progressive ovarian cancer. In Lund's series, the variables most commonly associated with intestinal obstruction included initial stage III or IV disease, suboptimal tumor debulking at initial surgery (greater than 2 cm tumor nodules), and the presence of intestinal carcinomatosis at initial surgical exploration (3). However, intestinal obstruction may also result from prior treatment, such as adhesions caused by previous surgery or intraperitoneal chemotherapy, or radiation injury caused by abdominal or pelvic external beam therapy or intraperitoneal administration of chromic phosphate (^{32}P). It is clearly necessary to identify those patients with intestinal obstructions caused by treatment, because they may not have active cancer and can be salvaged with appropriate management. The incidence of obstruction resulting from causes other than cancer has been reported to range from 5% to 24% (3–7). The management goals for patients with intestinal obstruction are aimed at obtaining the highest quality of life for the longest period. Obviously, the ovarian cancer patient who has intestinal obstruction due to surgical adhesions (but who is free of disease) should undergo immediate surgical correction, because this will relieve the obstruction and result in prolonged survival. These patients, as noted earlier, make up only a small portion of all series of patients reported. It is then clear that, to avoid denying a patient who could be successfully treated for intestinal obstruction, surgical exploration is mandatory if the diagnosis of active carcinoma cannot be established.

However, the majority of patients who are known to have ovarian cancer and subsequently develop an intestinal obstruction do, in fact, have recurrent ovarian cancer. It is in this group of patients that management decisions become more difficult. First, it is clear that medical management is extremely likely to be unsuccessful. Krebs and Goplerud (2) reported their experience with 96 women who had 165 episodes of small bowel obstruction. Management plans were individualized, with some patients being medically stabilized before surgery and others managed medically with the intention of avoiding surgery if possible. Of 43 patients who were thus managed by intestinal intubation (usually with a long intestinal tube) and intravenous replacement of fluid and electrolytes, only 14 (32%) had sufficient improvement of symptoms to allow hospital discharge. The hospital stay ranged from 2 to 30 days (mean, 5 days). Of these 14 patients, 12 returned to the hospital with recurrent intestinal obstruction within a mean of 5.5 weeks. In another group of 28 patients who were managed medically, only 12 (42%) improved sufficiently to allow hospital discharge (8), and we suspect that symptom-free survival was relatively short. Finally, Beattie reported that medical management of intestinal obstruction failed in 63% of patients in his institution (9).

Medical management, therefore, offers little to provide for prolonged palliation of symptoms. The only exception is the occasional patient who has not received an adequate trial of effective chemotherapy. For example, Tunca (5,10) and Krebs and Goplerud (2) reported on a group of 10 women with intestinal obstruction after initial treatment with a single-agent alkylator. With medical management using nasogastric suction, intravenous hydration, total parenteral nutrition

(TPN), and intravenous cisplatin chemotherapy, 9 patients had resolution of their intestinal obstruction. This sort of patient, however, is infrequently encountered today, because almost all patients have received multiagent chemotherapy, including cisplatin or carboplatin, and therefore would be unlikely to respond to other standard chemotherapy regimens. There may be two exceptions to this statement. First, women who develop a recurrence of ovarian cancer at least 6 months after an initial complete response to platin-based therapy have an approximately 50% chance of responding to subsequent platin regimens (11). The other hope for successful medical management of intestinal obstruction due to recurrent ovarian cancer lies in the potential efficacy of new chemotherapy regimens (12). However, the expectations for success using this strategy are very limited given that the most active agents (topotecan, Doxil, etoposide, Taxotere) result in response rates of only 10% to 20% in platin-resistant patients.

The majority of cases of ovarian cancer with intestinal obstruction cannot be managed successfully by medical means, and the option of surgical treatment must be seriously considered because it may be the only option for longer symptom-free survival. However, the decision to operate to correct intestinal obstruction is difficult and rests on the surgeon's estimate that the patient will recover from surgery and survive long enough with her progressive malignancy to enjoy the benefits of surgical relief of the obstruction. This decision must be balanced against the estimate of the patient's risks for surgical complications, operative mortality, and the possibility of resumption of adequate intestinal function to resume oral feedings outside of the hospital. Determining which patients will "benefit" from surgery is difficult and has been addressed by a number of authors who have used different definitions of successful surgical outcome. The estimation of surgical "benefit" was initially proposed by Castaldo and associates to denote any patient who survived 2 months after surgery (13); in their small series of 25 patients, 80% survived for at least 60 days postoperatively. Rubin and colleagues proposed that successful surgery should be defined as the ability to leave the hospital eating a regular or low-residue diet (14); 63% of their patients achieved successful recovery of GI function postoperatively. Another definition of success was put forward by Zoetmulder, who measured "bowel obstruction–free survival" (8). Other definitions might be proposed to document success of surgery; an important contribution would be quality-of-life measurements. In any case, it should be remembered that for patients who do not respond to medical management and do not undergo surgery, the expected median survival time is 13.5 days (range, 3 to 32 days) (2), and most of these women never leave the hospital.

The results of surgery for intestinal obstruction in ovarian cancer patients have been reported by a number of authors, who usually reported outcomes by noting median postoperative survival time (2–9,13–19). In total, more than 800 patients undergoing surgical procedures to correct intestinal obstruction have been analyzed. The most common anatomic sites of obstruction were the small intestine (57%), followed by colonic obstruction (30%) and a combined small and large bowel obstruction (13%). Overall "benefit" (defined as survival for longer than 60 days postoperatively) was achieved in 32% to 80% of these patients, with a median postoperative survival time of 10 to 33 weeks. Approximately 70% to 80% of the patients left the hospital eating a regular diet.

Several authors have attempted to analyze the clinical factors most likely to be associated with successful outcome and to identify factors that might portend surgical failure. Krebs and Goplerud were the first to systematically evaluate clinical variables associated with benefit of surgical procedure (16). They adopted the definition of "benefit" proposed by Castaldo (survival of 2 months postoperatively). Of 98 patients undergoing 118 surgical procedures for intestinal obstruction, 14 cases were found to be inoperable, there were 25 (22%) postoperative deaths, and 65% benefited from surgery. The overall median survival time was 12.5 weeks (range, 1 to 78 weeks). Prognostic factors including increasing age, nutritional deprivation, advanced tumor status, ascites, and previous chemotherapy and radiation therapy predicted a group of patients

TABLE 18.1. *Prognostic parameters in ovarian carcinoma complicated by bowel obstruction*

Parameter	No benefit from surgery (%)	p value	Assigned risk score
Age (y)			
<45	23		0
45–65	36		1
>65	75	<.025	2
Nutritional deprivation			
None or minimal	12		0
Moderate	33		1
Severe	62	<.001	2
Tumor status			
No palpable intraabdominal masses	11		0
Palpable intraabdominal masses	41		1
Liver involvement or distant metastases	58	<.005	2
Ascites			
None or mild (asymptomatic, not distended)	17		0
Moderate (distended)	42		1
Severe (symptomatic, frequent paracenteses)	81	<.001	2
Previous chemotherapy			
None or inadequate trial	11		0
Failed single agent	20		1
Failed combination drug therapy	49	<.025	2
Previous radiation therapy			
None	24		0
Pelvic	40		1
Whole abdomen	63	<.025	2

From Krebs HB, Goplerud DR. Surgical management of bowel obstruction in an advanced ovarian carcinoma. *Obstet Gynecol* 1983;61:327–330, with permission.

who were less likely to benefit from surgery (Table 18.1). Using these factors, Krebs and Goplerud developed a scoring system that assigned 0 to 2 points for each variable. Patients who had a risk score of 7 or greater had only a 20% chance of surviving 8 weeks postoperatively. On the other hand, 84% of patients with a score of 6 or less benefited from surgery. Larson and colleagues applied this prognostic scoring system to 33 patients in their institution and also found statistically significant correlation with survival (17). Unfortunately, the statistical analysis performed by Krebs did not take into account the possible interactions among the five variables. This may explain why other authors, including Rubin (14), Lund (3), and their coworkers, found that the risk scoring system proposed by Krebs and Goplerud was not predictive of survival at 60 days when applied to their patient populations. Rubin also found that there was no correlation between survival time and the following factors: age, prior radiation therapy, number of prior laparotomies, site of intestinal obstruction, and number of intestinal procedures performed.

In contrast, in the patient population studied by Lund and associates, risk factors associated with postoperative survival of less than 60 days included nodules larger than 2 cm at completion of initial surgery ($p = .005$) and colonic obstruction or a combination of small and large bowel obstruction ($p = .002$) (3). Zoetmulder, using "bowel obstruction–free survival" as the definition of success, found that patients whose intestinal obstruction developed less than 6 months after completing therapy and those who had ascites were significantly less likely to have a successful outcome from surgery (8). In fact, this group of patients fared no better than those who were medically managed.

Survival for 12 months after surgery for intestinal obstruction was evaluated by Fernandes and colleagues (19). Twenty clinical and laboratory variables in 64 patients with ovarian cancer and intestinal obstruction were evaluated. Factors associated with survival at 1 year included age at diagnosis of ovarian cancer (but not at time of obstruction); time from primary diagnosis to obstruction; tumor stage; prior radiation therapy; presence of ascites; radiographic findings; and abnormal serum levels of albumin, blood urea nitrogen, and alkaline phosphatase. This was a univariate analysis and did not attempt to control or adjust for potential interaction among the variables.

Clarke-Pearson and colleagues (20) evaluated 21 preoperative variables, 7 nutritional parameters, and 8 intraoperative and postoperative factors to ascertain any association with postoperative survival of less than 60 days. Significant individual factors included clinically detected ascites, low serum albumin, low lymphocyte count, clinical tumor status, and residual cancer volume at the end of surgery for intestinal obstruction. The score proposed by Krebs was also significantly predictive of survival ($p = .02$). These authors went on to control for potential interactions among variables by performing a multivariate logistic regression analysis. They found that the Krebs and Goplerud score was significant but predominantly due to the influence of clinical tumor status ($p = .008$) and serum albumin levels ($p = .02$). These two factors were also associated with overall survival. The other risk factors proposed by Krebs and Goplerud were not found to be important in the patient population of Clarke-Pearson and associates when subjected to logistic regression analysis. Using these two preoperative factors, an equation to estimate postoperative survival of greater than 60 days was created (Table 18.2). The validity of this equation has not been tested on another set of data. Despite the lack of a validated risk scoring system, it seems reasonable to use tumor status and nutritional status as two determinants that might influence the surgeon's judgment as to which patients should be considered surgical candidates.

Tumor status has been defined as the clinical detection of extent of recurrent tumor. Because no author has suggested otherwise, it must be assumed that the clinical status of tumor in all studies has been based on routine physical examination and chest radiographs. Despite the fact that computed tomography scanning, ultrasonography, and magnetic resonance imaging might improve the ability to detect the extent of recurrent cancer, no data yet exist to suggest that they might add to a refinement of the evaluation and serve as additional prognostic factors. It seems reasonable to assume, however, that patients with clinical ascites and clinically advanced tumor spread might be better detected with more sophisticated imaging techniques or the use of serum CA-125 in order to more accurately predict surgical outcome.

Although tumor status cannot be modified, nutritional depletion may be aided significantly by preoperative and postoperative TPN. An objective assessment of overall nutritional status can be made by incorporating a number of parameters, including serum albumin, transferrin, anthropometric evaluation, creatinine-height index, and total lymphocyte count. The commonly used guidelines recommended by Dudrick and coworkers characterize nutritional deficits as mild, moderate, or severe if measurements of body weight, serum albumin, and/or total lymphocyte count are less than 90%, 75%, or 60% of normal, respectively (21). Serum transferrin level has also been reported to be a more accurate measure of a patient's current nutritional status (22,23). Nutritional status can also be assessed with clinical examination in a fairly accurate and reproducible fashion. In fact, in a prospective evaluation, objective data collected in histories and physical examinations was found to correlate very well with the laboratory values traditionally used to assess nutritional status (24).

Data regarding the beneficial effect of nutritional support in the perioperative setting in

TABLE 18.2. *Equation to estimate the probability of postoperative survival for at least 60 days*

$$P = \frac{\mathrm{Exp}(-0.014 - 2.307\,\mathrm{Tumor} + 1.257\,\mathrm{Albumin})}{1 + \exp(-0.014 - 2.307\,\mathrm{Tumor} + 1.257\,\mathrm{Albumin})}$$

Tumor, tumor status score (0 = no clinical evidence of ovarian cancer; 1 = clinical evidence of ovarian cancer limited to abdomen and/or pelvis; 2 = clinical evidence of chest involvement); Albumin, actual value in grams per deciliter.

From DL Clarke-Pearson, Delong ER, Chin R, et al, Intestinal obstruction in patients with ovarian cancer: variables associated with surgical complications and survival. *Arch Surg* 1988;123:42–45, with permission.

ovarian cancer patients are inconclusive. Although nutritional support has been shown to correct metabolic derangements and improve body weight in cancer patients, it is unclear whether overall functional status and survival can be improved simply by correcting plasma levels of nitrogen, trace metals, or vitamins (24–27). Furthermore, although body fat stores are easily replaced with parenteral nutrition, protein reserves are more difficult to augment. Published prospective randomized studies evaluating TPN in patients undergoing abdominal surgery for GI malignancies have suffered from small numbers of patients, making it difficult to conclusively demonstrate a beneficial effect of nutritional support in regard to overall surgical outcome, morbidity, and mortality. One study that deserves special mention was reported by the Veterans Affairs Total Parenteral Nutrition Cooperative Study Group (28). This study evaluated the surgical morbidity and mortality in a series of 395 malnourished patients who were randomly assigned to receive TPN for 7 to 15 days before surgery and 3 days after surgery (the treatment group), or no perioperative TPN (the control group). Patients were monitored closely for overall outcome for 3 months postoperatively. There was no difference in the two groups of patients in regard to major postoperative complications or postoperative mortality rate at 90 days. Overall, there was a higher rate of infectious complications in the TPN group compared with controls, although there was no difference among those patients with severe malnutrition. Noninfectious complications were significantly less common in the group of severely malnourished patients given TPN. The overall rate of postoperative complications was therefore lower in the patients receiving TPN who were severely malnourished. The authors of the study concluded that preoperative and perioperative TPN should be limited to patients who are severely malnourished, unless there are other specific indications.

In ovarian cancer patients, data regarding the feasibility and beneficial effect of nutritional support perioperatively and its relation to clinical outcome exist only in retrospective form. The feasibility and safety of perioperative parenteral nutrition in patients with ovarian cancer was first documented by Ford and associates (29). Subsequently, numerous retrospective papers have been published evaluating the prognostic significance of nutritional status and nutritional support in patients managed surgically for a small bowel obstruction. Krebs and Goplerud reported on the selective use of hyperalimentation in 118 patients who underwent surgical management of bowel obstruction secondary to advanced ovarian carcinoma (16). They reported successful surgical palliation in 75% of cases in which hyperalimentation was employed, compared with 56% of the cases in which hyperalimentation was not administered ($p < .0025$). However, their study was retrospective in nature and spanned two decades. Changes in the management of ovarian cancer, the introduction of automatic surgical stapling devices, improved antibiotic therapies, decreased use of radiation therapy for ovarian cancer, and the introduction of more efficacious chemotherapy regimens over the 20-year period of the study could have accounted for the improved survival in patients receiving hyperalimentation.

Clarke-Pearson and colleagues reported on a series of ovarian cancer patients with intestinal obstruction of whom approximately half had either moderate or severe nutritional deficit before surgery (6,20). Only four of the patients received perioperative TPN. Overall, the rates of survival, operative mortality, and serious complications were similar to those reported from other series in which aggressive use of TPN was incorporated. In a subsequent multivariate logistic regression analysis, the authors reported that the preoperative serum albumin level and overall nutritional score were predictive of postoperative survival, even after accounting for tumor status (20). Although the role of TPN was not evaluated in this series, it did suggest that preoperative nutritional status could have prognostic significance. Researchers from the McGill University in Montreal reported on their experience with bowel obstruction in patients with ovarian cancer (19). Twenty variables were considered as possible prognostic factors to estimate 1-year survival probability in 62 patients with advanced ovarian cancer. Patients were stratified into one of three groups regarding the mode of nutrition at the time of admission for obstruction (nothing or small amounts per mouth, enteral feeding with nutritional supplements, or TPN required). There was no statistically significant difference in survival according to the mode of nutritional intake preoperatively. However, a statistically significant increase in survival was noted in those patients who had normal levels of serum albumin and blood urea nitrogen. This was a preliminary study involving only a univariate analysis, but it is consistent with other studies using more elaborate statistical methods.

Clearly, appropriate indications for the perioperative use of TPN in patients with ovarian cancer must await the results of a prospective, randomized trial. Undoubtedly, there is a subset of patients who stand to benefit from perioperative parenteral nutrition. Severely malnourished patients who are candidates for salvage therapies and who are expected to experience long surgical convalescences may benefit from nutritional support during their recovery.

Prevention of complications is a major goal of the surgeon attempting palliation in an ovarian cancer patient with intestinal obstruction. All series reported have had serious complication rates of 30% to 64% and operative mortality rates between 14% and 32%. In general, these complications can be classified as problems with anastomosis and wound healing, infection, and other complications generally encountered with major surgery in this age group of patients.

Prevention of postoperative death and nonfatal complications has been linked to good preoperative preparation, meticulous surgical technique, and excellent postoperative care. Again, patient selection is the most critical element in the prevention of postoperative death. Probably the most important single factor linked to postoperative death is whether the patient is able to receive a definitive surgical procedure to relieve the obstruction. Although some series have reported that all patients were able to undergo a definitive surgical procedure (5,6,15) others have reported that between 12% and 24% of patients were found to be inoperable and had only an exploratory laparotomy. Postoperative survival is significantly reduced in the group of women with inoperable disease. For example, in the experience of Rubin and associates, 5 (45.5%) of 11 patients who were inoperable died before leaving the hospital (14). Krebs noted that all 14 of the patients for whom corrective surgery could not be carried out died within 4 weeks of surgery, compared with a postoperative mortality rate of only 12% in patients in whom bowel surgery was actually performed (16). It would be ideal to identify patients who have such extensive intraperitoneal disease that surgical correction of intestinal obstruction is impossible. However, Rubin and associates specifically undertook an evaluation of clinical factors that might be associated with inoperability and were unable to identify any that distinguished the operable from the inoperable group of patients (14). At present, therefore, surgical judgment must prevail in the selection of patients who are thought to be operable.

Factors associated with major postoperative complications might also influence preoperative preparation and patient selection. Several authors have noted that serious complications are increased in certain groups, including those with poor nutrition (6,13,16), prior radiation therapy (13), or small intestinal obstruction (as opposed to colonic obstruction) (6,13). Clarke-Pearson and colleagues undertook a detailed statistical evaluation of factors possibly associated with major postoperative complications (20). They found that the scoring system proposed by Krebs and Goplerud did not predict the risk of surgical complications. Factors that Clarke-Pearson and coworkers found to be associated with complications included clinically detected ascites ($p = .01$), ovarian cancer involving intestine at prior surgery ($p = .01$), and prior platin-containing chemotherapy ($p = .02$). Two additional factors, low serum albumin ($p = .03$) and advanced tumor burden ($p = .03$), were statistically associated with postoperative mortality.

GI contrast studies (upper GI series with small bowel follow-through and retrograde studies of the colon) should be performed preoperatively in most patients. This is especially important in surgical planning, because an unsuspected obstruction of the colon may be detected, necessitating relief of both a small bowel obstruction and a colonic obstruction at the same operation. The incidence of concurrent obstruction of the small intestine and colon is approximately 15%.

In patients with clinical small bowel obstruction, the GI series rarely points to the site of obstruction. In fact, most patients demonstrate a patent upper GI tract despite obstructive symptoms. Tunca and associates suggested that those patients who have ovarian carcinomatosis that is encasing the bowel may be detected by a slowly emptying small bowel series (5). They believe that it is this group of patients who may not be served by surgical exploration. This observation has not been supported by others, however.

Selection of the specific surgical procedure to perform on a particular patient requires individualization, which cannot be determined until intraoperative exploration has been performed. The individualized approach is reflected in the experience of Clarke-Pearson and associates, who performed 10 different operations to provide relief of small bowel obstruction for 30 patients (6). Although there is no "standard" operation in the setting of intestinal obstruction and progressive ovarian cancer, most authors advise an intestinal bypass procedure rather than resection and reanastomosis. In general, bypass procedures require less time and do less to compromise blood supply to the newly formed anastomosis. Nonetheless, the surgeon must be prepared to perform the entire spectrum of intestinal surgery depending on the intraoperative findings. Resection of tumor at this operation is not the primary objective; however, in our multivariate analysis, the volume of residual tumor at the end of the surgery for intestinal obstruction was significantly associated with survival (20). It seems reasonable to consider resection of ovarian carcinoma obstructing the intestine if such a procedure can reduce tumor volume to less than 1-cm nodules and be performed without undue difficulty.

In several series it was noted that a small portion of patients are inoperable in that nothing can be done to relieve the intestinal obstruction. In most cases, the bowel and its mesentery are extensively encased in tumor, precluding any logical or safe intestinal operation. Although these patients may have a very short life expectancy, palliation may be partially achieved by the placement of a large gastrostomy tube to provide drainage of the stomach and thus eliminate the need for a chronic nasogastric tube (30–32). It has become our practice to place a gastrostomy tube at the completion of almost all procedures for small bowel obstruction. The advantages enjoyed by the patient are the fact that a nasogastric tube is not required, thereby providing more comfort for the patient in the immediate postoperative period while awaiting return of intestinal function. Further, there are some patients who, despite a definitive surgical procedure, never fully regain intestinal function. For example, Rubin and associates reported that 9 (21%) of 43 patients who had definitive surgical procedures did not regain adequate bowel function to consume a diet adequate to sustain the patient (14). Four of these patients never regained intestinal function and died before hospital discharge. Chronic gastrostomy drainage may provide palliation for this group of patients. For those in whom intestinal function returns, the gastrostomy tube can be clamped or removed without difficulty.

A gastrostomy tube should also be considered in patients who are not thought to be candidates for surgery. Several authors have reported methods for placement of percutaneous gastrostomy (30–32). In Malone and colleagues' series of 10 ovarian cancer patients who had percutaneous gastrostomies placed, 3 patients were alive at 77 and at 150 days. Of the 7 patients who died, the average survival time was 35 days (range, 25 to 56 days). Therefore, percutaneous gastrostomy may offer effective palliation by avoiding the prolonged use of a nasogastric tube during the last weeks of an ovarian cancer patient's life.

Clearly, the management of ovarian cancer with intestinal obstruction is a complex problem requiring the total breadth of skills of a gynecologic oncologist. Experience and data published in the literature offer some guidance, although all issues addressed are based on retrospective, biased patient selection. Nonetheless, we suggest an evaluation and management algorithm similar to that shown in Figure 18.1.

ASCITES

Ascites is commonly present in women with ovarian cancer, and it is especially associated with advanced-stage disease. In patients with primary ovarian cancer, reasonable control of

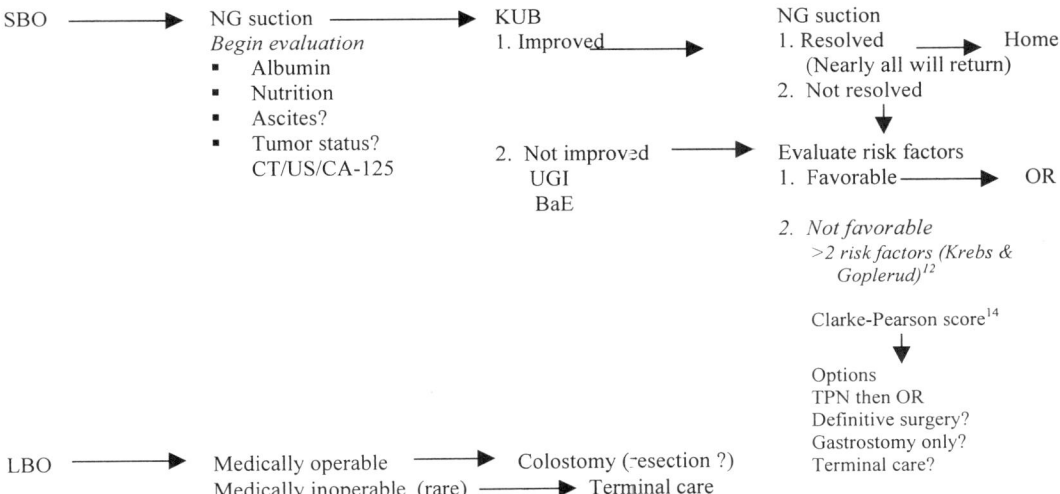

FIG. 18.1. Algorithm for managing intestinal obstruction in ovarian cancer patients.

ascites can usually be achieved through surgical extirpation of tumor followed by the administration of platin-based chemotherapy. However, the development of ascites after primary therapy is an ominous sign and is much more difficult to control. Small volumes of ascites can be ignored, but massive ascites and the associated abdominal distention, anorexia, nausea, vomiting, and respiratory difficulties can all compromise a patient's quality of life, justifying palliative attempts at ascites control.

Factors involved in the pathogenesis of ascites formation include (a) increased production secondary to a damaged peritoneal membrane, (b) decreased absorption due to obstructed lymphatics, and (c) plasma oncotic abnormalities that result in loss of vascular fluids into the interstitial spaces and peritoneal cavity. In a murine ovarian tumor model, Feldman eloquently demonstrated impaired egress of ^{51}Cr-labeled erythrocytes through the subdiaphragmatic lymphatic channels before ascites development (33). Obstruction of omental lymphatics due to metastasis from ovarian cancer undoubtedly also contributes to ascites formation. In addition, damage to the peritoneal membrane and peritoneal capillary endothelial barrier from carcinomatous implants increases capillary permeability and ascites formation. Hypoalbuminemia, which is commonly present as a result of malnutrition, results in a low plasma oncotic pressure, which further aggravates the problem. Occasionally, obstruction or transection of a major lymphatic channel, either by tumor or as a result of surgical injury during a retroperitoneal lymphadenectomy, results in chylous ascites (34). Although the chemical composition of ascitic fluid can be studied in detail, it is not necessary in the patient with a known diagnosis of advanced ovarian cancer. Elevated total protein or lactic acid dehydrogenase (LDH) levels in ascitic fluid, relative to serum, are suggestive but not diagnostic of a malignant etiology (35). Clearly, the diagnostic gold standard for verification of a malignant origin for ascites is demonstration of malignant cells on cytologic examination of ascitic fluid. However, the false-negative rate for cytology can be as high as 50% (36). A variety of palliative surgical approaches can be employed in the management of severe ascites. To date, there are no well-controlled studies comparing alternate therapeutic modalities for the management of recurrent ascites secondary to advanced ovarian cancer. Adjuncts reported to be successful in the treatment of benign causes for ascites have little impact on ascites caused by malignant disease. Alteration of diet, particularly restriction of fluid and sodium intake, can at best provide modest improvement and is largely unsuccessful in alleviating discomfort in most patients. Limited success has been reported with the use of large doses of potassium-sparing diuretics.

Acute palliation of severe ascites can be achieved through paracentesis. However, without a therapeutic approach that incorporates treatment of the ovarian cancer, ascites usually reaccumulates within several days. Repeated paracentesis procedures carry the hazards of iatrogenic injury to abdominal viscera and of peritoneal infection. Furthermore, removal of large volumes of ascites over a period of time can result in electrolyte imbalances and protein depletion. Nonetheless, despite the use of other treatments for ascites, paracentesis is often the only effective method of palliation.

A therapeutic approach that incorporates treating the ovarian cancer, either locally in the peritoneal cavity or systemically, is more likely to effect a sustained improvement in malignant ascites. Patients who are suitable candidates for chemotherapy should be offered a trial of systemic chemotherapy. If there has been prior evidence of response to platin-based chemotherapy, a platin regimen should be strongly considered. Alternatively, patients can be offered entry into clinical trails investigating new drug therapies or offered second-line salvage regimens. A number of investigators have reported variable success in the palliation of malignant ascites of ovarian carcinoma using intraperitoneal administration of radioactive colloids, chemotherapeutic agents, or biologic response modifiers (37–47). However, palliative benefit in most patients is of brief duration.

Peritoneovenous shunting of ascitic fluid has received renewed interest because of the development of pressure-sensitive peritoneovenous valves. In general, the peritoneovenous shunts connect the peritoneal cavity to the superior vena cava by way of plastic catheters placed into the peritoneal cavity, which are then tunneled subcutaneously in a cephalad direction and inserted into a neck vein. Unidirectional flow valves prevent backup of blood from the venous system into the peritoneum. Two relatively simple and reasonably effective peritoneovenous shunts (Leveen and Denver) are available and have been used extensively over the past two decades. The Denver shunt differs from the Leveen shunt in that it contains a valve that can be manually squeezed to clear it of accumulated debris or to pump fluid from the peritoneal cavity. A number of studies (48–54) have demonstrated that peritoneovenous shunting can be an affective method for palliation of malignant ascites. Success rates are reported to be as high as 60% to 70%. Technical problems with the shunts are common, resulting in shunt malfunction in up to 40% of cases. In patients with very short life expectancies, however, the shunts often function long enough to provide effective palliation. In one series the mean duration of shunt function was longer than 10 weeks, while the mean survival time after shunt placement was 11.6 weeks (49). Less frequent complications associated with shunts have included fluid overload, respiratory compromise, and disseminated intravascular coagulation. In order to avoid delivering malignant cells to the venous circulation, Stehman and Ehrlich reported a peritoneocystic shunt for treatment of malignant ascites (55). This shunt did achieve some palliation, but it subsequently became ineffective due to the absence of a pressure gradient between the peritoneal cavity and the bladder.

In summary, the limited life expectancy of ovarian cancer patients with refractory advanced disease dictates a therapeutic approach aimed toward improving the quality of life. Some palliation of massive ascites can be achieved through dietary modification, diuretics, paracentesis, peritoneovenous shunts, chemotherapy, and intraperitoneal radiopharmaceuticals or biologic response modifiers. Without effective cytotoxic therapy for the ovarian cancer, patients with recurrent ascites have a very limited life expectancy. Palliation of ascites, therefore, must avoid iatrogenic morbidity and maximize quality of life.

PLEURAL EFFUSIONS

Although ovarian cancer is a highly metastatic disease, most patients have disease confined to the abdominal cavity at the time of diagnosis.

The pleural space is a common site for extraabdominal metastases, which typically occur as a late manifestation of disease. Fortunately, in most of the patients with malignant pleural effusions, effective palliation can be achieved with current therapeutic techniques. Malignant pleural effusions in patients with primary stage IV ovarian carcinoma can often be successfully eradicated with intensive platin-based systemic chemotherapy. In patients with persistent or recurrent ovarian carcinoma, treatment of malignant pleural effusions can be more difficult and often requires direct treatment of the pleural space.

A clear understanding of the pathophysiology regarding the formation of a hydrothorax is essential for comprehension of the rationale for various treatment modalities for malignant effusions. Pleural fluid homeostasis is governed by the Starling principle and is based on the relation between the capillary and interstitial hydrostatic and plasma protein oncotic pressures. In the normal state, the capillary hydrostatic pressure of the parietal pleura is greater than the capillary hydrostatic pressure in the visceral pleura, resulting in a flow of fluid from the parietal to the visceral capillary bed. Approximately 90% of the fluid moving across the pleural space is absorbed by the visceral capillary pleural bed, with the remainder absorbed by lymphatics. Carcinomatous involvement of the parietal and visceral pleura creates an inflammatory response and direct injury to capillary endothelia, resulting in increased fluid egress from the plasma compartment into the pleural space. Cancers in the pleural space obstruct the pleural lymphatic drainage, thus impairing reabsorption of lymphatic fluid. With more advanced disease, lymphangitic spread throughout the lung parenchyma results in obstruction of pulmonary venous flow, thus increasing capillary hydrostatic pressure in the lung. The hydrostatic pressure gradient between the parietal and visceral pleura is reduced, which further impedes the flow of fluid in the appropriate direction. Hypoalbuminemia and hypoproteinemia, common in patients with advanced ovarian cancer, can further impair the plasma oncotic pressure and increase the interstitial osmotic pressure, permitting further loss of fluids from the vascular compartment into the third space, including the pleural space (56).

Most small pleural effusions are asymptomatic. With large pleural effusions, the most common symptoms are dyspnea, cough, and pleuritic chest pain. Symptoms seem to be more directly related to the rate of development of pleural effusions, rather than to the amount of pleural fluid present (57). Physical examination usually reveals decreased breath sounds and dullness to percussion at the lung base. Radiographically, a posterior-anterior chest film denotes a pleural effusion, as manifested by blunting of the costophrenic angle when at least 200 mL of pleural fluid is present. Lateral decubitus chest films are more sensitive and can detect small pleural effusions containing as little as 100 mL of fluid (58).

In addition to malignant causes, pleural effusions can occur in a number of nonmalignant diseases including cardiac disease, liver disease, renal disease, systemic lupus erythematosus, pulmonary infarction, pulmonary embolism, and pneumonia. Pleural effusions secondary to nonmalignant and noninfectious causes are usually transudative rather and exudative. If the cause of the pleural effusion is in question, the diagnostic workup should include a thoracentesis to determine the chemical and cytologic characteristics of the pleural fluid. Malignant effusions are classically exudative, with a protein content greater than 3 g/dL, a pleural protein/serum protein ratio greater than 0.5, a pleural LDH/serum LDH ratio of greater than 0.6, and a specific gravity greater than 1.015. In addition, malignant effusions are often heavily infiltrated with lymphocytes. The presence of a bloody effusion is highly predictive of malignancy (59).

The gold standard for the diagnosis of a malignant effusion is demonstration of malignant cytology. The sensitivity of cytology obtained by blind needle biopsy for diagnosis of malignant pleural effusions in patients with known malignancy ranges from 42% to 90% in selected series (59–62). Various immunologic and surgical techniques have been used to increase the diagnostic yield of pleural cytology. Monoclonal antibodies directed against the TAG-72 antigen were shown to have a sensitivity approaching 100% for the diagnosis of malignant pleural effusions in small series of patients with breast, ovarian, and lung cancers (63,64). Furthermore, techniques incorporating thoracoscopy for identification of pleural abnormalities and direct guidance of pleural biopsies were shown to have a sensitivity greater than 90% for identification of malignant cells (65,66).

Most women who present with stage IV ovarian cancer with malignant pleural effusions respond to platin-based chemotherapy, and in most of these patients resolution of the pleural effusion occurs. In women with advanced recurrent ovarian cancer with malignant effusions, local therapeutic modalities are often required, including thoracentesis, chest tube placement combined with sclerotherapy, or intracavitary instillation of antineoplastic agents, radioisotopes, or biologic response modifiers. Surgical interventions, including pleural peritoneal shunting and pleurectomy, are also potential options in carefully selected patents.

In general, before administration of sclerosing or antineoplastic agents, the entire pleural effusion should be removed by simple thoracentesis or by a large-bore thoracostomy tube. After 24 hours, sclerotherapy or intrapleural chemotherapy can be administered if a chest radiograph shows good lung expansion and complete evacuation of the pleural effusion. If there is a large volume of residual pleural fluid present, dilution of the sclerosing agent will increase the likelihood of treatment failure. To avoid this problem, we have found that placement of a chest tube most effectively drains the pleural effusion. Once the drainage from the tube is less than 200 mL in a 24-hour period, we instill a sclerotic agent such as talc or tetracycline.

Tetracycline is a highly effective agent and has been shown in prospective trials to be superior to placebo, chest tube drainage, and the antimalarial agent quinacrine (67–70). Tetracycline offers the additional advantages of being inexpensive and easily administered as a one-time treatment, and it is associated with little morbidity. Talc produces an intense pleuritis that obliterates the pleural space and is successful in 80% to 90% of patients. Side effects frequently include fever and chest pain, both of which are self-limited (71). A number of antineoplastic agents have been used with success.

In light of the fact that second-line chemotherapy regimens are associated with low response rates in patients with ovarian cancer, the most likely mechanism of action of the chemotherapeutic agents used for the treatment of pleural effusions is the intense inflammatory response that these agents induce in the pleural space. Of these agents, bleomycin has been used extensively and with consistently high success rates. Finally, a number of radioimmunoconjugates, consisting of monoclonal antibodies directed against tumor-associated antigens conjugated with alpha- and beta-emitting radioisotopes, *Corynebacterium parvum*, β-interferon, recombinant interleukin-2, streptococcal OK-432 preparation, and BCG (cell wall skeleton) have all been used with some success in the treatment of malignant pleural effusion (72–75). Although there are encouraging preliminary data, these new modalities should still be considered investigational.

Surgical management of malignant pleural effusions is usually reserved for patients in whom prior medical management has failed and reasonable palliation is expected. Martini and associates reported that pleurectomy controlled malignant pleural effusions in 87% to 100% of a selected group of patients with slow-growing malignancies (76). However, a 23% complication rate and a 9% mortality rate severely limit the use of this modality. Pleural peritoneal or pleural atrial shunts have also been successfully used (77–79). Although there is a potential risk for malignant seeding from these devices, it is probably of little consequence because the majority of the patients in whom these devices are used have terminal disease. The Denver pleural peritoneal shunt can be placed under local anesthesia, and the complications in experienced hands are minimal. Before widespread use of these devices can be advocated, a comparison with the use of intrapleural tetracycline should be done in a prospective, randomized trial.

URETERAL OBSTRUCTION

Clinically evident ureteral obstruction does not often occur in women with ovarian malignancy, which is surprising considering that most patients eventually develop extensive intraperitoneal disease. Undoubtedly, a significant number of cases of ureteral obstruction occur silently and escape detection. Gynecologic tumors, such as ovarian neoplasms, obstruct the ureter in the pelvis, either throughout its course along the pelvic sidewall or as it courses through the cardinal ligament. Occasionally, extensive periaortic lymphatic metastases can obstruct the ureter outside of the pelvis.

Much of the gynecologic literature regarding palliation of ureteral obstruction has focused on the management of ureteral obstruction in patients with cervical cancer (80,81). In patients with ovarian cancer, important factors to consider in the management of ureteral obstruction include whether there is infection in the obstructed urinary tract, the overall extent of tumor burden, and whether any effective salvage regimens are available.

Ureteral obstruction in women with advanced ovarian cancer often occurs asymptomatically without any clinical or laboratory evidence of urinary tract compromise. Occasionally, patients present with symptoms of renal colic or with pyelonephritis. Acute elevation in the serum creatinine concentration may lead the clinician to suspect renal obstruction. However, increased serum creatinine levels are often difficult to interpret in patients who have experienced fluid loss or who have previously been treated with renal toxic drugs such as cisplatin. Furthermore, serum creatinine often remains normal so long as one kidney has good renal function. Symptoms of renal colic or a clinical presentation of pyelonephritis can be suggestive of ureteral obstruction, but these symptoms are nonspecific and can certainly occur in the absence of urinary tract compromise.

The gold standard test for diagnosis of ureteral obstruction is intravenous pyelography, which can reliably image urinary tract anatomy. Intravenous pyelography may be contraindicated, however, in patients who are receiving renal toxic drugs or who have compromised renal function. In these patients, an intravenous pyelogram carries a significant risk for inducing acute tubular necrosis. Renal ultrasonography has been found to be an excellent alternative to intravenous pyelography for detecting ureteral obstructions. One large series evaluating more than 400 kidneys reported sensitivities and specificities both greater than 96% and a positive predictive value of 88% for detection of ureteral obstruction by renal ultrasound (82). The renal lasix scan can also be used to diagnose ureteral obstruction and can be further useful in evaluating function in an obstructed kidney before considering urinary diversion.

Once the diagnosis of ureteral obstruction is established, an attempt should be made to determine the cause of the obstruction. The differential diagnosis includes extrinsic compression of the ureter by primary or recurrent cancer and fibrosis caused by prior surgery or radiation therapy. Careful correlation of physical examination, CA 125 measurements, and computed tomography scanning of the abdomen can often be helpful in determining the cause of the obstruction.

The management of ureteral obstruction in women with advanced ovarian cancer varies greatly and must be individualized to each patient's unique circumstances. One healthy, well-functioning kidney can supply all of the renal function that is necessary. In the absence of a ureteral obstruction complicated by pyelonephritis, and with one good functioning kidney, operative intervention unilaterally to divert the urinary stream on the obstructed side is not mandatory, especially in terminal patients not actively under treatment. In these patients, the use of dexamethasone can sometimes relieve tumor-induced ureteric obstruction. Such intervention is not always appropriate, but it may be of great value in symptomatic control (83). The use of corticosteroids in the palliative care of patients with advanced ovarian cancer should be individualized and is appropriate only in a selected group of patients.

Aggressive surgical debulking to relieve ureter obstruction secondary to advanced recurrent ovarian cancer can be performed on selected patients who are suitable candidates for salvage chemotherapy. In terms of survival, the benefit of surgery in this setting is controversial. Retrograde ureteral stent placement or percutaneous nephrostomy placement may be necessary preoperatively to correct the uremia and fluid electrolyte abnormalities before proceeding with operative decompression of the urinary tract.

Furthermore, chemoreduction of tumor occasionally relieves ureteral obstruction sufficiently to allow subsequent removal of ureteral stents or percutaneous nephrostomy tubes. Initially, cystoscopic retrograde placement of ureteral stents should be attempted to relieve ureteral obstruction. If cystoscopic retrograde placement of stents is unsuccessful, or if it is deemed unlikely that retrograde stents can be passed based on preoperative radiographic studies, unilateral or bilateral percutaneous nephrostomies can be placed with acceptable morbidity. Silastic catheters can be left indefinitely in the urinary tract with acceptable morbidity. Soper and associates (80) reported a series of 34 patients in whom percutaneous nephrostomies were used to treat ureteral obstruction secondary to gynecologic malignancy. One patient in the series sustained a perinephric hematoma, and another patient had a perinephric abscess. One patient in the series died from sepsis, and four patients with significant intrinsic renal disease failed to achieve normalization of renal function after placement of percutaneous nephrostomies.

Finally, a viable management approach in selected patients who have unilateral ureteral obstruction with a normally functioning remaining kidney, or in patients who have advanced terminal disease with bilateral ureteral obstruction, is to manage the patient expectantly, with maximal attempts at comfort care and without diverting the urinary stream. Patients can function perfectly well with one viable kidney as long as the obstructed kidney does not suffer from recurrent episodes of pyelonephritis, and in women with advanced terminal ovarian cancer who have exhausted all surgical and chemotherapeutic attempts at palliation, uremic coma can provide a comfortable death.

REFERENCES

1. Rubin SC. Intestinal obstruction in advanced ovarian cancer: what does the patient want? *Gynecol Oncol* 1999;75:311–312.
2. Krebs HB, Goplerud DR. The role of intestinal intubation in obstruction of the small intestine due to carcinoma of the ovary. *Surg Gynecol Obstet* 1984;158:467–471.
3. Lund B, Hansen M, Lundrael F, et al. Intestinal obstruction in patients with advanced carcinoma of the ovaries treated with combination chemotherapy. *Surg Gynecol Obstet* 1989;169:213–218.
4. Solomon HJ, Atkinson KH, Coppleson JV, et al. Bowel complications in the management of ovarian cancer. *Aust N Z J Obstet Gynecol* 1983;23:65–68.
5. Tunca JC, et al. The management of ovarian cancer-caused bowel obstruction. *Gynecol Oncol* 1981;12:186–192.
6. Clarke-Pearson DL, et al. Surgical management of intestinal obstruction in ovarian cancer: clinical features, postoperative complications and survival. *Gynecol Oncol* 1987;26:11–18.
7. Redman CWE, Shafi MI, Ambrose S, et al. Survival following intestinal obstruction in ovarian cancer. *Eur J Surg Oncol* 1988;14:383–386.
8. Zoetmulder FAN, Helmerhorst ThJM, v.Coevorden F, et al. Management of bowel obstruction in patients with advanced ovarian cancer. *Eur J Cancer* 1994;30A:1625–1628.
9. Beattie GJ, Leonard RCF, Smyth JF. Bowel obstruction in ovarian carcinoma: a retrospective study and review of the literature. *Palliat Med* 1989;3:275–280.
10. Tunca JC. Impact of cis-platinum multiagent chemotherapy and total parenteral hyperalimentation on bowel obstruction caused by ovarian cancer. *Gynecol Oncol* 1981;12:219–221.
11. Markman M, et al. Second-line platinum therapy in patients with ovarian cancer previously treated with cisplatin. *J Clin Oncol* 1991;9:389–393.
12. McGuire WP, Rowinsky EK, Rosenstein NB, et al. Taxol: a unique antineoplastic agent with significant activity in advanced ovarian epithelial neoplasms. *Ann Intern Med* 1989;111:273–279.
13. Castaldo TW, et al. Intestinal operations in patients with ovarian carcinoma. *Am J Obstet Gynecol* 1981;139:80–84.
14. Rubin SC, Hoskins WJ, Benjamin I, et al. Palliative surgery for intestinal obstruction in advanced ovarian cancer. *Gynecol Oncol* 1989;34:16–19.
15. Piver MS, et al. Survival after ovarian cancer induced intestinal obstruction. *Gynecol Oncol* 1982;13:44–46.
16. Krebs HB, Goplerud DR. Surgical management of bowel obstruction in advanced ovarian carcinoma. *Obstet Gynecol* 1983;61:327–330.
17. Larson JE, Podczaski ES, Manetta A, et al. Bowel obstruction in patients with ovarian carcinoma: analysis of prognostic factors. *Gynecol Oncol* 1989;35:61–65.
18. Pecorelli S, Sartori E, Santin A. Followup after primary therapy: management of the symptomatic patient—surgery. *Gynecol Oncol* 1994;55:S138–S142.
19. Fernandes JR, Seymour RJ, Suissa S. Bowel obstruction in patients with ovarian cancer: a search for prognostic factors. *Am J Obstet Gynecol* 1988;158:244–249.
20. Clarke-Pearson DL, et al. Intestinal obstruction in patients with ovarian cancer: variables associated with surgical complications and survival. *Arch Surg* 1988;123:42–45.
21. Dudrick SJ, Jensen TG, Rowlands BJ. Nutritional support: assessment and indications. In: Deitel M, ed. *Nutritional and clinical surgery*. Baltimore: Williams & Wilkins, 1980:19–27.
22. Cerra FB. Assessment of nutritional and metabolic status. In: Cerra FB, ed. *Surgical nutrition*. St. Louis: CV Mosby, 1984:24–28.

23. Albina JE, Iorouda MJ, Rombeau JL. Perioperative total parenteral nutrition. In: Rombeau JL, Caldwell MD, eds. *Parenteral nutrition*. Philadelphia: WB Saunders, 1986:370–379.
24. Baker JP, Detsky AS, Wesson DE. Nutritional assessment: a comparison of clinical judgement and objective measurements. *N Engl J Med* 1982;306:969–972.
25. Lowry SF, Smith JC, Brennan MF. Zinc and copper replacement during total parenteral nutrition. *Am J Clin Nutr* 1981;34:1853.
26. Kirkemo AK, Burt ME, Brennan MJ. Serum vitamin level maintenance in cancer patients on TPN. *Am J Clin Nutr* 1982;35:1003.
27. Shike M, et al. Changes in body composition in patients with small cell lung cancer: the effect of TPN as an adjunct for chemotherapy. *Ann Intern Med* 1984;101:303.
28. Veterans Affairs Total Parenteral Nutrition Study Group: perioperative total parenteral nutrition in surgical patients. *N Engl J Med* 1991;325:525–532.
29. Ford JH, et al. Parenteral hyperalimentation in gynecologic oncology patients. *Gynecol Oncol* 1972;1:70.
30. Hopkins MP, Roberts JA, Morley GW. Outpatient management of small bowel obstruction in terminal ovarian cancer. *J Reprod Med* 1987;32:827–829.
31. Malone JM, et al. Palliation of small bowel obstruction by percutaneous gastrostomy in patients with ovarian carcinoma. *Obstet Gynecol* 1986;68:431–433.
32. Ponsky JL, Ganderer MWL, Stellato TA. Percutaneous endoscopic gastrostomy: review of 150 cases. *Arch Surg* 1983;116:913–914.
33. Feldman GB, et al. The role of lymphatic obstruction in the formation of ascites in a murine ovarian carcinoma. *Cancer Res* 1972;32:1663–1666.
34. Herz J, et al. Chylous ascites following retroperitoneal lymphadenectomy: report of 2 cases with guidelines for diagnosis and treatment. *Cancer* 1978;42:349–352.
35. Garrison RN, et al. Malignant ascites: clinical and experimental observations. *Ann Surg* 1986;203:644–651.
36. Menard S, et al. Sensitivity enhancement of the cytologic detection of cancer cells in effusions by monoclonal antibodies. *Am J Clin Pathol* 1985;83:571–576.
37. Ariel IM, Oropeza R, Pack GT. Intracavitary administration of radioactive isotopes in the control of effusions due to cancer; results in 267 patients. *Cancer* 1966;19:1096–102.
38. Paladine W, et al. Intracavitary bleomycin in the management of malignant effusions. *Cancer* 1976;38:1903–1908.
39. Kefford RF, Woods RL, Fox RM, et al. Intracavitary Adriamycin nitrogen mustard and tetracycline in the control of malignant effusions: a randomized study. *Med J Aust* 1980;2:447–448.
40. Jackson GL, Blosser NM. Intracavitary chromic phosphate (^{32}P) colloidal suspension therapy. *Cancer* 1981;48:2596–2598.
41. Ozols RF, et al. Phase I and pharmacological studies of Adriamycin administered intraperitoneally to patients with ovarian cancer. *Cancer Res* 1982;42:4265–4269.
42. Currie JL, et al. Intracavitary Corynebacterium parvum for treatment of malignant effusions. *Gynecol Oncol* 1983;16:6–14.
43. Bitran JD. Intraperitoneal bleomycin: pharmacokinetics and the results of a phase II trial. *Cancer* 1985;56:2420–2423.
44. Stewart JS, et al. Intraperitoneal ^{131}I- and ^{90}Y- labelled monoclonal antibodies for ovarian cancer: pharmacokinetics and normal tissue dosimetry. *Int J Cancer* 1988,3:71–76.
45. Kamada M, Sakamoto Y, Furumoto H, et al. Treatment of malignant ascites with allogeneic and autologous lymphokine-activated killer cells. *Gynecol Oncol* 1989;34:34–37.
46. Bezwoda WR, Seymour L, Dansey R. Intraperitoneal recombinant interferon-alpha 2b for recurrent malignant ascites due to ovarian cancer. *Cancer* 1989;64:1029–1033.
47. Cherchi PL, et al. Endocavitary beta-interferon in neoplastic effusions. *Eur J Gynecol Oncol* 1990;11:477–479.
48. Oosterlee J. Peritoneovenous shunting for ascites in cancer patients. *Br J Surg* 1980;67:663–666.
49. Straus AK, Roseman DL, Shapiro TM. Peritoneovenous shunting in the management of malignant ascites. *Arch Surg* 1979;114:489–491.
50. Lokich J, et al. Complications of peritoneovenous shunt for malignant ascites. *Cancer Treat Rep* 1980;64:305–309.
51. Sonnefeld T, Tyden G. Perioneovenous shunts for malignant ascites. *Acta Chir Scand* 1986;152:117–121.
52. Souter RG, et al. Surgical and pathologic complications associated with peritoneovenous shunts in management of malignant ascites. *Cancer* 1985;55:1973–1978.
53. Li KW, Wong WS. Double valve Denver peritoneal venous shunt used in ovarian malignant ascites: a case report. *Chin Med J (Engl)* 1989;102:300–302.
54. Battaglia GB, et al. Preliminary experience in the treatment of rebel ascites from ovarian cancer with the peritoneo-venous shunt of Leveen. *Eur J Gynecol Oncol* 1982;3:88–90.
55. Stehman FB, Ehrlich CE. Peritoneo-cystic shunt for malignant ascites. *Gynecol Oncol* 1984;18:402–407.
56. Leininger BJ, Barker WL, Langston HT. A simplified method for management of malignant pleural effusion. *J Thorac Cardiovasc Surg* 1969;58:758–763.
57. Zehner LC, Hoogstraten B. Malignant effusions and their management. *Semin Oncol Nurs* 1985;1:259–268.
58. Austin EH, Flye MW. The treatment of recurrent malignant pleural effusion. *Ann Thoracic Surg* 1979;28:190–203.
59. Martensson G, Pettersson K, Thiringer G. Differentiation between malignant and non-malignant pleural effusion. *Eur J Respir Dis* 1985;67:326–334.
60. Jarvi OH, et al. The accuracy and significance of cytologic cancer diagnosis of pleural effusions. *Acta Cytol* 1972;16:152–158.
61. Johnson WD. The cytological diagnosis of cancer in serous effusions. *Acta Cytol* 1986;10:161–172.
62. Ceelen GH. The cytologic diagnosis of ascitic fluid. *Acta Cytol* 1984;8:175–185.
63. Johnston WD, Szpak CA, Lottich SC, et al. Use of a monoclonal antibody (B72.3) as an immunocytochemical adjunct to diagnosis of adenocarcinoma in human effusions. *Cancer Res* 1985;45:1894–1900.
64. Martin SE, et al. Identification of adenocarcinoma in cytospin preparations of effusions using monoclonal antibody B72.3. *Am J Clin Pathol* 1986;86:234–237.
65. Lodden Kemper R, et al. Diagnostic yield of blind needle biopsy and of thoracoscopy in pleural effusion: an intra-individual comparison. *Endoscopy* 1978;10:143–147.

66. Boutin, Viallat JR, Cargnino P, et al. Thorascopy in malignant pleural effusions. *Am Rev Respir Dis* 1981;124:558–592.
67. Zaloznik AJ, Oswald SG, Langin M. Intrapleural tetracycline in management of pleural effusions: a randomized study. *Cancer* 1983;51:752–755.
68. O'Neill W, et al. A prospective study of chest tube drainage and tetracycline sclerosis vs. chest tube drainage alone in the treatment of malignant pleural effusion. *Proc Am Assoc Cancer Res Clin Oncol* 1980;21:349–352.
69. Bayly TC, Kisner DL, Sybert A, et al. Tetracycline and quinacrine in the control of malignant pleural effusions: a randomized trial. *Cancer* 1978;41:1188–1192.
70. Wallach HW. Intrapleural tetracycline for malignant pleural effusions. *Chest* 1975;68:510–512.
71. Kennedy L, Rusch VW, Strange C, et al. Pleurodesis using talc slurry. *Chest* 1994;106:342–346.
72. Leahy BC, Honey Bourne D, Brear SE, et al. Treatment of malignant pleural effusions with intrapleural *Corynebacterium parvum* or tetracycline. *Eur J Respir Dis* 1985;66:50–54.
73. Hillerdal G, et al. *Corynebacterium parvum* in malignant pleural effusion: a randomized prospective study. *Eur J Respir Dis* 1986;69:204–206.
74. Cherchi PL, Campiglio A, Rubatti A, et al. Endocavitary beta-interferon in neoplastic effusions. *Eur J Gynaecol Oncol* 1990;11:447–479.
75. Li DJ, et al. A new approach to the treatment of malignant effusion. *Chin Med J (Engl)* 1990;103:998–1002.
76. Martini N, Bains MS, Beattie EJ Jr. Indications for pleurectomy in malignant effusion. *Cancer* 1975;35:734–738.
77. Pollock AV. The treatment of resistant malignant ascites by insertion of a peritoneo-atrial Holter valve. *Br J Surg* 1975;62:104–107.
78. Little AG, Fergnson MK, Coloumb HM, et al. Pleuroperitoneal shunting for malignant pleural effusions. *Cancer* 1986;58:2740–2743.
79. Cimochowski GE, et al. Pleuroperitoneal shunting for recalcitrant pleural effusions. *J Thorac Cardiovasc Surg* 1986;92:866–870.
80. Soper JT, Blaozczyk TM, Oke E, et al. Percutaneous nephrostomy in gynecologic oncology patients. *Am J Obstet Gynecol* 1988; 158:1126–1131.
81. Dudley BS, et al. Percutaneous nephrostomy catheter use in gynecologic malignancy. *Gynecol Oncol* 1986;24:273–278.
82. Frohlich EP, Bex P, Nissenbaum MM, et al. Comparison between renal ultrasonography and excretory urography in cervical cancer. *Int J Gynaecol Obstet* 1991;34:49–54.
83. Walsh TD, West TS. Malignant ureteric obstruction relieved by dexamethasone. *Postgrad Med J* 1984;60:437–438.

19
Radiotherapy in the Management of Epithelial Ovarian Cancer

Higinia R. Cardenes and Marcus E. Randall

INTRODUCTION

Ovarian carcinoma (OC) is the second most common gynecologic cancer and is the leading cause of death from gynecologic malignancy. It is overall the fourth leading cause of cancer death in women, behind lung, breast, and colorectal cancer, with 25,400 new cases and 14,500 deaths projected in 1998 (1). Although important advances in surgery, chemotherapy (CT), and radiation therapy (RT) have been made, the overall survival for patients with OC has not changed significantly—even for those with early-stage disease—over the past 20 years. More than 70% of the patients with OC have stage III or IV disease at the time of diagnosis. With the introduction of platinum compounds in the late 1970s and the introduction of paclitaxel in the early 1990s, response rates to CT increased significantly (2). However, after almost 15 years of experience with these new drugs there has not been a clear improvement in survival, particularly in patients with suboptimal debulking, and only a modest survival benefit has been shown in patients with optimally debulked disease. Therefore, although response to initial therapy is expected, most patients eventually develop progressive disease or relapse and die from their disease.

Despite its long history in the treatment of OC and its proven curative role in patients with microscopic or minimal residual disease, the proper role of RT in the management of OC is not clearly established. Similarly, the potential roles of RT in consolidative treatment, as salvage therapy after CT failure, and as palliative therapy remain controversial. However, it is clear that RT techniques and equipment have significantly improved in the last 20 years. Furthermore, although RT administered in many of the earlier trials was inadequate by today's standards, the results were often comparable to those achieved with modern CT combinations.

EARLY-STAGE OVARIAN CANCER: ADJUVANT/PRIMARY THERAPY

The role of adjuvant treatment in patients with early epithelial OC (stage I or II) after comprehensive surgical staging is still controversial. Data from the Gynecologic Oncology Group (GOG) (3) have established a group of "good prognosis" patients who have a low risk for recurrence. These include patients with stage IA and IB disease (disease confined to one or both ovaries, intact ovarian capsule, no adhesions or extracystic tumor, no ascites, and negative peritoneal washings) and well or moderately differentiated tumors (diploid tumors). These patients have an excellent prognosis (5-year survival rate, 94% to 98%) which does not seem to be improved with adjuvant therapy (melphalan). In contrast, patients with poorly differentiated tumors (and grade 1 aneuploid tumors) or more advanced stage I or II disease (rupture of the capsule, dense adhesions, clear cell histology, extraovarian spread, or positive peritoneal washings) have poorer outcomes (5-year survival rate, 70% to 80% among the treated patients; relapse rate, 25% to 40%). For these "high-risk" early OC patients, the majority of the gynecologist oncologists would advise adjuvant therapy. Historically, both intraperitoneal (IP) radiocolloids and

TABLE 19.1. *Procedure for administration of intraperitoneal radioactive phosphate suspention (^{32}P)*

1. Patient is admitted to the hospital the day before or the same day of the administration. Patient needs to be NPO after midnight.
2. Two multiperforated peritoneal dyalisis catheters (e.g., Tenckhoff) are placed in the right and left lower quadrants, respectively.
3. Patient is transported to the nuclear medicine department, where approximately 2 mCi of ^{99m}Tc is inserted into the right catheter, followed by approximately 250 mL of NS.
4. Patient is instructed to roll from side to side and preferably to lie on the abdomen in order to distribute the radioisotope. Small detectable external markers should be placed on the patient's skin to identify the xiphoid process and the pubic symphysis.
5. The abdomen is then scanned, anteroposterior and lateral, after the right side injection.
6. The left catheter is injected with approximately 5 mCi of ^{99m}Tc and the abdomen is scanned as before.
7. If the distribution is poor on both sides, the procedure is terminated and no ^{32}P is administered.
8. 10 to 15 mCi of ^{32}P is injected into the NS (catheter) intravenous line (running full flow) that demonstrated good intraperitoneal distribution on the ^{99m}Tc scan.
9. Approximately 250 mL of NS in then injected into each catheter after the radioisotope administration. The total intraperitoneal infusion is approximately 1000 mL.
10. Intraperitoneal catheters are removed at the completion of the procedure. The catheter insertion site should be closed with a purse-string suture.
11. The patient is transported to her room and instructed to turn to her left side, onto her back in Trendelenburg and reverse Trendelenburg positions, onto her right side and onto her abdomen every 10 minutes for about 2 hours.
12. Intramuscular prochlorperazine may be given routinely for the first 24 hours to prevent the occurrence of nausea and vomiting.
13. The patient is confined to her room and is observed for approximately 24 hours after the administration of ^{32}P.
14. Radiation precautions are recommended within the patient's room regarding linens saved and room decontamination procedures.

NPO, nothing by mouth; ^{99m}Tc, technetium Tc 99m-labeled agent; NS, normal saline.

external whole-abdomen irradiation (WAI) have been used.

Intraperitoneal Radioactive Chromic Phosphate Suspension

Radioactive phosphorous P 32 (^{32}P) seems to be the most attractive radiocolloid for IP administration because it is a pure β-emitter, which avoids the hazard of γ-radiation. ^{32}P has a half life of 14.3 days, average tissue penetration of 1.4 to 3.0 mm, and maximum and average β energies of 1.71 and 0.69 MeV, respectively. Chromic phosphate is a blue-green, chemically inert colloidal form of ^{32}P used for intracavitary instillation. The precise distribution and dose delivered by ^{32}P to the peritoneal surface is unknown and often unpredictable. The IP isotope distribution should be tested before instillation with radioactive technetium sulfur colloid or after radiocolloid administration with scintigraphic imaging of Bremsstrahlung photons. The protocol of instillation and distribution of ^{32}P is complex but well worked out, and it is outlined in Table 19.1.

The best available data supporting the theory that 10 to 15 mCi of ^{32}P delivers superficial but therapeutic dosages to the peritoneal surfaces is from Currie and colleagues (4). There appears to be predominantly an abdominal distribution, with much smaller systemic absorption. The majority of the ^{32}P is either absorbed by the peritoneal surface, by the macrophages lining the peritoneal cavity, or phagocytized by free floating macrophages. The rest of the ^{32}P is carried by the abdominal current to the right hemidiaphragm, where it passes through the diaphragmatic lymphatics and enters the mediastinal lymphatics. It then passes to the right subclavian vein via the right thoracic trunk and enters the general circulation, where it is rapidly cleared by the liver and deposited to a lesser extent in other tissues (spleen and bone marrow). Pelvic and paraaortic lymph nodes receive relatively low, nontherapeutic doses. Several studies using imaging techniques confirm that the distribution of chromic ^{32}P is dynamic for the first 6 to 24 hours but thereafter is fixed. Boye and associates (5) reported that the estimated peritoneal surface dose from 10 mCi of ^{32}P is approximately 30 Gy, although the uptake and distribution of ^{32}P in the peritoneal cavity often shows significant inhomogeneity. They noted an increase in the measurable level of ^{32}P in the blood for 7 days, after which it declined; the estimated maximum dose to the peripheral blood even at its peak was 1.2 cGy. The dose to the bone marrow was higher by two to five times, but the maximum dose was still very low, on the order of 6 cGy.

Randomized Trials Using Intraperitoneal Radioactive Phosphorus

Table 19.2 shows the results of randomized trials using IP-^{32}P in the adjuvant setting for early-stage OC. Young and coworkers (3) reported in 1990 the results of a GOG trial in which 141 eligible patients with International Federation of Gynecology and Obstetrics (FIGO) stage IC and II, or poorly differentiated tumors FIGO stage IA or IB after accurate and comprehensive surgical staging, were randomly allocated to receive either ^{32}P (15 mCi) at the time of surgery or melphalan (0.2 mg/kg/day for 5 days, repeated every 4 to 6 weeks for up to 12 cycles). The outcomes for the two treatment groups, with a median follow-up of more than 6 years, were similar with respect to 5-year disease-free survival (DFS) (80% in both groups) and overall survival (81% with melphalan versus 78% with ^{32}P; $p = .48$). Seven percent of the patients could not receive the prescribed ^{32}P because of catheter difficulties, and 6% subsequently required surgery for bowel obstruction. However, although there was no observation arm, the GOG concluded that the added cost, inconvenience, and risk of alkylating agent–induced leukemia were not justified, and ^{32}P was chosen as the control arm for the next GOG trial. It is unclear whether any benefit resulted from the use of ^{32}P. The observed survival could be attributed to favorable tumor characteristics rather than the therapy employed. In this study, 17% of the patients entered had grade I or borderline tumors.

The second major GOG trial included a similar high-risk group of patients with early-stage OC (stage IC and II with no macroscopic residua and stage IA and IB poorly differentiated tumors). After complete surgical staging, patients were randomly assigned to receive either IP-^{32}P (15 mCi) or cyclophosphamide (1 g/m^2 IV) plus cisplatin (100 mg/m^2 IV) every 21 days for three cycles (CP). The trial was closed in 1994 and now has a minimum follow-up of 3 years and a median follow-up of 5 years. A total of 204 evaluable patients with high-risk OC were accrued over 7 years. Ninety-eight patients received ^{32}P and 106 received CP; 78% of the latter group were

TABLE 19.2. *Early-stage ovarian cancer: intraperitoneal-^{32}P prospective randomized trials*

Series (ref. no.)	High risk	No. patients	Study design	5-year DFS (%)	5-year survival (%)
GOG (3)	IA, IB, G3 IC-II OpD	141	^{32}P vs. Melphalan	80 80	78 81
GOG (6)	IA, IB, G3 IC-II OpD	204	^{32}P vs. CTX + CDDP	66[a] 78[a]	76 83
Norwegian Radium Hospital (8)	I-III OpD	347	CDDP vs. ^{32}P	75[b] 81[b]	81 83
GICOG Italy (10)	IC	161	CDDP vs. ^{32}P	81 66	83 79

DFS, disease-free survival; G3, grade 3; OpD, optimally debulked; CTX, cyclophosphamide; CDDP, cisplatin.
[a]After adjusting for stage and histologic grade, the estimated recurrence rate was 1% less for CP than for ^{32}P ($p = 0.08$).
[b]Five-year DFS rates in patients with stage I by treatment subgroups were 86%, 95%, and 83% for ^{32}P, whole abdomen irradiation (WAI), and cisplatin, respectively.

recurrence free at 5 years, compared with 66% of those receiving ^{32}P. After adjusting for stage and histologic grade, the estimated recurrence rate was 31% less for CP than for ^{32}P ($p = .08$). Survival at 5 years was 83% for CP and 76% for ^{32}P. Eight patients randomly assigned to the ^{32}P arm were unable to receive the treatment, and two patients had small bowel perforations during catheter insertion. Although there were no statistically significant differences between the two arms, the better progression-free interval for CP and the problems with adequate distribution and late toxicities associated with ^{32}P made the platinum-based combination the preferred standard treatment for patients with early-stage high-risk OC (6).

The current GOG trial has omitted ^{32}P and randomly assigns a similar group of patients with early OC (stage IC and II and poor-prognosis IA and IB), after complete surgical staging, to receive three versus six cycles of intravenous carboplatin (area under the time-versus-concentration curve [AUC], 7.5) and paclitaxel (175 mg/m^2 infusion over 3 hours), administered every 21 days. As in the previous trial, the endpoints for this investigation will be DFS, survival, and comparative toxicity.

The National Cancer Institute of Canada Clinical Trials Group (7) randomly assigned 257 eligible patients with high-risk stage I to IIA disease (high grade, capsular penetration, positive cytology, cyst rupture) or completely resected stage IIB or III disease to receive either WAI by moving-strip technique (2,250 cGy, 20 fractions), oral melphalan (8 mg/m^2/day for 4 days, every 4 weeks for 18 cycles), or IP-^{32}P (10 to 15 mCi); these treatments were administered after pelvic irradiation (2,250 cGy before WAI or 4,500 cGy before melphalan or ^{32}P). All patients had abdominal hysterectomy, but comprehensive surgical staging was not mandatory. With a median follow-up of 8 years, no difference in actuarial 5-year survival rate was observed among the three study arms (62%, 61%, and 66% for WAI, melphalan, and ^{32}P, respectively). The ^{32}P plus pelvic RT arm was closed prematurely because of a high incidence of bowel complications. Interestingly, protocol violations in covering the whole-abdomen target volume correlated with reduced survival in the multivariate analysis.

In the Norwegian Radium Hospital study (8), adjuvant IP-^{32}P (7 to 10 mCi) was compared with six cycles of cisplatin (50 mg/m^2) in a group of 347 patients with stage I to III OC without residual tumor after primary surgical debulking. Patients with extensive adhesions randomly assigned to the ^{32}P arm were treated with WAI (17%). The median follow-up was 62 months. No difference in actuarial survival or DFS was seen between the two treatment groups. The estimated 5-year rates of crude survival and DFS in the ^{32}P group were 83% and 81%, respectively, compared with 81% and 75%, respectively, for those patients receiving cisplatin. When the patients randomly assigned to receive ^{32}P were subgrouped into those who actually received it and those who were treated with WAI, the estimated 5-year DFS rates in patients with stage I disease were 86%, 95%, and 83% for patients treated with ^{32}P, WAI, and cisplatin, respectively (differences not statistically significant). The 5-year DFS rate was 55% for stage II patients randomly assigned receive ^{32}P compared with 68% in the cisplatin group. Late bowel obstruction requiring surgery occurred more often in the group treated with ^{32}P (4%) or WAI (11%), compared with the cisplatin group (1%). The authors recommended that cisplatin be used as standard adjuvant treatment for subsequent controlled studies, although this group had an inferior median survival time, a shorter median time to recurrence, and a greater percentage of patients relapsing. In 1993, the same authors (9) reported on 313 patients with OC who received IP-^{32}P as primary adjuvant treatment (245 patients), as consolidating therapy after negative second-look laparotomy (SLL) (59 patients), or after positive SLL with minimal residuum (9 patients). The actuarial 5-year crude survival was 81% in the group treated adjuvantly and 79% in the group treated after SLL. However, the morbidity rate was substantial: 2 patients died of treatment complications attributed to ^{32}P, and small bowel obstruction without tumor recurrence occurred in 22 (7%) of the patients (13 treated surgically and 9 medically). The authors concluded that, without an untreated observation group, it was unclear whether adjuvant ^{32}P conferred a survival advantage.

The Gruppo Italiano Colaborativo Oncologica Ginecologica (GI-COG) performed two multicenter randomized clinical trials (10). After surgical staging and stratification by center, eligible patients in study 1 ($n = 92$; eligible, 83; stage IA and IB, grades 2 and 3) were randomly assigned to receive either cisplatin (50 mg/m^2 every 28 days for 6 cycles) or no further treatment (control). Patients in study 2 ($n = 186$; eligible, 176: stage IC, any grade) were randomly assigned to cisplatin (50 mg/m^2 every 28 days for 6 cycles) or IP-^{32}P (15 mCi). The median follow-up was 76 months in each study. The 5-year DFS in study 1 was 83% for cisplatin and 64% for the control group ($p = .09$), but no difference in overall survival could be detected (the 5-year survival rates were 87% and 81% for the cisplatin and control groups, respectively). But when the control group patients were treated with cisplatin at relapse, they had the same 5-year survival rate as the group treated with cisplatin immediately. In study 2, the 5-year DFS was 81% for the cisplatin group and 66% for the ^{32}P group ($p = .008$). Again, there was no difference in overall survival (83% and 79% at 5 years for the cisplatin and ^{32}P groups, respectively). These two studies also demonstrated that the cisplatin-treated patients had a poorer outcome at relapse than the noncisplatin-treated patients. In both trials the difference in relapse pattern was primarily the result of a reduction in relapses in the pelvis only. The fact that there was no difference in the overall survival either of the two trials may be related to (a) the limited impact of this adjuvant therapy; (b) the relatively low doses of cisplatin used; (c) the impact of salvage treatment at the time of recurrence; or (d) simply a power of the study that was too low. Since the above-mentioned studies for high-risk patients lacked a control group, the optimal adjuvant therapy for this group of patients with intermediate prognosis remains subject to question, particularly in stage I disease. The trend in the United States is to treat patients with high-risk stage I and II OC with systemic CT, primarily platinum/paclitaxel combinations.

One possible explanation for failure to demonstrate a therapeutic benefit for ^{32}P is the relatively low radiation dose delivered to sites of possible tumor involvement. With the average energy of the β particles being 0.6 MeV and the rapid falloff in dose below the surface, doses at a depth of more than 2 mm are negligible. Furthermore, dosimetric studies have shown an uneven distribution of the colloid throughout the abdominal cavity, resulting in a variable and unpredictable radiation dose through the peritoneal surface, with up to 10-fold differences (11). No randomized trials of ^{32}P versus observation alone in patients with early-stage OC have been performed.

For early-stage OC, long-term survival is the most appropriate endpoint; therefore, it would important to perform a large prospective, multicenter study with long-term follow-up to resolve the question of whether any up-front adjuvant therapy contributes significantly to survival. There are currently three ongoing randomized trials in Europe trying to determine whether adjuvant CT in high-risk stage I and II OC significantly improves long-term survival. The outcome of these trials, coupled with the results from the GOG trial of cisplatin and paclitaxel, should allow us to reach more definitive conclusions regarding the benefits of adjuvant therapy in poor-prognosis early OC.

Whole-Abdomen Irradiation

The tendency of OC to remain localized to the abdomen throughout its natural history led to the frequent use of external abdominal and/or pelvic RT more than 25 years ago. The theoretical and practical advantages of WAI over ^{32}P administration are mainly a more homogeneous dose distribution, better coverage of the pelvic and periaortic lymph nodes, and the ability to treat all of the peritoneal surfaces without limitations caused by the presence of postoperative adhesions. However, WAI is associated with a higher incidence of acute and late toxicity, primarily related to dose-limiting organs including the liver, kidneys, and small bowel.

The use of external beam RT in the treatment of OC began to decline significantly after publication of the M.D. Anderson Cancer Center randomized trial in 1975 (12). This trial, which

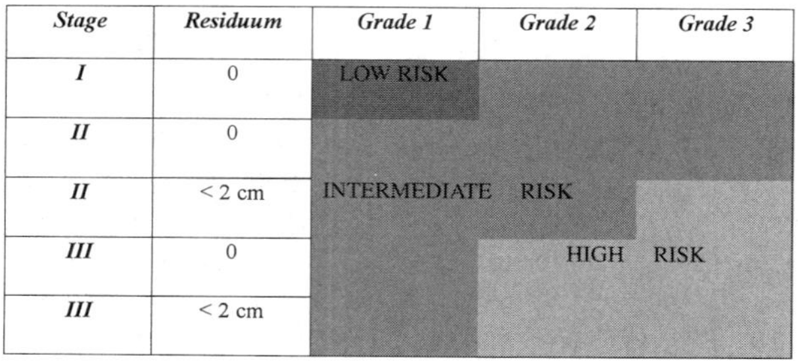

Stage	Residuum	Grade 1	Grade 2	Grade 3
I	0	LOW RISK		
II	0			
II	< 2 cm		INTERMEDIATE RISK	
III	0			
III	< 2 cm			HIGH RISK

FIG. 19.1. Prognostic subgroupings according to stage, residuum, and grade in patients with stages I through III ovarian cancer. (From Dembo AJ, Bush RS. Choice of postoperative therapy based on prognostic factors. *Int J Radiat Oncol Biol Phys* 1982;8:893–897, with permission.)

included 108 evaluable patients with stage I or II OC, randomly assigned patients to 12 cycles of single-agent treatment with oral melphalan (0.2 mg/kg/day for 5 days) versus WAI (2,600 to 2,800 cGy, using moving-strip technique with liver shielding, and 2,000 cGy pelvic boost). The two therapies were equally efficacious. The overall actuarial 2-year survival rates for patients with stage I and II disease were 85% and 90%, respectively, for WAI treatment and 55% and 58% for melphalan. However, this study has been criticized for not irradiating the diaphragm adequately, providing low RT doses to the liver and kidney areas, an imbalance in stage distribution between the two arms (significant preponderance of more advanced-stage IIB versus I to IIA cases in the RT arm), and short follow-up. In addition, even though the findings did not show CT to be superior to WAI in terms of treatment outcome, it was clear that WAI involved greater acute morbidity and cost. However, RT equipment and technique have improved significantly since that time, resulting in decreased acute and late toxicity, whereas the toxicity and cost of the currently used platinum/paclitaxel CT are significantly greater than for single-agent melphalan.

Only in the past decade has a clear appreciation emerged of the risk factors within FIGO stages. In 1977 early-stage disease was subdivided into a high-risk group (all stage II, all stage IC, and stage IA and IB with high-grade tumors) and a low-risk group (all other types). Traditional clinical and pathologic prognostic factors in early-stage disease include FIGO substage, histologic type and grade, amount of residual tumor after primary surgery, presence of dense adhesions, large-volume ascites, age, and performance status (13–14). Based on the analysis performed at the Princess Margaret Hospital, Dembo and associates (13), and Lederman and colleagues (14) defined several risk groups in order to select those patients most suitable for primary postoperative adjuvant RT. Ideal patients had optimal debulking with no macroscopic residual disease in the abdomen and up to 2 cm residual disease in the pelvis, which can be safely boosted. Dembo and Bush (15,16) recommended adjuvant WAI for patients in the intermediate-risk group (stage I to II grade 2 to 3 and stage III grade 1, with less than 2 cm residual disease) (Figure 19.1). In this group the rate of freedom from relapse at 5 years was approximately 70% after RT. The rate for patients in the high-risk group, including stage III grade 2 to 3 and stage II grade 3 with small residuum, was only 20%. The latter patients were subsequently treated with combined CT and RT.

Randomized Trials of Whole-Abdomen Irradiation in Early-Stage Disease

Table 19.3 shows the results of large, randomized trials of WAI as adjuvant therapy in the management of early-stage OC (stage I and II). Dembo and colleagues (17) published results of a randomized trial comparing WAI (22.5 Gy in 10 fractions, moving-strip, followed by pelvic boost) versus pelvic RT (45 Gy in 20 fractions), either alone or followed by chlorambucil (6 mg/day for 2 years). With an accrual of 147 patients who had stage I to III OC with minimal (less than 2 cm) or no residual disease, the study demonstrated a 10-year survival advantage of 64% versus 40%, in favor of WAI ($p = .0007$). No survival benefit was seen for patients with

TABLE 19.3. Early-stage ovarian cancer: whole-abdomen irradiation (WAI)–randomized studies

Series (ref. no.)	Patient population (stage)	No. patients	Study design	Outcome
Klaassen et al. (7)	I–III	107	Randomized: WAI vs. Pelvic RT + Melphalan	62%-5 y RFS
		106		61%-5 y RFS
Smith et al. (12)	I	14	Randomized: WAI vs. Melphalan	85%-2 y RFS
		28		90%-2 y RFS
Smith et al. (12)	II	37	Randomized: WAI vs. Melphalan	55%-2 y RFS
		29		58%-2 y RFS
Sell et al. (19)	I	60	Randomized: WAI vs. Pelvic RT + CTX	63%-4 y survival
		58		55%-4 y survival
Chiara et al. (20)	I–II	44	Randomized: CDDP + CTX vs. WAI	73%-5 y survival
		25		68%-5 y survival

Differences not statistically significant except for Dembo's series; ($p = .0007$).
OpD, optimally debulked; RT, radiotherapy; WAI, whole-abdomen irradiation; CDDP, cisplatin; CTX, cyclophosphamide; RFS, relapse-free survival.

gross residual disease (more than 2 cm). Therefore, it appears that WAI, when administered in appropriate volumes with adequate techniques to patients with OC and minimal residual disease, results in treatment outcomes comparing favorably with those obtained by modern CT regimens (18).

Three other randomized trials have been reported comparing WAI with CT, although only one study involved cisplatin-based CT (7,19,20). None of these trials demonstrated a significant difference between the WAI and CT arms. Sell and coworkers (19) randomly assigned patients to receive WAI versus pelvic RT plus cyclophosphamide, observing 4-year overall survival rates of 63% and 55%, respectively. When the analysis was restricted to intermediate-risk patients (as defined by Dembo), a survival advantage for WAI was not shown.

In 1985, the Northwest Oncologic Cooperative Group of Italy (20) initiated a prospective randomized trial in high-risk patients with early-stage disease (stage IA or IB grade 3, stage IC, and stage II). Patients were randomly assigned to receive either CT (cisplatin, 50 mg/m^2, plus cyclophosphamide, 600 mg/m^2, on day 1 every 28 days for 6 cycles) or WAI (43.2 Gy to the pelvis, 30.2 Gy to the abdomen). For the entire series, the 5-year survival rates were 71% and 53% ($p = .16$) for CT and WAI, respectively, while the rate of relapse-free survival (RFS) was 74% and 50% ($p = .07$). The trial was closed prematurely because of poor accrual, and 15% of the patients did not have complete surgical staging. The high toxicity associated with WAI could be explained by the higher dose per fraction used in this trial (130 cGy/day). When the data were analyzed according to treatment received rather than treatment assigned, no significant differences could be detected in RFS (73% versus 60%) or overall survival (73% versus 68%) between the patients receiving CT versus WAI.

In 1986, the GOG activated a randomized protocol to compare WAI versus platinum-based CT. This trial asked a crucial question, namely which therapy given adjuvantly produced better survival and DFS. However, the trial was closed because patient accrual was inadequate, and the question remains answered.

It is unclear whether pelvic RT, when given with CT, has any impact on final outcome based on the results of various clinical trials. However, two randomized trials conducted by the GOG and Princess Margaret Hospital compared pelvic RT versus observation in stage I OC and failed to demonstrate any impact on recurrence rate (21,22). The GOG randomly assigned surgically debulked (not surgically staged) patients with stage I OC to observation, melphalan, or pelvic RT (21). Although 186 patients were enrolled in the study, only 86 were evaluable. Neither of the adjuvant treatment arms significantly reduced the recurrence rate compared with the observation arm. Similarly, in the randomized trial from Princess Margaret Hospital, pelvic RT had no impact on the rates of relapse or survival when compared with observation in stage I patients (22).

The available data make a compelling argument in favor of a rigorous reinvestigation of the role of WAI in OC. Unfortunately, prevailing biases have precluded the completion of randomized trials directly comparing WAI with state-of-the-art CT regimens (cisplatin/paclitaxel) as adjuvant therapy in patients with high-risk stage I and II disease.

The recommendations given by the National Institutes of Health (NIH) Consensus Development Conference Statement in 1994 (23) included the following statements:

1. Patients with stage IA grade 1 and most IB grade 1 tumors do not require adjuvant therapy.
2. All patients with grade 3 tumors require adjuvant therapy.
3. Patients with clear cell carcinoma require adjuvant therapy.
4. Many but not all women with stage IC disease require adjuvant therapy.
5. Consensus on the need for postoperative adjuvant therapy in the remaining subsets of patients with stage I epithelial cancer could not be reached.
6. Although it is clearly acknowledged that many subsets of women with stage I OC have a substantial likelihood for recurrence and mortality, the most effective adjuvant therapy has not been established. Ideally, patients with these high-risk stage I cancers should be enrolled in clinical trials to identify adjuvant therapy that will optimally improved survival.

ADVANCED-STAGE OVARIAN CANCER: ADJUVANT/PRIMARY THERAPY

Whole-Abdomen Irradiation in Patients with Limited Residual Disease

In the United States there has not been a randomized trial evaluating state-of-the-art WAI alone versus "standard" CT regimens (cisplatin/paclitaxel) in "optimally debulked" stage III ovarian cancer (OC). The NIH consensus conference in 1994 (23) indicated that "the role of RT in advanced epithelial OC is controversial. Long-term relapse-free survival (RFS) have been demonstrated for stages II and III after optimal debulking and postoperative RT, but no prospective trials of whole abdomen irradiation (WAI) compared with chemotherapy (CT) have been performed." They also recommended that "WAI should be reevaluated and newer RT techniques evaluated in the treatment of optimally debulked stage II and III disease."

Several studies of WAI in advanced-stage OC with minimum residuum have been published (Table 19.4). Dembo (15,16,24) reported 5-year survival rates of 58% and 43% for stage II and III OC, respectively, in patients who had optimal debulking (less than 2 cm residuum) and were treated with WAI (Table 19.4). Goldberg and Peschel (25) reviewed the Yale experience with adjuvant WAI (17.5 to 25 Gy, with a pelvic boost to 40 to 46 Gy) in 74 OC patients with stage I to III disease and limited (less than 2 cm) or no residual disease. The rates of actuarial survival and DFS at 10 years were 77% and 79%, respectively, for the favorable group. The actuarial 10-year survival rate for the unfavorable group was only 7%. Severe late toxicity occurred in 7% of the patients and consisted largely of small bowel obstruction. Weiser and colleagues (26) reported on 68 stage II and III patients who were treated with WAI after cytoreductive surgery at Walter Reed Army Medical Center. Patients with no residual disease had a 10-year actuarial survival rate of 59% and a median survival time in excess of 10 years. Those with less than 2 cm residual disease had a 10-year survival rate of 42% and a median survival time of 6 years. Seventeen percent of the patients experienced late severe toxicity, probably as a result of the higher dose delivered to the entire abdomen when compared with other series (40 Gy in 20 fractions).

Fuller and associates (27) published the results of postoperative WAI in 106 patients with stage I to III OC. Those patients who had stage I to IIIA disease with no postoperative residual tumor, or less than 0.5 cm abdominal disease and/or less

TABLE 19.4. *Whole-abdomen irradiation (WAI) in advanced-stage ovarian cancer with minimum residuum*

Series (ref. no.)	Patient population (stage)	No. patients	Study design	Outcome
Dembo (24)			Nonrandomized	
	II	36	≤2 cm	58%-5 y survival
	III	101	≤2 cm	43%-5 y survival
Goldberg and Peschel (25)	II-III	74	Nonrandomized	
			Intermediate-risk group (none or <2 cm residuum)	Favorable group
				77%-10 y survival
				79%-10 y survival
Weiser et al. (26)	II-III	68	Nonrandomized	
			No residual disease	59%-10 y survival
			≤2 cm	42%-10 y survival
Fuller et al. (27)	I-III	106	Nonrandomized	
			≤0.5 cm in the abdomen	71%-10 y RFS (WAI)
			≤2 cm in the pelvis	

RFS, relapse-free survival; DFS, disease-free survival.

than 2 cm pelvic residual disease, formed a favorable group in whom the WAI resulted in a 10-year RFS of 71%, compared with 40% RFS when subtotal abdominopelvic techniques were used. The survival benefit was even more pronounced when the comparison was adjusted for differences in stage, grade, and volume of residual disease. Surgical bowel complications were similar for WAI (7.1%) and for subtotal abdominopelvic techniques (8.1%).

ADVANCED-STAGE OVARIAN CANCER: CONSOLIDATION/SALVAGE RADIOTHERAPY

Published data frequently fail to distinguish between planned sequential combined modality therapy (CMT) using CT and RT and salvage irradiation. However, these are distinctly different approaches. With CMT, many patients have no demonstrable disease but are at high risk for recurrence; with salvage therapy, all patients have clinical or pathologic evidence of disease. Planned CMT permits the omission of SLL in selected patients, probably limiting late toxicity. Finally, planned sequential CMT often incorporates a reduction in CT duration, providing improved tolerance to RT, permitting appropriate RT doses to be given, and potentially limiting the emergence of platinum-RT cross-resistance.

Although approximately 33% to 50% of patients with negative SLL would experience recurrent disease, the value of consolidation therapy remains controversial. The risk of recurrence in this situation has been shown to be related to the amount of tumor residual after the primary surgery, the initial stage of the disease, the histologic grade and type, and the patient's age (28,29). After the work of Dembo and colleagues (17), which showed that WAI was an effective adjuvant treatment for patients with early OC with minimal residual disease, it was believed that WAI might prolong survival of patients with advanced OC in whom surgery and CT have successfully reduced bulky stage II or III disease to a minimal residuum (30). A phase II trial was conducted at the Princess Margaret Hospital (14) in which six cycles of cyclophosphamide, doxorubicin, and cisplatin CT followed by WAI were given to patients with stage III, high-grade histology or macroscopic residual disease. The results were compared with those of a matched control group with similar prognostic features who received WAI alone. The median survival time was extended from 2.4 to 5.7 years with the combined therapy, and 43% of the patients were free of relapse at 5 years, compared with 22% of those treated with WAI alone ($p = .03$). Tolerance and toxicity of the combined approach was acceptable, although SLL was not part of the treatment plan.

TABLE 19.5. *Planned sequential salvage radiotherapy in ovarian cancer*

Series (ref. no.)	Patient population (stage)	Study design	Outcome
Lambert et al. (31)	IIB-IV (<2 cm residuum at SLL)	Randomized consolidation WAI vs. consolidation CT	<30% 5-year DFS and overall survival for both groups
Bruzzone et al. (32)	III-IV (path CR or <2 cm residuum at SLL)	Randomized consolidation WAI vs. consolidation CT	55% (disease progression) WAI vs. 28.5% (disease progression)
Lawton et al. (33)	"Advanced stages," minimum residuum at SLL	Randomized consolidation WAI vs. consolidation CT	No difference in outcome between arms
Hoskins et al. (34)	I-III (minimum residuum after primary surgery)	Nonrandomized Adjuvant CT alone Adjuvant CT + WAI (between cycles 3 and 4)	5-y survival-64% 5-y survival-78%
Reid et al. (35)	III (<1 cm residuum after primary surgery)	Nonrandomized phase II sequential CT + WAI	3-y survival-26% 3-y DFS-20%
Wong et al. (40)	I-III (optimally debulked)	Nonrandomized sequential CT + WAI	3-y survival-91% 3-y DFS-78%
Randall et al. (GOG) (42)	III	Nonrandomized: phase II primary CT + S + WAI	40% progression during CT Median survival-24 mo Median DFS-46 mo

SLL, second-look laparotomy; CT, chemotherapy; WAI, whole-abdomen irradiation; RFS, relapse-free survival; DFS, disease-free survival.

Planned sequential CMT has shown some promise (Table 19.5). Lambert and coworkers (31), from the North Thames Ovary Group Study, reported in 1993 the results of a randomized trial in patients with advanced OC (stage IIB or IV with less than 2 cm residual disease at SLL) designed to determine whether consolidation therapy with WAI after CT improved survival and DFS compared with continued CT. A total of 254 patients were entered in the study, which consisted of five monthly courses of 400 mg/m² of carboplatin; 117 patients with residual disease less than 2 cm at SLL or laparoscopy were then randomly assigned to receive consolidation therapy with either five further courses of carboplatin or WAI (24 Gy at 120 cGy per fraction without pelvic boost). No statistical difference was found in either survival or DFS between both arms (less than 30% 5-year survival and DFS), even if only patients with negative SLL were analyzed. One of the 58 patients who received consolidation WAI died from septicemia secondary to small bowel obstruction/perforation. The authors concluded that there is no significant advantage for consolidation WAI compared with continuation of the same CT, even when no macroscopic residual disease is apparent at the time of the SLL.

Bruzzone and associates (32) conducted a randomized trial of platinum-based CT versus RT (WAI 30.2 Gy, pelvis 43.2 Gy) in the management of 41 patients with stage III and IV OC with pathologic complete response or minimal residual disease (less than 2 cm) at SLL, after primary surgery and three courses of platinum-based CT. Of the 41 patients randomized, with a median follow-up of 22 months, disease progression was observed in 55% and 28.5% of those receiving RT versus CT, respectively. Because of the overall survival and progression-free survival advantage for the patients in the CT consolidation arm, the trial was stopped prematurely. However, the authors admitted that the two arms were not well balanced (no residual disease at SLL in 71% and 50% of the CT and RT patients, respectively). Lawton and colleagues (33) reported the results of the West Midlands Ovarian Cancer Group Trial II, which compared consolidation with WAI versus chlorambucil for 1 year after primary cytoreductive surgery, five courses of cisplatin, and SLL. No significant differences were shown between the two consolidative treatment arms, although only about 50% of those patients randomized had minimal residual disease at SLL and were able to complete the consolidation therapy.

Hoskins and associates (34) reported on a series of OC patients with tumors of stage I and II grade 3, or stage III any grade, who received either six cycles of CT alone or the same platinum-based CT with abdominal RT between cycles 3 and 4. Five-year survival rates were 78% and 64%, favoring the group receiving RT. Reid and coworkers (35) conducted a prospective phase II clinical trial of 13 patients with previously untreated, optimal surgically resected (1 cm or less), stage III OC at the University of Michigan Hospitals. After primary surgery, four courses of CT consisting of cisplatin (50 mg/m^2) and cyclophosphamide (1,000 mg/m^2) were administered, followed by WAI (30 Gy with a pelvic boost of 20 Gy). Six of the 13 patients received a paraaortic radiation boost. Thirty-eight percent of patients developed small bowel obstruction, and 2 patients died after SLL was performed. Actuarial 3-year survival and progression-free survival rates were 26% and 20%, respectively. The authors indicated that because survival was not superior to that reported for CT alone, such delayed toxicity is not justified. One explanation for such high toxicity could be the use of pelvic boosts in all patients, as well as paraaortic boosts in 50% of the cases. Thomas and Dembo (36,37) reported disappointing results in a review of 28 trials of sequential WAI (both for consolidation and for salvage) after CT in advanced OC. A strong association was found between tumor residuum before WAI and survival (76% for those patients with no residuum, 49% for those with microscopic or less than 5 mm residuum, and 17% for patients with macroscopic gross residual disease). Similar results have published by MacGibbon and associates (38).

A European study (39) evaluated the effect of consolidation RT after carboplatin-based CT on RFS and overall survival in patients with advanced optimally debulked OC. Sixty-four of 94 patients with OC (stage IC to IV), "radically operated", without surgical evidence of gross residual disease after six courses of CT (carboplatin 400 mg/m^2 on day 1, epirubicin 70 mg/m^2 on day 1, and prednimustine 100 mg/m^2 on days 3 through 7) were randomly assigned to receive either consolidation WAI (30 Gy), followed by boost to the paraaortic region and pelvis (12 Gy and 21 6 Gy, respectively) or no further therapy. The RFS and overall survival rates of patients who received adjuvant CT and RT were significantly higher than those of patients who received adjuvant CT only (RFS, 68% versus 56% at 2 years, 49% versus 26% at 5 years, respectively; overall survival, 87% versus 61% at 2 years, 59% versus 33% at 5 years, respectively). The differences were more pronounced in patients with stage III disease (RFS, 77% versus 54% at 2 years, 45% versus 19% at 5 years, respectively; overall survival, 88% versus 58% at 2 years, 59% versus 26% at 5 years, respectively). Cox multivariate analysis showed a positive prognostic value of additional RT. However, residual disease, stage, grade, and pelvic lymph node involvement were not unfavorable prognostic factors. The authors concluded that sequential combination of platinum-based CT with open-field WAI is a promising adjuvant regimen for selected patients with advanced OC without gross residual disease after adjuvant CT.

Wong and colleagues (40) reported 3-year DFS rates of 83% and 59%, respectively, for low/intermediate- and high-risk OC patients with stage I to III optimally cytoreduced disease who received adjuvant cisplatin-based CT and WAI. Although no benefit in outcome could be demonstrated in patients with low/intermediate risk as defined by Dembo (15), there was a trend toward improved DFS with CMT in the high-risk patients (3-year DFS, 62% versus 25%, respectively; $p = .21$).

Whelan and coworkers (41) reviewed the records of 105 patients with advanced OC treated with cisplatin combination CT followed by WAI at the Princess Margaret Hospital, in order to define the morbidity of this approach and identify those factors predictive of toxicity. Nine (8.6%) of the 105 patients required surgery for bowel obstruction that was not caused by recurrent disease, 3 had a bowel obstruction treated conservatively, and 5 underwent surgery for obstruction secondary to recurrent tumor. WAI dose greater than 2,250 cGy and SLL before RT were factors associated with an increased risk of serious bowel complications.

The GOG conducted a phase II multimodality trial using three courses of CT (three cycles of cisplatin + cyclophosphamide) followed by surgical reassessment and hyperfractionated WAI (80 cGy per fraction, administered twice daily, total dose 30.4 Gy), in 42 patients with optimal stage III disease (less than 1 cm residual disease) (42). Five patients progressed while receiving CT, could not be effectively cytoreduced, and were not eligible for WAI. Of the remaining 37 patients, 35 received WAI. Based on the measurements recorded after initial laparotomy and surgical reassessment, progression during CT was noted in 40%, stable disease in 37%, and objective response in 23%. In addition, the authors reported that, after limited CT, hyperfractionated WAI was acutely well tolerated; late radiation-related toxicity was noted in only 3 patients (8.6%) in the absence of recurrent disease, and late gastrointestinal morbidity was significantly associated with the administration of pelvic RT boost. The median survival time for all patients entered was 39 months, and the median DFS time was 18 months. For patients completing CT and WAI, the median survival and DFS times were 47 and 24 months, respectively.

Although the optimal intensity and duration of CT given before surgical reassessment and consolidation WAI remains unclear, it seems that the ability to deliver potentially tumoricidal doses of RT to the abdomen is compromised in patients heavily pretreated with myelotoxic CT. Lith and associates (43) reported that patients receiving 3 rather than 6 to 12 cycles of platinum-based CT before WAI would be expected to have less myelosuppression during the RT. Another potential advantage of limiting the amount of CT administered is that emergence of cisplatin-radiation cross-resistance might be limited. Ensley and coworkers (44) found a strong correlation between cisplatin resistance and subsequent response to RT in patients with head and neck cancers. In an OC cell line, Louie and colleagues (45) demonstrated the emergence of radiation resistance simultaneously with cisplatin resistance during chronic cisplatin exposure. In a human OC cell line, Britten and associates (46) demonstrated a three-fold reduction in radiation sensitivity in cells that had developed cisplatin resistance compared with the cisplatin-naïve parent cell line. Silver and coworkers (47) demonstrated *in vitro* that RT not only had a direct cytotoxic effect but also sensitized a cisplatin-resistant OC cell line to cisplatin, with doses of radiation low enough to suggest a potential clinical role in treating platinum-resistant OC. Because some data suggests a substantial cross-resistance between cisplatin and radiation (47,48), it is possible that prolonged exposure to cisplatin renders residual tumor cells less radiosensitive. In addition to a reduction in myelosuppression, this observation provides an additional rationale for limiting the amount of CT administered before WAI in patients managed with CMT. Furthermore, this concept should be considered in the design of clinical trials that use both CT and RT. This concept must be considered in light of data supporting a synergistic effect between cisplatin and RT (*vide infra*). Possibly, cross-resistance is facilitated by sequential exposure while synergism results from concomitant exposure.

Salvage Therapy after Chemotherapy with or without Second-Look Laparotomy: Whole-Abdomen Irradiation

Favorable experiences with salvage RT in CT refractory OC continue to be reported, although the published studies offer widely differing experiences with regard to response rates, duration of response, and toxicity. Eifel and associates (49) published the M.D. Anderson experience in 37 patients with OC and positive SLL after platinum-based CT, or recurrent disease after initial complete response to CT, who received WAI using a hyperfractionated split regimen (1 Gy per fraction to a total of 30 Gy, with a 3-week break after 15 Gy). A pelvic boost was given only if gross residual disease was present. Their results were disappointing, with 3-year RFS rates of 10% and 14% for patients with grade II and III OC, respectively, and microscopic residual disease. Twelve patients with gross residual disease had rapid recurrences (median time to relapse, 4.9 months), and all died from their disease. Although 38% of the patients experienced small bowel obstruction, this was found to be related to recurrent abdominal disease at the time.

Reddy and colleagues (50) published a retrospective evaluation of the feasibility, efficacy, and toxicity of WAI (25 Gy) as salvage therapy in 44 patients with OC for whom one or more CT regimens had failed. Eleven percent of patients were unable to complete the planned therapy secondary to acute toxicity. The 4-year actuarial survival and RFS rates for the entire group were 23% and 22%, respectively. For the group with microscopic residual disease before WAI, the same endpoints were 37% and 42%, compared with 9% and 5% for patients with macroscopic residual disease. Patients with disease limited to the pelvis only had a RFS rate of 56%, compared with 0% when the upper abdomen was involved. Eight patients (18%) developed bowel complications, 5 of which necessitated surgical intervention.

Baker and coworkers (51) updated this experience and analyzed the efficacy of WAI (25 Gy) as a salvage modality in 51 patients with epithelial OC who had failed one or more CT regimens and had undergone a second- or third-look laparotomy. Seventy-eight percent of patients had stage III to IV disease. In 22 patients (43%) macroscopic disease was present after laparotomy, while the remaining 29 patients (57%) had only microscopic disease present; 39% had residual disease limited to the pelvis, and 61% had upper abdominal involvement. Median follow-up for surviving patients was 66 months. Ten percent were unable to complete the therapy secondary to acute toxicity, and 27% of patients required a treatment break of 1 to 5 weeks, usually secondary to prolonged cytopenias. Four-year actuarial overall survival and RFS rates for the entire group of patients were 32% and 23%, respectively. For the patients with microscopic residual disease the overall survival and RFS rates were 48% and 37%, respectively, compared with 11% and 5% for patients with macroscopic residual disease. Those patients with disease limited to the pelvis after laparotomy had a 4-year actuarial overall survival rate of 60% and a 4-year RFS rate 54%. Conversely, when upper abdominal involvement was present, survival and RFS rates were 16% and 4%, respectively. Eleven patients (22%) experienced bowel complications, six of which (12%) required surgery. The authors concluded that WAI is an effective salvage treatment in patients with OC who have microscopic residual disease or disease limited to the pelvis after SLL.

Fein and associates (52) reported the experience from the University of Florida in 28 patients with stage III OC found to have persistent disease at laparotomy after platinum-based CT (6 to 28 cycles, mean 12), who received hyperfractionated WAI (0.8 Gy per fraction, administered twice daily, total dose 30.4 Gy). Twenty patients received additional pelvic boost (14.54 Gy). All patients had undergone two to four laparotomies before WAI. The absolute 5-year survival and DFS rates were 21% and 19%, respectively. For the 11 patients without evidence of residual disease at SLL, the 5-year survival rate was 27%, compared with 18% for those with gross residual disease. Fourteen percent of the patients developed small bowel obstruction, and 2 patients died from treatment-related complications.

Cmelak and Kapp (53), from Stanford University, evaluated the efficacy and toxicity of WAI in 41 patients with persistent or recurrent OC after initial treatment with surgical debulking and CT. Thirty-one patients had received platinum-based regimens, and 22 of these had failed within 6 months after completion of CT (platinum-refractory). Before WAI, 11 patients (27%) had microscopic residual disease, 21 (51%) had gross residual disease up to 1.5 cm, and 9 (22%) had residual tumors greater than 1.5 cm in maximal diameter. Median doses of 28 Gy to the abdomen and 48 Gy to the pelvis were delivered using open-field techniques with liver and kidney shielding. They observed a 47% 5-year actuarial disease-specific survival rate in all 41 patients treated with salvage WAI, and a 50% rate in the 22 patients deemed platinum-refractory. Both residual tumor size at the time of WAI and initial stage were of prognostic value. The 5- and 10-year rates of disease-specific survival for all patients with stages I to III, nonbulky (less than 1.5 cm) disease before WAI were 53%

and 40%, respectively, compared with 0% for those patients with residual disease greater than 1.5 cm. Twenty-nine percent of patients failed to complete the planned course of WAI due to acute toxicity (mostly thrombocytopenia). Three patients experienced severe late bowel toxicity. The authors concluded that "WAI should be considered in selected patients who fail initial CT, especially in patients who can or have been debulked to small amounts of residual disease; salvage WAI can be delivered with acceptable toxicity and the results appear to be as good as or better than second-line CT, particularly in platinum-refractory patients." Similarly, high response rates were reported by Suzuki and associates (54) in patients with platinum-refractory disease, most of whom had already received taxane-based second-line CT.

Sedlaceck and colleagues (55) reported on 27 patients who had failed aggressive cytoreductive surgery followed by multiple-drug platinum-based CT and were given WAI (30 to 35 Gy at 100 to 150 cGy per fraction, with a pelvic boost to 45 Gy). The 5-year survival rate was 15%. Residual disease at initiation of RT strongly correlated with length of survival (63 months for patients with microscopic disease, 24 months for those with residuum less than 1 cm, 19 months with less than 2 cm residuum, and 9 months with residual disease larger than 2 cm). Eight patients experienced grade 3 or 4 toxicity, primarily hematologic and gastrointestinal, but there were no deaths related to toxicity.

Overall, the review of the published series report a response rate to salvage RT of 30% to 40% in patients with microscopic residual disease, compared with less than 10% for those patients with gross disease. However, the definition of long-term response varies and is sometimes calculated from the initiation of treatment and other times from initiation of the salvage RT. Nevertheless, it appears that the subset of patients with microscopic or less than 1 cm residual disease at the time of the SLL often respond well to WAI, with a long-term survival rate of approximately 35%.

CMT and salvage RT remain controversial due to limited knowledge regarding patient selection, conflicting data, and the lack of comparisons to other consolidative or salvage treatments such as platinum reinduction in patients with tumors previously sensitive to platinum, paclitaxel in "naïve" patients, IP CT, IP-^{32}P, phase I or II agents or combinations, and high-dose CT with bone marrow or stem cell rescue.

Consolidation/Salvage Therapy after Chemotherapy with or without Second-Look Laparotomy: Radioactive Phosphorus

^{32}P has been considered by several authors as possible adjuvant therapy for patients with negative or microscopic residual disease at SLL, after cisplatin-based CT. In the Duke experience (56), patients with only microscopic residual or resected macroscopic residual disease had a median DFS time of 24 months and 3- and 4-year DFS rates of 36% and 27%, respectively. Vergote and coworkers (9) in 1993 reported on 68 patients who received ^{32}P as consolidation therapy after SLL (59 with no residual disease and 9 with microscopic or gross residual disease). In addition, 50 patients without residual tumor after primary surgery and negative SLL were randomly assigned to receive either ^{32}P or no treatment (only 12% of the patients had stage III disease). The estimated 5-year crude and DFS rates were 79% and 66%, respectively. No survival difference was observed between the group of patients receiving adjuvant ^{32}P (245 patients) and the group treated with ^{32}P after SLL. In patients with SLL, the estimated 5-year DFS rate was 92% in stage I, 53% in stage II, and 67% in stage III or IV. Among patients with residual tumor after primary surgery and negative SLL, the 5-year DFS rate was 62%, compared with 81% among patients with no residual tumor. In the 50 patients randomly assigned to receive ^{32}P or no further therapy after negative SLL, the 5-year DFS rates were 82% and 97%, respectively (difference not significant statistically). ^{32}P was associated with a considerable number of bowel complications.

In analyzing the patient and treatment factors that influence gastrointestinal complications, some authors have recommended instillation of ^{32}P during the immediate postoperative period, preferably within 12 hours, before formation of adhesions. In the series of Spanos and associates (57), which included 56 patients who received ^{32}P after CT and SLL or as the only postsurgical management, a significant reduction in complications (from 21% to 4.1%) was noted among those patients who received ^{32}P within 12 hours after surgery. A limited boost of external beam RT to residual disease did not increase the complication rate. It seems that with adequate technique of administration and patient selection, ^{32}P can be delivered effectively with minimal long-term toxicity. The 5-year survival rates after SLL were 75% for negative, 48% for microscopic, and 32% for gross residual disease.

Rogers and associates (58) reported results in 51 patients with stage I to III invasive epithelial OC who were found to have no evidence of disease al SLL and received 15 mCi of IP-^{32}P. They compared the results with those of a group of 35 patients, otherwise eligible for ^{32}P, who did not receive it primarily because of other treatment protocols, peritoneal adhesions, or the recommendation that no further therapy be given after a negative SLL. Patients in both groups were comparable with regard to stage, histology, grade, median age, residual disease after initial surgery, and CT regimen. The 5-year actuarial DFS rate from the date of the SLL was 86% for those receiving ^{32}P and 67% for those not receiving ^{32}P ($p = .05$). The corresponding 5-year overall survival rates were 90% and 78%, again favoring the patients treated with ^{32}P. Late adverse effects were similar in both groups. Bowel complications were seen in 3 of 51 patients receiving ^{32}P and in 1 of 18 patients not receiving ^{32}P. The authors concluded that ^{32}P confers a survival advantage to patients with pathologically negative SLL and that administration immediately after SLL seems to be a safe and well-tolerated therapy. In 1996 the GOG completed a prospective, randomized trial comparing ^{32}P with no additional therapy for patients with stage III OC after negative SLL. Results are still pending from this study, which accrued 201 patients.

Patillo and colleagues (59) studied the *in vitro* enhancement of ^{32}P cytotoxicity by cisplatin in cultured human ovarian adenocarcinoma (CHOA) cell lines and in a fibroblast cell strain. In addition, they combined fractionated low-dose IP-^{32}P instillations (5 mCi, eight administrations) with up to eight monthly cycles of cisplatin (100 mg/m^2) or carboplatin (360 mg/m^2) in 30 patients with advanced disease. Of note, 16 of 25 patients with stage III or IV disease had residual IP disease measuring more than 2 cm. Complete and partial response rates were 47% and 40%, respectively. Therapy was well tolerated. The 3-year survival rate was 63%, with a mean survival time of 17 months. For the 16 patients with residual disease measuring more than 2 cm in greatest diameter, the median survival time (18.8 months) was not significantly different from that experienced by the other 14 patients included in the study (15.2 months). Based on their laboratory and clinical data, the authors concluded that cisplatin enhances the tumor cell killing effect of ^{32}P with a supraadditive effect.

Alvarez and coworkers (60) administered radiolabeled tumor-reactive antibodies in an effort to better target the cytotoxic effects of the radiocolloid. Although follow-up was short, consistent tumor effects were noted in patients with refractory disease, warranting further investigation of this therapeutic approach.

PALLIATIVE RADIOTHERAPY

Patients with grossly recurrent and metastatic OC after CT often have significant symptoms that are not responsive to further systemic therapy. Symptoms are most commonly caused by recurrent disease in the pelvis that results in pain and/or bleeding, but recurrences in the brain, chest, groins, and other areas can become management problems. Corn and associates (61) reviewed the use of RT in 33 such patients, finding an overall symptomatic response rate of 79%, with complete palliative response in 51%. Symptoms remained palliated until death in 90%. Patients with high performance status who received a biologically effective dose of at least 44 Gy appeared to derive the greatest benefit. Davidson and colleagues (62) reported their experience in 35 patients with persistent or recurrent OC limited to the pelvis, retroperitoneum, or vaginal cuff who were treated with salvage pelvic or paraaortic RT. The median actuarial and progression-free survival times from the beginning of the RT were 40 and 14 months, respectively. At least 62% of the recurrences involved the treatment field. They found limited-field RT in patients with localized persistent or recurrent disease to be well tolerated, with limited acute or late morbidity, even in patients heavily pretreated with systemic and IP CT. Suzuki and associates (63) reported an overall response rate of 86.2% to moderate doses of RT in 17 patients with measurable localized relapsed or refractory OC after CT. They also noted significantly better response in metastatic lymph nodes compared with other sites (100% versus 66.7%).

With increasingly effective systemic therapy, some authors have reported an increasing incidence of brain metastases, presumably owing to the ability of the central nervous system to act as a "sanctuary site." Although the median survival time of this group of patients is only 4 to 6 months when treated with whole-brain RT, certain subsets appear to enjoy longer survival. Corn and colleagues (64) published a series of 32 patients who received RT for symptomatic cerebral metastases, finding clinical responses in 23 patients, which were maintained until death in 71%.

WHOLE-ABDOMEN IRRADIATION

Technique

Surgical staging information, as well as analysis of patterns of failure, suggests that RT for OC must include all peritoneal surfaces. Furthermore, the ability of WAI to alter failure patterns by decreasing upper abdominal relapse compared to no or smaller-volume RT has been clearly demonstrated (7,15,17,28,65). Dembo and associates (15,17) emphasized the necessity of covering the diaphragm with adequate margin during all phases of normal respiration. This requires that liver shielding be limited or absent. Appropriate kidney localization and blocking should be undertaken to keep total doses within tolerance. To further exploit the role of RT in OC, consideration should be given to use of three-dimensional treatment planning techniques or CT-simulation for precise shielding of the kidneys and liver (when indicated) (Figures 19.2 and 19.3). The moving-strip technique for WAI has been replaced by open-field technique antero-posterior/postero-anterior (AP/PA). Dembo and

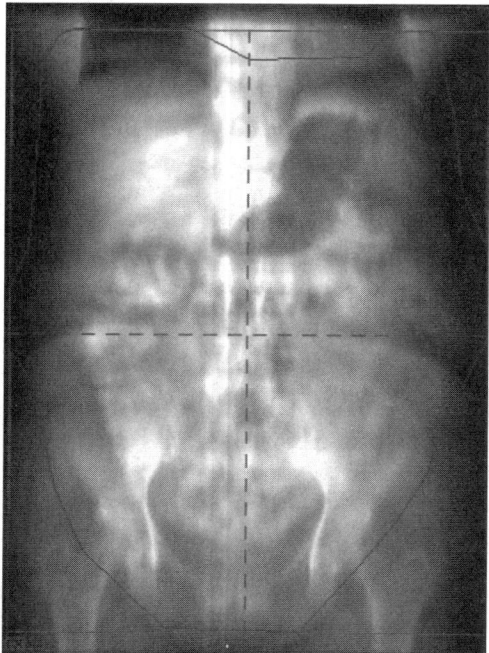
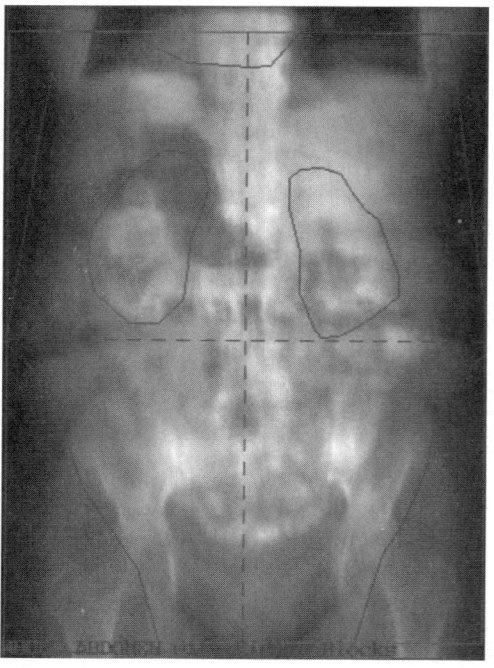

FIG. 19.2A,B. Digital reconstructed radiographs (DRRs): whole abdomen antero-posterior/postero-anterior (AP/PA) fields.

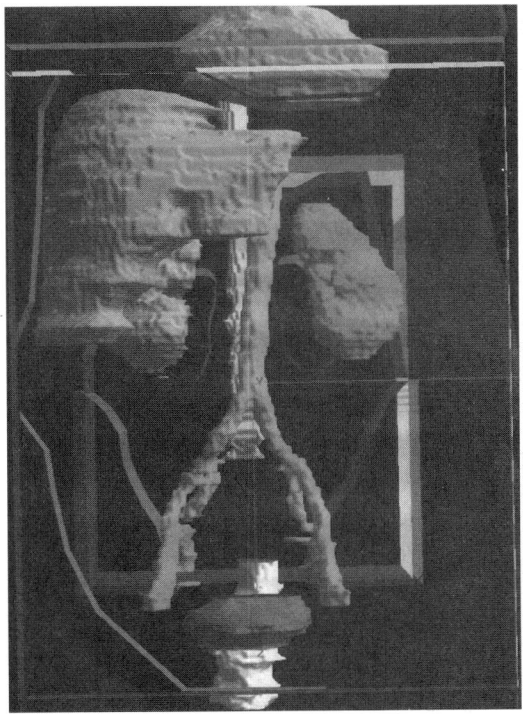

FIG. 19.3. Coronal projection, three-dimensional reconstruction, and "beam's-eye" view of the wholeabdomen irradiation, AP/PA fields.

colleagues (66) showed the therapeutic equivalence of these techniques in a prospective, randomized trial.

Fyles and coworkers (67) published in 1998 the results of a randomized study performed in Princess Margaret Hospital to determine whether an increased dose of WAI (27.5 Gy in 27 fractions) resulted in improved disease control and survival compared with the standard WAI dose (22.5 Gy in 22 fractions). A pelvic boost dose of 22.5 Gy was used in both arms. One hundred and twenty-five patients with early-stage OC (optimally debulked, intermediate-risk: stage I to III, with no gross residual disease in the abdomen or less than 2 cm residual disease in the pelvis) were entered in the study. No difference was found between the low-dose and high-dose arms in 5-year overall survival (83% and 72%, respectively) or 5-year DFS (74% and 67%, respectively). There were no differences in patterns of relapse, hematologic toxicity, or late complications between the two arms. The authors concluded that high-dose WAI is unlikely to be associated with an increase in overall survival.

WAI doses of 22.5 to 25 Gy (at 130 to 150 cGy per fraction) administered over 4 weeks appear be associated with a favorable long-term toxicity profile while maintaining considerable therapeutic efficacy in appropriately selected patients. Periaortic boost is usually recommended in those patients without complete lymph node sampling or in the presence of completely debulked retroperitoneal lymphadenopathy (median dose, 45 Gy) (Figures 19.4 and 19.5). Additional pelvic boost is given to those patients at high risk for pelvic recurrence (gross residual disease, defined intraoperatively or radiographically) (Figure 19.6). In these cases three-dimensional conformal therapy, using a multiple-beam arrangement with limited margins, should be used in an attempt to decrease long-term toxicity. Figure 19.7 demonstrates the isodose distribution for the composite plan in the axial, coronal, and sagittal planes. Furthermore, stereotactic techniques and intraoperative RT or brachytherapy implants would allow "conformal" boosts to areas of gross disease while keeping the dose to limiting structures within tolerance.

Although there has been some promising experience with the use of hyperfractionated WAI in advanced OC (42,52), it is unlikely that these regimens will prove therapeutically superior to once-per-day regimens, and they are difficult to use because of patient convenience issues. Therefore, such approaches are unlikely to be widely adopted.

A basic question regarding WAI concerns whether these limited RT doses can be effective since they are considerably below doses conventionally used in epithelial malignancies. Tumor sterilization at these dose levels is a long-recognized clinical phenomenon and was validated in Fletcher's work on dose-response relationships in subclinical disease (68). More recently, theoretical bases for this observation have been presented by Marks (69) and by Withers and Suwinski (70). Marks (69) illustrated the importance of the absolute risk of occult disease at any one site, the number of sites at risk, the

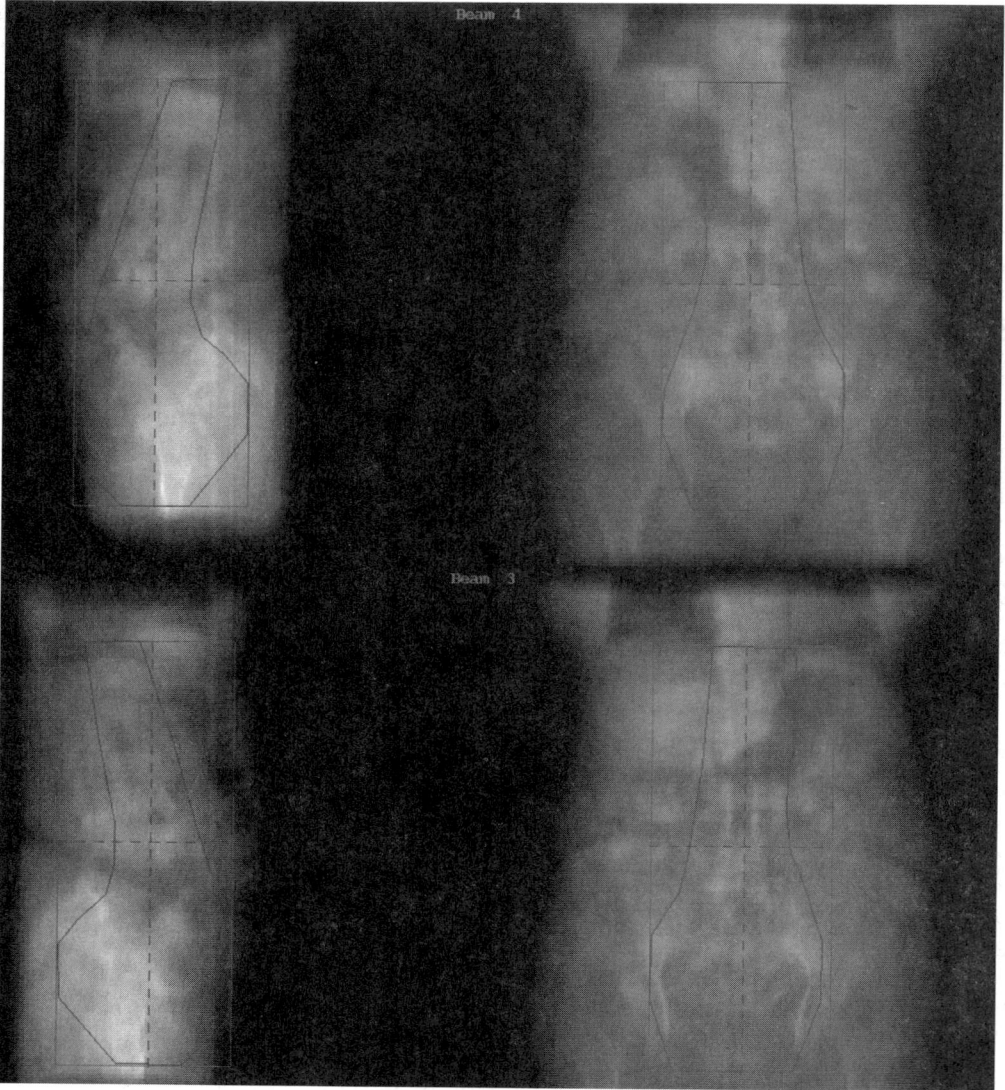

FIG. 19.4. Digital reconstructed radiographs (DRRs): pelvis and periaortic AP/PA, right and left lateral fields.

number of clonogens present in a given site, and their radiation sensitivity in determining the dose required to treat a site of potential occult disease electively. In addition, the model designed by Withers and Suwinski (70) assumed that not all patients with microscopic residuum have 10^8 or 10^9 clonogenic cells and that the radiation dose-response curve for microscopic residual disease is more shallow than for gross disease. Therefore, it appears that WAI dose levels within limits of tolerance should be able to sterilize limited deposits of OC in many cases. Evidence in support of this concept is found in the clear evidence of alterations in failure patterns as a function of RT volume (7,16,28,65).

Toxicity

The initiation of WAI generally results in immediate toxicity. Fyles and coworkers (71)

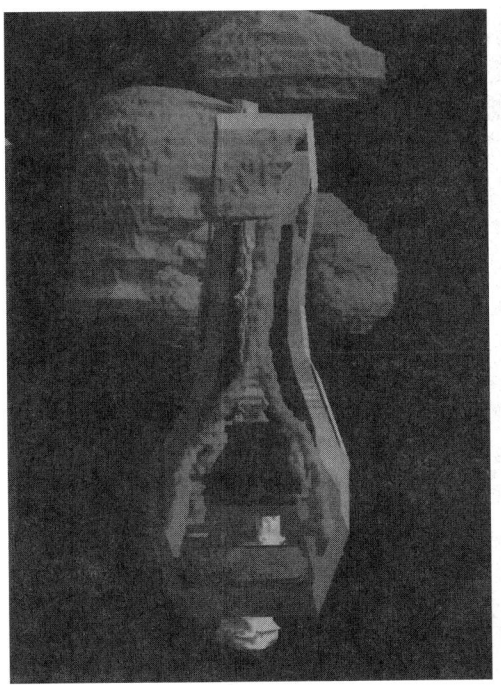 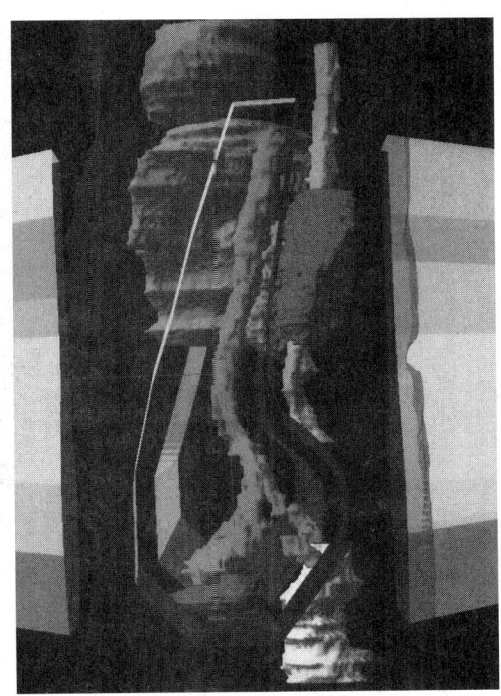

FIG. 19.5A,B. Coronal and sagittal projections of the three-dimensional reconstruction of the pelvis and periaortic cone-down.

reported the WAI toxicity in 598 patients. Acute complications included nausea and vomiting in 61% (severe in 10%), diarrhea in 68% (severe in 10%), leukopenia (11%), and thrombocytopenia (11%). Treatment interruptions occurred in 23%, and 10% of the patients did not complete the treatment. Late complications included chronic diarrhea (14%), transient hepatic enzyme elevation (44%), and symptomatic basal pneumonitis (4%). Severe late bowel complications were infrequent, with 25 (4%) patients developing bowel obstruction, 16 requiring surgery. In multivariate analysis, the moving-strip technique was associated with a significantly higher risk of chronic complications compared with the open technique. Although the gastrointestinal side effects can generally be managed, the associated myelosuppression (neutropenia and thrombocytopenia) can result in a deleterious protraction of treatment. Efforts to ameliorate neutropenia with growth factors (e.g., granulocyte colony-stimulating factor) have not been successful in limiting treatment breaks because thrombocytopenia becomes the dose-limiting toxicity (72).

A possible strategy to limit WAI acute toxicity is to initiate RT first to a pelvic field in patients in whom a pelvic boost is planned, since bone marrow toxicity is limited. Therefore, patients with failures limited to or predominantly in the pelvis are given pelvic RT, allowing considerable dose to be delivered over an appropriate period. The abdominal irradiation follows, potentially allowing overall treatment time to be shortened. An additional benefit of this approach is that patients with measurable disease in the pelvis can be evaluated for response. Patients not demonstrating symptomatic or clinical response are spared the acute and possible late toxicities of WAI, improving overall results from salvage RT because of better patient selection. Baker and associates (51) used this approach in 51 patients who had failed one or more CT regimens and received WAI after second- or third-look laparotomy. These investigators found actuarial 4-year survival and RFS rates of 48% and 37%,

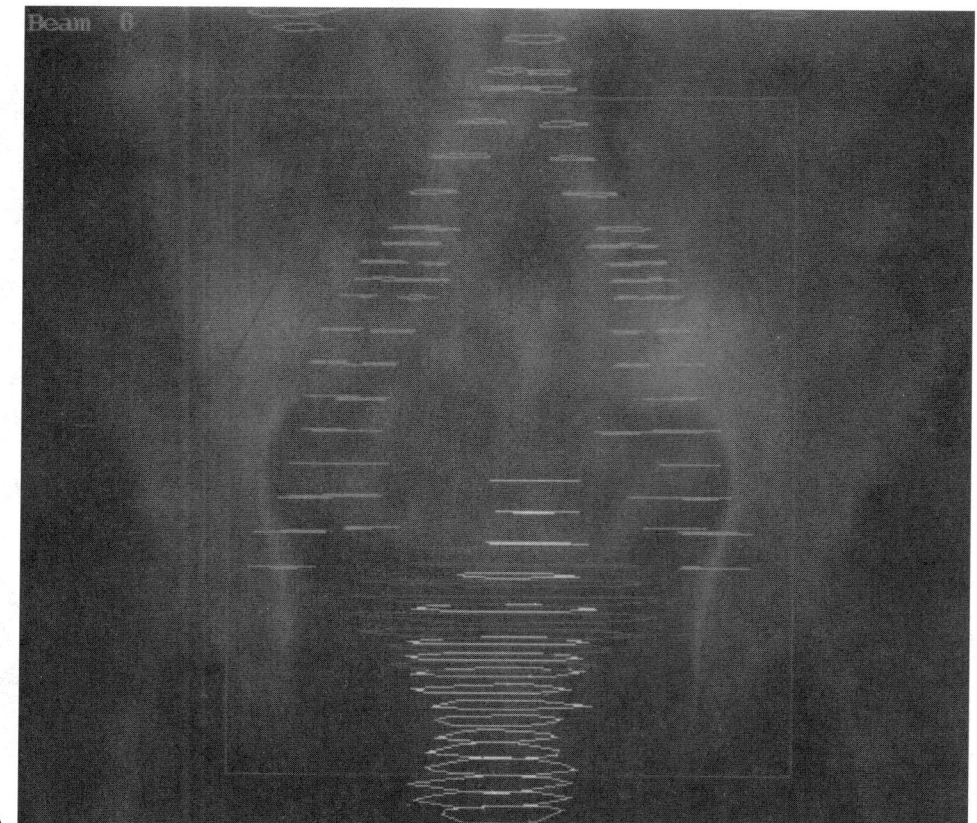
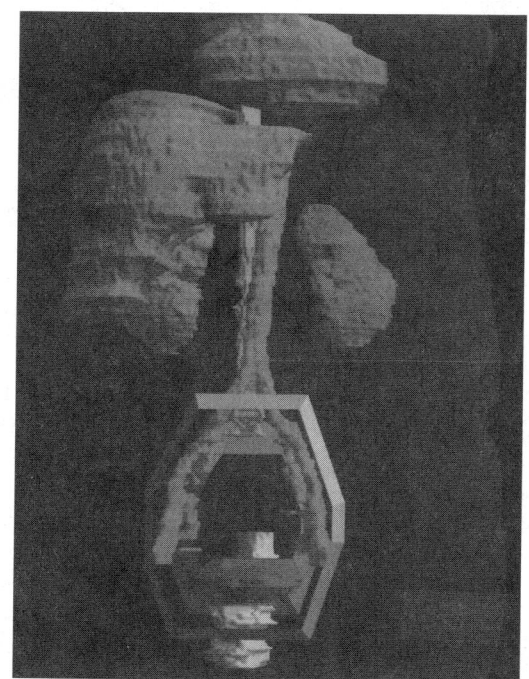
FIG. 19.6A,B. Digital reconstructed radiograph, final AP/PA pelvis cone-down, coronal projection of the three-dimensional reconstruction of final pelvis cone-down.

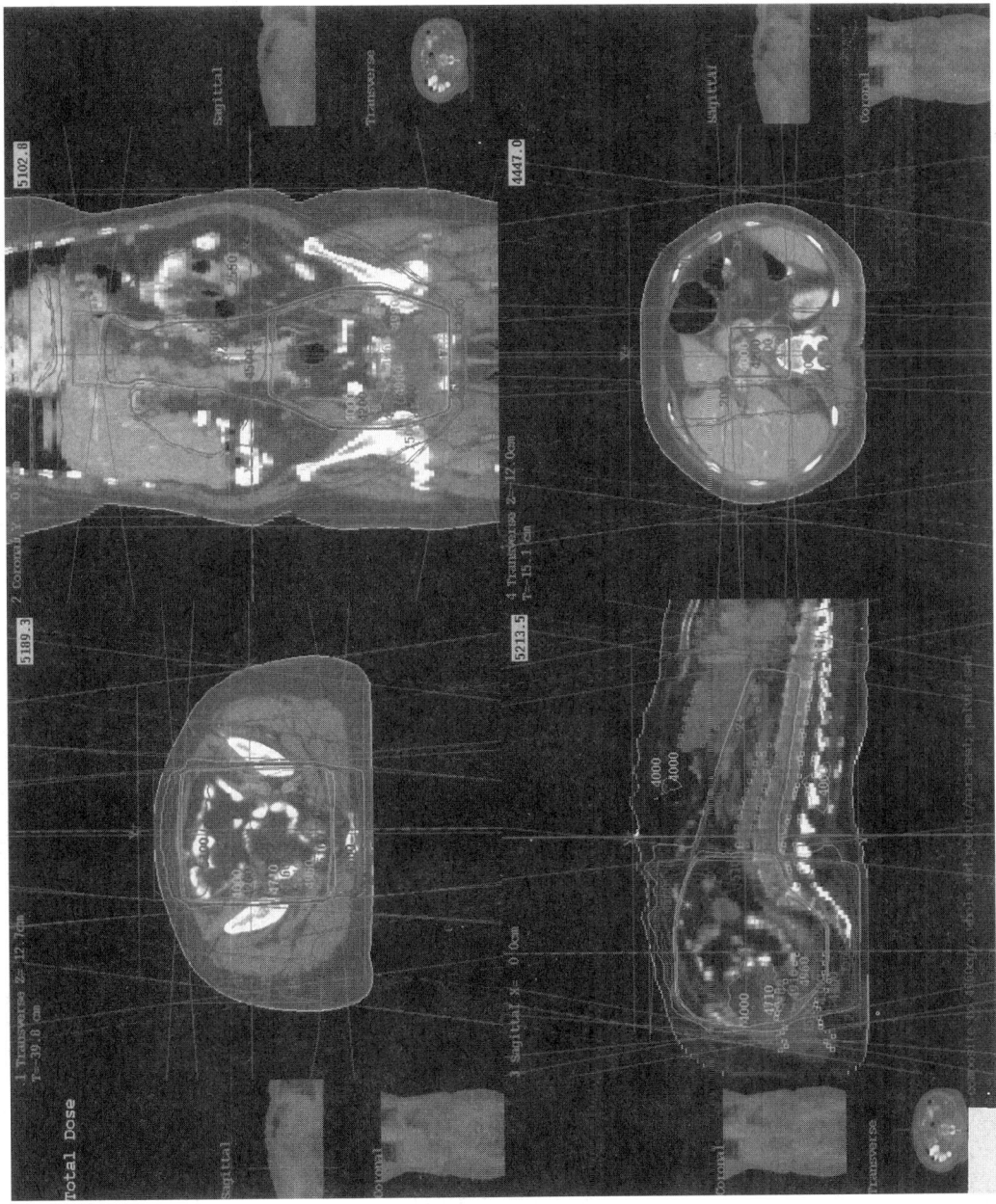

FIG. 19.7. Axial, coronal and sagittal isodose distribution, composite plan, whole-abdomen irradiation, including pelvic and periaortic boosts.

respectively. Among patients with disease confined to the pelvis (including gross disease), the same endpoints were 60% and 54%, respectively.

In addition, a possible means of decreasing late toxicity from WAI is limiting or eliminating arbitrary pelvic boosts in patients with no or minimal residual disease. This seems reasonable given that, for many patients, active tumor clonogens are equally likely to exist in the upper abdomen as in the pelvis. Although most RT series describe routine administration of the pelvic boost, this is not universally true. Kuten and coworkers (73) reported the efficacy of combined CT with WAI and no pelvic boost, resulting in minimal chronic bowel toxicity. In the GOG study published by Randall and colleagues (42) the authors reported a 50% incidence of late bowel toxicity in 22 of 35 patients who received a pelvic boost in addition to hyperfractionated WAI, whereas none of the 13 patients not receiving the pelvic boost developed gastrointestinal morbidity.

Toxicities of Chemotherapy and Whole-Abdomen Irradiation

A review of 598 patients treated at the Princess Margaret Hospital with WAI for OC revealed severe gastrointestinal toxicity in 6% of the cases. Only 10% did not complete WAI (most frequently due to myelosupression), and 4.2% developed bowel obstruction (2.7% requiring surgery). No patients died from radiation-induced second malignancies (71). This is in contrast to patients treated with CT (especially melphalan), in whom a high incidence of second cancers have been reported (74). In the standard "dose-intense" arms of the GOG Protocol 97 using cisplatin and cyclophosphamide, the incidences of grades 3 and 4 myelotoxicity were 39% and 82%, respectively. Randall and associates (42) found that the toxicity of short-duration CT and WAI was associated with a lower rate of grade 3 and 4 toxicities compared with standard-duration CT. In an article by Travis (75), the relative risk of leukemia among 28,971 women who received platinum-based CT for OC was 4.0 (95% confidence interval, 1.4 to 11.4). The relative risks for treatment with carboplatin and cisplatin were 6.5 and 3.3, respectively. RT without CT did not increase the risk of leukemia.

FUTURE DIRECTIONS

Primary Chemotherapy–Surgery–Radiation Therapy

Neoadjuvant CT for advanced OC has been investigated by a number of authors. Schwartz and coworkers (76) published the experience at Yale University in 49 patients with advanced OC treated with neoadjuvant platinum-based CT; 41 patients subsequently underwent cytoreductive surgery. No statistical difference was observed in overall survival or in progression-free survival between this group and a group of 206 patients with stage IIIC and IV OC who were treated with conventional cytoreductive surgery followed by platinum-based CT during the same era. This approach, if validated, presents an opportunity to combine CT with WAI in patients, selected on the basis of surgical findings, who have had only one laparotomy. Potentially, this represents another opportunity to decrease morbidity from WAI, since multiple surgeries are probably causally related to late toxicity after RT.

Concurrent Chemotherapy and Radiation Therapy

Silver and associates (47) demonstrated that *in vitro* RT not only had a direct cytotoxic effect but also sensitized a cisplatin-resistant OC cell line to cisplatin, with doses of radiation low enough to suggest a potential clinical role in treating platinum-resistant OC. King and colleagues (77) published a pilot study to assess the feasibility of concomitant WAI (20 Gy) and IP cisplatin followed by additional IP cisplatin after debulking surgery. Eleven patients with OC, stage III and IV, were included in the study. Hematologic and gastrointestinal toxicities were significant. Therapeutic efficacy was considered to be comparable with standard CT regimens, and no therapeutic (survival) advantage could be demonstrated. In order to minimize hematologic toxicity and facilitate timely deliverance of WAI, the employment of colony-stimulating factors should be considered in future prospective trials.

Reisinger and coworkers (78) published the results of a GOG trial using WAI (30 Gy followed by pelvic boost) in combination with weekly cisplatin (15 mg/m^2) as adjuvant treatment in patients with advanced endometrial cancer, finding the combination to be well tolerated at this dose level. A similar approach was reported by Dowlatshahi and colleagues (79) in 49 patients with stage IIIC CT-refractory OC. They delivered

30 Gy WAI in 30 fractions with concomitant weekly IP cisplatin (5 mg/m^2) as a radiosensitizer. All of these patients had residual disease at the time of the SLL. With a median follow-up of 32 months, the projected 5- and 10-year survival rates were 44% and 35%, respectively. Thirty-five percent of patients could not complete treatment because of side effects. There is a compelling need to build on such pilot studies with broad-based clinical trials in order to investigate, and hopefully validate, these promising approaches.

Integration of Radiation Therapy with New Cytotoxic Agents

Extensive evidence suggests that the platinum and taxane compounds are excellent radiosensitizers as well as effective cytotoxic agents for OC. However, there have been no studies in OC examining the potential role of a taxane combined with WAI. Steren and associates (80) demonstrated in a human ovarian cell line that the combination of a nontoxic dose of paclitaxel and RT resulted in a large cell arrest in G_2-M. Therefore, the effect of concurrent paclitaxel, administered intravenously or intraperitoneally, with WAI should be explored. Furthermore, both altered fractionation schedules and sensitizing CT agents could be exploited together.

REFERENCES

1. Landis SH, Murray T, Bolden S, Wingo PA. Cancer Statistics, 1998. *CA: Cancer J Clin* 1998;48:6–30.
2. McGuire WP, Hoskins WJ, Brady MF, et al. Cyclophosphamide and cisplatin compared with paclitaxel and cisplatin in patients with stage III and stage IV ovarian cancer. *N Engl J Med* 1996;334:1–6.
3. Young RC, Walton LA, Ellenberg SS, et al. Adjuvant therapy in stage I and stage II epithelial ovarian cancer: results of two prospective randomized trials. *N Engl J Med* 1990;322:1021–1027.
4. Currie JL, Bagne F, Harrix C, et al. Radioactive chromic phosphate suspension: studies on distribution, dose absorption, and effective therapeutic radiation in phantoms, dogs and patients. *Gynecol Oncol* 1981;12:193–218.
5. Boye E, Lindergaad MW, Paus E, et al. Whole-body distribution of radioactivity after intraperitoneal administration of ^{32}P colloids. *Br J Radiol* 1984;57:395–402.
6. Young RC, Brady MF, Nieberg RM: Randomized clinical trial of adjuvant treatment of women with early (FIGO I–IIA, high risk) ovarian cancer—GOG #95 [Abstract 47]. *Int J Gynecol Oncol* 1997;7:17.
7. Klaasen D, Shelley W, Starreveld A, et al. Early stage ovarian cancer: a randomized clinical trial comparing whole abdominal radiotherapy, melphalan, and intraperitoneal chromic phosphate. A National Cancer Institute of Canada Clinical Trials Group report. *J Clin Oncol* 1988;6:1254–1263.
8. Vergote IB, Vergote-DeVos LN, Abeler VN, et al. Randomized trial comparing cisplatin with radioactive phosphorus or whole abdomen irradiation as adjuvant treatment of ovarian cancer. *Cancer* 1992;69:741–749.
9. Vergote IB, Winderen M, De Vos LN, Trope CG. Intraperitoneal radioactive phosphorus therapy in ovarian carcinoma: analysis of 313 patients treated primarily or at second-look laparotomy. *Cancer* 1993;71:2250–2260.
10. Bolis G, Colombo N, Pecorelli S, et al. Adjuvant treatment for early epithelial ovarian cancer: results of two randomized clinical trials comparing cisplatin to no further therapy or chromic phosphate. *Ann Oncol* 1995;9:887–893.
11. Ott RJ, Flower MA, Jones A, McCready VR. The measurement of radiation doses from ^{32}P chromic phosphate therapy of the peritoneum using SPECT. *Eur J Nucl Med* 1985;11:305–308.
12. Smith JP, Rutledge FN, Delclos L. Postoperative treatment of early cancer of the ovary: a random trial between postoperative irradiation and chemotherapy. *J Natl Cancer Inst* 1975;42:149–153.
13. Dembo AJ, Davy M, Stenwig AE, et al. Prognostic factors in patients with stage I epithelial ovarian cancer. *Obstet Gynecol* 1990;75:263.
14. Lederman, JA, Dembo AJ, Sturgeon JFG, et al. Outcome of patients with unfavorable optimally cytoreduced ovarian cancer treated with chemotherapy and whole abdominal radiation. *Gynecol Oncol* 1991;41:30–35.
15. Dembo AJ, Bush RS. Choice of postoperative therapy based on prognostic factors. *Int J Radiat Oncol Biol Phys* 1982;8:893–897.
16. Dembo AJ. Abdominopelvic radiotherapy in ovarian cancer: a 10-year experience. *Cancer* 1985;55:2285–2290.
17. Dembo AJ, Bush RS, Beale FA. Ovarian carcinoma: improved survival following abdominopelvic irradiation in patients with a complete pelvic operation. *Am J Obstet Gynecol* 1979;134:793–800.
18. Carey M, Dembo AJ, Simm JE, et al. Testing the validity of a prognostic classification in patients with surgically optimal ovarian carcinoma: a 15 years review. *Int J Gynecol Cancer* 1993;3:24–35.
19. Sell A, Bertelsen K, Andersen JE, et al. Randomized study of whole abdomen irradiation versus pelvic irradiation plus cyclophosphamide in treatment of early ovarian cancer. *Gynecol Oncol* 1990;37:367–373.
20. Chiara S, Pierfranco C, Franzone P. High-risk early-stage ovarian cancer: randomized trial comparing cisplatin plus cyclophosphamide versus whole abdominal radiotherapy. *Am J Clin Oncol* 1994;17:72–76.
21. Hreshchyshyn MM, Park RC, Blessing JA. The role of adjuvant therapy in stage I ovarian cancer. *Am J Obstet Gynecol* 1980;138:139–145.
22. Bush RS, Allt WEC, Beale FA. Treatment of carcinoma of the ovary: operation, irradiation and chemotherapy. *Am J Obstet Gynecol* 1977;127:692–704.
23. National Institutes of Health Consensus Development Conference Statement. Ovarian cancer: screening, treatment and follow-up. *Gynecol Oncol* 1994;5S:S4–S14.

24. Dembo AJ. Radiotherapeutic management of ovarian cancer. *Semin Oncol* 1984;11:238–250.
25. Goldberg N, Peschel RE. Postoperative abdominopelvic radiation therapy for ovarian cancer. *Int J Radiat Oncol Biol Phys* 1988;14:425–429.
26. Weiser EB, Burke TW, Heller PB, et al. Determinants of survival of patients with epithelial ovarian carcinoma following whole abdominal irradiation (WAR). *Gynecol Oncol* 1988;30:201–208.
27. Fuller DB, Sause WT, Plenk HP, Menlove RL. Analysis of postoperative radiation therapy in stage I through III epithelial ovarian carcinoma. *J Clin Oncol* 1987;5:897–905.
28. Vergote IB, Kaern J, Abeler VM. Analysis of prognostic factors in stage I epithelial ovarian cancer: importance of the degree of differentiation and DNA ploidy in predicting relapse. *Am J Obstet Gynecol* 1993;169:40.
29. Rubin SC, Hoskins WJ, Saigo PE, et al. Prognostic factors for recurrence following negative second-look laparotomy in ovarian cancer patients treated with platinum-based chemotherapy. *Gynecol Oncol* 1991;42:137–141.
30. Fuks Z, Rizel S, Anteby SO. The multimodal approach to the treatment of stage III ovarian carcinoma. *Int J Radiat Oncol Biol Phys* 1982;8:903–908.
31. Lambert HE, Rustin GJS, Gregory WM, Nelstrop AE. A randomized trial comparing single-agent carboplatin with carboplatin followed by radiotherapy for advanced ovarian cancer: a North Thames Ovary Group Study. *J Clin Oncol* 1993;11:440–448.
32. Bruzzone M, Repetto L, Chiara S, et al. Chemotherapy versus radiotherapy in the management of ovarian cancer patients with pathological complete response or minimal residual disease at second-look. *Gynecol Oncol* 1990;38:392–395.
33. Lawton F, Luesley D, Blackledge G, et al. A randomized trial comparing whole abdominal radiotherapy with chemotherapy following cisplatinum cytoreduction in epithelial ovarian cancer: West Midlands Ovarian Cancer Group Trial II. *Clin Oncol* 1990;2:4–9.
34. Hoskins PJ, Swenerton KD, Wong F, et al. Platinum plus cyclophosphamide plus radiotherapy is superior to platinum alone in "high risk" epithelial ovarian cancer (residual negative and either stage I or II, grade 3, or stage III, any grade). *Int J Gynecol Cancer* 1995;5:134–142.
35. Reid GC, Roberts JA, Hopkins MP, et al. Primary treatment of stage III ovarian carcinoma with sequential chemotherapy and whole abdominal radiation therapy. *Gynecol Oncol* 1993;49:333–338.
36. Thomas GM, Dembo AJ. Integrating radiation therapy into the management of ovarian cancer. *Cancer* 1993;71:1710–1718.
37. Thomas GM. Is there a role for consolidation or salvage radiotherapy after chemotherapy in advanced epithelial ovarian cancer? *Gynecol Oncol* 1993;51:97–103.
38. MacGibbon A, Bucci J, MacLeod C, et al. Whole abdominal radiotherapy following second-look laparotomy for ovarian carcinoma. *Gynecol Oncol* 1999;75:62–67.
39. Pickel H, Lahousen M, Petru E, et al. Consolidation radiotherapy after carboplatin-based chemotherapy in radically operated advanced ovarian cancer. *Gynecol Oncol* 1999;72:215–219.
40. Wong R, Milosevic M, Sturgeon J, et al. Treatment of early epithelial ovarian cancer with chemotherapy and abdominopelvic radiotherapy: results of a prospective treatment protocol. *Int J Radiat Oncol Biol Phys* 1999;45:657–665.
41. Whelan TJ, Dembo AJ, Bush RS, et al. Complications of whole abdominal and pelvic radiotherapy following chemotherapy for advanced ovarian cancer. *Int J Radiat Oncol Biol Phys* 1992;22:853–858.
42. Randall ME, Barrett RJ, Spirtos NM, et al. Chemotherapy, early surgical reassessment and hyperfractionated abdominal radiotherapy in stage III ovarian cancer: results of a Gynecologic Oncology Group study. *Int J Radiat Oncol Biol Phys* 1996;34:139–147.
43. Van Lith JMM, Bouma J, Aalders JG. Role of an early second-look laparotomy in ovarian cancer. *Gynecol Oncol* 1989;35:255–260.
44. Ensley JF, Jacobs RJ, Weaver A, et al. Correlation between response to cisplatinum combination chemotherapy and subsequent radiotherapy in previously untreated patients with advanced squamous cell cancers of the head and neck. *Cancer* 1984;54:811–814.
45. Louie KG, Behrens BC, Kinsella TJ, et al. Radiation survival parameters of anti-neoplastic drug-sensitive and resistant human ovarian cancer cell lines and their modification by buthionine sulfoxime. *Cancer Res* 1985;45:2110–2115.
46. Britten RA, Peacock J, Warenious HM. Collateral resistance to photon and neutron irradiation is associated with acquired cisplatinum resistance in human ovarian tumor cells. *Radiother Oncol* 1992;23:170–175.
47. Silver DF, Wheeless CR, Dubin NH. Radiotherapy as a cisplatin-sensitizer in a resistant ovarian carcinoma cell line. *Cancer* 1996;77:1850–1853.
48. Schwartz JL, Rotmensch J, Beckett MA. X-ray and cis-diammine dichoroplatinum cross-resistance in human tumor cell lines. *Cancer Res* 1988;48:5133–5135.
49. Eifel PJ, Gershenson DM, Delclos L, et al. Twice-daily, split-course abdominopelvic radiation therapy after chemotherapy and positive second-look laparotomy for epithelial ovarian carcinoma. *Int J Radiat Oncol Biol Phys* 1991;21:1013–1018.
50. Reddy S, Lee M-S, Yordan E, et al. Salvage whole abdomen radiation therapy: its role in ovarian cancer. *Int J Radiat Oncol Biol Phys* 1993;27:879–884.
51. Baker K, Reddy S, Lee M-S, et al. Salvage whole abdominal radiation therapy for ovarian cancer: a twelve year experience [Abstract]. *Int J Radiat Oncol Biol Phys* 1996;36[Suppl 1]:176.
52. Fein DA, Morgan LS, Marcus RB, et al. Stage III ovarian carcinoma: an analysis of treatment results and complications following hyperfractionated abdominopelvic irradiation for salvage. *Int J Radiat Oncol Biol Phys* 1994;29:169–176.
53. Cmelak AJ, Kapp DS. Long-term survival with whole abdominopelvic irradiation in platinum-refractory persistent or recurrent ovarian cancer. *Gynecol Oncol* 1997;65:453–460.
54. Suzuki S, Fujiwara K, Yamauchi H, et al. Efficacy of radiation therapy for chemo-resistant ovarian cancers [Abstract]. *Int J Gynecol Cancer* 1997;7[Suppl 2]:80.
55. Sedlaceck TV, Spyropoulus P, Cifaldi R, et al. Whole-abdomen radiation therapy as salvage treatment for epithelial ovarian carcinoma. *Cancer J Sci Am* 1997;3:358–363.
56. Soper JT, Wilkinson RH Jr, Bandy LC, et al. Intraperitoneal chromic phosphate (^{32}P) as salvage therapy for

persistent carcinoma of the ovary after surgical restaging. *Am J Obstet Gynecol* 1987;156:1153–1158.
57. Spanos WJ, Day T, Jose B, et al. Use of ^{32}P in stage III epithelial carcinoma of the ovary. *Gynecol Oncol* 1994;54:35–39.
58. Rogers L, Varia M, Halle J, et al. ^{32}P following negative second-look laparotomy for epithelial ovarian cancer. *Gynecol Oncol* 1993;50:141–146.
59. Patillo RA, Collier BD, Abdel-Dayem H, et al. Phosphorous-32-chromic phosphate for ovarian cancer: I. Fractionated low-dose intraperitoneal treatments in conjunction with platinum analog chemotherapy. *J Nucl Med* 1995;36:29–36.
60. Alvarez RD, Partridge EE, Khazaeli MB, et al. Intraperitoneal radioimmunotherapy of ovarian cancer with 177-Lu-CC49: a phase I/II study. *Gynecol Oncol* 1997;65:94–101.
61. Corn BW, Lanciano RM, Boente M, et al. Recurrent ovarian cancer: effective radiotherapeutic palliation after chemotherapy failure. *Cancer* 1994;74:2979–2983.
62. Davidson SA, Rubin SC, Mychalczak B, et al. Limited-field radiotherapy as salvage treatment of localized persistent or recurrent epithelial ovarian cancer. *Gynecol Oncol* 1993;51:349–354.
63. Suzuki S, Fujiwara K, Yamauchi H, et al. *Focal radiation therapy for localized relapsed or refractory ovarian cancer.* American Society of Clinical Oncology, 1999.
64. Corn BW, Greven KM, Randall ME, et al. The efficacy of cranial irradiation in ovarian cancer metastatic to the brain: analysis of 32 cases. *Obstet Gynecol* 1995;86:955–959.
65. Martinez A, Schray MF, Howes AE, Bagshaw MA. Postoperative radiation therapy for epithelial ovarian cancer: the curative role based on 24-year experience. *J Clin Oncol* 1985;3:901–911.
66. Dembo AJ, Bush RS, Beale FA, et al. A randomized clinical trial of moving strip versus open field whole abdominal irradiation in patients with invasive epithelial cancer of the ovary. *Int J Radiat Oncol Biol Phys* 1983;9:97.
67. Fyles AW, Thomas GM, Pintilie M, et al. A randomized study of two doses of abdominopelvic radiation therapy for patients with optimally debulked stage I, II and III ovarian cancer. *Int J Radiat Oncol Biol Phys* 1998;41:543–549.
68. Fletcher GH. *Textbook of radiotherapy,* 3rd ed. Philadelphia: Lea & Febiger, 1980.
69. Marks LB. A standard dose of radiation for "microscopic disease" is not appropriate. *Cancer* 1990;66:2498–2502.
70. Withers HR, Suwinski R. Radiation dose response for subclinical metastases. *Semin Radiat Oncol* 1998;8:224–228.
71. Fyles AW, Dembo AJ, Bush RS, et al. Analysis of complications in patients treated with abdomino-pelvic radiation therapy for ovarian carcinoma. *Int J Radiat Oncol Biol Phys* 1992;22:847–851.
72. Fyles AW, Manchul L, Levin W, et al. Effect of filgrastim (G-CSF) during chemotherapy and abdomino-pelvic radiation therapy in patients with ovarian carcinoma. *Int J Radiat Oncol Biol Phys* 1998;41:843–847.
73. Kuten A, Stein M, Steiner M, et al. Whole abdominal irradiation following chemotherapy in advanced ovarian carcinoma. *Int J Radiat Oncol Biol Phys* 1988;14:273–279.
74. Einhorn N, Nilsson B, Holmberg K. Risk of second tumors in a cohort of patients with ovarian carcinoma. *Int J Gynecol Cancer* 1996;6:313.
75. Travis LB. Risk of leukemia after platinum-based chemotherapy for ovarian cancer. *N Engl J Med* 1999;340:351–357.
76. Schwartz PE, Rutherford TJ, Chambers JT, et al. Neoadjuvant chemotherapy for advanced ovarian cancer. *Gynecol Oncol* 1999;72:93–99.
77. King LA, Downey GO, Potish RA. Concomitant whole-abdominal radiation and intraperitoneal chemotherapy in advanced ovarian carcinoma: a pilot study. *Cancer* 1991 67:2867–2871.
78. Reisinger SA, Asbury R, Liao S-Y, Homesley HD. A phase I study of weekly cisplatin and whole abdominal radiation for the treatment of stage III and IV endometrial carcinoma: a Gynecological Oncology Group pilot study. *Gynecol Oncol* 1996;63:299–303.
79. Dowlatshahi M, Miller M, Semrad N, et al. Use of concomitant low dose cisplatinum and whole abdominal radiation (WARP) as salvage therapy for persistent ovarian carcinoma after positive second look procedure: a pilot study [Abstract]. *Cancer J Sci Am* 1999;5:123.
80. Steren A, Sevin BU, Perras J, et al. Taxol as a radiosensitizer: a flow cytometric study. *Gynecol Oncol* 1993;50:89–93.

20
Ovarian Germ Cell Tumors

Jean A. Hurteau and Steven J. Williams

Germ cell tumors of the ovary comprise fewer than 5% of ovarian cancers (1). They occur in young women and adolescent girls and despite their aggressive nature are generally curable if treated with appropriate chemotherapy. Although surgery plays an important role in diagnosis and initial treatment, complete resection of the reproductive organs is rarely necessary in this group of young women who desire to maintain their reproductive capabilities. Most patients now survive free of cancer because of the development of improved chemotherapy regimens. However, the role of appropriate surgical staging and tumor reductive surgery cannot be overlooked. The information acquired at surgical-pathologic assessment often guides the clinician in the use of adjuvant therapy.

CLASSIFICATION

The primitive malignant germ cell tumors can be divided into dysgerminomas and nondysgerminomatous tumors. The latter group includes yolk sac tumors, immature teratomas, embryonal carcinomas, choriocarcinomas, polyembryomas, mixed germ cell tumors, and gonadoblastomas. Table 20.1 represents the World Health Organization (WHO) classification of germ cell tumors of the ovary (2).

CLINICAL PROFILE

Malignant germ cell tumors of the ovary occur principally in adolescent girls and young women. The median age is 16 to 20 years, with a range from 6 to 46 years. Because these tumors have a rapid growth rate, most patients present with an abdominal mass and pain. Approximately 10% of patients present with an acute abdomen secondary to intracapsular hemorrhage, torsion, and/or rupture. This finding may be somewhat more common in patients with endodermal sinus tumors or mixed germ cell tumors, and it is frequently misdiagnosed as an acute appendicitis or another abdominal emergency, with the true diagnosis being made at the time of surgery. Other, less common symptoms include vaginal bleeding, fever, and isosexual precocity thought to be related to human chorionic gonadotropin (hCG) production by the tumor.

Given the age group associated with primitive germ cell tumors, it is predictable that these tumors are overrepresented in pregnancy, accounting for approximately 25% of all malignant tumors diagnosed during pregnancy (3).

While the search for biologic markers continues for many other malignancies, germ cell tumors have a unique property in that most secrete tumor-associated antigens that can be detected in serum. This has allowed accurate diagnosis, comprehensive monitoring during treatment, and detection of recurrence. Both hCG and α-fetoprotein (AFP) have been identified as sensitive markers that can be measured in the serum of most patients with ovarian germ cell tumors. These markers are usually elevated at diagnosis, and serial measurements usually reflect the clinical course of the disease. AFP is most often elevated in yolk sac tumors but also has been detected in immature teratomas. hCG is often elevated in choriocarcinomas, embryonal carcinomas, and polyembryomas (4). It has also been detected in dysgerminomas that harbor multinucleated syncytiotrophoblastic giant cells. Serum lactate dehydrogenase (LDH) is another biologic marker that is increased in dysgerminomas (5–7). LDH is composed of multiple isoenzymes, of which the LDH-1 and LDH-2 isoenzymes are

TABLE 20.1. World health organization classification of ovarian germ cell tumors

Dysgerminoma
  Variant: with syncytiotrophoblast cells
Yolk sac tumor (endodermal sinus tumor)
  Variant: polyvesicular vitteline tumor
    Hepatoid
    Glandular
      Variant: endometrioid
Embryonal carcinoma
Polyembryoma
Choriocarcinoma
Teratomas
  Immature
  Mature
    Solid
    Cystic (dermoid cyst)
      With secondary tumor formation (specify type)
      Fetiform (homunculus)
  Monodermal and highly specialized
    Struma ovarii
      With thyroid tumor (specify type)
    Carcinoid
      Insular
      Trabecular
    Strumal carcinoid
    Mucinous carcinoid
    Neuroectodermal tumors
    Sebaceous tumors
    Others
  Mixed (specify types)
Mixed (specify types)

TABLE 20.2. Serum tumor markers in malignant germ cell tumors of the ovary

Histology	α-Fetoprotein	β-Human chorionic gonadotropin
Dysgerminoma	−	±
Yolk sac tumor	+	−
Immature teratoma	±	−
Mixed germ cell tumor	±	±
Choriocarcinoma	−	+
Embryonal carcinoma	±	+
Polyembryoma	±	+

thought to be selectively elevated (8). This may account for the nonspecific fluctuation of this biologic marker during follow-up periods when selective isoenzymes are not measured. Macrophage colony-stimulating factor (M-CSF) was also noted to be elevated in 16 patients with stage 1 dysgerminoma (9) and in 44 of 49 patients with germ cell tumors (9). Further evaluation of M-CSF as a biologic marker for germ cell tumors, specifically dysgerminomas, is needed to confirm these preliminary findings (Table 20.2).

Neuron-specific enolase (10) and the antigen CA 125 (11) have also been identified in the serum of patients with ovarian germ cell malignancies, but their roles are not well defined.

Dysgerminomas

Dysgerminomas are the most common ovarian germ cell malignancy, accounting for 50% of all cases. The diagnosis of dysgerminoma requires a normal AFP value; however, an elevation in hCG is not inconsistent with this diagnosis. Dysgerminomas are grossly bilateral in 10% to 15% of cases and involve a contralateral grossly normal ovary on microscopic examination in an additional 10%. Dysgerminomas have a predilection for lymphatic spread compared with other germ cell tumors. They can be associated with gonadoblastomas in a small proportion of patients. These patients usually present with primary amenorrhea, virilization, or developmental abnormalities of the genitalia with or without a pelvic mass. Sex chromatin studies are important because they reveal whether the Y chromosome is present, thereby requiring bilateral oophorectomy.

Currently, the approach to dysgerminomas includes a thorough staging laparotomy as performed in epithelial ovarian cancers. Sixty percent to 70% of patients are diagnosed with stage I disease. Because most of these patients are in the reproductive age group, early-stage disease can be managed by unilateral salpingo-oophorectomy with conservation of the uterus and contralateral ovary. The procedure should be performed through a vertical midline incision and should include peritoneal washings, upper abdominal exploration with cytology and biopsies, omentectomy, biopsies of pelvic peritoneum, and pelvic and periaortic lymph node sampling. All suspicious areas should be biopsied, and random biopsies as performed in epithelial ovarian cancer staging should be obtained. The contralateral ovary should be carefully inspected and should not be bivalved or biopsied if normal in size, shape, and consistency.

In patients with advanced disease, it is recommended that the same principles of cytoreductive surgery that are applied to epithelial ovarian cancer be followed, with resection of as much tumor as is safe and technically possible (12). Because of the rarity of these tumors, however, the benefit of cytoreductive surgery has not been clearly defined. Support for the concept of cytoreductive surgery in germ cell tumors may be found in two studies by the Gynecologic Oncology Group (GOG) (13,14). The first, by Slayton and colleagues (13), found that 15 (28%) of 54 patients with completely resected disease at primary surgery failed chemotherapy with a combination of vincristine, actinomycin D, and cyclophosphamide (VAC), as opposed to 15 (68%) of 22 patients with incompletely resected disease treated with the same regimen. Furthermore, they also found that a higher percentage of patients with bulky residual disease (82%) failed chemotherapy compared with those with minimal residual disease (55%). In a second GOG study reported by Williams and associates (14), patients receiving a combination of cytoplastin, vinblastine, and bleomycin (PVB) for tumors other than dysgerminoma were more likely to remain progression free if they were clinically without evidence of disease (65%, versus 34% for patients with measurable disease). In addition, patients with optimal surgical resection had an outcome intermediate between that of patients with suboptimal disease and patients with optimal disease without surgical resection. Overall, patients with stage II or III completely resected dysgerminomas followed by effective chemotherapy may have a cure rate as high as 95% to 98%.

Germ cell tumors, especially dysgerminomas, are generally very chemosensitive, and, in selected patients with advanced disease, preservation of reproductive function remains an option as long as the uterus and contralateral ovary are not grossly involved with tumor (15–17). Even with involvement of the contralateral ovary, Schwartz and colleagues has reported four patients with metastasis to the contralateral ovary managed with preservation of that ovary followed by subsequent chemotherapy. When the data were last revised, all were alive at 14 to 56 months from diagnosis (15).

Patients with completely staged IA dysgerminomas may be observe closely without adjuvant treatment. The overall 10-year survival rate for these patients approaches 100%. About 15% to 25% of tumors recur, but they can be retreated successfully with a high likelihood of cure. Patients with more advanced disease should receive adjuvant therapy with either radiotherapy or chemotherapy (18). Although dysgerminomas are exquisitely sensitive to radiotherapy, loss of reproductive function due to ovarian failure usually results. Therefore, radiation therapy for dysgerminomas has been replaced by effective and less toxic chemotherapy regimens (12).

Experience with chemotherapy in dysgerminomas was in the past limited because of the efficacy of radiation therapy (18). However, because these patients are young and fertility is an issue, chemotherapy has been pushed into the forefront and radiotherapy has fallen out of favor as primary therapy (19–25). Reports of efficacious and less toxic multiagent chemotherapy regimens consisting of bleomycin, etoposide, and cisplatin (BEP) in the treatment of testicular seminomas have stimulated interest in the use of these agents in patients with dysgerminomas. Gershenson first reported sustained remissions in two patients treated with BEP (17). In a follow-up study in which 9 of 14 patients has advanced or recurrent disease, all 14 patients were found to be free of disease with a median follow-up of 23 months (26). Currently, the group at M.D. Anderson Cancer Center has treated 17 patients with BEP, of whom 12 had advanced disease, and all have had a sustained remission (12). The GOG reported on 20 patients with advanced incompletely resected dysgerminomas on two consecutive protocols. Treatment was PVB in the first protocol and BEP followed by consolidation with VAC in the second. To date, 20 dysgerminoma patients have been evaluable on these protocols. All had stage II or IV disease and most had greater than 2-cm residual tumor. Overall, 19 were alive and disease-free with follow-up of 6 to 68 months (median, 26 months) (27). Fourteen second-look procedures were done, and all were negative.

TABLE 20.3. *BEP chemotherapy regimen*

Bleomycin	20 units/m^2 I.V. (max. 30 units) weekly
Etoposide (VP-16)	100 mg/m^2 I.V. on days 1–5
Cisplatin	20 mg/m^2 I.V. on days 1–5

These studies led the GOG to recommend BEP (Table 20.3) as the preferred adjuvant treatment for patients with dysgerminomas because of its high cure rate, its presumed minimal impact on fertility, and its reasonable toxicity (28). The optimal number of cycles remains to be defined; however, most authors recommend three cycles in patients who have had a complete resection of their tumor and four cycles in patients with incomplete resection (12). Therefore, considering the relatively low toxicity and ease of treatment, chemotherapy has replaced radiation therapy as the preferred adjuvant modality even when fertility is not an issue.

The follow-up of patients with early disease who require no adjuvant therapy has not been defined. Because these are rapidly growing tumors and 15% to 25% recur, with most recurrences within the first 2 years, we recommend initial follow-up at 4- to 6-week intervals for the first 2 years. Tumor markers, LDH, and hCG should be measured in all patients. After 2 years, follow-up can be extended to 8- to 12-week intervals until 3 years, then 3- to 4-month intervals until 5 years. After 5 years, late recurrences are rare but have been documented. A recent report described a relapse of ovarian dysgerminoma 20 years after the initial diagnosis. Patients with late recurrences of ovarian dysgerminomas are paradoxically thought to be less responsive to chemotherapy.

Nondysgerminomatous Tumors

The nondysgerminomatous tumors include the yolk sac tumors (endodermal sinus tumors), immature teratomas, mixed germ cell tumors, choriocarcinomas, embryonal carcinomas, and polyembryomas. Collectively, they account for 50% of ovarian germ cell tumors. Of these, the yolk sac tumors are the second most common germ cell tumors, after dysgerminomas, comprising 25% of all cases. They are followed in frequency by immature teratomas (20%) and mixed germ cell tumors (8%).

The yolk sac tumors differ from dysgerminomas in that they are bilateral in fewer than 5% of cases. Pathologically, they are characterized by Schiller-Duval bodies, which are single papillae lined by tumor cells and containing a central vessel. Yolk sac tumors are derived from primitive gut (glandular yolk sac tumor) and primitive liver (hepatoid yolk sac tumor) and therefore secrete AFP as a tumor marker.

Immature teratomas are the third most common germ cell tumor. They are bilateral in fewer than 5% of the cases and can be associated with benign mature teratoma (dermoid cyst) in the contralateral ovary in 10% of cases. Pathologic examination reveals that immature teratomas are derived from tissues representing all three embryonic germ cell layers (ectoderm, mesoderm, and endoderm). The immature teratomas are graded from 1 to 3 based on the amount of primitive neuroectodermal tissue present. The grade has been correlated with prognosis and dictates the mode of therapy. For stage I tumors, immature teratomas as well as mature teratomas can be complicated by peritoneal implants composed exclusively of mature glial tissue. The presence of such tissue does not change the stage or alter prognosis, but the implants can grow slowly and require surgical intervention for diagnosis and symptoms.

The mixed primitive germ cell tumors are the fourth most common malignant germ cell tumors, accounting for approximately 19% of all cases. Dysgerminomas and yolk sac tumors are the most common combination encountered. Bilaterality of mixed germ cell tumors is dependent on the presence of dysgerminoma elements; when they are present, the contralateral ovary can be involved in 10% of cases. It is important for the pathologist to carefully sample germ cell tumors that have the potential to be treated conservatively, such as stage IA dysgerminomas and stage I and grade 1 immature teratomas. The detection of other germ cell elements in these tumors necessitates adjuvant chemotherapy.

Embryonal carcinomas and choriocarcinomas are extremely rare in pure forms and are most likely to be seen as components of mixed primitive germ cell tumors. Choriocarcinomas are characterized by a nest of cytotrophoblasts and intermediate trophoblasts surrounded by syncytiotrophoblasts. Both choriocarcinomas and embryonal carcinomas may secrete hCG that can be detected in serum samples. These germ cell tumors have also been associated with endocrine changes such as sexual precocity and abnormal uterine bleeding.

Polyembryomas are extremely rare tumors that are characterized by numerous embryo-like bodies resembling morphologically normal embryos. They are most often associated with mixed primitive germ cell elements, of which the immature teratoma is the most common.

In the past, nondysgerminomatous tumors had a poor prognosis, with only 5% to 20% of patients surviving after treatment with surgery alone (12). These tumors were not radiosensitive, and it was only with the introduction of chemotherapy that the survival of patients improved. Initial trials with chemotherapy began in the 1960s and progressed to efficacious combination chemotherapy in the 1970s with the use of VAC (29). The treatment regimen was originally recommended for 2 years and was later modified to 12 cycles or 1 year (29). Schwartz and colleagues recommended treatment courses ranging from 3 cycles in patients with early disease to 12 cycles in patients with advanced nondysgerminomatous tumors with immature teratomatous elements (15). However, reports detailing sustained remission rates of less than 50% with VAC chemotherapy in the treatment of patients with advanced nondysgerminomatous tumors led to a search for more effective agents (15,25,29,30).

The VPB regimen has been considered more toxic than the VAC regimen, but its effectiveness in advanced disease has outweighed its potential risks (31–35). De Palo and associates reported a failure rate of 42% of patients with advanced disease treated with VPB (36). The GOG, using VPB, reported that 47 (53%) of 89 patients were disease free with a median follow-up period of 52 months; 4-year survival was about 70%. About one third of the patients entered on this trial had had previous chemotherapy. However, 27% of patients in this trial had no prior treatment and nonmeasurable disease and yet failed.

Regimens substituting etoposide for vinblastine have been used successfully in testicular germ cell cancers. Early reports with etoposide-containing regimens in the treatment of ovarian germ cell tumors have described excellent results (37–40). Gershenson and coworkers (26) and the GOG (29,41) reported a 96% sustained remission rate with the BEP regimen. Both studies confirmed the effectiveness of cisplatin-based chemotherapy given as a short course of the BEP regimen in completely resected germ cell tumors.

A study from Australia also concluded that platinum-based therapy was effective for nondysgerminomatous ovarian germ cell tumors (42). The authors found, in multivariate analysis, that relapse was generally seen in patients with yolk sac tumors who had elevated AFP (more than 1,000 kU/L) compared with lower AFPs (30% versus 3% relapse), as well as patients who received nonplatinum-based chemotherapy. In univariate analysis of only those patients who received platinum-based treatment, elevated AFP in yolk sac tumors was still associated with higher relapse rates.

Several trials in patients with advanced disease treated with this regimen have shown that about 60% to 80% of patients will be long-term survivors. However, in advanced disease, results with this regimen were less favorable than in the testicular cancer group, and it was thought that further improvement is possible. Therefore, GOG Protocol 90 evaluated patients with advanced, incompletely resected to recurrent disease with three cycles of BEP followed by three cycles of VAC. Results are still pending.

Germa and colleagues described a short-term sequential chemotherapy regimen consisting of nine agents: cisplatin, vincristine, methotrexate, bleomycin, etoposide, actinomycin-D, cyclophosphamide, Adriamycin, and vinblastine (POMB-ACE-PAV). The rationale for this combination was to reduce the total dose of each agent, therefore limiting toxicity. A 97% sustained remission rate with limited toxicity has been described (43,44).

In summary, patients who have undergone complete surgical staging and have a stage IA grade 1 immature teratoma need no further treatment and may be observed closely. All other patients require adjuvant chemotherapy. Current treatment recommendations for nondysgerminomatous germ cell tumors include three cycles of BEP for completely resected tumors and four cycles for incompletely resected tumors. The treatment should be given at full dose and on schedule because of presumptive evidence in testicular cancer that the timeliness of chemotherapy may be associated with outcome. With the advent of hematopoietic growth factors, dose reduction for patients with previous neutropenic fevers can be avoided. It is important that these patients receive the chemotherapy as soon as possible after surgery because of the risk of early relapse. We prefer to initiate therapy within 7 to 10 days of surgery. Furthermore, in testicular cancer the data suggest that bleomycin is an important component of the treatment regimen, particularly if only three courses of therapy are given, and should not be omitted.

The current recommendations for adjuvant chemotherapy in patients with immature teratomas were developed at a time when comprehensive surgical staging was not routine. Investigators are now reevaluating the role of adjuvant chemotherapy in patients who have undergone comprehensive surgical staging and complete surgical resection of immature teratomas of grades 2 and 3 confined to the ovary (stage I). It is conceivable that patients with grade 2 or 3 immature teratomas were understaged and that their high risk of recurrence was not entirely due to the biology of the disease but secondary to incomplete staging. Support for this rationale is based on three studies in which surveillance of patients with grades 2 and 3 immature teratomas offered interesting but not conclusive results.

The largest of these studies was an intergroup study at the Pediatric Oncology Group and the Children's Cancer Group. Investigators followed 41 young female patients with a median age of 10 years after surgical resection of ovarian immature teratoma. Of 41 patients, 31 had pure immature teratoma (18 grade 1, 9 grade 2, 4 grade 3), and 10 patients had mixed immature teratomas with elements of yolk sac tumor. Details regarding staging were not recorded, but 40 of the 41 patients remained free of disease with a median follow-up of 33 months in the immature teratoma group and 24 months in the mixed group (45). There was only one recurrence, and that patient was successfully salvaged with BEP chemotherapy. Two other studies, one from Mt. Vernon and Charing Cross Hospital in England and one from the University of Milan, reported a total of 18 patients with grades 2 or 3 stage I immature teratomas treated with careful observation after initial strategy. Only two patients developed recurrent disease, of which one was salvaged with surgery alone and the other with chemotherapy. At last review, all patients were free of disease (46,47).

Although these three studies combined 49 patients with pure immature teratomas and only 3 recurrences were documented, the results are too premature to draw definitive conclusions. Further study is needed before we can recommend omission of adjuvant chemotherapy in these patients. In addition, it is not known whether the biology of germ cell tumors in pediatric patients is different from that in the adult population.

SECOND-LOOK LAPAROTOMY

The concept of second-look laparotomy was introduced by Wagensteen and associates in 1951 for the assessment of disease in patients who had previously undergone primary surgical resection for colon cancer (48). This approach was later adopted and modified by Rutledge and Burns to evaluate the status of intraabdominal disease in epithelial ovarian cancer patients who had undergone a prescribed course of systemic chemotherapy and were thought to be free of disease (49). This concept has recently been extrapolated into the management of malignant ovarian germ cell tumors.

Williams and associates and the GOG reviewed their experience with the second-look surgery in malignant ovarian germ cell tumor (50). Forty-five patients underwent complete surgical resection followed by three courses of BEP. Second-look surgery in these patients revealed no tumor or mature teratoma in 43, and 2 patients had immature teratoma elements. In the 2 patients with immature teratoma elements, 1 underwent further salvage chemotherapy and 1 did not; all 45 patients reportedly were free of disease. In the same study, 72 patients underwent incomplete tumor resection for advanced germ cell tumors followed by four cycles of BEP or PVB. Forty-eight of these patients did not have immature teratoma elements in the primary tumor. Second-look surgery revealed that 45 patients had no residual disease and 3 patients had persistent yolk sac tumors or embryonal carcinomas. The latter 3 patients died despite salvage chemotherapy. Immature teratoma elements were found in the primary tumor of 24 patients. At second-look surgery in these 24 patients, 16 were found to have mature teratoma elements. In 7, the mature teratoma elements were bulky or progressive. Fourteen of the total 16 and 6 of the 7 with bulky residual tumor remained disease free after surgical resection.

It is concluded from this study that second-look surgery is of no benefit to patients who initially undergo complete tumor resection or incomplete resection when there are no elements of immature teratoma in the primary tumor. Second-look surgery is, however, recommended for patients who undergo an initial incomplete resection of tumor containing elements of immature teratoma, because they are the group most likely to benefit from the procedure.

INCOMPLETE SURGICAL STAGING

Because germ cell tumors grow rapidly, they can manifest as a acute abdomen in a young patient. The initial surgical intervention may be performed in the community-based hospital to alleviate symptoms. Diagnosis of a germ cell tumor brings about a referral to a tertiary care center without comprehensive surgical staging. The management of these tumors can be challenging, but a rational approach can be outlined based on current data.

Dysgerminomas

These tumors are extremely chemosensitive, and even patients with bulky residual tumors can be salvaged with current BEP therapy. Although 10% to 15% of dysgerminomas are bilateral, recommendation for biopsy of the contralateral ovary is based on an abnormal or enlarged ovary. Furthermore, 65% to 70% of these tumors are stage I at diagnosis, and most of these data were derived before the era of comprehensive surgical staging.

The current recommendation for no adjuvant therapy includes all patients with stage IA dysgerminoma after comprehensive surgical staging. This implies that patients with incomplete staging require a further laparotomy for completion of surgical staging. Restaging can be offered to patients either in a limited (laparoscopy) or comprehensive (laparotomy) fashion. However, based on current data, we recommend obtaining measurements of tumor markers, hCG, LDH, and AFP (elevation of AFP excludes a dysgerminoma) followed by computed tomographic (CT) scans of the abdomen and pelvis with ultrasound studies of the contralateral ovary. Should these parameters be negative, it would be appropriate to monitor these patients at 4- to 6-week intervals as described earlier, without administering chemotherapy. We also recommend CT scanning every 3 to 4 months for the first year. Follow-up should decrease in frequency after 2 years, since most relapses occur within this time period and by 4 years.

If tumor markers are elevated but radiologic imaging is negative, we would recommend the following approach. Elevation of the hCG concentration implies residual tumor that requires further therapy. An intercurrent pregnancy should be ruled out by pelvic ultrasonography. LDH elevations can be nonspecific unless LDH-1 and LDH-2 isoenzyme concentrations are determined. Elevation of the AFP would indicate germ cell elements other than dysgerminoma and mandate chemotherapy. We would not consider a formal laparotomy, because these tumors are extremely chemosensitive and virtually all these patients can be salvaged with chemotherapy.

Should markers be negative with imaging studies suspicious for metastatic disease, we would recommend confirmation by CT-guided biopsy or laparoscopy before initiation of therapy.

In summary, patients with dysgerminomas that are incompletely staged do not require a formal second laparotomy for comprehensive surgical staging. These patients can be closely monitored. Seventy percent will have stage I disease based on data obtained before the era of comprehensive surgical staging. Furthermore, 15% to 25% of stage I tumors will recur, and these patients can be cured by current chemotherapy regimens.

Nondysgerminomatous Tumors

Nondysgerminomatous tumors had a poor prognosis, with only 5% to 20% of patients surviving, after treatment with surgery alone (12). With the addition of BEP chemotherapy, 60% to 80% of patients with advance disease can be long-term survivors; however, improvements can be made.

Because the only group of patients among those with nondysgerminomatous tumors who require no further adjuvant therapy are those with grade 1 immature teratomas, these would be the only patients, if incompletely staged, that we would consider for repeat laparotomy and completion of comprehensive surgical staging.

A conservative approach with no adjuvant therapy has been advocated in some centers for completely staged grade 2, grade 3, and stage II immature teratoma. However, the data are limited, and we continue to advocate adjuvant therapy in these patients and all others with nondysgerminomatous tumors.

Therefore, in patients with incompletely staged nondysgerminomatous tumors, other than grade 1 immature teratomas, we recommend obtaining measurements of tumor markers, AFP, and hCG as well as a CT scan of the abdomen and pelvis followed by initiation of BEP chemotherapy.

SALVAGE THERAPIES

Currently, little information regarding salvage therapies for recurrent or persistent ovarian germ cell tumors exists in the literature. The treatment of these patients is usually described in reports of failures of adjuvant chemotherapy. In addition, because germ cell tumors are so uncommon, their response to chemotherapy in the adjuvant setting continues to be defined. The first salvage regimens described were in response to failure of the VAC regimen. These patients underwent salvage chemotherapy with PVB or etoposide-containing regimens (12,22,25,51). Because most of the adjuvant chemotherapy regimens are now platinum based, the issue of salvage therapy remains to be determined. In patients who have failed PVB, a durable remission can be attained with VAC or etoposide/cisplatin chemotherapy (25). In the GOG study that evaluated the efficacy of PVB in patients with advanced ovarian germ cell tumors, 5 of 12 patients were salvaged with VAC and 3 of 7 with etoposide and cisplatin (25). Because the initial therapy is now generally BEP, salvage regimens with combinations of ifosfamide, vinblastine, and cisplatin are recommended (52).

Undoubtedly the most useful information regarding salvage chemotherapy for ovarian germ cell tumors has come from the experience in treating testicular cancer. In these studies, the single most important prognostic factor was whether the patient's disease was platin resistant (defined as no response or progression of disease within 6 weeks after completion of treatment). Data from the testicular germ cell tumor literature strongly support the role of high-dose chemotherapy with carboplatin, etoposide with or without cyclophosphamide, or ifosfamide followed by stem cell rescue as superior to standard-dose salvage therapy. Generally, one course of standard-dose therapy, usually cisplatin, vinblastine, and ifosfamide, is administered. If an initial response is noted, two subsequent courses of high-dose chemotherapy, each followed by stem cell rescue, are given (53). Because these are similarly derived cancers in men and women, we would recommend this approach for recurrent ovarian germ cell tumors even though a paucity of data exist at this time.

In patients with truly cisplatin-refractory disease, the likelihood of long-term survival and cure after high-dose chemotherapy is less than 5%. Therefore, the appropriateness of this management option is debatable. On the other hand, the likelihood of cure with high-dose salvage chemotherapy in patients with relapse from a complete remission after initial therapy may be as high as a 50% (53).

LATE EFFECTS

Because ovarian germ cell tumors are now potentially curable cancers in young women, our attention has focused on the potential side effects of the treatment modalities that have been used to achieve these results. Although the testicular cancer literature has a significant body of information regarding the side effects of chemotherapy and reproduction function, there is paucity of data regarding ovarian germ cell tumors.

Because ovarian germ cell tumors are diagnosed in young women of reproductive age, fertility issues are of concern. We now have a greater understanding of the biology of this disease and its potential sensitivity to platinum-based chemotherapy. Because most of these tumors are diagnosed as stage I disease, fertility-sparing unilateral salpingo-oophorectomy with staging biopsies has become a more common surgical intervention.

Of further concern has been the gonadal function and fertility potential of these young women after chemotherapy. Studies of patients with a variety of cancers suggest that, although ovarian dysfunction or failure is a risk of chemotherapy, the majority of survivors can anticipate normal menstrual and reproductive function. Factors such as older age at initiation of therapy, greater cumulative drug dose, and longer duration of therapy have an adverse effect on the future gonadal function. On the other hand, oral contraceptives are known to cause ovarian suppression and could protect the ovarian follicles from the toxic effects of chemotherapeutic agents. Although studies have failed to confirm this hypothesis (54,55), it seems reasonable to start these young women on oral contraceptives during chemotherapy to prevent an inadvertent pregnancy.

Successful pregnancies after treatment with combination chemotherapy have been well documented in other types of malignancies, including Hodgkin's disease, non-Hodgkin's lymphoma, and leukemia. There are many anecdotal reports of successful pregnancy in patients with malignant ovarian germ cell tumors (56,57).

Data regarding ovarian dysfunction and fertility were recently updated in a study from M.D. Anderson (58). Researchers identified 16 patients with pure dysgerminomas who underwent fertility-sparing unilateral salpingo-oophorectomy followed by three cycles of BEP chemotherapy. Two were lost to follow-up, one premenarchal and one when pregnant. Of the 14 patients left for evaluation, 10 (71%) retained their normal menstrual function during and after chemotherapy. Thirteen (93%) returned to their normal prechemotherapy menstrual pattern. Two patients have had difficulty conceiving, but five pregnancies had been achieved at the time of this writing.

In an earlier study from M.D. Anderson, 27 (68%) of 40 patients who retained a normal contralateral ovary and uterus after successful treatment with combination chemotherapy for ovarian germ cell tumors maintained regular menses consistently after completion of chemotherapy, and 33 (83%) were having regular menses at the time of follow-up (59). Of the 16 patients who had attempted to become pregnant, 12 were successful. One patient had an elective first-trimester abortion, and the other 11 patients delivered 22 healthy infants. The majority of these patients were not treated with cisplatin-based chemotherapy.

A more recently recognized effect of chemotherapy used in the treatment of germ cell tumors is the risk of secondary malignancy (60). Most of the data from the testicular cancer literature involve etoposide and its association with the development of acute leukemia. In respect to the epipodophyllotoxins, this treatment complication may be dose and schedule dependent. The Indiana University Cancer Center experience in testicular cancer revealed that, of 348 male patients with germ cell tumor who received three to four courses of BEP as first-line therapy, 2 developed etoposide-related leukemia. None of the 67 patients who received only three courses developed this complication (61). In a study by Pederson-Bjergaard, 5 of 212 patients developed acute leukemia or myelodysplastic syndrome after etoposide therapy (60). All of these patients had received more than 2,000 mg/m^2 of etoposide. Patients receiving less than 2,000 mg/m^2 did not develop myelodysplastic syndromes.

Of considerable interest and concern has been the report of platinum-induced leukemia in ovarian cancer patients (62). In this case-control study of a population-based cohort of 28,971 women who received platinum-based chemotherapy for ovarian cancer, 96 developed leukemia. The relative risk for development of leukemia was 3.3 (95% confidence interval [CI], 1.1 to 9.4) after cisplatin chemotherapy and 6.5 (95% CI, 1.2 to 36.6) after carboplatin chemotherapy. A dose-response relation was noted when the dose of platinum increased above 1,000 mg total dose ($p \leq .001$). Considering that four cycles of BEP at a maximal body surface area of 2 square meters would give a maximum dose of cisplatin equaling 800 mg, we conclude that the dose would be well below the dose-response relationship described. The same logic can be followed for etoposide-related dose-response effects.

Because the dosages of BEP used for ovarian germ cell tumors are below the threshold for documented chemotherapy-induced leukemia and the potential for cure is high, we continue to favor this regimen as the standard of care.

SUMMARY

Comprehensive surgical staging and complete resection of tumor followed by effective chemotherapy with BEP is now the cornerstone of therapy for ovarian germ cell tumors. Young patients in their reproductive years can now be cured from these cancers and maintain their fertility. Patients with stage IA dysgerminoma and stage I grade 1 immature teratoma require no further adjuvant therapy. All other patients should be treated with three to four cycles of BEP chemotherapy depending on residual disease status. Most dysgerminoma patients will be cured, as will 60% to 80% of those with other cell types. However, further study is needed to improve on the survival rate of patients with nondysgerminomatous tumors. Continued vigilance for better salvage therapies and study of the testicular cancer patient population may improve on current results.

REFERENCES

1. Creasman WT, Soper JT. Assessment of the contemporary management of germ cell malignancies of the ovary. *Am J Obstet Gynecol* 1985;153:828–835.
2. Talerman A. Germ cell tumors of the ovary. In: Kurman RJ, ed. *Blaustein's pathology of the female tract*. New York: Springer-Verlag, 1987:659–721.
3. Krepart G, Smith JP, Rutledge F, Delclos L. The treatment of dysgerminoma of the ovary. *Cancer* 1978;41:986–990.
4. Kawai M, Kano T, Kikkawa F, Morikawa Y, et al. Seven tumor markers in benign and malignant germ cell tumors of the ovary. *Gynecol Oncol* 1992;45:248–253.
5. Zondag HA. Enzyme activity in dysgerminoma and seminoma: a study of lactic dehydrogenase isoenzymes in malignant diseases (the 1963 Fiske essay). *R I Med J* 1964;47:273–281.
6. Awais GM. Dysgerminoma and serum lactic dehydrogenase levels. *Obstet Gynecol* 1983;61:99–101.
7. Sheiko MC, Hart WR. Ovarian germinoma (dysgerminoma) with elevated serum lactic dehydrogenase: case report review of literature. *Cancer* 1982;49:994–998.
8. Schwartz PE, Morris JM. Serum lactic dehydrogenase: a tumor marker for dysgerminoma. *Obstet Gynecol* 1988;72:511–515.
9. Suzuki M, Kobayashi H, Ohwanda M, et al. Macrophage coony-stimulating factor as a marker for malignant germ cell tumors of the ovary. *Gynecol Oncol* 1998;68:35–37.
10. Kawata M, Sekiya S, Hatadeyama R, Takamizawa H. Neuron-specific enolase as a serum marker for immature teratoma and dysgerminoma. *Gynecol Oncol* 1989;32:191–197.
11. Altaras MM, Goldberg GL, Levin W, et al. The value of cancer antigen-125 as a tumor marker in malignant germ cell tumors of the ovary. *Gynecol Oncol* 1986;25:150–159.
12. Gershenson DM. Update on malignant ovarian germ cell tumors. *Cancer Suppl* 1993;71:1581–1590.
13. Slayton RE, Park RC, Silverberg SG, et al. Vincristine, dactinomycin, and cyclophosphamide in the treatment of malignant germ cell tumors of the ovary: a Gynecologic Oncology group study (a final report). *Cancer* 1985;56:243–248.
14. Williams SD, Blessing JA, Moore DH, et al. Cisplatin, vinblastine, and bleomycin in advanced recurrent ovarian germ-cell tumors. *Ann Intern Med* 1989;111:22–27.
15. Schwartz PE, Chambers SK, Chambers JT, et al. Ovarian germ cell malignancies: the Yale University experience. *Gynecol Oncol* 1992;45:26–31.
16. Wu P, Huang R, Lang J, et al. Treatment of malignant ovarian germ cell tumors with preservation of fertility: a report of 28 cases. *Gynecol Oncol* 1991;40:2–6.
17. Gershenson DM, Wharton JT, Kline RC, et al. Chemotherapeutic complete remission in patients with metastatic ovarian dysgerminomas: potential for cure and preservation of reproductive capacity. *Cancer* 1986;58:2594–2599.
18. Thomas GM, Dembo AJ, Hacker NF, DePetrillo AD. Current therapy for dysgerminoma of the ovary. *Obstet Gynecol* 1987;70:268.
19. Creasman WT, Fetter BF, Hammond CB, Parker RT. Germ cell malignancies of the ovary. *Obstet Gynecol* 1979;53:226–230.
20. Krepart G, Smith JP, Rutledge F, Delclos L. The treatment for dysgerminoma of the ovary. *Cancer* 1978;41:986–990.
21. Weinblatt ME, Ortega JA. Treatment of children with dysgerminoma of the ovary. *Cancer* 1982;49:2608–2611.
22. Jacobs AJ, Harris M, Deppe G, et al. Treatment of recurrent and persistent germ cell tumors with cisplatin, vinblastine, and bleomycin. *Obstet Gynecol* 1982;59:129–132.

23. Vriesendrop R, Aalders JG, Sleijfer DT, et al. Treatment of malignant germ cell tumors of the ovary with cisplatin, vinblastine, and bleomycin (PVB). *Cancer Treat Rep* 1984;68:779–781.
24. Willemse PHB, Aalders JG, Bouma J, et al. Long-term survival after vinblastine, bleomycin and cisplatin treatment in patients with germ cell tumors of the ovary: an update. *Gynecol Oncol* 1987;28:268–277.
25. Williams SD, Blessing JA, Moore DH, et al. Cisplatin vinblastine, and bleomycin in advanced and recurrent ovarian germ cell tumors: a trial of the Gynecologic Oncology Group. *Ann Intern Med* 1989;111:22–27.
26. Gershenson DM, Morris M, Cangir A, et al. Treatment of malignant germ cell tumors of the ovary with bleomycin, etoposide, and cisplatin (BEP). *J Clin Oncol* 1990;8:715–720.
27. Williams SD, Blessing JA, Hatch KD, Homesley HD. Chemotherapy of advanced dysgerminoma: trials of the Gynecologic Oncology Group. *J Clin Oncol* 1991;9:1950–1955.
28. Williams SD, Blessing JA, Liao S-Y, et al. Adjuvant therapy of ovarian germ cell tumors with cisplatin, etoposide and bleomycin: a trial of the Gynecologic Oncology Group. *J Clin Oncol* 1994; 12:701–706.
29. Gershenson DM, Copeland LJ, Kavanagh JJ, et al. Treatment of malignant nondysgerminomatous germ cell tumors of the ovary with vincristine, dactinomycin and cyclophosphamide. *Cancer* 1985;56:2756–2761.
30. Slayton RE, Park RC, Silverberg SG, et al. Vincristine, dactinomycin and cyclophosphamide in the treatment of malignant germ cell tumors of the ovary. *Cancer* 1985;56:243–248.
31. Julian CG, Barrett JM, Richardson RL, Greco FA. Bleomycin, vinblastine, and cis-platinum in the treatment of advanced endodermal sinus tumor. *Obstet Gynecol* 1979;56:396–401.
32. Wiltshaw E, Stuart-Harris R, Barker GH, et al. Chemotherapy of endodermal sinus tumor (yolk sac tumor) of the ovary: preliminary communication. *J R Soc Med* 1982;75:888–892.
33. Carlson RW, Sikic BI, Turbow MM, Ballon SC. Combination cisplatin, vinblastine, and bleomycin (PVB) for malignant germ cell tumors of the ovary. *J Clin Oncol* 1983;1:645–651.
34. Taylor MH, DePetrillo AD, Turner AR. Vinblastine, bleomycin and cisplatin in malignant germ cell tumors of the ovary. *Cancer* 1984;56:1341–1349.
35. Gershenson DM, Kavanagh JJ, Copeland LJ, et al. Retreatment of malignant nondysgerminomatous germ cell tumors of the ovary with vinblastine, bleomycin and cisplatin. *Cancer* 1986;57:1731–1737.
36. De Palo G, Zambetti M, Pilotti Rottoli L, et al. Nondysgerminomatous tumors of the ovary treated with cisplatin, vinblastine and bleomycin: long-term results. *Gynecol Oncol* 1992;47:239–246.
37. Williams SD, Birch R, Einhorn LH, et al. Treatment of disseminated germ-cell tumors with cisplatin, bleomycin, and either vinblastine or etoposide. *N Engl J Med* 1987;316:1435–1440.
38. Smith EB, Clark-Pearson DL, Creasman WT. A VP-16-213 and cisplatin containing regimen for treatment of refractory ovarian germ cell malignancies. *Am J Obstet Gynecol* 1984;150:927–931.
39. Smales E, Peckman MJ. Chemotherapy of germ cell ovarian tumors: first-line treatment with etoposide, bleomycin and cisplatin or carboplatin. *Eur J Cancer Clin Oncol* 1987;23:469–474.
40. Williams S, Blessing J, Slayton R, et al. Ovarian germ cell tumors: adjuvant trials of the Gynecologic Oncology Group (GOG) [Abstract]. *Proc Am Soc Clin Oncol* 1989;8:150–155.
41. Segelov E, Campbell J, Ng M, et al. Cisplatin-based chemotherapy for ovarian germ cell malignancies: the Australian experience. *J Clin Oncol* 1994;12:378–384.
42. Mitchell PL, Al-Nasiri N, A'Hern R, et al. Treatment of nondysgerminomatous ovarian germ cell tumors. *Cancer* 1999;85:2232–2244.
43. Germa JR, Izquierdo MA, Sequi MA, et al. Malignant ovarian germ cell tumors: the experience at the hospital de la Santa Creu I Sant Pau. *Gynecol Oncol* 1992;45:153–159.
44. Germa JR, Piera JM, Barnadas A, Badia J. Sequential combination chemotherapy for malignant germ cell tumors of the ovary. *Cancer* 1988;61:913–918.
45. Marina NM, Cushing B, Giller R, et al. Complete surgical excision is effective treatment for children with immature teratomas with or without malignant elements: a Pediatric Oncology Group/Children's Cancer Group intergroup study. *J Clin Oncol* 1999;17:2137–2143.
46. Dark CG, Bower M, Newlands ES, et al. Surveillance policy for stage I ovarian germ cell tumors. *J Clin Oncol* 1997;15:620–624.
47. Bonazzi C, Peccatori F, Columbo N, et al. Pure ovarian immature teratoma, a unique and curable disease: 10 year's experience of 32 prospectively treated patients. *Obstet Gynecol* 1994;84:598–604.
48. Wangensteen OH, Lewis FJ, Tongen LA. The second-look in cancer surgery. *Lancet* 1951;71:303.
49. Rutledge F, Burns B. Chemotherapy for advanced ovarian cancer. *Am J Obstet Gynecol* 1966;96:761.
50. Williams SD, Blessing JA, DiSaia PJ, et al. Second-look laparotomy in ovarian germ cell tumors: the Gynecologic Oncology Group experience. *Gynecol Oncol* 1994;52:287–291.
51. Jacobs AJ, Harris M, Deppe G, et al. Treatment of recurrent germ cell tumors with cisplatin, vinblastine, and bleomycin. *Obstet Gynecol* 1982;59:129–132.
52. Loehrer PJ, Gonin R. Nichols GR, et al. Vinblastine plus ifosfamide plus cisplatin as initial salvage therapy in recurrent germ cell tumor. *J Clin Oncol* 1998;16:2500–2506.
53. Beyer J, Kramar A, Mandanas R, et al. High-dose chemotherapy as salvage treatment in germ cell tumors: a multivariate analysis of prognostic variables. *J Clin Oncol* 1996;14:2638–2645.
54. Whitehead E, Shalet SM, Blackledge G, et al. The effect of combination chemotherapy on ovarian function in women treated for Hodgkin's disease. *Cancer* 1983;52:988–993.
55. Specht L, Hansen MM, Geisler C. Ovarian function in young women in long-term remission after treatment for Hodgkin's disease stage I or II. *Scand J Haematol* 1984;32:265–270.
56. Siris E, Leventhal BG, Vaitukaitis JL. Effects of childhood leukemia and chemotherapy on puberty and reproductive function in girls. *N Engl J Med* 1976;294:1143.
57. Horning SJ, Hoppe RT, Kaplan HS, Rosenberg SA. Female reproductive potential after treatment for Hodgkin's disease. *N Engl J Med* 1981;304:1377.

58. Brewer M. Gershenson DM, Herzog CE, et al. Outcome and reproduction function after chemotherapy for ovarian dysgerminoma. *J Clin Oncol* 1999;17;2670–2675.
59. Gershenson DM. Menstrual and reproductive function after treatment with combination chemotherapy for malignant ovarian germ cell tumors. *J Clin Oncol* 1998;6:270–275.
60. Pedersen-Bjergaard J, Hansen SW, Larsen SO, et al. Increased risk of myelodysplasia and leukemia after etoposide, cisplatin, and bleomycin for germ-cell tumours. *Lance* 1991;338:359–363.
61. Nichols CR, Breeden ES, Loehrer PJ, et al. Secondary leukemia associated with a conventional dose of etoposide: review of serial germ cell tumor protocols. *J Natl Cancer Inst* 1993;85:36–40.
62. Travis LB, Holoway EJ, Bergfeldt K, et al. Risk of leukemia after platinum-based chemotherapy for ovarian cancer. *N Engl J Med* 1999;4:340:351–357.

21
Management of Ovarian Stromal Tumors

Peter E. Schwartz, Fredric V. Price, and Melanie K. Snyder

Tumors derived from primitive sex cords and gonadal stromal tumors make up the third most common class of neoplasms of the ovary. They represent only about 6% of ovarian tumors, but they are the most common hormonally active neoplasms (1). Although rare, they are of special interest because they exhibit distinct histologic features, produce steroid hormones, and often affect children and young women (2). Early-stage sex cord–stromal tumors are usually managed by conservative surgery. Treatment for advanced-stage disease remains controversial, mainly because of the limited number of patients seen in any single institution over a short period (3). This chapter reviews the clinical features and current therapy for patients with sex cord–stromal and steroid-cell tumors of the ovary. The classification of these tumors is given in Chapter 7.

SEX CORD–STROMAL TUMORS

Granulosa Cell Tumors

Clinical Features

Granulosa cell tumors represent less than 2% of all ovarian tumors, but they account for 6% of all ovarian cancers (1). They can be found in any age group, although reports from single institutions suggest that they occur most frequently in postmenopausal women (1,3,4). Ohel and coworkers (5) reported an epidemiologic study of granulosa cell tumors from Israel. Over a 15-year period, 172 cases were diagnosed, for an incidence of 0.9 cases per 100,000 women per year. The incidence in women of European or American background was almost twice that of women of African or Asian descent (0.98 versus 0.552 per 100,000 per year). The calculated incidence of granulosa cell tumors is 0.99 per 100,000 white women the United States (5). Fewer than 5% of these tumors occur before puberty (1,6). Three fourths of prepubertal granulosa cell tumors are associated with isosexual pseudoprecocity caused by estrogen secretion from the tumor (1,6). Stimulation of the endometrium by unopposed estrogen can lead to hyperplasia, which is frequently reported in association with granulosa cell tumors. Up to 13% of these patients develop well-differentiated adenocarcinoma of the endometrium (7–9). Breast swelling, tenderness, and pain can also be associated with unopposed estrogen secretion by granulosa cell tumors. Rarely, virilizing effects have been observed, usually in association with very large unilocular or multilocular thin-walled cystic masses (10,11). Patients with granulosa cell tumors have not demonstrated an increased incidence of infertility, despite the association with excessive hormone production (5). A four-fold increased incidence of breast cancer has been reported among Israeli patients with granulosa cell tumors.

The most common presenting symptoms of granulosa cell tumors are abnormal uterine bleeding and pain. Women in their reproductive years often experience amenorrhea, and postmenopausal women may present with vaginal bleeding. In older patients, the symptoms of granulosa cell tumors may mimic those of common epithelial cancer, such as vague abdominal discomfort, increasing abdominal girth, and weight loss. In a series of 51 patients treated at a single institution, Schwartz and Smith (3) noted that most of the patients with granulosa cell tumors were in their fifth and sixth decades of life. The most common presenting symptoms were postmenopausal bleeding, the presence of a mass, and pelvic or abdominal pain. Similar presenting symptoms were observed in the series of Fox and colleagues (8) and Ohel and associates (5). In approximately 10% of patients, the tumor is either discovered at the time of surgery for abnormal bleeding or found only after histologic examination of the specimen (1).

The juvenile variant of granulosa cell tumor usually occurs before the normal age of puberty and is associated with microscopic features that distinguish it from the adult granulosa cell tumor (2). Patients with juvenile granulosa cell tumors often present with isosexual precocity (1). An association has been found with Potter syndrome (12), multiple congenital anomalies (13), Ollier disease (multiple enchondromatosis) (14,15), and Maffucci syndrome (Ollier disease with hemangiomas) (16). Approximately 90% of granulosa cell tumors found in prepubertal patients, and many tumors found in women younger than 30 years of age, are juvenile granulosa cell tumors (17). Of 124 patients in the series by Young and colleagues (17), 121 had stage I lesions and 3 had stage II lesions. Eleven tumors ruptured preoperatively, and 2 ruptured intraoperatively. Only 4 of the patients were older than 30 years of age at the time of diagnosis.

Rupture of adult granulosa cell tumors was reported by Stenwig and colleagues (18) to occur in 10% of patients. In the series of Schwartz and Smith (3), 35% of the tumors (13/37) ruptured. Five of these ruptured within 24 hours of surgery, and 8 ruptured at the time of surgery. Torsion can produce acute abdominal signs and symptoms (8), but huge hemorrhagic granulosa cell tumors may be relatively asymptomatic (19). Spread of these tumors is by local, direct extension and intraperitoneal seeding. They rarely spread hematogenously. Diddle (20) found that only 8% of 110 cases had lymph node metastasis at postmortem examination.

Granulosa cell tumors are the most classic late-recurring malignancies in gynecology. Recurrence may not be detected for more than 5 years after the original diagnosis. Hines and associates reported a recurrence after 37 years, and their review of the literature depicted 16 cases with recurrence from 13 to 37 years after original diagnosis (21). However, 14 of 19 patients with recurrent granulosa cell tumors were identified within 3 years after the original diagnosis in the Schwartz and Smith series (3), and more than half of the recurrences were identified within 2 years in the series of Fox and colleagues (8).

Experiments (22) using a laboratory strain of mice with a propensity to develop granulosa cell tumors have increased understanding of the pathogenesis of these tumors. Progression of granulosa cells through abnormal folliculogenesis to frank metastatic granulosa cell tumors has been seen, suggesting that granulosa cell tumors may result from abnormal follicles. A granulosa cell susceptibility gene has been identified in these mice (23,24). An association with trisomy 12 in humans has been reported (25,26), but the clinical significance is unclear. Contrary to earlier reports linking trisomy 12 to granulosa cell tumors, Shashi and colleagues (27) reported a stronger correlation between trisomy 12 and thecoma-fibroma tumors rather than granulosa cell tumors. There has been research into DNA ploidy of granulosa cell tumors and clinical prognosis. Despite a correlation between DNA ploidy and prognosis of epithelial ovarian tumors, granulosa cell tumor data reveal ambiguous results (28,29,30).

Management

The management of granulosa cell tumors is based on important prognostic factors, such as the International Federation of Gynecology and Obstetrics (FIGO) stage of the tumor, age of the patient, and volume of residual tumor after the initial operation (2–4,8,18,31). The microscopic pattern of granulosa cell tumors does not appear to correlate with prognosis. One half of the tumors in several series contained the diffuse growth pattern without any apparent effect on prognosis (3,18,22). Mitotic activity was of prognostic significance in two series (18,32) and in the experience of Bjorkholm and Silfversward (4). A high degree of nuclear atypia was also shown to be a bad prognostic finding. Flow cytometry has been used to study granulosa cell tumors, and the percentage of cells in S phase may provide a means for determining which patients are likely to benefit from adjuvant therapy (33–35).

TABLE 21.1. *Potential circulating tumor markers for stromal tumors of the ovary*

Granulosa cell tumors
  Inhibin (30B,30C,31,32)
  Müllerian Inhibiting Subs (32D)
  Follicle regulatory protein (33)
Sertoli-Leydig cell tumors
  Alpha-fetoprotein (77–83)
  Inhibin (84)
  Testosterone and dihydrotestosterone (70)
  Androstenedione (70)
Steroid-cell tumors
  Testosterone and dihydrotestosterone (96,97,103)
  Dehydroepiandrosterone (103)

Progress has been made toward identifying a circulating tumor marker for granulosa cell tumors of the ovary (Table 21.1). Inhibin has come to attention as such a marker. Inhibin is a glycoprotein hormone that inhibits the production and/or secretion of pituitary gonadotropins, specifically follicle-stimulating hormone (FSH) (36); it has been detected in ovarian tumor tissue by immunohistochemistry (37). Inhibin has been postulated to be biologically active in granulosa cell tumors, as evidenced from the inverse relation between elevated inhibin concentrations and FSH levels (38). Serum inhibin levels have been found to be increased seven times above the normal premenopausal level in women with granulosa cell tumors, and increased serum levels presage clinical recurrence (38,39). Elevated serum concentrations of the peptide hormone inhibin have been shown to return to normal after resection of granulosa cell tumors and appear to correlate with tumor burden found at laparotomy (40,41). Immunohistochemically, inhibin may be helpful in identifying extraovarian metastases in patients with primary granulosa cell tumors of the ovary and subsequent distant recurrence (42).

Antimüllerian hormone (AMH) has also been reported to be a tumor marker for granulosa cell tumors (43). Rey and coworkers showed in a study of 16 patients that AMH is a reliable marker for disease with less fluctuation from normal levels than inhibin during clinical remission (44). Follicle regulatory protein, which is secreted by normal granulosa cells, may also be useful as a tumor marker (45).

Surgical staging at the time of the initial operation is important for determining which patients are likely to have recurrence and to require adjuvant therapy (46). The initial operation should be performed through a vertical midline or paramedian incision to allow adequate exposure of the upper abdomen and the pelvis. On entry into the peritoneal cavity, ascites or free fluid should be aspirated and sent for cytology and cell block analysis. If no fluid is present, approximately 100 mL of normal saline should be instilled into the pelvis and each lateral paracolic space. The irrigant should be aspirated and sent for cytology and cell block analysis. The involved ovary should be excised, and the nature of the tumor should be confirmed histologically by frozen section. If the patient is young, desires to preserve fertility, and appears to have disease confined to one ovary, a wedge biopsy of the opposite ovary should be performed and sent for frozen section to rule out the presence of microscopic disease. An omentectomy and samples of multiple intraperitoneal sites should be taken, including the diaphragm peritoneum, lateral paracolic peritoneum, small and large bowel serosa, cul-desac, and pelvic sidewall peritoneum; and paraaortic and pelvic lymph nodes should be biopsied. If all biopsy specimens and washings are free of disease, no further therapy is recommended (Figure 21.1).

The management of patients with ruptured granulosa cell tumors remains controversial. Bjorkholm and Silfversward (4) reviewed a 50-year experience and found that patients with clinical stage I disease whose tumors ruptured did significantly worse than those whose tumors were removed intact. However, the staging for most of these patients was probably incomplete. A more recent review by Kietlinska and colleagues confirms that stage IA disease carries a significantly better survival rate within 20 years of diagnosis than does stage IC (47). They also noted that radical surgery rather than fertility-preserving surgery gave patients a better 5-year rate survival without recurrence, but this finding was not statistically significant and patient number was small. In a young patient with a ruptured tumor who has undergone proper operative staging and wishes to preserve fertility, we believe

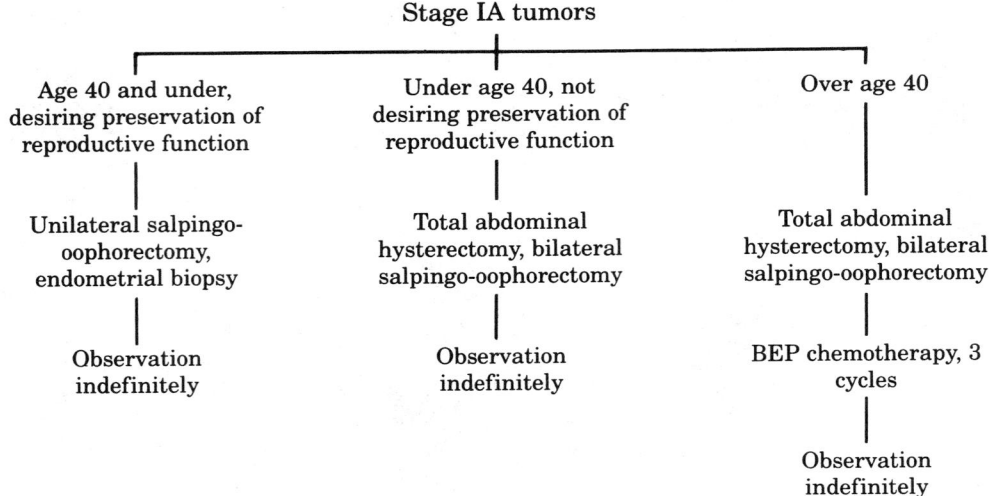

FIG. 21.1. Management of early stromal tumors.

that three courses of combination chemotherapy with bleomycin, etoposide, and cisplatin (BEP) should be offered (Figure 21.2). The recommended dosages are given in Table 21.2.

Disease that involves both ovaries or has metastasized to the pelvis or upper abdomen requires more aggressive therapy. Debulking surgery should be performed to remove as much gross tumor as possible. Patients with suspected advanced disease should have a preoperative bowel preparation. A preoperative intravenous pyelogram is extremely helpful in identifying ureteral obstruction, deviation, or duplication, and it can sometimes identify bladder infiltration. A barium enema can rule out primary bowel disorders such as carcinoma or diverticulitis with abscess, and it may identify sites of extrinsic compression. Alternatively, a computed tomographic (CT) scan of the abdomen and pelvis with intravenous and oral contrast can yield even more information about the nature of the primary tumor and sites of metastases.

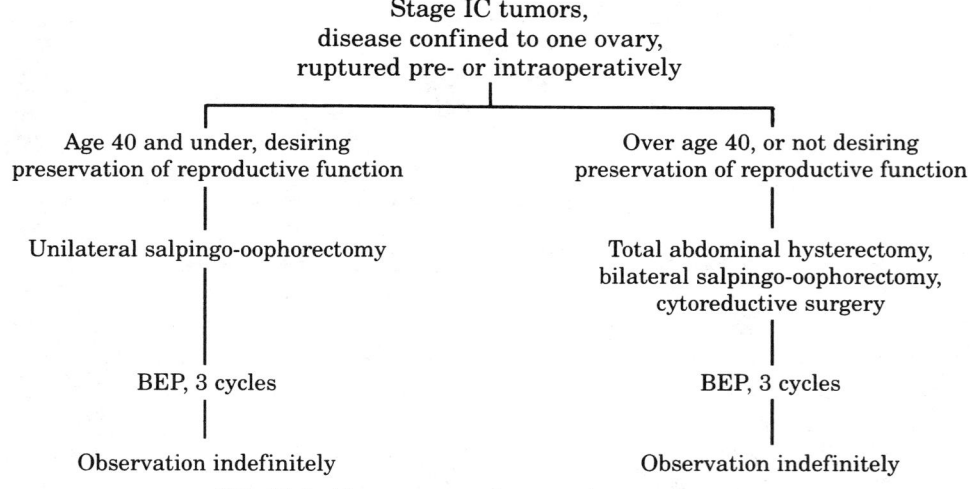

FIG. 21.2. Management of ruptured stromal tumors.

TABLE 21.2. Chemotherapy regimens for stromal tumors

BEP	
Cisplatin	Day 1: 100 mg/m^2 continuous infusion over 24 h
Etoposide (VP-16)	Days 1 to 4: 100 mg/m^2 bolus
Bleomycin	Days 3 to 5: 10 units/m^2 over 96 h
VAC	
Vincristine	1.5 mg/m^2 (max. dose 2.5 mg) IV q.d. × 5 days, q. 4 weeks
Actinomycin D	0.5 mg IV q.d. × 5 days, q. 4 weeks
Cyclophosphamide	5 to 7 mg/kg (max. single dose 500 mg) IV q.d. × 5 days, q. 4 weeks

Postoperative adjuvant therapy remains controversial because of the small number of patients in any reported series. Combination chemotherapies (Table 21.2) include VAC (vincristine, dactinomycin, and cyclophosphamide); PVB (cisplatin, vinblastine, and bleomycin); and BEP. Such combinations have been extremely successful in the management of germ cell malignancies (46–50). PVB is active in patients with previously untreated granulosa cell tumors (51,52), but some dose-limiting neurotoxicity and fatalities have been reported. The BEP regimen, which substitutes etoposide for vinblastine, is better tolerated. BEP is currently recommended for adjuvant postoperative chemotherapy at Yale University School of Medicine, based on its acceptable toxicity and activity against germ cell tumors of the testis and ovary (53). This regimen is offered to women with stage IA granulosa cell tumors who are older than 40 years of age and to all women with stages IB to IV granulosa cell tumors (Figures 21.2 and 21.3). Gershenson and colleagues reported a series of nine patients with a response to BEP chemotherapy, but the data were not from a large sample size (54). A Gynecologic Oncology Group trial of BEP chemotherapy has produced results for the largest series of stromal malignancies thus far published (55). The series comprised 75 patients, of whom 38 had evaluable disease, and BEP was shown to be an active chemotheraputic regimen, although it did have significant myelotoxicity (56). In this study, 69% of patients with advanced primary disease and 51% of those with recurrent disease remained progression free with BEP.

A schema for follow-up of patients with granulosa cell tumors is presented in Table 21.3. Patients must be monitored carefully for the rest of their lives so that recurrence can be detected early. The Yale University School of Medicine advocates examining patients every 3 months for the first year after diagnosis of a stage IA granulosa cell tumor, every 4 months

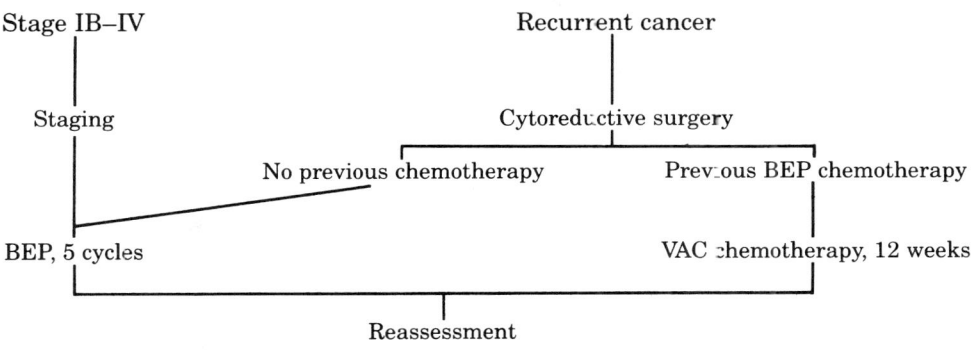

FIG. 21.3. Management of advanced or recurrent stromal tumors.

TABLE 21.3. *Recommendations for follow-up of patients with stromal tumors*

Physical examination including pelvic exam
  First year: every 3 months
  Second to fifth year: every 4 months
  After fifth year: every 6 months
Computed tomography (CT) scan
  After completion of therapy as baseline study
  For unexplained abdominal symptoms or hormonal changes
Chest x-ray
  Annually
Tumor markers
  As available

for the second year, and every 6 months until 5 years from diagnosis, after which the patients are examined annually. At each follow-up visit, a routine physical examination, including pelvic examination, is performed. A chest radiograph is obtained annually. Patients who are treated with chemotherapy are evaluated every 4 weeks during therapy. Patients who receive adjuvant radiation therapy are monitored in a similar manner. Second-look laparotomy should be reserved for patients in formal experimental protocols. Tumor markers inhibin and müllerian inhibiting substance may be measured with each visit.

Patients treated only with surgery may develop recurrent cancer (3). Management of recurrence should involve aggressive debulking surgery followed by combination chemotherapy (Figure 21.3). Most recurrent granulosa cell tumors occur in the peritoneal cavity, although liver, lung, and skeletal metastases can also occur (8,57). Transient responses to doxorubicin-based combination regimens have been reported (58–61), but the first choice for management of recurrent granulosa cell tumors at the Yale University School of Medicine is presently the BEP regimen. For patients previously treated with BEP, the VAC regimen is offered (Figure 21.3).

Radiation therapy, although often overlooked in favor of chemotherapy, may play a role in the treatment of residual primary disease or recurrent granulosa cell tumor. A retrospective study by Wolf and coworkers reported on 14 patients with measurable disease treated with irradiation (62). Overall response rate was 43% with 6 of the 14 patients completely responding and follow-up ranging from 5 to 21 years. Radiation may also play a role in the treatment of a recurrent granulosa cell tumor if the patient is found to have an isolated metastasis that can be completely resected. A small field of intense radiation therapy has been associated with prolonged survival. A case has been reported of a 4-year-old with juvenile granulosa cell tumor treated with regional deep hyperthermia for a liver metastasis, along with chemotherapy and adjuvant radiation (63). Margolin and colleagues (57) noted that intraabdominal hemorrhage is a frequent preterminal event in advanced recurrent granulosa cell tumors.

Recurrent disease may also be managed with hormone therapy, but experience is limited. Schwartz and associates (65) reported the presence of cytosol estrogen receptors in one of three granulosa cell tumors, with increased levels of cytosol progestin receptors in two of the three tumors (the remaining tumor had borderline levels of cytosol progestin receptors). One patient with a progestin receptor–positive tumor was treated for advanced recurrent disease with oral progestins, and her disease was stable for 10 months. It was again stabilized for 4 months with oral antiestrogen therapy (tamoxifen). Malik and Slevin (66) reported on two patients treated with high doses of medroxyprogesterone acetate who responded with prolonged remissions after documented widespread recurrence. Treatment with a gonadotropin-releasing hormone (GnRH) analog achieved a transient partial response in one patient who had a recurrence after cytotoxic chemotherapy (67).

Management of juvenile granulosa cell tumors is based on the same prognostic factors as that of the adult tumors. Young and colleagues (17) demonstrated that stage was overwhelmingly the most important prognostic factor. Only 1 of 70 patients with juvenile granulosa cell tumor confined to one ovary died from the disease, and 1 of 10 patients with ruptured capsules and 2 of 10 with ascites died from their disease. However, each of 2 patients with stage IIB lesions and the only patient with a stage IIC lesion died from the disease.

Tumors in the Thecoma-Fibroma Group

Tumors in this group of sex cord–stromal neoplasms represent a spectrum that ranges from the benign thecoma to the fibrosarcoma, including a group of "unclassified tumors" that have cells characteristic of both types (1,2). The sclerosing stromal tumor is also in this category.

Thecomas

Clinical Features

Thecomas account for fewer than 1% of all ovarian tumors. They are rare before puberty and occur most often in perimenopausal and postmenopausal women (1,6). Fewer than 10% of the cases are diagnosed in patients younger than 30 years of age. Accurate statistics about the frequency of tumors in this group are difficult to obtain because of similarities between thecomas and fibromas and between thecomas and lipid-containing nodules of stromal hyperplasia (6). Often, the distinctions between these benign entities are arbitrary, and the term fibrothecoma has been used to describe tumors with characteristics of both fibromas and thecomas (1).

Thecomas are seldom malignant (68), are usually smaller than granulosa cell tumors, and are less likely to be palpable. In many cases, surgery is undertaken for reasons other than expected ovarian pathology, and the diagnosis is made incidentally (69). Most thecomas are associated with estrogen production, and uterine bleeding is a frequent presenting symptom (1,69). These tumors may also be associated with endometrial hyperplasia and, occasionally, adenocarcinoma. Because morphologic criteria for distinguishing thecomas from fibromas are inexact and each tumor may contain intracytoplasmic lipids, Young and Scully (70) reserve the designation of "thecoma" for stromal tumors that are associated with evidence of steroid hormone production. Roth and Sternberg (71) reported four cases of partly luteinized theca cell tumors of the ovary, two of which were associated with endometrial hyperplasia. The partly luteinized theca cell tumor tends to occur in young women and to have a benign course.

Four cases of benign, densely calcified thecomas in young women were reported by Young and colleagues (72). These tumors were palpable and visible on plain radiographs of the abdomen. Dense calcification was the most prominent histologic feature, with adipose metaplasia in one case. These tumors produced characteristic menstrual irregularities due to estrogen secretion.

Management

Unilateral oophorectomy is adequate treatment for a thecoma. Secondary endocrine manifestations are reversed with excision of the tumor (71). Sampling of the endometrium should be performed routinely in patients with a thecoma treated by unilateral oophorectomy to be certain that endometrial hyperplasia or carcinoma is not present. In older women, a total abdominal hysterectomy and bilateral salpingo-oophorectomy is recommended.

Fibromas

Clinical Features

Fibromas represent approximately 4% of all ovarian tumors. Ovarian fibromas have an appearance that is distinct from that of fibromas occurring elsewhere in the body (1). The average age at presentation is 48 years (6), and fewer than 10% of fibromas are reported to occur before age 30. The characteristic findings of multinodular, bilateral, and calcified fibromas are associated with the basal cell nevus syndrome that develops in young women (73). Fibromas are also well known for their association with ascites and right hydrothorax (Meigs syndrome) (74). However, fewer than 1% of all fibromas are associated with this syndrome. Ascites is associated with tumors greater than 10 cm in diameter in 40% of the cases (75).

Management

Oophorectomy is required for management of the typical fibroma or cellular fibroma. A total abdominal hysterectomy and bilateral salpingo-oophorectomy is recommended for patients who are older than 40 years of age. The rare fibrosarcoma should be treated with BEP chemotherapy (Table 21.2). Patients with fibromas of uncertain malignant potential should be examined frequently for signs of recurrent cancer (Table 21.3).

Sclerosing Stromal Tumor

In contrast to the other tumors in the thecoma-fibroma group, 80% of sclerosing stromal tumors occur in women younger than 30 years of age (70,76,77). Endocrine manifestations are infrequent. Only 5% of sclerosing stromal tumors have been associated with endometrial hyperplasia. Androgen production has been reported in two cases (77,78), and secretion of estradiol, progesterone, and testosterone was demonstrated in a sclerosing stromal tumor by Yuen and colleagues (79). Definitive production of hormonal activity, however, has not been consistently reported (80). No bilateral or malignant cases of sclerosing stromal tumor have yet been reported (1), and most tumors occur on the right adnexa (80). Reversal of endometrial hyperplasia and infertility has been reported after tumor removal (81).

Current management is limited to unilateral oophorectomy in young women and removal of the uterus and both ovaries in older women. Endometrial sampling is appropriate for women treated by removal of only the involved ovary. Reversal of primary infertility in a patient with a functioning sclerosing stromal tumor has been accomplished by oophorectomy (79).

"Unclassified" and Stromal Tumors with Minor Sex Cord Elements

Fibromas or thecomas that are found to contain up to 5% sex cord components on any slide examined are called "stromal tumors with minor sex cord elements" (1). Unclassified tumors are defined by the presence of cells that are intermediate between thecomas and fibromas. These tumors occur in the same age distribution as tumors in the thecoma-fibroma group. Scully (6) suggested that rare cellular tumors that are reported to be malignant thecomas possibly belong in this category.

Removal of the involved ovary is satisfactory treatment for patients who desire preservation of reproductive function. Most patients with unclassified tumors, however, are older than 30 years of age, and total abdominal hysterectomy with bilateral salpingo-oophorectomy is recommended (Figure 21.1). A large review by Seidman confirmed the difficulty with regard to classification of this tumor (82). He agreed that prognosis is good, with a 5-year survival rate of 92%. Many of these tumors are not formally staged, however, and the rarity of the diagnosis precludes prospective studies.

Sertoli-Leydig Cell Tumors (Androblastomas)

Clinical Features

Sertoli-Leydig cell tumors are rare sex cord–stromal tumors of the ovary that contain cells that resemble Sertoli cells, Leydig cells, and indifferent stromal cells of the testes in their cytologic features and growth pattern. The older term of "arrhenoblastoma" is no longer used because it connotes masculinization, which is an inconstant feature. Many Sertoli-Leydig cell tumors are associated with virilization, but some are inactive, and others are estrogenic (83). These tumors can be responsible for isosexual pseudoprecocity, and they can secrete progesterone and simulate pregnancy (84). Sertoli-Leydig cell tumors account for fewer than 0.2% of ovarian neoplasms (6). The average age of patients with Sertoli-Leydig cell tumors is 25 years. Fewer than 5% of these tumors occur in prepubertal girls, and approximately 10% occur in women over 50 years of age. Seven examples of familial occurrence of Sertoli-Leydig cell tumors have been reported to date (85). An association with Peutz-Jeghers syndrome was found in two sisters. The tumors are unilateral and almost always have a benign course (86). Virilization has been reported in approximately half of the collected pathology reports of Sertoli-Leydig cell tumors (2). Young and Scully (85) reported that one third of their series of 207 patients with Sertoli-Leydig cell tumors had unequivocal virilization, but an additional 10% had histories that suggested androgen excess. In one series of 64 patients with intermediate and poorly differentiated Sertoli-Leydig cell tumors, the most commonly occurring symptoms (46%) were nonspecific. The most frequent symptoms were a palpable abdominal mass, abdominal distention, and pain (87). Five patients in that series presented with an acute abdomen due to torsion of the involved ovary. Menstrual disorders and virilization were noted in 24 (38%) of the 63 patients. Ollier disease (enchondromatosis), usually associated with granulosa cell tumors, has been reported in association with a Sertoli-Leydig cell tumor (88).

Virilization does not appear to be related to tumor differentiation (83,86,87). Usually, oligomenorrhea is followed by amenorrhea and then by defeminization, which is manifested by breast atrophy and loss of body contours. Acne and hirsutism proceed to frank virilization. Virilized patients have clitoromegaly, deepening of the voice, and temporal recession of the hairline. Menses returns to normal after removal of the tumor. Some loss of excess hair occurs, but voice changes and regression of clitoromegaly may not occur (2). Characteristically, Sertoli-Leydig cell tumors make large quantities of testosterone, androstenedione, or both, but levels of dehydroepiandrosterone (DHEA) may be normal or slightly elevated (88–90). The differential diagnosis of virilization includes adrenal tumors, which are typically associated with high serum levels of dehydroepiandrosterone sulfate (DHEAS). Adrenal tumors are essentially excluded by a normal serum DHEAS level. In general, suppression of ovarian and adrenal androgen production is not useful for distinguishing tumors in these sites (91). CT canning of the adrenals and ovaries should be done if DHEAS levels are normal and there is no palpable adnexal mass. Magnetic resonance imaging (MRI) may also be valuable in diagnosing small androgen-secreting ovarian tumors (92) and distinguishing them from adrenal neoplasms. Although it rarely is necessary, localization of functioning ovarian and adrenal tumors may be accomplished with the use of radiolabeled norcholesterols such as [^{131}I]-iodomethylnorcholesterol (93) or [^{75}Se]-selenomethylnorcholesterol (94), which localize lesions according to their biologic activity rather than their size or anatomic characteristics.

Sertoli-Leydig cell tumors may be estrogenic and can be associated with isosexual precocity, menometrorrhagia, or postmenopausal bleeding. No specific cell type dominates such tumors. Scully (6) suggested that these estrogenic manifestations may be related to the ovarian tumor in several ways. Androgen levels may be sufficient to prevent ovulation but insufficient to completely inhibit the release of gonadotropins, follicular activity, and estrogen secretion. The tumor itself may produce estrogen in either the Sertoli or Leydig cells. Androgens may be converted to estrogens by other tissues. Tseng and others (95) demonstrated that endometrial cancer cells have aromatase activity that can result in conversion of circulating androgens to estrogens. There are no histologic or immunocytochemical features of Sertoli-Leydig cell tumors that consistently correlate with virilization (87).

Management

In the series of Young and Scully (85), Sertoli-Leydig cell tumors had a malignant course in 18% of the cases. The most important indicators of prognosis are FIGO stage and degree of differentiation (86). Complete surgical staging is important for deciding whether adjuvant therapy is necessary. The surgical staging approach that is recommended for patients with granulosa cell tumors is also used for patients with Sertoli-Leydig cell tumors (46). Patients with only one involved ovary, a smooth capsule, no ascites, and an unruptured tumor may be treated with unilateral oophorectomy alone if preservation of fertility is important. Ten of 22 patients with malignant Sertoli-Leydig cell tumors in the series reported by Young and Scully (86) had unruptured tumors confined to one ovary. The completeness of surgical staging did not seem to relate to outcome. Women older than 40 years of age are advised to undergo a total abdominal hysterectomy and bilateral salpingo-oophorectomy (Figures 21.1 and 21.2) (3). For FIGO stage IA tumors, histology is an important prognostic factor. Approximately 10% of 200 patients in a collected series of Sertoli-Leydig cell tumors had well-differentiated tumors, and each was treated successfully by oophorectomy alone. No recurrences were noted in the 21 patients in Young and Scully's series (86), and none have been reported elsewhere in the literature.

Zaloudek and Norris (87) reported on a collected series of 64 intermediate and poorly differentiated neoplasms in which 62 of 64 patients had stage IA disease (2 patients had stage III lesions). The 5- and 10-year actuarial survival rates (92%) supported the role of unilateral oophorectomy in the management of stage IA tumors. Metastatic disease in this series was associated with poor differentiation, the presence of heterologous mesenchymal elements (e.g., cartilage, striated muscle), frequent mitotic figures in stromal cells (more than five per 10 high-power fields), and tumor rupture. Tumor size and the presence of heterologous mucinous elements were not of prognostic significance. Seven additional patients reported by Zaloudek and Norris (87) had well-differentiated tumors, and each was alive and well 1 to 12.2 years after diagnosis.

Patients with FIGO stages IB to IV disease should undergo total abdominal hysterectomy, bilateral salpingo-oophorectomy, and tumor debulking (Figure 21.3). Sertoli-Leydig cell tumors usually do not spread by hematogenous dissemination. Adjuvant VAC, PVB, or BEP chemotherapy has been recommended for patients with significant residual disease (Table 21.2). Schwartz and Smith (3) reported that two patients treated with VAC responded to this regimen. Zaloudek and Norris (87) reported a similar response with VAC therapy. Pride and colleagues (96) reported a complete response to BV-CAP (vincristine, bleomycin, cyclophosphamide, doxorubicin, and cisplatin) in a pregnant patient with metastatic Sertoli-Leydig cell tumor. Patients with stages IB to IV or recurrent Sertoli-Leydig cell tumors are routinely recommended for adjuvant therapy (Figure 21.3). The current treatment recommendation at the Yale University School of Medicine is the BEP regimen (Table 20.2), based on its acceptable toxicity and documented activity against germ cell tumors of the testis and ovary.

Several cases of elevated α-fetoprotein levels in the serum of patients with Sertoli-Leydig cell tumors have been reported (Table 21.1) (97–101). This marker can be demonstrated by immunohistochemical techniques within the tumor (102,103). The serum inhibin level, which is a marker of early recurrence for granulosa cell tumors, may also be increased by Sertoli-Leydig cell tumors (Table 21.1) (104). These circulating markers may be useful for monitoring Sertoli-Leydig cell tumors and for early diagnosis of recurrent disease.

Gynandroblastoma

The gynandroblastoma is an extremely rare tumor that contains substantial elements of both Sertoli-Leydig and granulosa-stromal cell tumors. Scully (6) noted that it is common for sex cord–stromal tumors to contain cells that are normally associated with gonads of the opposite sex. Granulosa-stromal cell tumors may have Sertoli-Leydig cell elements, and Sertoli-Leydig cell tumors may have granulosa-stromal cell elements. However, such findings are insufficient to place these tumors in the gynandroblastoma category; they should be included in pure categories. For a tumor to be called a gynandroblastoma, it must contain at least 10% of the minor element (1). Using this criterion, Scully (6) suggested that almost all published cases of gynandroblastomas can be categorized as granulosa-stromal tumors, Sertoli-Leydig cell tumors, or unclassified tumors. The presence of both male and female elements in the same tumor suggests that the granulosa-stromal cell and Sertoli-Leydig cell tumors have a common origin. Treatment recommendations would be the same as for other sex cord–stromal tumors, and would be based on adequate surgical staging (Tables 21.1 and 21.2). Patients in whom fertility is a consideration may be treated with conservative surgery (Figure 21.1).

Sex Cord Tumors with Annular Tubules

Clinical Features

Sex cord tumors with annular tubules have been regarded as granulosa cell tumors by some pathologists (105) and as Sertoli-Leydig cell tumors by others (106). One third of the cases have been reported in association with Peutz-Jeghers syndrome (gastrointestinal polyposis with oral and cutaneous hyperpigmentation) and minimal deviation carcinoma of the cervix (1,107). Young and colleagues (107) reported that almost all patients with Peutz-Jeghers syndrome have sex cord tumors with annular tubules.

In 40% of patients with these tumors, signs of increased estrogen secretion are present (107). Secretory hyperplasia of the endometrium has also been seen, which suggests that some sex cord tumors with annular tubules may secrete progestins (108). These tumors tend to be multifocal, bilateral, and less than 3 cm in diameter, and they are frequently associated with calcification. Sex cord tumors with annular tubules have never been reported to be malignant when associated with Peutz-Jeghers syndrome, but they may be malignant when associated with minimal deviation adenocarcinoma of the cervix (adenoma malignum) (107,108). These tumors, when seen in Peutz-Jeghers syndrome, are usually incidental findings at the time of surgery for other indications (109).

Sex cord tumors with annular tubules not associated with Peutz-Jeghers syndrome are usually large, unilateral lesions. Only 1 of 50 patients reported by Young and colleagues (107) had microscopic disease. Forty percent of these patients show clinical manifestations of excessive estrogen production. Calcifications are not present in these tumors (1).

Management

Stage IA sex cord tumors with annular tubules that do not arise in association with Peutz-Jeghers syndrome may be successfully managed by unilateral oophorectomy. However, at least 20% of these tumors are malignant. Experience in the management of these tumors is limited, but the recommendation would be the same as for granulosa cell tumors (Figures 21.1 through 21.3).

Sex cord tumors with annular tubules that caused isosexual precocity in association with Peutz-Jeghers syndrome in two young girls were reported by Young and colleagues (110). Each patient had a single large tumor, which differed from the small, multiple, bilateral tumors usually found in association with Peutz-Jeghers syndrome. The tumors had a complex histologic pattern, with diffuse areas, foci of hollow tubular differentiation, microcysts, and papillae. Two predominant epithelial cell types were seen, one with scant and the other with abundant cytoplasm. Unilateral oophorectomy was apparently curative in these cases.

Unclassified Sex Cord–Stromal Tumors

In approximately 5% to 10% of sex cord–stromal tumors, classification as a Sertoli-Leydig cell tumor or granulosa-stromal cell tumor is not possible because the features are suggestive but not characteristic of either tumor (1). The cells fail to differentiate clearly into male or female elements. These tumors tend to be poorly differentiated and presumably are more malignant than classified granulosa-stromal cell or Sertoli-Leydig cell tumors. Pregnancy makes the diagnosis of sex cord–stromal tumors more difficult. Edema and differential maturation of the underlying granulosa cells cause up to 17% of sex cord–stromal tumors to remain "unclassified" in pregnancy (111).

STEROID-CELL TUMORS

Because 40% of what are called "lipid" and "lipoid" cell tumors do not contain intracellular fat, Young and colleagues advocated the more general term "steroid-cell tumors" to describe this rare group. This category is further divided into the three subcategories of stromal luteoma, Leydig cell tumor (hilar and nonhilar types), and steroid-cell tumor not otherwise specified (NOS) (112).

Stromal Luteoma

Twenty percent of steroid-cell tumors are stromal luteomas. These are small tumors that presumably arise from the adjacent ovarian stroma. They typically develop after menopause, with an average age of 58 years at presentation. Approximately 60% of stromal luteomas are associated with hyperestrogenism, and 12% are androgenic (113). The designation of stromal luteoma is reserved for grossly visible tumors that are completely confined to the ovarian stroma. They are well-circumscribed and rarely exceed 3 cm (113). Microscopically, a mass of luteinized cells arranged in cords or nests is usually seen, with eosinophilic cytoplasm and scant lipid content. Ninety percent of stromal luteomas are associated with stromal hyperthecosis, which may partially explain their hormonal manifestations (113).

Leydig (Hilus) Cell Tumor

Leydig cell tumors are classified according to the location of their cells of origin. They are rare ovarian neoplasms that are diagnosed only if crystalloids of Reinke are present in the cytoplasm. Leydig cell tumors may originate in the hilus or within the ovarian stroma. Hilus cells are present in association with nonmyelinated nerve fibers in 80% to 85% of normal ovaries. The majority of Leydig cell tumors develop in these cells (1) and are often called hilus cell tumors. Only four Leydig cell tumors arising from within the ovarian stroma have been reported (6,114). Hilus cells and Leydig cells are morphologically identical (115), and the distinction between hilar and nonhilar Leydig cell tumors is based on location only. In the majority of cases, crystalloids of Reinke can be identified only by electron microscopy, and many unclassified sex cord–stromal tumors may actually be from this group of steroid-cell tumors. Sometimes cells from steroid-cell tumors NOS exhibit morphologic similarity to Leydig cells, but crystalloids of Reinke cannot be identified. These tumors are sometimes called "crystal-negative" hilus cell tumors (112).

Clinical Features

Approximately 40 cases of Leydig (hilus) cell tumors have been reported (115). Seventy-five percent of these tumors are associated with some degree of virilization (1), although it is milder than what is usually seen in patients with Sertoli-Leydig cell tumors. Estrogenic manifestations such as endometrial hyperplasia or cancer may be seen, as may obesity, hypertension, diabetes, and erythrocytosis. Leydig (hilus) cell tumors tend to secrete primarily testosterone, and peripheral blood levels may be greater than 300 ng/dL (116,117). Patients with Leydig (hilus) cell tumors are almost always premenopausal or postmenopausal.

Management

These tumors are almost invariably unilateral and benign, and they are treated adequately with unilateral oophorectomy. Two cases of malignant hilus cell tumor have been reported (116–118). They were associated with both local spread and distant metastases, but unequivocal documentation of crystalloids of Reinke was lacking (8,112).

Steroid-Cell Tumors Not Otherwise Specified

In general, steroid-cell tumors NOS are composed of large, round, or polyhedral cells that resemble Leydig, lutein, and adrenal cortical cells, but they cannot be identified specifically as any of the three. Their cytogenesis is not well understood (112).

Clinical Features

Steroid-cell tumors NOS accounted for 56% of steroid-cell tumors in the series of Hayes and Scully (119). They can occur in any age group and are associated with steroid production. Although they are often virilizing, they can also be estrogenic, and rare cases of isosexual pseudoprecocity have been reported. Steroid secretion by these tumors may vary considerably. Most tumors produce testosterone, androstenedione, and dehydroepiandrosterone, with serum levels similar to those of a virilizing adrenal tumor (120). Four cases of frank Cushing syndrome have been reported (1,121).

Although most tumors are found confined to a single ovary, 40% behave in a malignant fashion. Metastasis is an inconstant feature that is most commonly associated with larger tumors (greater than 7 cm), older age, and nuclear atypia with high mitotic rate.

Management

Most steroid-cell tumors are confined to one ovary, and unilateral oophorectomy is considered adequate surgical management. However, the recommendations for adjuvant therapy are not consistent because of the rarity of these tumors. In the series of Taylor and Norris (122), more than 20% of patients with lipid-cell tumors developed intraabdominal metastases or recurrences. Tumors greater than 8 cm in diameter were more likely to be malignant. Patsner and Piver (123) reported a patient who presented to them with persistent disease after therapy. The patient had been treated initially with whole-abdomen irradiation followed by six courses of 5-fluorouracil, cyclophosphamide, and megestrol acetate. After complete debulking, the patient was treated with BV-CAP. After a positive second-look laparotomy, the patient was treated with VAC chemotherapy. The disease remained stable for a short time but then progressed, and the patient died. Serum dihydrotestosterone and testosterone were effective markers of tumor recurrence and response to therapy. At the Yale University School of Medicine, the current treatment recommendation for steroid-cell tumors is debulking surgery followed by adjuvant BEP therapy (Table 21.2).

REFERENCES

1. Young RH, Clement PB, Scully RE. The ovary. In: Stemberg SS, Mills SE, eds. *Surgical pathology of the female reproductive system and peritoneum.* New York: Raven Press, 1991:169–248.
2. Schwartz PE. Sex cord-stromal tumors of the ovary. In: Piver MS, ed. *Ovarian malignancies: diagnostic and therapeutic advances.* New York: Churchill Livingstone, 1987:251–271.
3. Schwartz PE, Smith JP. Treatment of ovarian stromal tumors. *Am J Obstet Gynecol* 1976;125:402.
4. Bjorkholm E, Silfversward C. Prognostic factors in granulosa cell tumors. *Gynecol Oncol* 1981;11:261.
5. Ohel G, Kaneti H, Schenker JG. Granulosa cell tumors in Israel: a study of 172 cases. *Gynecol Oncol* 1983;15:278.
6. Scully RE. *Tumors of the ovary and maldeveloped gonads,* 2nd Series. Washington, DC: Armed Forces Institute of Pathology, 1979:32–33,152–225.
7. Bennington JL, Ferguson BR, Haber SL. Incidence and relative frequency of benign and malignant ovarian neoplasms. *Obstet Gynecol* 1968;32:627.
8. Fox H, Agrawal K, Langley IA. A clinicopathologic study of 92 cases of granulosa cell tumor of the ovary with special reference to the factors influencing prognosis. *Cancer* 1975;35:231.
9. Evans AJ III, Gaffey TA, Markasian GD, et al. Clinicopathologic review of 118 granulosa and 82 theca tumors. *Obstet Gynecol* 1980;55:231.
10. Nakashima N, Young RH, Scully RE. Androgenic granulosa cell tumors of the ovary: a clinicopathologic analysis of 17 cases and review of the literature. *Arch Pathol Lab Med* 1984;108:786.
11. Lack EE, et al. Granulosa theca cell tumors in premenarchal girls: a clinical and pathological study in ten cases. *Cancer* 1981;48:1346.
12. Roth LM, Nicholas TR, Ehrlich CE. Juvenile granulosa cell tumor: a clinicopathologic study of three cases with ultrastructural observations. *Cancer* 1979;44:2194.
13. Pysher TJ, Hitch DC, Krous HF. Bilateral juvenile granulosa cell tumors in a 4month-old dysmorphic infant: a clinical, histologic, and ultrastructural study. *Am J Pathol* 1981;5:789.
14. Tamini HK, Bolen J. Enchondromatosis (Ollier's disease) and juvenile granulosa cell tumor of the ovary. *Cancer* 1984;53:1505.
15. Velasco-Oses A, Alonso-Alvero A, Blanco-Pozo A, et al. Ollier's disease associated with ovarian juvenile granulosa cell tumor. *Cancer* 1988;62:222.
16. Lewis RJ, Ketcham AS. Maffucci's syndrome: functional and neoplastic significance. Case report and review of the literature. *J Bone Joint Surg Am* 1973;55:1465.
17. Young RH, Dickersin GR, Scully RE. Juvenile granulosa cell tumor of the ovary. *Am J Surg Pathol* 1984;8:575.
18. Stenwig JT, Hazelcamp JT, Beecham JB. Granulosa cell tumors of the ovary: a clinicopathological study of 118 cases with longterm follow-up. *Gynecol Oncol* 1979;7:136.
19. Choi CH, Pritchard JR. Large cystic granulosa cell tumor: case report. *Am J Obstet Gynecol* 1990;63:74.
20. Diddle AW. Granulosa and theca cell ovarian tumors: prognosis. *Cancer* 1952;5:215.
21. Hines JF, Khalifa MA, Moore JL, et al. Recurrent granulosa cell tumor of the ovary 37 years after initial diagnosis: a case report and review of the literature. *Gynecol Oncol* 1996;60:484.
22. Tennent BJ, Shultz KL, Snndberg JP, et al. Ovarian granulosa cell tumorigenesis in SWR-derived F1 hybrid mice: preneoplastic follicular abnormality and malignant disease progression. *Am J Obstet Gynecol* 1990;163:625.
23. Beamer WG, Shultz KL, Tennent BJ. Induction of ovarian granulosa cell tumors in SWXJ-9 mice with dehydroepiandrosterone. *Cancer Res* 1988;48:2788.
24. Beamer WG, et al. Gene for ovarian granulosa cell tumor susceptibility, Gct, in SWXJ recombinant inbred strains of mice revealed by dehydroepiandrosterone. *Cancer Res* 1988;48:5092.
25. Leung WY, et al. Trisomy 12 in benign fibroma and granulosa cell tumor of the ovary. *Gynecol Oncol* 1990;38:28.
26. Fletcher JA, Gibas Z, Donoven K, et al. Ovarian granulos astromal cell tumors are characterized by trisomy 12. *Am J Pathol* 1991;138:515.
27. Shashi V, Golder WL, von Kap-Herr C, et al. Interphase fluorescence in situ hybridization for trisomy 12

28. Evans MP, Webb MJ, Gaffey TA, et al. DNA ploidy of ovarian granulosa cell tumors. *Cancer* 1995;75:2295.
29. Hitchcock CL, Norris HJ, Khalifa MA, Wargotz ES. Flow cytometric analysis of granulosa tumors. *Cancer* 1989;64:2127.
30. Roush GR, El-Naggar AK, Abdul-Karim FW. Granulosa cell tumor of ovary: a clinicopathologic and flow cytometric DNA analysis. *Gynecol Oncol* 1995;56:430.
31. DiSaia PJ, Saltz A, Kagan AR, et al. A temporary response of recurrent granulosa cell tumor to Adriamycin. *Obstet Gynecol* 1978;52:355.
32. Scharl A, et al. Zur Klinik und Prognose von Granulosazelltumoren des Ovars. *Geburtshilfe Frauenheilkd* 1988;48:567.
33. Kjemi PJ, Joensuu H, Salmi T. Prognostic value of flow cytometric DNA content analysis in granulosa cell tumor of the ovary. *Cancer* 1990;65:1189.
34. Suh KS, et al. Granulosa cell tumor of the ovary: histopathologic and flow cytometric analysis with clinical correlation. *Arch Pathol Lab Med* 1990;114:496.
35. Chadha S, Cornelisse CJ, Schaberg A. Flow cytometric DNA ploidy analysis of ovarian granulosa cell tumors. *Gynecol Oncol* 1990;36:240.
36. Burger HG. Inhibin. *Reprod Med Rev* 1992;1:1.
37. Gurusinghe CJ, Healy DL, Mamers P, Burger HG. Inhibin and activin are demonstrable by immunohistochemistry in ovarian tumor tissue. *Gynecol Oncol* 1995;57:27.
38. Jobling T, Mamers P, Healy DL, et al. A prospective study of inhibin in granulosa cell tumors of the ovary. *Gynecol Oncol* 1994;55:285.
39. Lappohn RE, Burger HG, Bouma J, et al. Inhibin as a marker for granulosa cell tumors. *N Engl J Med* 1989;321:790.
40. Nishida M, et al. Juvenile granulosa cell tumor in association with a high serum inhibin level. *Gynecol Oncol* 1991;40:90.
41. Boggess JF, Soules MR, Goff BA, et al. Serum inhibin and disease status in women with ovarian granulosa cell tumors. *Gynecol Oncol* 1997;64:64.
42. Flemming P, Wellmann A, Maschek H, et al. Monoclonal antibodies against inhibin represent key markers of adult granulosa cell tumors of the ovary even in their metastases. *Am J Surg Pathol* 1995;19:927.
43. Gustafson ML, Lee MM, Scully RE, et al. Mullerian inhibiting substance as a marker for ovarian sex-cord tumor. *N Engl J Med* 1992;326:466.
44. Rey RA, Lhomme C, Marcillac I, et al. Antimullerian hormone as a serum marker of granulosa cell tumors of the ovary: comparative study with serum inhibin and estradiol. *Am J Obstet Gynecol* 1996;174:958.
45. Rodgers KE, et al. Follicle regulatory protein: a novel marker for granulosa cell cancer patients. *Gynecol Oncol* 1990;37:381.
46. Schwartz PE. Surgical management of ovarian cancer. *Arch Surg* 1981;116:99.
47. Kietlinska Z, Pietrzak K, Drabik M. The management of granulosa-cell tumors of the ovary based on long-term follow up. *Eur J Gynaecol Oncol* 1993;392:118.
48. Slayton RE, Park RC, Silverberg SG, et al. Vincristine, dactinomycin, and cyclophosphamide in the treatment of malignant germ cell tumors of the ovary: a Gynecologic Oncology Group study (a final report). *Cancer* 1985;56:243.
49. Smith JP, Rutledge F. Advances in chemotherapy for gynecologic cancer. *Cancer* 1975;36:669.
50. Schwartz PE. Combination chemotherapy in the management of germ cell malignancies. *Obstet Gynecol* 1985;64:564.
51. Colombo N, Sessa C, Landoni F, et al. Cisplatin, vinblastine, and bleomycin combination chemotherapy in metastatic granulosa cell tumor of the ovary. *Obstet Gynecol* 1986;67:265.
52. Zambetti M, et al. Cis-platinum/vinblastine/bleomycin combination chemotherapy in advanced or recurrent granulosa cell tumors of the ovary. *Gynecol Oncol* 1990;36:317.
53. Peckham MJ, et al. The treatment of metastatic germ cell testicular tumors with bleomcyin, etoposide, and cisplatin (BEP). *Br J Cancer* 1983;47:613.
54. Gershenson DM, Morris M, Burke TW, et al. Treatment of poor-prognosis sex cord-stromal tumors of the ovary with the combination of bleomycin, etoposide, and cisplatin. *Obstet Gynecol* 1996;8:527.
55. Homesley HD, Bundy BN, Hurteau JA, Roth LM. Bleomycin, etoposide, and cisplatin combination therapy of ovarian granulosa cell tumors and other stromal malignancies: a Gynecologic Oncology Group study. *Gynecol Oncol* 1999;72:131.
56. Colombo N, Parma G, Franchi D. An active chemotherapy regimen for advanced ovarian sex cord-stromal tumors [Editorial]. *Gynecol Oncol* 1999;72:129.
57. Margolin K, et al. Hepatic metastasis in granulosa cell tumor of the ovary. *Cancer* 1985;56:691.
58. Gershenson DM, Copeland LJ, Kavanagh JJ, et al. Treatment of metastatic stromal tumor of the ovary with cisplatin, doxorubicin, and cyclophosphamide. *Obstet Gynecol* 1987;70:765.
59. DiSaia PJ, et al. A temporary response of recurrent granulosa cell tumor to Adriamycin. *Obstet Gynecol* 1978;52:355.
60. Barlow JJ, et al. Adriamycin and bleomycin, alone and in combination, in gynecologic tumors. *Cancer* 1973;32:735.
61. Jacobs AJ, Deppe G, Cohen CJ. Combination chemotherapy of ovarian granulosa cell tumors with cis-platinum and doxorubicin. *Gynecol Oncol* 1982;14:294.
62. Wolf JK, Mullen J, Eifel PJ, et al. Radiation treatment of advanced or recurrent granulosa cell tumor of the ovary. *Gynecol Oncol* 1999;73:35.
63. Wessalowski R, Spaar HJ, Pape H, et al. Successful liver treatment of a juvenile granulosa cell tumor in a 4-year-old child by regional deep hyperthermia, systemic chemotherapy, and irradiation. *Gynecol Oncol* 1995;57:417.
64. Simmons RL, Sciarra JJ. Treatment of late recurrent granulosa cell tumors of the ovary. *Surg Gynecol Obstet* 1967;124:65.
65. Schwartz PE, et al. Steroid-receptor proteins in nonepithelial malignancies of the ovary. *Gynecol Oncol* 1983;15:305.
66. Malik ST, Slevin ML. Medroxyprogesterone acetate in advanced granulosa cell tumors of the ovary: a new therapeutic approach? *Br J Cancer* 1991;63:410.
67. Martikainen H, et al. Gonadotropin-releasing hormone agonist analog therapy effective in ovarian granulosa cell malignancy. *Gynecol Oncol* 1989;35:406.

68. Waxman M, et al. Ovarian low grade stromal sarcoma with thecomatous features: a critical reappraisal of the so-called "malignant" thecoma. *Cancer* 1979;44:206.
69. Barrenetxea G, Schneider J, Centeno MM, et al. Pure theca cell tumors: a clinicopathologic study of 29 cases. *Eur J Gynaecol Oncol* 1990;11:429.
70. Young RH, Scully RE. Ovarian sex-cord stromal tumors: recent progress. *Int J Gynecol Pathol* 1982;1:101.
71. Roth LM, Sternberg WH. Partly luteinized theca cell tumor of the ovary. *Cancer* 1983;51:1697.
72. Young RH, Clement PB, Scully RE. Calcified thecomas in young women: a report of four cases. *Int J Gynecol Pathol* 1988;7:343.
73. Gorlin RJ, Sedano HO. The multiple nevoid basal cell carcinoma syndrome revisited. *Birth Defects* 1971;7:140.
74. Meigs JV, Cass JW. Fibroma of the ovary with ascites and hydrothorax with a report of seven cases. *Am J Obstet Gynecol* 1937;33:249–267.
75. Samanth KK, Black WC. Benign ovarian stromal tumors associated with free peritoneal fluid. *Am J Obstet Gynecol* 1970;107:538.
76. Suit PF, Hart WR. Sclerosing stromal tumor of the ovary: an ultrastructural study and review of the literature to evaluate hormonal function. *Cleve Clin J Med* 1988;55:189.
77. Damjanov I, Drobnjak P, Grizeij V, et al. Sclerosing stromal tumor of the ovary: a hormonal and ultrastructural analysis. *Obstet Gynecol* 1975;45:675.
78. Quinn MA, Oster AA, Fortune D. Sclerosing stromal tumor: case report with endocrine studies. *Br J Obstet Gynaecol* 1981;88:555.
79. Ho Yuen B, Robertson DI, Clement PB, et al. Sclerosing stromal tumor of the ovary. *Obstet Gynecol* 1982;60:252.
80. Marelli G, Carinelli S, Mariani A, et al. Sclerosing stromal tumor of the ovary: report of eight cases and review of the literature. *Eur J Obstet Gynecol Reprod Biol* 1998;76:85.
81. Gee DC, Russel P. Sclerosing stromal tumor of the ovary. *Histopathology* 1979;3:367.
82. Seidman JD. Unclassified ovarian gonadal stromal tumors. *Am J Surg Pathol* 1996;20:699.
83. Roth LM, Anderson MC, Govan AD, et al. Sertoli-Leydig cell tumors: a clinicopathologic study of 34 cases. *Cancer* 1981;48:187.
84. Tracy SL, et al. Progesterone secreting Sertoli cell tumor of the ovary. *Gynecol Oncol* 1985;22:85.
85. Young RH, Scully RE. Ovarian Sertoli-Leydig cell tumors: a clinicopathologic analysis of 207 cases. *Am J Surg Pathol* 1985;9:543.
86. Young RH, Scully RE. Well-differentiated ovarian Sertoli-Leydig cell tumors: a clinicopathologic analysis of 23 cases. *Int J Gynecol Pathol* 1984;3:277.
87. Zaloudek C, Norris HJ. Sertoli-Leydig cell tumors of the ovary: a clinicopathologic study of 64 intermediate and poorly differentiated neoplasms. *Am J Surg Pathol* 1984;8:405.
88. Weyl-Ben Arush M, Oslander L. Ollier's disease associated with ovarian Sertoli-Leydig cell tumor and breast adenoma. *Am J Pediatr Hematol Oncol* 13:49, 1991.
89. Goslar HG, et al. Steroid biosynthesis in the Sertoli-Leydig cell tumor tissue of the human ovary: enzymhistochemical and immunohistochemical studies. *Acta Histochem Suppl* 1984;29:175.
90. Van Dessel T, Heineman MJ. Endocrinological aspects of a Sertoli-Leydig cell tumour: case report. *Br J Obstet Gynaecol* 1990;97:1054.
91. Speroff L, Glass RH, Kase NG. Hirsutism. In: , ed. *Clinical gynecologic endocrinology and infertility,* 4th ed. Baltimore: Williams & Wilkins, 1989:240–244.
92. Ayalon D, Graif M, Hetman-Peri M, et al. Diagnosis of a small ovarian tumor (androgen secreting) by magnetic resonance imaging: a new noninvasive procedure. *Am J Obstet Gynecol* 1988;159:903.
93. Taylor L, Ayers JW, Gross MD, et al. Diagnostic considerations in virilization: Iodomethyl-norcholesterol scanning in the localization of androgen secreting tumors. *Fertil Steril* 1986;46:1005.
94. Younis JS, et al. Lipid cell tumor of the ovary: steroid hormone secretory pattern and localization using 75 Se-selenomethylcholesterol. *Gynecol Obstet Invest* 1989;7:110, 87.
95. Tseng L, et al. Preliminary studies of aromatase in human neoplastic endometrium. *Obstet Gynecol* 1984;63:150.
96. Pride GL, Pollock WJ, Norgard MJ. Metastatic Sertoli-Leydig cell tumor of the ovary during pregnancy treated by BV-CAP chemotherapy. *Am J Obstet Gynecol* 1982;143:231.
97. Benfield GFA, Tapper-Jones L, Stont TV. Androblastoma and raised serum AFP with familial multinodular goiter: case report. *Br J Obstet Gynaecol* 1982;89:323.
98. Tetu B, Ordonez NG, Silva EG. Sertoli-Leydig cell tumor of the ovary with alpha-feto-protein production. *Arch Pathol Lab Med* 1986;110:65.
99. Mann WJ, et al. Elevated serum alpha-fetoprotein associated with Sertoli-Leydig cell tumors. *Obstet Gynecol* 1986;67:141.
100. Chumas JC, Rosenwaks Z, Mann WJ, et al. Sertoli-Leydig cell tumor of the ovary producing alpha-fetoprotein. *Int J Gynecol Pathol* 1984;126:213–219.
101. Chadha S, Honnebier WJ, Schaberg A. Raised serum alpha-fetoprotein in Sertoli-Leydig cell tumor (androblastoma) of the ovary: report of two cases. *Int J Gynecol Pathol* 1987;6:82
102. Gagnon S, et al. Frequency of alpha-fetoprotein production by Sertoli-Leydig cell tumors of the ovary: an immunohistochemical study of eight cases. *Mod Pathol* 1989;2:63.
103. Motoyama I, et al. Ovarian Sertoli-Leydig cell tumor with elevated serum alpha-fetoprotein. *Cancer* 1989;63:2047.
104. Ohashi M, Hasegawa Y, Haji M, et al. Production of immunoreactive inhibin by a virilizing ovarian tumor (Sertoli-Leydig cell tumor). *Clin Endocrinol (Oxf)* 1990;33:613.
105. Hart WR, Kumar N, Crissman JD. Ovarian neoplasms resembling sex cord tumors with annular tubules. *Cancer* 1980;45:2352.
106. Tavassoli FA, Norris HJ. Sertoli tumors of the ovary: a clinicopathologic study of 28 cases with ultrastructural observations. *Cancer* 1980;46:2281.
107. Young RH, et al. Ovarian sex cord tumor with annular tubules: review of 74 cases including 27 with Peutz-Jeghers syndrome and four with adenoma malignum of the cervix. *Cancer* 1982;50:1384.
108. Czernobilsky B, Gaedecke G, DallenbachHellweg G. Endometrioid differentiation in ovarian sex cord tumor

with annular tubules accompanied by gestagenic effect. *Cancer* 1985;55:738.
109. Benagiano G, Bigotti G, Bnzzi M, et al. Endocrine and morphological study of a case of ovarian sex cord tumor with annular tubules in a woman with Peutz-Jeghers syndrome. *Int J Gynecol Obstet* 1988;26:441.
110. Young RH, Dickersin GR, Scully RE. A distinctive ovarian sex cord-stromal tumor causing sexual precocity in the Peutz-Jeghers syndrome. *Am J Surg Pathol* 1983;7:233.
111. Young RH, Dudley AG, Scully RE. Granulosa cell, Sertoli-Leydig cell and unclassified sex cord-stromal tumors associated with pregnancy: a clinicopathologic analysis of thirty-six cases. *Gynecol Oncol* 1984; 18:181.
112. Paraskevas M, Scully RE. Hilus cell tumor of the ovary: a clinicopathological analysis of 12 Reinke crystal-positive and nine crystal-negative cases. *Int J Gynecol Pathol* 1989;8:299.
113. Hayes MC, Scully RE. Stromal luteoma of the ovary: a clinicopathologic analysis of 25 cases. *Int J Gynecol Pathol* 1987;6:313.
114. Sternberg WH, Roth LM. Ovarian stromal tumors containing Leydig cells: 1. Stromal Leydig cell tumor and non-neoplastic transformation of ovarian stroma to Leydig cells. *Cancer* 1973;32:940.
115. Baramki TA, Leddy AL, Woodruff JD. Bilateral hilus cell tumor of the ovary. *Obstet Gynecol* 1983;62:128.
116. Stewart RS, Woodward DE. Malignant ovarian hilus cell tumor: the first reported case. *Arch Pathol* 1962; 73:91.
117. Raaf JH, Bajourunas DR, Smith DN, et al. Virilizing hilus (Leydig) cell tumor of the ovary: the challenge of an accurate preoperative diagnosis. *Surgery* 1983; 94:951.
118. Echt CR, Hadd HE. Androgen excretion patterns in a patient with a metastatic hilus cell tumor of the ovary. *Am J Obstet Gynecol* 1968;100:1055.
119. Hayes MC, Scully RE. Ovarian steroid cell tumors, not otherwise specified (lipid cell tumors): a clinicopathologic analysis of 63 cases. *Am J Surg Pathol* 1987; 11:835.
120. Barkan AL, et al. Steroid and gonadotropin secretion in a patient with a 30 year history of virilization due to a lipoid-cell ovarian tumor. *Obstet Gynecol* 1984; 64:287.
121. Marieb NJ, Cassorla F, Loriaux DL, et al. Cushing's syndrome secondary to ectopic cortisol production by an ovarian carcinoma. *J Clin Endocrinol Metab* 1983;57:737.
122. Taylor HB, Norris HJ. Lipid cell tumors of the ovary. *Cancer* 1967;20:1953.
123. Patsner B, Piver MS. Treatment of metastatic lipid cell tumor of the ovary with BVCAP and VAC chemotherapy, using serum testosterone and dihydrotestosterone as tumor markers. *Eur J Gynaecol Oncol* 1988;9:441.

22
Ovarian Tumors of Low Malignant Potential

Gregory P. Sutton

HISTORY

In 1929 Taylor (1) published the first report of an ovarian tumor that had some of the histologic features of malignancy yet did not behave in a malignant fashion in the other respects. In a review of ovarian tumors from the Gynecological Division of Roosevelt Hospital from 1910 to 1927, he characterized such ovarian tumors, which were neither benign nor malignant, as follows:

> Of the hyperplastic variety, 3 were bilateral and each of these had implants scattered diffusely over the peritoneum or in the intestine or omentum, one other had ascites and external papillae on the surface of the cyst, while a fifth had external papillae alone. In spite of this, 2 of the patients have lived 14 years, another 6, one other 4, and the 3 others are alive and well less than that time.
> It is the hyperplastic type of papillary cyst, which we believe is the one involved in the spectacular reports of regression of carcinomata of the ovary following incomplete operation.... If we regard this type of papillary cyst with implants upon the peritoneum as hyperplasia of a peritoneal endometriosis or of a tissue with similar functional status, the explanation of the regression following castration becomes more simple. In our entire series we have no case of a true cancer showing any sign of spontaneous regression, although some pathologists might classify our hyperplastic papillary cysts as carcinoma.

In 1961, the International Federation of Gynecology and Obstetrics (FIGO) acknowledged the importance of this intermediate group of epithelial tumors and suggested a system that subdivided ovarian tumors into three types: benign cystadenomas, cystadenocarcinomas of low malignant potential, and cystadenocarcinomas. This classification became effective in 1971. In 1973, the World Health Organization (WHO) adopted a classification that included a "borderline" or "carcinoma of low malignant potential" group of epithelial tumors (2). These possessed the malignant characteristics of epithelial hyperplasia or stratification, mitotic activity, and cellular and nuclear atypia but did not have evidence of stromal invasion.

TERMINOLOGY

Other terms applied to these neoplasms include proliferative tumors, borderline carcinomas, borderline tumors, questionably or potentially malignant tumors, and well-differentiated or grade 1 carcinomas (3). The term *tumor of low malignant potential* (LMP) is preferred by many pathologists (3,4) because it neither implies frank malignancy nor presupposes an entirely benign growth. Others prefer the term *carcinoma of low malignant potential,* because it is more consistent with WHO terminology (5). The term *borderline* is thought to be ambiguous and is generally discouraged, although it is occasionally used (6).

PATHOLOGY

Norris and Mount (4) summarized the need for appropriate testing of the epithelial tumors of the ovary:

> Thorough sampling of each neoplasm is required because wide variation in histology is frequent in epithelial tumors. The determination of benign, LMP, or malignant is based on the least differentiated area. To obtain reasonable sampling, a block of tissue for microscopic examination should be taken for each 1 to 2 cm of maximal tumor diameter. Solid areas, the base of papillary processes, and regions adjacent to the surface should be given special attention.

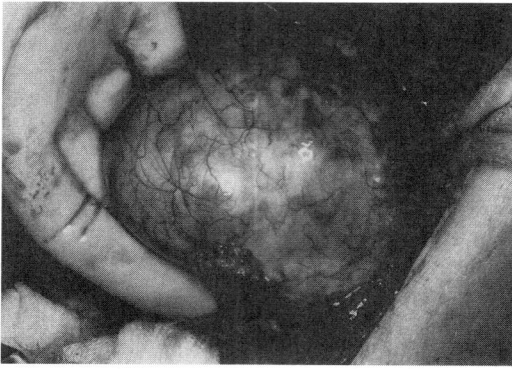

FIG. 22.1. External appearance of a serous low malignant tumor (LMP) tumor arising in the left ovary of a 19-year-old woman.

LMP tumors have been identified in all epithelial subtypes, including endometrioid, clear cell, and proliferative Brenner tumors. Serous and mucinous histologies are most common and are therefore better understood.

Serous Tumors

Grossly, serous LMP tumors resemble benign serious cystadenomas with solid and cystic areas lined with papillary projections generally more profuse than those found in the benign variant (Figures 22.1 and 22.2). It is impossible to differentiate among benign, malignant, and LMP tumors on gross examination, however.

Microscopically, the epithelium resembles that of the fallopian tube and may be present on the ovarian surface or within cystic or solid

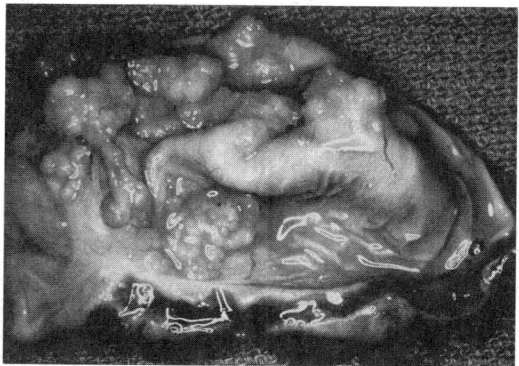

FIG. 22.2. Internal papillations visible when the cystic tumor seen in Figure 22.1 is opened.

areas. This epithelium may include branching, complex papillary fronds with stratification, and tufting. Katzenstein and coworkers (7) suggested that buds of many cells without a central stalk, lacking epithelial polarity, could occur. Cellular atypia, hyperchromatism, nuclear enlargement, and conspicuous nucleoli may also be features of these lesions. Necrosis, stromal infiltration by inflammatory cells, epithelial bridging, and psammoma bodies may all be present in the absence of stromal invasion. However, necrosis, cribriform change, mitotic activity, and papillary change are less extensive than in invasive serous carcinomas (7).

Cribriform glands situated in the stroma do not typify invasion, which is characterized by irregular infiltration by tongues or sheets of cells that may be destructive (edema, inflammation, and fibrosis of the stroma) (4).

Microcystic Tumors and Microinvasion

Among tumors of LMP, the histologic patterns referred to as "micropapillary" or "cribriform" have been the focus of some attention. Kurman's group (8) evaluated 65 patients with stage II and III tumors of LMP and classified them as typical (9), with invasive implants (3), or with micropapillary serous cancers (10). The latter were characterized as having "a filigree pattern of highly complex micropapillae arising directly from large, bulbous papillary structures" (11). In this series, 2 (4%) of 51 patients with LMP tumors developed invasive cancer and 1 died. Two of the 3 patients with invasive implants and 7 of the 11 patients with "micropapillary" cancers had recurrence or death. In a contrasting study, Eichorn and colleagues (12) identified patients with 40 such tumors and compared them with 44 control patients in whom micropapillary lesions were not identified. Advanced stage, bilaterality, and surface growth were more common among micropapillary tumors than controls, but prognosis was similar in both groups. Patients with micropapillary tumors who died from their disease were more often found to have invasive peritoneal implants, a known risk factor.

Other methods of diagnosis, including flow cytometry, morphometric analysis, and other techniques, are discussed in later sections.

Mucinous Tumors

Mucinous LMP tumors were first studied in a comprehensive way by Hart and Norris (13) in 1973. In a series of 97 borderline mucinous tumors referred to the Armed Forces Institute of Pathology, they excluded cases where a coexistent adenocarcinoma of another organ system was present, because metastases to the ovary are difficult to differentiate from primary mucinous tumors. On gross examination, most of the mucinous LMP tumors were multicystic, with smooth exteriors and thickened cyst linings that contained solid elements in about 50% of the cases. Neither surface nor internal papillary structures were seen frequently in comparison with serous tumors of LMP. The authors described a histologic pattern similar to that seen in hyperplastic or adenomatous polyps of the colon. There was either a diffuse or local overgrowth of the mucinous epithelium with stratification of two to three layers of cells. They suggested that mucinous tumors with four or more epithelial strata, or with evidence of cribriform growth or epithelial bridging, be considered malignant.

Rutgers and Scully (14) introduced the concept of müllerian mucinous papillary borderline tumors with features more closely resembling those of endocervical epithelium than the typical intestinal differentiation seen in common mucinous LMP tumors. These represented about 15% of the mucinous tumors in their referral population. The tumors often had excessive epithelial stratification, were associated with endometriosis in 30% of cases, and tended to be bilateral.

Superficial stromal invasion or "microinvasion" up to 2 mm may be identified in many typical serous and mucinous tumors of LMP. Several authors (15,16) have suggested that these findings are clinically insignificant. In mucinous tumors, invasion of up to 5 mm apparently had no detrimental effect on survival in one study (17).

Other Histologic Types

Most endometrioid tumors of the ovarian epithelium are malignant, and reports of endometrioid LMP tumors are few (4). Both a solid or fibrous variety, resembling an adenofibroma, and a predominantly epithelial type were recognized by Norris and Mount (4). The epithelium of the latter resembled adenomatous endometrial hyperplasia. Of the 34 total endometrioid LMP tumors reported by Russell (18) and by Bell and Scully (10), there were only 2 cases of extraovarian spread and 1 bilateral tumor.

Clear cell LMP tumors, like other clear cell neoplasms, contain cytoplasmic glycogen that is mucicarmine positive. This histologic subtype is extremely rare, with a total of only nine cases summarized in the review by Norris and Mount (4).

Roth and associates (19) subdivided Brenner tumors into benign, proliferative, metaplastic, LMP, and malignant. These lesions are similar to transitional tumors of the bladder. Proliferation is characterized by highly stratified epithelium, and LMP tumors have high-grade cellular atypia in addition. These rare tumors are almost always unilateral and occasionally are quite large (4).

Additional Discriminatory Studies

Differentiating between LMP tumors and well-differentiated malignancies solely on the basis of light-microscopic criteria may be difficult. Hernandez and coworkers (20) conducted a study in which 68 histologic sections from 34 patients were independently reviewed by two pathologists. Of the 23 diagnostic disparities, 5 (23%) were between LMP and invasive tumors. Several techniques to enhance or improve on light microscopic diagnosis have been proposed.

Baak and Vanderley (21) introduced the use of a scoring system with five morphometric criteria in the differentiation of LMP and invasive tumors. The criteria were mitotic index, epithelium to stroma ratio, nuclear perimeter, area, and axis. The authors were able to retrospectively assign a majority of cases to the correct clinical group, but prospective information on their system is lacking. Erhardt and coworkers (22) assessed DNA content cytophotometrically in 54 LMP or malignant ovarian tumors acquired by the Karolinska Hospital. Nine were reclassified as benign tumors, but DNA levels alone produced no clearcut intergroup boundaries. Similarly, Fu and associates (23) evaluated 16 LMP serous tumors and 7 grade 1 invasive carcinomas using Feulgen microspectrophotometry to determine DNA ploidy. Only 1 (11%) of the LMP tumors was aneuploid, whereas 4 (57%) of the carcinomas contained aneuploid DNA. None of the LMP tumors was triploid, although five of the carcinomas had greater than triploid stem cell modal DNA values. Again, no obvious means of distinction was presented.

The technique of flow cytometry has enabled investigators to study not only DNA content but also ploidy, DNA-synthetic phase (S-phase) fraction, and a variety of oncogene-related proteins. Using flow cytometry, Freidlander and coworkers (24) found 2 aneuploid serous LMP tumors in a group of 44 patients, the remainder being diploid. Both patients had peritoneal implants with invasive qualities, and 1 died from metastatic disease. Iverson and Skarrdland (25) identified six women with serious LMP tumors, all of which were diploid and clinically benign. Klemi and associates (26) reported aneuploidy in 3 (11%) of 43 serous LMP tumors, as well as in 7 of 27 benign cystadenomas. None of the patients with an aneuploid LMP or benign lesion died from the disease.

DNA ploidy was found to be the most important prognostic discriminator in a large study by Kaern and associates (27); 91% (293/321) of their patients had diploid tumors and 9% (28/321) had aneuploid tumors. Patients with aneuploid tumors had a 19-fold increase in the risk of dying from their disease. Other important negative prognostic features among patients in this study were advanced age, residual tumor after surgery, advanced stage, and nonserous histology.

Kotylo and coworkers (28) found both aneuploid and diploid stemlines in tumors of LMP. They also found that the oncogene-related protein ras p21 was expressed more commonly in invasive cancers or LMP tumors than in benign tumors or normal ovaries.

Several authors have evaluated oncogenes and tumor suppressor genes in tumors of LMP. Berchuck and colleagues (29) demonstrated P53 overexpression, common in invasive ovarian cancers, in only 2 (4%) of 49 tumors of LMP. Both cases were stage III tumors. Van Haaften-Daly and coworkers (30) observed similar findings for P53 and also reported that epidermal growth factor receptor was expressed in 18% of LMP tumors compared with 69% of invasive cancers ($p < .004$).

Microsatellite instability and loss of heterozygosity at a variety of chromosomal loci were observed in 87% of invasive cancers of the ovary and 60% of tumors of LMP in a study by Haas and colleagues (31). Microsatellite instability in LMP tumors occurred at more than one locus, whereas it was sporadic in invasive cancers. The authors concluded that the mechanism of tumorigenesis of at least some tumors of LMP was different than for invasive cancers. Cheng and associates (32) found that both LMP tumors and ovarian cancers commonly had loss of heterozygosity (LOH) at 6q, 17p, and 17q. LOH at 13q was seen only in invasive cancers. Half of the LMP tumors showed LOH at Xq, most due to interstitial deletions, and all involving the inactive copy of the X chromosome only. Losses in the X chromosome were not observed in benign ovarian tumors or carcinomas, supporting the idea that tumors of LMP are *not* precursors of invasive cancers.

Electron microscopy has been a helpful tool in differentiating invasive from LMP tumors. Both demonstrate pronounced infolding of the nuclear membrane, but the epithelial cells of malignant tumors lack cilia, which are preserved in LMP tumors and in those which are benign (33).

EPIDEMIOLOGY

Incidence

Russell (18) and Purola (34) reported a 15% incidence of LMP lesions among epithelial ovarian tumors. Subsequent estimates are similar, although the actual frequency may reflect the population under study. At the Norwegian Radium Hospital from 1945 to 1964, 161 (16.3%) of 990 epithelial tumors were LMP tumors (35). In a series from the same institution conducted from 1968 to 1974, 88 (21.1%) of 418 stage I and II epithelial neoplasms were LMP tumors (36). This difference most likely reflects the propensity for LMP tumors to be of low stage. Although 32.2% of stage I lesions in the latter study were LMP tumors, only 3.2% of stage II tumors were not frankly malignant.

Nikrui (37) and Nation and Krepart (38) reported rates of 9.2% and 9.4% in large studies of ovarian epithelial tumors from the Massachusetts General Hospital (1962 to 1979) and the University of Manitoba (1976 to 1984), respectively. Hopkins and associates (39) described a group of 68 patients with LMP tumors, representing 12.6% of all ovarian tumors and 22% of serous and mucinous tumors at the University of Michigan from 1970 to 1985. A report of 76 LMP tumors among 300 epithelial tumors (25.3% incidence) from the Royal Women's Hospital in Melbourne may include several patients with colorectal primaries (40). Among patients with stage IIIA or IIIB ovarian lesions, 7.3% were found to have LMP tumors at the time of pathologic review in a study conducted by the Gynecologic Oncology Group (GOG) (41).

Age

Several studies have indicated that the mean age of patients with LMP tumors of the ovary is less than that of those with frankly invasive neoplasms. In the large series of Aure and associates (35), the mean age of patients with LMP tumors was 45.7 years, which is 6.8 years younger than the average age of 52.5 years for patients with epithelial cancer. In Hopkins' collection of patients, those with LMP tumors of serous histology had a mean age of 37.9 years, compared with 51.6 years for those with cancer. However, among patients with mucinous tumors, the mean ages of those with LMP tumors and cancer were quite similar. Patients with LMP tumors had a mean age of 44.3 years, and those with invasive lesions, 46.3 years. There were 3 patients each with endometrioid and endometrioid/serous tumors with mean ages of 48.6 and 56.0 years, respectively (39). Kliman and coworkers (40) also reported that women with serous LMP tumors were younger than those with mucinous lesions. In 76 cases, the ages ranged from 19 to 82 years, with a cumulative mean of 46.6 years. Patients with serous tumors had an average age of 40.0 years, compared with a mean of 50.5 years among those with mucinous tumors ($p < .01$). The ages of the few patients with endometrioid tumors in this series averaged 55 years. In contrast, Bostwick and coworkers (42) found mean ages of 40.5 and 41 years among 79 patients with serous and 30 patients with mucinous tumors, respectively. They reported a bimodal frequency distribution, with peak ages at 30 to 34 and 50 to 54 years in patients ranging in age from 10 to 79 years. Hart and Norris (13) found a median age of 35 years in their large series of patients with mucinous LMP tumors.

The majority of patients with LMP tumors are younger than 50 years of age. In Nikrui's study (37), 65% of 36 women with serous tumors and 56% of 25 women with mucinous lesions were younger than 50 years of age. Nation and Krepart (38) also found that 53.8% of the subjects in their study were less than 50 years old.

Parity

Nulliparity has been reported in 23%, 27%, and 43.1% (40,42,43) of women with ovarian LMP tumors, and nulligravidity in 29%, 38%, and 39% (6,37,39). In the series of Chambers and associates (6), the mean gravidity of 94 cases was 1.9. Four tumors (4.3%) were diagnosed during pregnancy, and 2 of them were discovered at the time of cesarean section. Hart and Norris (13) found that 56 (55.7%) of 97 patients with mucinous LMP tumors (4.1%) were diagnosed during gestation and 7 (7.2%) in the postpartum period.

Race

No conclusions can be drawn from racial data. Most patients in the two large studies from the University of Michigan (39) and Stanford University (42) (83% and 95%, respectively) were Caucasian. In the latter study, 1 Asian and 3 black patients were included among 78 patients with serous tumors. Hart and Norris (13) identified 6 Asian subjects among 85 with known racial extraction.

Other Factors

As a group, women with LMP tumors are relatively healthy. In the GOG series of stages IIIA and IIIB tumors, 22 of 32 patients had no impairment of performance status, and all but 1 of the remainder had minimal functional impairment

(41). In one series (42), 16 of 109 patients had a history of estrogen use. In no reports was a family history of ovarian epithelial malignancy described.

A variety of associated malignancies have been reported, most often endometrial adenocarcinoma (6,37,40). Gastrointestinal malignancies were reported in the series of Nikrui (37) and Chambers and colleagues (6) and were associated with mucinous ovarian lesions in two of the patients in the report by Kliman and colleagues (40).

Pregnancy

Three of 427 patients seen at M.D. Anderson Cancer Center in the 50 years before 1994 had tumors of LMP diagnosed during pregnancy. Several additional patients were identified from pathology referrals. All but two tumors were stage I, and most were associated with marked epithelial proliferation and multiple areas of microinvasion.

One patient had disease in a supraclavicular lymph node and did well after resection and chemotherapy. Two patients had resections during pregnancy with residual disease; in both, marked regression was observed after delivery. All patients were alive and disease free at the time of the report. The authors suggested that LMP tumors diagnosed during pregnancy may have histologic and clinical features suggesting poor prognosis that regress in the postpartum interval (43a).

SYMPTOMS

The most common symptom associated with serous LMP tumors has been abdominal discomfort or pain (37–39). In women with mucinous tumors, abdominal fullness or the perception of a mass was the most common complaint (13). Abnormal premenstrual bleeding was reported by Hopkins and coworkers (39) in 39.5% of cases, and by Hart and Norris (13) in 15% of cases. Up to 25% of patients remain asymptomatic, presenting with masses on physical or pelvic examination (13) or at the time of an operation such as tubal litigation. Bostwick and coworkers (42) included one patient in whom the diagnosis was suspected when psammoma bodies were identified on vaginal cytologic examination. Also reported infrequently were torsion (43), intraperitoneal hemorrhage (13), weight loss (41), and dyspareunia (44).

Early-Stage Disease

One of the most significant advances of the 1980s was the demonstration by investigators including Young and associates (45) and Piver (46) that extraovarian metastases could be identified in 30% of patients with apparent stage I epithelial ovarian carcinoma if exhaustive surgical staging was employed. Undiscovered metastases may explain in part the relatively low (70%) 5-year survival rates reported earlier for stage I cancers. These studies also provided a basis for subsequent clinical trials, which demonstrated that surgery alone could cure almost all patients with genuine stage I tumors.

Although extraovarian spread has been described in only 16% to 18% of LMP ovarian tumors at the time of diagnosis (18,35), two studies have suggested that accurate surgical staging may disclose metastases in 25% to 30% of patients with these neoplasms. Yazigi and colleagues (44) reviewed 38 cases of presumed stage I LMP tumors and found gross extraovarian spread in only 2 cases (5.3%). In 29 of the remaining 36 patients, some effort at surgical staging was made. Fourteen (48.3%) had complete surgical procedures including biopsy of the contralateral ovary, omentum, diaphragm, pelvic and paraaortic lymph nodes, peritoneal surfaces, and peritoneal cytologic washings. In the final analysis, 7 patients were found to have stage III disease, leaving only 76.3% in stage I.

In a similar study, Kliman and coworkers (40) showed that only 2 (5.7%) of 35 LMP tumors reported before 1977 were stage III, whereas 12 (29.3%) of 41 patients presenting in 1977 or later had stage III disease. This difference was statistically significant ($p < .02$, chi-square test) and was attributed to more effective staging in the second group of patients.

Table 22.1 outlines the proportion of patients with stage I LMP tumors reported by some

TABLE 22.1. *Relative proportion of stage I tumors*

Author	Year	N	Stage I	% Stage I
Aure	1971	197	168	85.3
Julian	1972	64	34	53.1
Nikrui	1970	62	44	71.0
Barnhill	1985	94	47	50.0
Bostwick	1986	109	87	79.8
Kliman	1986	76	62	81.6
Nation	1986	65	55	84.0
Hopkins	1987	68	34	50.0
Chambers	1988	94	73	77.7
Font	1988	48	29	60.4
Yazigi	1988	38	29	76.3
Massad	1991	31	18	58.1
TOTAL		946	771	79.8

investigators. The surgical staging efforts in these studies were variable.

The size of the primary tumor varies widely. In a study from the University of Michigan (39), half of 62 tumors were between 10 and 20 cm in diameter. One fourth were less than 10 cm and one fourth greater than 20 cm in diameter. Bostwick and associates (42) reported a mean tumor diameter of 17.6 cm, with a range of 8 to 60 cm. And in the GOG study of stage III LMP tumors (41), the mean diameter was 12.5 cm (range, 3 to 30 cm).

PATTERNS OF SPREAD

Contralateral Ovary

In the reports of Snider and coworkers (47), Bell and Scully (10), and Bostwick and colleagues (42), there was involvement of the contralateral ovary in 10% of the cases. Williams and Dockerty (48) found evidence of metastatic neoplasia in 4 (6%) of 70 patients with apparently normal contralateral ovaries and suggested that biopsy was unnecessary. Yazigi and associates (44) identified contralateral metastases in 4 (15%) of 27 patients by either wedge biopsy or oophorectomy. Hopkins and coworkers (39) reported increasing bilaterality with stage: 35% in stage I, 46% in stage II, and 57% in stage III.

In the GOG study of 32 patients with stage III disease (41), most of whom had serous tumors, there was bilateral involvement in 27 (84.3%). Although removal after childbearing of the ovary retained during surgery for early-stage disease is advocated by several authors, Bostwick and colleagues (42) "do not feel that salpingo-oophorectomy and hysterectomy is indicated for removal of the residual ovary after fertility is no longer required."

Tazelaar and associates (49) reported a case of recurrent and LMP tumor in an ovary previously shown to be uninvolved by biopsy, and Hart and Norris (13) identified 2 neoplasms occurring in the residual ovary among 53 patients treated for mucinous tumors of LMP with conservative surgery. One was benign and the other a tumor of LMP.

Uterus and Fallopian Tubes

In the studies of LMP tumors with extraovarian spread (14) and of stage III disease (41), spread to the serosa of the uterus was identified in 33 (40.2%) of 82 and 12 (37.5%) of 32 patients, respectively. In the same two studies, fallopian tube metastases were identified in 31.7% and 53.6% of cases, respectively. Figure 22.3 illustrates a stage III tumor of LMP.

Peritoneal Involvement

In the GOG study of 32 women with early stage III tumors, the pelvic and upper abdominal peritoneum were respectively implicated in 56.3%

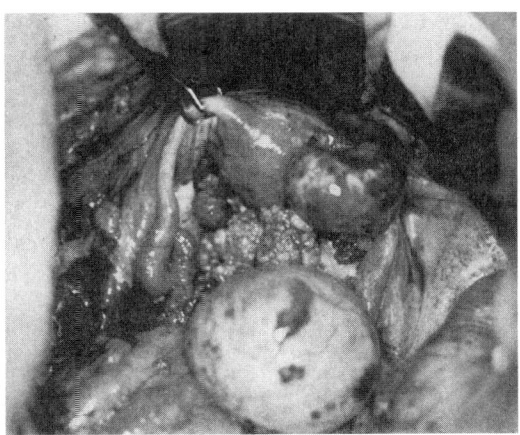

FIG. 22.3. Stage III ovarian serious LMP tumor. Note massive cul-de-sac disease.

and 37.5% of the cases. Some authors have suggested more than a single type of peritoneal involvement. In one type of lesion, Tazelaar and associates (49) described gross thickening of peritoneal surfaces, with microscopic prominence of fibrous connective tissue and psammoma bodies. In the second type, which appeared grossly normal, there were dilated, bland glands lined with single-layer tubal epithelium consistent with endosalpingiosis. Other authors (50) have distinguished between invasive and noninvasive (endosalpingiosis) peritoneal implants. Gershenson and Silva (51) reported the presence of endosalpingiosis in one third of 72 serous LMP tumors and "noninvasive" implants in about one half. In addition, 13 subjects (18%) in their study had peritoneal implants that were histologically invasive. Patients with endosalpingiosis or noninvasive peritoneal implants survived without disease in 132 (89.8%) of 147 cases collected from this and five other studies (40,52–55).

In a subsequent report, Gershenson and colleagues (56) identified 39 patients with serous tumors of LMP and invasive peritoneal implants. Twelve patients (31%) developed either progressive disease or recurrence at a median of 24 months, many despite chemotherapy. None of these patients developed invasive low-grade cancers. The most important predictor of recurrence was residual microscopic disease at the end of primary resection. This underscores the importance of complete surgical resection and a meticulous exploration for occult implants in patients with tumors of LMP.

Lymph Node Metastases

In addition to metastases from malignancies or LMP tumors, lymph nodes may harbor benign epithelial inclusions, epithelial papillae, and psammoma bodies, all of which are benign (57). Although the histologic distinction is important in malignant ovarian tumors, nodal metastases from LMP tumors may not affect clinical outcome. Leake and colleagues (50) described pelvic lymph node involvement in 3 (21.4%) of 14 patients with LMP tumors undergoing surgical staging. Paraaortic nodes were involved in 6 (18%) of 33 patients. All nodal metastases were associated with serous tumors and all were noninvasive; 4 of 21 patients with apparent stage I disease were upstaged based on the finding of lymph node involvement. Recurrence was more common among those patients with disease confined to the pelvis and lymph node spread, but no decrement in survival was observed.

Omentum

Omental involvement has been described in 3 (13%) of 24 patients (44) and in 6 (17.6%) of 34 patients (38) with clinical stage I disease, as well as 33 (40.2%) of 82 patients (51) with stage III tumors.

Ascites

Among patients with other peritoneal spread, Gershenson and Silva (51) found that 36 (43.9%) of 82 had ascites. In the GOG study of patients with stage III disease (41), 12 (37.5%) of 32 had ascites with an average volume of 1,700 mL (range, 20 to 6,000 mL). Malignant ascites or malignant peritoneal washings were found in 22 patients (68.8%). Nation and Krepart (38) found that 5 (7.6%) of 65 patients had cytologically malignant ascites, and 4 (17.6%) of 23 patients with early-stage disease undergoing lavage had malignant cells. Similarly, Yazigi and coworkers (44) reported positive washings in 2 (7.4%) of 27 patients undergoing surgical staging for apparent stage I tumors. Julian and Woodruff (43) reported ascites in nine patients, all with stage II tumors or greater, five of whom had persistent carcinoma; four of these five died from their disease. Tumor spill at the time of surgery did not influence outcome in six patients with early-stage disease who received no adjuvant therapy, as reported by Hopkins and associates (39).

Extraperitoneal Spread

Stage IV LMP tumors are exceedingly rare. Although Julian and Woodruff (43) reported 5 cases, or 7.7% of their total, only 4 additional cases (1.5%) were gleaned from a total of 613 reported by seven other authors

(6,37,38,40,42,58,59). All but 1 case were serous lesions. Julian and Woodruff (43) did not specify the sites of metastases but did report 60% tumor-free survival. Of the other four cases, two involved the lung or pleura, one the abdominal viscera, and the other was not specified.

Other Sites of Spread

Among the 32 women with stage III disease in the GOG study (41), 14 (43.8%) had biopsy-proven diaphragmatic metastases and 10 (31.3%) and 17 (53.1%) had spread to small and large bowel, respectively. In Gershenson and Silva's study of patients with extraovarian spread (51), only 2.4% had diaphragmatic metastases, and 7.3% and 25.6% had spread to the large and small bowel, respectively.

TUMOR MARKERS

Little has been written in this area. Chambers and colleagues (6) obtained serum CA 125 levels in 18 patients with LMP tumors and found elevation above 35 U/mL in only 4 (22.2%). Elevations did not exceed 100 U/mL. One patient who later developed an invasive ovarian cancer did have an abnormally high CA 125 (96 U/mL) at the time of the malignancy, indicating a potential role for CA 125 in monitoring.

THERAPY FOR PATIENTS WITH STAGE I DISEASE

Generally, the diagnosis of an LMP ovarian tumor is followed by abdominal hysterectomy and bilateral salpingo-oophorectomy, except in patients with approximately-staged early disease (IA) in whom childbearing is incomplete. Staging is important, but perhaps not as important in determining therapy as it is in patients with invasive cancer. Survival rates for patients with stage I LMP tumors are excellent whether or not the stage is determined by exhaustive surgery. It appears unnecessary to reexplore patients with early LMP tumors in order to perform biopsies that may have been omitted during the primary laparotomy.

Conservative Therapy

Ovarian Cystectomy

Lim-Tan and colleagues (60) studied the rates of persistence or recurrence of disease in 35 patients with serous tumors of LMP who were treated with unilateral cystectomy, bilateral cystectomy, or unilateral cystectomy and contralateral oophorectomy or salpingo-oophorectomy. Although tumor persisted or recurred in only two ovaries subjected to cystectomy (6%), there were also bilateral recurrences and subsequent involvement of the opposite ovary in one patient each (total failure rate, 12%). Positive surgical margins or multiple cystectomies in a single ovary were always associated with recurrence. These authors noted that survival was 100% at the median time of 6.5 years after surgery despite the recurrences and reported 8 pregnancies among 16 patients treated conservatively. They cautioned that, because a number of patients underwent tumor-related surgery after cystectomy, the excellent outcome in this study does not reflect the use of ovarian cystectomy alone.

Chambers and coworkers (6) noted recurrences after cystectomy in a patient who subsequently developed an invasive serous cancer. This is one of only five patients in the literature known to have developed an invasive cancer subsequent to therapy for an LMP tumor. Nikrui presented one case (37), and the three other patients reported by Fort and associates (59) and by Gershenson and coworkers (51) had stage III disease at the time of initial diagnosis. The risk of developing an ovarian malignancy at a later time, calculated from the five series including this phenomenon, is 1 in 57, or about 1.8%.

Ovarian cystectomy in the management of LMP tumors is not widely embraced and must be limited to exceptional cases.

Unilateral Oophorectomy or Salpingo-oophorectomy

Among the many authors who have published accounts of favorable outcomes after unilateral removal of an affected ovary, Julian and Woodruff (43) documented a 100% survival rate at 5 years among 15 patients who underwent unilateral

TABLE 22.2. Conservative therapy in stage I tumors

Therapy and author	N	Recurred	Died
Cystectomy			
Chambers	5	2	0
Lim-Tan	35	4	0
TOTAL	40	6 (15.0%)	0
Adnexectomy			
Hart	53	1	0
Chambers	14	0	0
Bostwick	24	3	0
Julian	15	0	0
Kliman	19	1	1
Fort	7	1	0
TOTAL	132	6 (4.5%)	1 (0.8%)

TABLE 22.3. Complete surgery without adjuvant therapy in stage I

Author	N	Recurred	Died
Creasman	25	0	0
Hart	34	2	2
Kliman	37	0	0
Chambers	50	3	1
Massad	11	1	0
Barnhill	24	0	0
Bostwick	56	3	0
Julian	10	0	0
Katerstein	19	0	0
Fort	7	0	0
Hopkins	26	1	0
Nation	34	0	0
TOTAL	333	10 (3.0%)	3 (0.9%)

adnexectomy, and Tazelaar and colleagues (49) reported that 17 of 20 patients were disease-free after unilateral salpingo-oophorectomy with or without wedge biopsy of the contralateral gonad. On the other hand, Munell (61) published an absolute 5-year survival rate of 58% among 12 patients with low-grade serous tumors who underwent conservative therapy. Other authors who reported isolated recurrences in retained ovaries include Hart and Norris (13) (1 benign and 1 LMP mucinous tumor), Russell and Merkur (62) (3 recurrences in 122 cases treated conservatively), and Hopkins and colleagues (39) (1 recurrence successfully resected).

Results of conservative surgery for stage I LMP tumors are summarized in Table 22.2.

Patients who develop recurrent neoplasia after conservative therapy may do quite well. Bostwick and associates (42) described relapses in 6 of 14 patients undergoing unilateral ovarian surgery. After subsequent surgical resection (and radiotherapy in 2), all were alive at 47 to 156 months (median, 69 months) after diagnosis.

As stated previously, there is no certain guideline for "completion surgery" in these patients after childbearing. Buttini and colleagues (63) reported a single contralateral recurrence among 29 patients undergoing conservative surgery (3.5%), and Kennedy and Hart (15) had 1 of 18 patients with a similar recurrence. Lu and associates (64) demonstrated that in 25% of patients with bilateral tumors, different androgen receptor alleles were inactivated in each ovarian tumor, indicating independent derivation. They suggested that advanced tumors of LMP and those with bilateral or sequential ovarian involvement may be of multifocal origin, in contrast to invasive cancers of the ovary.

Abdominal Hysterectomy and Bilateral Salpingo-oophorectomy

Removal of the reproductive organs must be considered standard therapy in women with stage I LMP tumors who have completed childbearing. Table 22.3 summarizes the outcome of 333 patients with stage I disease treated with extirpative surgery without adjuvant therapy. Recurrences were observed in only 10 patients (3.0% of the series), and only 3 of these patients (0.9%) died. Two had mucinous tumors that exceeded 25 cm in diameter and in which the histologic sampling may have been incomplete (13).

Adjuvant Therapy in Stage I Disease

Radiotherapy

Colgan and Norris (3) suggested that "adjuvant therapy has nothing to offer in patients with stage IA and IB tumors of LMP," but conceded without giving a reason that "in patients with stage IC disease, intraperitoneal radioactive colloids may be useful."

The role of adjuvant therapy in stage I LMP tumors has been studied prospectively only by Kolstad and coworkers (36). Eighty-three patients with stage I "potentially malignant" tumors were randomly assigned to receive either 5,000-cGy whole-pelvis radiotherapy or 3,000-cGy whole-pelvis radiotherapy plus 100 mCi of intraperitoneal radioactive gold 198 after hysterectomy, salpingo-oophorectomy, and omentectomy. One patient from each treatment arm died from recurrent disease, and two who received radiogold died from complications of therapy. Five-year survival rates were 92.5% and 87.2%, respectively. The use of combined radiogold and external pelvic radiotherapy resulted in more deaths from therapy than from disease in this study.

Massad and colleagues (65) and Fort and coworkers (59) contributed 10 patients with stage I disease successfully treated with radioactive chromic phosphate. The above-cited excellent results with surgery alone suggest a limited role, if any, for radioisotopes in the treatment of this disease (Table 22.4).

Creasman and associates (9) published a study of 55 patients randomly assigned to treatment with surgery alone, adjuvant pelvic radiotherapy, or adjuvant melphalan chemotherapy as part of a study designed to evaluate these treatments in women with frankly invasive cancer. All had undergone abdominal hysterectomy and bilateral adnexectomy. Median follow-up was 36 months. There was only 1 disease-related death in this study. A patient with a 34-cm primary tumor and 3,000 mL ascites received pelvic radiotherapy postoperatively; she developed recurrent cancer in 3 months and died 6 months later.

TABLE 22.4. Radiotherapy in stage I tumors

Author	N	Recurred	Died
External therapy			
Hart	2	0	0
Barnhill	9	0	0
Bostwick	5	2	0
Creasman	13	1	1
Kolstad	46	1	1
Subtotal	75	4 (5.3%)	2 (2.7%)
^{32}P			
Massad	7	0	0
Fort	3	0	0
Subtotal	10	0	0
^{198}Au			
Kolstad	37	1	1
Subtotal	34	1 (2.7%)	1 (2.7%)
TOTAL	122	5 (4.1%)	3 (2.5%)

TABLE 22.5. Complete surgery and chemotherapy in stage I tumors

Author	N	Recurred	Died
Chambers	15	0	0
Hart	5	1	1
Barnhill	13	0	0
Creasman	17	0	0
Fort	11	0	0
Hopkins	6	0	0
O'Quinn	2	1	1
Nation	5	0	0
TOTAL	74	2 (2.7%)	2 (2.7%)

Chemotherapy

Chemotherapy appears to be of limited value in the treatment of patients with stage I tumors of LMR. Table 22.5 summarizes the outcomes of 74 patients treated with a variety of cytotoxic agents. The two relapses and deaths represent a risk of only 3.4% in this group of patients, which is very similar to the results observed in patients treated with surgery alone. Conversely, the literature concerning LMP ovarian tumors is replete with cases of acute leukemia arising after prolonged therapy with alkylating agents such as melphalan. Several authors (6,39,41,59) have each reported one case, and O'Quinn and Hannigan (66) and Gershenson and associates (51) reported a total of seven leukemia-related deaths. Although the risk of leukemia is decreased with short-term therapy and with combinations containing cisplatin, other toxicities preclude the use of chemotherapy in tumors of early stage.

THERAPY FOR ADVANCED-STAGE OR RECURRENT TUMORS OF LOW MALIGNANT POTENTIAL

Therapy for Stage IV Tumors

It appears that all patients except the five reported by Julian and Woodruff (43) received adjuvant chemotherapy. Three clearly died from disease despite therapy (Table 22.6), for a tumor-related mortality rate of 33.3%.

Therapy for Stage II and III Tumors

Although there may be an inclination among oncologists to treat patients found to have

TABLE 22.6. Stage IV LMP tumors

Author	Adjuvant Therapy	Histology	Outcome (mo)
Barnhill	Chemo, ^{32}P	Serous	NED (32)
Nikrui	Chemo	Mucinous	DOD (54)
Fort	RT, Chemo	Serous	NED
Nation	Chemo	Serous	DOD
Julian	None	Serous	2 NED, 1 DOD, 1 AWD, 1 DOC
Disease-related mortality			3/9 (33.3%)

LMP, low malignant potential; Chemo, chemotherapy; RT, radiation therapy; AWD, alive with disease; DOC, dead of other causes; DOD, dead of disease; NED = no evidence of disease.

advanced-stage LMP tumors with adjuvant therapy, there is no compelling evidence in the literature that such treatment improves survival. Table 22.7 summarizes results from eight series in which patients with stages II and III tumors were treated with surgery alone. Of 58 patients, 14 (24.1%) developed recurrent disease, but only 5 (8.6%) died from progressive tumor. When the data from a number of studies are collected, it does not appear that either adjuvant radiotherapy (Table 22.8) or adjuvant chemotherapy (Table 22.9) offers more protection against recurrence or death than surgery alone.

Response to Chemotherapy

It is difficult to assess the efficacy of chemotherapy in women with tumors of LMP. Patients with advanced recurrent, clinically measurable disease are relatively rare, and no traditional prospective phase II or III studies are available. This observation itself suggests that the majority of patients with these tumors do well. Several authors have described outcomes in patients treated with chemotherapy. Nikrui (37)

TABLE 22.7. Surgery alone in stages II and III tumors

Author	N	Recurred	Died
Chambers	2	0	0
Bostwick	8	1	0
Conrad	25	8	3
Kliman	8	0	0
Massad	3	0	0
Fort	1	0	0
Hopkins	10	5	2
Nation	1	0	0
TOTAL	58	14 (24.1%)	5 (8.6%)

TABLE 22.8. Adjuvant radiotherapy in stages II and III

Author	N	Recurred	Died
Chambers	1	0	0
Barnhill	13	1	1
Bostwick	3	0	0
Kliman	3	1	1
Hopkins	8	2	1
TOTAL	28	4 (14.3%)	3 (10.7%)

reported deaths in four patients with disease refractory to alkylating agents and 5-fluorouracil; no specific response data were reported. Massad and colleagues (65) reported death despite chemotherapy in a patient with progressive disease. Barnhill and associates (58) reported a measurable response in a single patient treated with cisplatin, doxorubicin, and cyclophosphamide (PAC) and three patients who failed to respond to chemotherapy; two of the latter group experienced tumor growth while receiving alkylating agents and one with the three-drug cisplatin combination. One of the patients failed both melphalan and PAC. Kliman and coworkers (40) also described three patients who failed to respond to chemotherapy.

Of great interest, Llerena and colleagues (67) reported a case of chemotherapy-resistant 1AT tumor which responded serologically to tamoxifen.

Second-Look Laparotomy to Evaluate the Activity of Chemotherapy

This operation was first employed to permit discontinuation of alkylating agent chemotherapy in patients with invasive ovarian cancer.

TABLE 22.9. Surgery and chemotherapy in stages II and III

Author	N	Recurred	Died
Chambers	26	2	1
Barnhill	18	4	1
Bostwick	2	0	0
Kliman	9	5	3
Sutton	32	0	0
Massad	6	1	1
Fort	18	5	3
Hopkins	6	2	2
O'Ouinn	9	3	3
Nation	8	0	0
TOTAL	134	22 (16.5%)	14 (10.5%)

Second-look surgery also provides information regarding the efficacy of chemotherapy in patients who have tumors that cannot be measured by examination or radiographic methods.

O'Quinn and Hannigan (66) described 13 second-look operations in women treated with melphalan. Seven of these patients had stage III disease before treatment, and 10 of the 13 had persistent tumor at the time of the second operation. Five of these 10 were treated with more melphalan and had a third laparotomy; all had disease. Barnhill and colleagues (58) also reported a patient with a stage III serous LMP tumor who had positive second- and third-look operations despite 24 courses of melphalan therapy. Nation and Krepart (38) documented 10 second-look operations, 4 in patients with stage III disease. In half of the operations, persistent tumor was found. No patient with visible disease remaining at the end of the primary operation was free of tumor at the second surgical procedure. These studies suggest that alkylating agents are not effective in the treatment of advanced-stage LMP tumors.

Other authors have commented on the surgical findings after chemotherapy, but there are few studies in which a chemotherapy regimen was used consistently. Barnhill and associates (58) found tumor at second-look surgery in four of five patients who had macroscopic residual disease at the end of primary surgery; conversely, Chambers and coworkers (6) found that only one of four patients with residual tumor had tumor at second look. Although the type of chemotherapy was not specified in these two reports, the range of surgically documented responses represented in these two papers was 20% to 75%. Massad and colleagues (65) related that only one of three patients treated with chemotherapy for stage III disease had a histologically confirmed complete response.

Gershenson and Silva (51) recounted 20 patients with macroscopic residual tumor who were treated with either an alkylating agent or combination chemotherapy before a second-look operation. There were eight partial and eight complete surgical responses, for a total surgical response rate of 80%. Fort and coworkers (59) found persistent tumor in 3 of 15 patients undergoing second-look operation for tumors of stage II or higher. In this study subjects were treated with a variety of chemotherapeutic agents with or without radiotherapy.

All patients received combination chemotherapy, including cisplatin, in a study of stage III disease conducted by the GOG (41). Of eight patients with residual macroscopic tumor, only two had pathologically confirmed complete responses. Conversely, two of six patients who were believed to have had all tumor removed at the first operation had histologic evidence of tumor at the second surgery. The findings of this study indicate a maximum response rate of 20%. One subject with persistent tumor at second look surgery died from leukemia after subsequent alkylating agent treatment and radiotherapy There was no disease at autopsy. In this study, there were no tumor-related deaths during a median follow-up interval of 31.7 months.

These analyses do not establish a clear benefit for the routine use of adjuvant chemotherapy or second-look surgery in patients with stages II and III LMP ovarian tumors. Many authors have echoed the need for prospective trials in these patients. The GOG is presently conducting a study that will serve as a model for the conservative treatment of LMP tumors. Initially, tissue from all subjects is submitted for central pathologic review. Those patients whose disease is completely resected will have periodic clinical examinations with no adjuvant therapy. Those women in whom residual disease is present will be treated with chemotherapy only in the event of clinical progression or evidence of growth at the time of second look surgery. The results of this study are not yet available.

The importance of long-term surveillance of patients with LMP tumors cannot be overstated. Nikrui (37) observed recurrences in patients at 10 and 12 years after diagnosis, and Hopkins and associates (39) described recurrences as late as 23 and 25 years after primary surgical therapy. Median time to recurrence in the latter study was 5 years. Silva and coworkers (68) described 11 patients with stage I disease who developed recurrences after radiotherapy or chemotherapy 7 to 39 years (mean, 16 years) after diagnosis.

In summary, LMP ovarian tumors are best treated with abdominal hysterectomy, bilateral salpingo-oophorectomy, and indicated biopsies for complete staging. In young women with

TABLE 22.10. *Overall recurrence and survival in LMP tumors*

	N	Recurred	Died
Stage I	686	29	9
Stages II and III	219	40	22
TOTAL	905	69 (7.6%)	31 (3.4%)

LMP, low malignant potential.

stage I lesions, unilateral adnexectomy may be acceptable. The use of adjuvant therapy in stage I tumors is unnecessary. In tumors of stage II through IV, chemotherapy is of unproven benefit but may be acceptable if used judiciously. Second-look surgery is certainly not indicated women with stage I disease, and it is of dubious value in more advanced stages. Long-term monitoring of these patients is important. Overall results of therapy are shown in Table 22.10.

PSEUDOMYXOMA PERITONEI

Definition

Pseudomyxoma peritonei is loculated gelatinous material that accumulates in the peritoneal cavity, sometimes in massive amounts (Figures 22.4 and 22.5). The finding is usually associated with mucinous neoplasms of the ovary or appendix. Characteristically, the abdominal viscera and extraperitoneal sites are spared. Albeit slowly progressive, this condition is often refractory to therapy, and frequently leads to death from bowel obstruction.

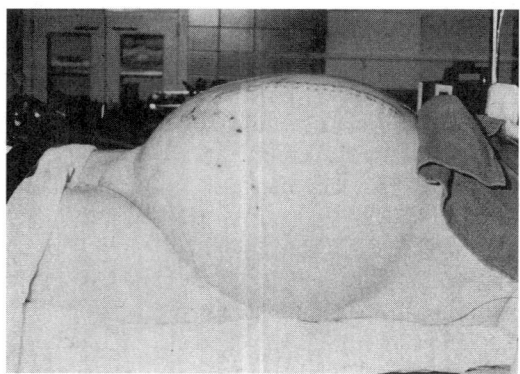

FIG. 22.4. Abdominal distension caused by pseudomyxoma peritonei.

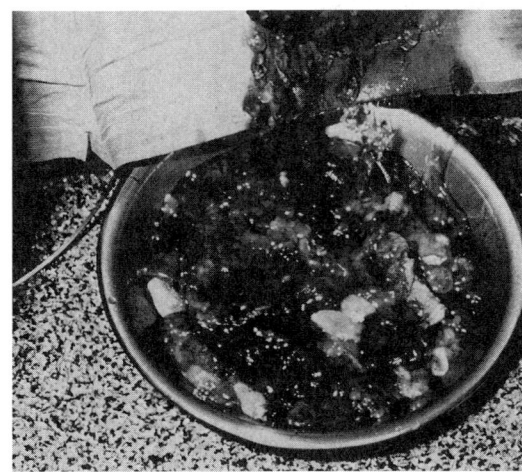

FIG. 22.5. Gross appearance of gelatinous ascites in pseudomyxoma peritonei.

History

Although Rokitansky described this condition in 1842, the term "pseudomyxoma peritonei" is ascribed to Werth, who presented a case associated with perforation of an ovarian cyst in 1844 (69). In 1901, Fraenkel (70) first reported pseudomyxoma peritonei in association with a mucocele of the appendix.

Incidence

Pseudomyxoma peritonei was diagnosed at the Ottawa General Hospital in 9 cases during a 20-year span in which 96,981 surgical specimens were accrued, for an incidence of 1 in 10,000 cases (71). Masson and Hamrick (72) found 30 cases of pseudomyxoma among 7,800 oophorectomies performed at the Mayo Clinic. Russell recorded pseudomyxoma peritonei in association with 5 (1.7%) of 293 benign mucinous ovarian tumors (18), 8 (15.4%) of 52 LMP tumors (73), and 5 (29.4%) of 17 frankly malignant tumors (74).

Gross and Microscopic Pathology

The ovarian neoplasms associated with pseudomyxoma peritonei may range from 4 to 40 cm (75,76), although the massive accumulation of mucoid material may preclude identification of an ovarian primary. Young and associates (77) found a median size of 16 cm in 22 patients. The volume of mucinous ascites may vary; from 1,000 mL to 15 kg of this material was described in one study (76). Histologically, the ovarian lesions usually have the characteristics of mucinous LMP tumors, although some benign-appearing epithelium may be seen. Manifestations of invasion such as desmoplasia, inflammation, and solid or cribriform areas are characteristically absent (75). Stromal mucin is present in varying amounts, and the quantity of ovarian epithelium or stroma may vary widely from case to case.

Etiology and Pathogenesis

Several theories have been advanced to explain the phenomenon of pseudomyxoma peritonei. Rupture of a mucinous tumor of the ovary or appendix with spread of cellular debris throughout the peritoneal cavity is often blamed for the development of pseudomyxoma peritonei. Although this is a plausible theory, mucoceles induced by appendiceal ligation in the rabbit do not lead to pseudomyxoma peritonei when perforated. Similarly, it has repeatedly been demonstrated that rupture of a mucinous ovarian neoplasm in humans does not lead to the development of pseudomyxoma peritonei (3,33,78,79). Additionally, pseudomyxoma peritonei may develop in instances in which mucinous tumors clearly have not ruptured (80). Sadenbergh and Woodruff (76) suggested that mucin released from the ovary induces a process of "mucinification" of the surrounding peritoneum through a kind of foreign body reaction. Peritoneal metaplasia, such as is suggested in peritoneal endometriosis or endosalpingiosis, seems an unlikely cause. These processes may be observed in the absence of a primary ovarian lesion, whereas pseudomyxoma peritonei is virtually always associated with a "primary" neoplasm in the ovary, appendix, or other site.

Michael and colleagues (75) observed that some mucinous neoplasms of the ovary contain acellular pools of mucin or "pseudomyxoma ovarii." Hart and Norris (13) indicated that the presence of these stromal collections imbued mucinous LMP tumors with more aggressive behavior. Michael and colleagues (75) surmised that when mucin dissected through the ovarian stroma and contained epithelial fragments, a form of invasion was present. In tumors of the ovary that otherwise could be characterized as LMP tumors, this indicated a poorer prognosis. They suggested the term "ovarian carcinoma with extracellular mucin production" to describe these lesions. This pattern of invasion of the stroma by mucin-containing epithelial fragments is recognized in the breast and gastrointestinal tract and is associated with malignant behavior.

Colonic differentiation of the peritoneal mesothelium may also play a role in the pathogenesis of pseudomyxoma peritonei. Epithelial goblet cells are commonly identified (18), and the gelatinous ascites contains large quantities of carcinoembryonic antigen (CEA), a marker strongly identified with colorectal neoplasms.

Biochemistry

Beller and associates (81) showed that this mucinous substance was 95.5% water, 1.6% lipid, and 2.9% acid sialomucopolysaccharide. In addition to containing large quantities of CEA, the material is rich in gamma globulin and possesses thromboplastic activity. It is also water soluble and readily dissolves in both glucose and dextran solutions.

Clinical Characteristics

The age distribution of patients with pseudomyxoma peritonei ranges from 16 to 81 years (75,76,82,83), with reported means of 49 to 63 years (75,82,83). Symptoms in order of frequency, as reported by Carter and associates (82), included abdominal mass, abdominal pain, distention, weight loss, and hernia. Umbilical hernias predominated in women, while inguinal hernias were more common in men with pseudomyxoma associated with appendiceal lesions. The average duration of symptoms was 11.5 months (range, 1 to 60 months).

Pseudomyxoma peritonei has been described in association with all types of mucinous ovarian tumors as well as appendiceal mucocele and appendiceal adenocarcinoma (84). There are diverse opinions regarding the predominance of different ovarian lesions. Masson and Hamrick (72) presented 30 cases, 13 associated with "low-grade" ovarian tumors and the remainder with benign mucinous cystadenomas. Similarly, Long and associates (85) and Woodruff and coworkers (78) reported a total of 11 cases occurring with benign ovarian tumors. Shanks (86) found 2 adenocarcinomas in 12 patients with pseudomyxoma peritonei, and Limber and associates (79) found mucinous ovarian malignancies in 5 of 10 patients with pseudomyxoma peritonei. In contrast to these reports, Cariker and Dockerty (80) reported that pseudomyxoma peritonei was always associated with malignant ovarian or appendiceal tumors.

In the survey of Carter and colleagues (82), a mucocele of the appendix was observed in 36 of 64 cases (56.3%), and the appendix was the apparent primary site of the lesion in 23 cases (35.9%). Of the mucoceles, 14 were associated with a primary appendiceal tumor. Cerame (84) identified pseudomyxoma in 18 (5.6%) of 316 cases of primary appendiceal adenocarcinoma.

Young and associates (77) found that the appendix and ovary were synchronously involved in 21 cases of pseudomyxoma peritonei. The group postulated that the appendix was the site of origin because of the frequency of bilaterality and the fact that the right ovary was involved more often than the left. Histologically, all 21 cases contained a mucinous LMP tumor of the appendix.

Other tumors associated with pseudomyxoma peritonei include mucinous carcinoma of the endometrium, colon, and common duct (82), ovarian teratomas (83), umbilical and urachal lesions, and LMP lesions of the fallopian tube.

Radiographic Studies

Radiographic studies in patients with pseudomyxoma peritonei typically demonstrate extrinsic compression of the large and small bowel. Ultrasound may exhibit multiloculated cystic masses within the abdomen. Computed tomography may be diagnostic. Large low-density intraperitoneal masses are visualized, and characteristic smooth scalloping of the liver surface differentiates this process from ascites or solid tumors (87).

Treatment and Survival

Because pseudomyxoma peritonei is uncommon, almost all trials of therapy have been small and retrospective in nature. No consensus on therapy exists.

Limber and coworkers (79) reported on 10 patients with pseudomyxoma peritonei who received no adjuvant therapy. All patients who were monitored for 3 or more years developed recurrence at a median time of 18 months. Michael and colleagues (75) reported two deaths within 1 year of diagnosis in untreated patients. Mann and colleagues (88) suggested that repeated surgical intervention was the only treatment that could prolong survival. Bernhardt and Young (89) described a patient in whom eight laparotomies were performed in a 15-year period. Green and associates (90) and Piver and coworkers (91) suggested the use of mucolytic agents such as sterile water or hyaluronidase. The latter group described a woman who survived without a recurrence for 3.5 years after tumor resection and lavage with 5% dextrose in water.

Radiotherapy has been advocated by a few authors. Fernandez and Daly (92) reported a 5-year survival rate of 75% in patients receiving radiotherapy, compared with 44% in those subjects who were treated with melphalan. Radioactive chromic phosphate was administered intraperitoneally by Sandenbergh and Woodruff (76) and by Ghosh and colleagues (93). Of four patients, two were alive at 1 year, and two had developed bowel obstructions within a few years. One obstruction was fatal.

Immunotherapy in the form of autogenous vaccines was discussed briefly by Graham and Graham (94), and Magell (95) described the creation of a mucous fistula through which the ascites could be drained.

Several authors have advocated chemotherapy in this disease. Jones and Homesley (96) attained

48 months of tumor-free survival in a single patient treated with cisplatin, doxorubicin, and cyclophosphamide. In our report (75) from Indiana University, chemotherapy was used initially in six patients and in one patient who had recurrent disease after treatment with intraperitoneal radiogold. Four patients had clinical complete responses (56%) and two had negative second-look laparotomies after melphalan therapy. Neither of these two patients had evidence of disease at 62 and 64 months, but one died from leukemia. One patient treated with cisplatin, doxorubicin, and cyclophosphamide had progression of disease 27 months after therapy. Overall survival in this report ranged from 8 months to 13.5 years, with a mean of 4.2 years. The 2-year survival rate was 45%. Mann and associates (88) treated seven patients with adjuvant chemotherapy that included cisplatin. Six had recurrence or progression of tumor, and no patient had a measurable response to therapy. One patient whose tumor was completely resected before chemotherapy was healthy at 6 years' time. These authors "found no evidence that cisplatin chemotherapy provides any benefit to patients with pseudomyxoma peritonei." Sugarbaker and associates (97) recommended the use of intraperitoneal 5-fluorouracil and systemic mitomycin C after aggressive surgical resection of pseudomyxoma peritonei. They reported that five of seven patients so treated were well at intervals from 2 to 4 years after therapy.

We have treated 10 patients at Indiana University with intraperitoneal 5-fluorouracil. Of 9 patients who had measurable tumors, 3 had growth at 7 to 9 months of therapy, and 1 had a complete clinical response but had evidence of progression at the time of second-look surgery. Four of the remaining five patients had second look surgery; two had no tumor and two had microscopic evidence of persistent disease. The last patient refused second look surgery and is doing well. Median survival for the entire group of patients was 46.8 months, similar to a group of historical controls.

Although surgical therapy may prove beneficial initially, the inexorable progress of this disease leads inevitably to morbidity and mortality. These facts warrant the development of innovative therapeutic approaches.

REFERENCES

1. Taylor HC. Malignant and semimalignant tumors of the ovary. *Surg Gynecol Obstet* 1929;48:702.
2. International Federation of Gynecology and Obstetrics. Classification and strategy of malignant tumors in the female pelvis. *Acta Obstet Gynecol Scand* 1977;50:1.
3. Colgan T, Norris H. Ovarian epithelial tumors of low malignant potential: a review. *Int J Gynecol Pathol* 1983;1:367.
4. Norris HJ, Mount PM. Pathology of ovarian tumors of low malignant potential. In: Rutledge F, Wharton T, Gershenson D, eds *Gynecologic cancer: diagnosis and treatment strategies.* Austin, University of Texas Press, 1987:171–192.
5. Czernobilsky B. Common epithelial tumors of the ovary. In: Kurman R, ed. *Blaustein's pathology of the female genital system.* New York: Springer-Verlag, 1990:560–569.
6. Chambers JT, et al. Borderline ovarian tumors. *Am J Obstet Gynecol* 1988;159:1088.
7. Katzenstein AA, et al. Proliferative serous tumors of the ovary. *Am J Surg Pathol* 1978;2:339.
8. Seidman JD, Kurman RJ. Subclassification of serous borderline tumors of the ovary into benign and malignant types: a clinical pathological study of 65 advanced stage cases. *Am J Surg Pathol* 1996;20:1331–1345.
9. Creasman WT, et al. Stage I borderline ovarian tumors. *Obstet Gynecol* 1982;59:93.
10. Bell DA, Scully RE. Clinical perspective on borderline tumors of the ovary. In: Hale RW, ed. *Current topics in obstetrics and gynecology.* New York: Elsevier, 1991:119–134.
11. Birks RT, Sherman MIE, Kurman RT. Micropapillary serous carcinoma of the ovary: a distinctive low-grade carcinoma related to serous borderline tumors. *Am J Surg Pathol* 1996;20:1319–1330.
12. Eichhorn J-H, Bell DA, Young RH, Scully RE. Ovarian serous borderline tumors of micropapillary and cribriform patterns: a study of 40 cases and comparison with 44 cases without these patterns. *Am J Surg Pathol* 1999;23:397–409.
13. Hart WR, Norris HJ. Borderline and malignant mucinous tumors of the ovary: histologic criteria and clinical behavior. *Cancer* 1973;31:1031.
14. Rutgers JL, Scully RE. Ovarian müllerian mucinous papillary cystadenomas of borderline malignancy. *Cancer* 1988;61:340.
15. Kennedy AW, Hart WR. Ovarian papillary serous tumors of low malignant potential (serous borderline tumors): a long-term follow-up study, including patients with microinvasion, lymph node metastasis, and transformation to invasive serous carcinomas. *Cancer* 1996;78:278.
16. Nayar R, Siliunkgul S, Robbins KM, et al. Microinvasion in low malignant potential tumors of the ovary. *Hum Pathol* 1996;27:521–527.
17. Riopel NIA, Ronnett BM, Kunnan RJ. Evaluation of diagnostic criteria and behavior of ovarian intestinal type mucinous tumors: atypical proliferative (borderline) tumors and intraepithelial, microinvasive, invasive, and metastatic carcinomas. *Am J Surg Pathol* 1999;23:617–635.

18. Russell P. The pathological assessment of ovarian neoplasms: I. Introduction to the common "epithelial" tumors and analysis of benign "epithelial" tumors. *Pathology* 1979;11:5.
19. Roth LM, Dallenbach-Hellweg G, Czernobilsky B. Ovarian Brenner tumors: I. Metaplastic, proliferating, and of low malignant potential. *Cancer* 1985;56:582.
20. Hernandez E, Bhagavan BS, Parmley TH, et al. Interobserver variability in the interpretation of epithelial ovarian cancer. *Gynecol Oncol* 1984;17:117.
21. Baak JPA, Vanderley G. Borderline or malignant ovarian tumor? A case report of decision making with morphometry. *J Clin Pathol* 1984;37:1110.
22. Erhardt E, et al. Combined morphologic and cytochemical grading of serous ovarian tumors. *Am J Obstet Gynecol* 1985;151:356.
23. Fu YS, Ro J, Reagan JW, et al. Nuclear deoxyribonucleic acid heterogeneity of ovarian borderline malignant serous tumors. *Obstet Gynecol* 1986; 67:478.
24. Friedlander ML, et al. Flow cytometric analysis of cellular DNA content as an adjunct to the diagnosis of ovarian tumors of borderline malignancy. *Pathology* 1984;16:301.
25. Iverson O, Skarrdland E. Ploidy assessment of benign and malignant ovarian tumors by flow cytometry. *Cancer* 1987;60:82.
26. Klemi PJ, et al. Clinical significance of abnormal nuclear DNA content in serous ovarian tumors. *Cancer* 1988;62:2005.
27. Kaern J, Trope CG, Kristensen GB, et al. DNA ploidy: the most important prognostic factor in patients with borderline tumors of the ovary. *Int J Gynecol Cancer* 1993;3:349.
28. Kotylo PK, Michael H, Fineberg N, et al. Flow cytometric analysis of DNA content and RAS p21 oncoprotein expression in ovarian neoplasms. *Int J Gynecol Pathol* 1992;11:30–37.
29. Berchuck A, Kohler W, Hopkins MP, et al. Overexpression of p53 is not a feature of benign and early stage borderline epithelial ovarian tumors. *Gynecol Oncol* 1994;52:232.
30. Van Haaften-Daly C, Russell P, Boyer CM, et al. Expression of cell regulatory proteins in ovarian borderline tumors. *Cancer* 1996;77:2092.
31. Haas CJ, Diebold J, Ferschmann A, et al. Microsatellite analysis in serous tumors of the ovary. *Int J Gynecol Pathol* 1999;18:158–162.
32. Cheng PC, Gosewehr JA, Kim TM, et al. Potential role of inactivated X chromosome in ovarian epithelial tumor development. *J Natl Cancer Inst* 1996;88:510.
33. Gondos B. Electron microscopic study of papillary serous tumors of the ovary. *Cancer* 1971;27:1455.
34. Purola E. Serous papillary ovarian tumors. *Acta Obstet Gynecol Scand* 1963;42[Suppl]:1.
35. Aure JC, Hoeg K, Kolstad P. Clinical and histologic studies of ovarian carcinoma. *Obstet Gynecol* 1971;37:1.
36. Kolstad P, Davy M, Hoeg K. Individualized treatment of ovarian cancer. *Am J Obstet Gynecol* 1977;128:617.
37. Nikrui N. Survey of clinical behavior of patients with borderline epithelial tumors of the ovary. *Gynecol Oncol* 1981;12:107.
38. Nation JG, Krepart GV. Ovarian carcinoma of low malignant potential: staging and treatment. *Am J Obstet Gynecol* 1986;154:290.
39. Hopkins MP, Kumar NB, Morley GW. An assessment of pathologic features and treatment modalities in ovarian tumors of low malignant potential. *Obstet Gynecol* 1987;70:923.
40. Kliman L, Rome RM, Fortune DW. Low malignant potential tumors of the ovary: a study of 76 cases. *Obstet Gynecol* 1986;68:338.
41. Sutton GP, Bundy BN, Omara GA, et al. Stage III ovarian tumors of low malignant potential treated with cisplatin combination therapy (a Gynecologic Oncology Group study). *Gynecol Oncol* 1991;41:230.
42. Bostwick DG, et al. Ovarian epithelial tumors of borderline malignancy. *Cancer* 1986;58:2052.
43. Julian CG, Woodruff JD. The biologic behavior of low-grade papillary serous carcinoma of the ovary. *Obstet Gynecol* 1972;40:860.
43a. Moorey J, Silva E, Tomos C, et al. Unusual features of serous neoplasms of low malignant potential during pregnancy. *Gynecol Oncol* 1997;65:30–35.
44. Yazigi R, Sandstad J, Munoz AK. Primary staging in ovarian tumors of low malignant potential. *Gynecol Oncol* 1988;31:402.
45. Young RC, et al. Staging laparotomy in early ovarian cancer. *JAMA* 1983;250:3072.
46. Piver MS. Ovarian carcinoma: a decade of progress. *Cancer* 1984;54:2706.
47. Snider DD, Stuart GC, Nation JG, et al. Evaluation of surgical staging in stage I low malignant potential ovarian tumors. *Gynecol Oncol* 1991;40:129–132.
48. Williams TJ, Dockerty MB. Status of the contralateral ovary in encapsulated low grade malignant tumors of the ovary. *Surg Gynecol Obstet* 1981;143:763–766.
49. Tazelaar HD, et al. Conservative treatment of borderline ovarian tumors. *Obstet Gynecol* 1985;66:417.
50. Leake JF, Radar JS, Woodruff JD, et al. Retroperitoneal lymphatic involvement with epithelial ovarian tumors of low malignant potential. *Gynecol Oncol* 1991;42:124–130.
51. Gershenson DM, Silva EG. Serous ovarian tumors of low malignant potential with peritoneal implants. *Cancer* 1990;65:578.
52. Michael H, Roth LM. Invasive and noninvasive implants in ovarian serous tumors of low malignant potential. *Cancer* 1986;57:1240–1247.
53. Russell P. Borderline epithelial tumors of the ovary: a conceptual dilemma. *Clin Obstet Gynecol* 1984;11:259–277.
54. McCanghey WT, Kirk ME, Lester W. Peritoneal epithelial lesions associated with proliferative serous tumors of the ovary. *Histopathology* 1984;8:195–208.
55. Bell DA, Weinstock MA, Scully RE. Peritoneal implants of ovarian serous borderline tumors. *Cancer* 1988;62:2212.
56. Gershenson DM, Silva EG, Levy L, et al. Ovarian serous borderline tumors with invasive peritoneal implants. *Cancer* 1998;82:1096–1103.
57. Malloy JJ, et al. Papillary ovarian tumors. *Am J Obstet Gynecol* 1965;93:867.
58. Barnhill D, et al. Epithelial ovarian carcinoma of low malignant potential. *Obstet Gynecol* 1985;65:53.
59. Fort MG, Piera VK, Saigo PE. Evidence for the efficacy of adjuvant therapy in epithelial ovarian tumors of low malignant potential. *Gynecol Oncol* 1989;32:269–272.

60. Lim-Tan SK, Cajigas HE, Scully RE. Ovarian cystectomy for serous borderline tumors: a follow-up study of 35 cases. *Obstet Gynecol* 1988;72:775.
61. Munnell EW. Is conservative therapy ever justified in stage I (IA) cancer of the ovary? *Am J Obstet Gynecol* 1969;103:641.
62. Russell P, Merkur H. Proliferative ovarian "epithelial" tumors: a clinicopathological analysis of 144 cases. *Aust N Z J Obstet Gynaecol* 1979;19:45.
63. Buttini M, Nicklin JL, Crandon A. Low malignant potential tumors: a review of 175 consecutive cases. *Aust N Z J Obstet Gynaecol* 1997;37:100.
64. Lu KH, Bell DA, Welch VR, Berkowitz RS. Evidence for the multifocal origin of bilateral and advanced human borderline ovarian tumors. *Cancer Res* 1998;58:2328.
65. Massad LS, et al. Epithelial ovarian tumors of low malignant potential. *Obstet Gynecol* 1991;78:1027.
66. O'Quinn AG, Hannigan EV. Epithelial ovarian neoplasms of low malignant potential. *Gynecol Oncol* 1985;21:177.
67. Llerena E, Kudelka A, Tomos C, et al. Remission of a chemotherapy-resistant tumor of low malignant potential with tamoxifen. *Eur J Gynecol Oncol* 1997;18:23–25.
68. Silva EG, Tomos C, Zehang Z, et al. Tumor recurrence in stage I ovarian serous neoplasms of low malignant potential. *Int J Gynecol Pathol* 1998;17:1–6.
69. Werth R. Pseudomyxoma peritonei. *Arch Gynecol Obstet* 1884; 24:100.
70. Fraenkel E. Uber das sogenannte pseudomyxoma peritonei. *Munch Med Wschr* 1901;48:965.
71. Campbell JS, et al. Pseudomyxoma peritonei et ovarii with occult neoplasms of the appendix. *Obstet Gynecol* 1973;42:897.
72. Masson JC, Hamrick RA. Pseudomyxoma peritonei of ovarian origin: an analysis of thirty cases. *Surg Clin North Am* 1930;10:61.
73. Russell P. The pathological assessment of ovarian neoplasms: II. The proliferating "epithelial" tumors. *Pathology* 1979;11:251.
74. Russell P. The pathological assessment of ovarian neoplasms: 111. The malignant "epithelial" tumors. *Pathology* 1979;11:493.
75. Michael H, Sutton G, Roth LM. Ovarian carcinoma with extracellular mucin production: reassessment of "pseudomyxoma ovarii et peritonei." *Int J Gynecol Pathol* 1987;6:298.
76. Sandenbergh HA, Woodruff JD. Histogenesis of pseudomyxoma peritonei. *Obstet Gynecol* 1977;49:339.
77. Young RH, Gilks CB, Scully RE. Mucinous tumors of the appendix associated with mucinous tumors of the ovary and pseudomyxoma peritonei. *Am J Surg Pathol* 1991;15:415.
78. Woodruff JD, Bie LS, Sherman RJ. Mucinous tumors of the ovary. *Obstet Gynecol* 1960;16:699.
79. Limber GK, King RE, Silverberg SG. Pseudomyxoma peritonei: a report of ten cases. *Ann Surg* 1973;178:587.
80. Cariker M, Dockerty M. Mucinous cystadenomas and mucinous cystadenocarcinomas of the ovary. *Cancer* 1951;7:302.
81. Beller FK, Zimmerman RE, Nienhaus H. Biochemical identification of mucus of pseudomyxoma peritonei as the basis for mucolytic treatment. *Am J Obstet Gynecol* 1986;155:970.
82. Carter J, et al. Pseudomyxoma peritonei: a review. *Int J Gynecol Cancer* 1991;1:243.
83. Osborne CL. Pseudomyxoma peritonei: a report of seven cases. *Gynecol Oncol* 1973;1:195.
84. Cerame MA. A 25-year review of adenocarcinoma of the appendix. *Dis Colon Rectum* 1988;31:145.
85. Long RT, Spratt JS, Dowling E. Pseudomyxoma peritonei: new concepts in management with a report of seventeen patients. *Am J Surg* 1969;117:162.
86. Shanks HGI. Pseudomyxoma peritonei. *Br J Obstet Gynaecol* 1961;68:212.
87. Hann L, Love S, Goldberg RP. Pseudomyxoma peritonei: preoperative diagnosis by ultrasound and computed tomography. *Cancer* 1983;52:642.
88. Mann WJ, Wagner J, Chumas J, et al. The management of pseudomyxoma peritonei. *Cancer* 1990;66:1636.
89. Bernhardt H, Young JM. Mucocele and pseudomyxoma peritonei: new concepts in management with a report of seventeen patients. *Am J Surg* 1969;117:162.
90. Green N, et al. Pseudomyxoma peritonei of appendiceal origin: clinicopathologic aspects. *Am J Surg* 1965;109:235.
91. Piver MS, Lele SB, Patsner B. Pseudomyxoma peritonei: possible prevention of mucinous ascites by peritoneal lavage. *Obstet Gynecol* 1984;64:95.
92. Fernandez RN, Daly JM. Pseudomyxoma peritonei. *Arch Surg* 1981;115:409.
93. Ghosh BC, Huvos AG, Whiteley HW. Pseudomyxoma peritonei. *Dis Colon Rectum* 1972;15:420.
94. Graham JB, Graham R. Pseudomyxoma peritonei treated with autogenous vaccine. *Clin Obstet Gynecol* 1969;12:955.
95. Magell J. Pseudomyxoma peritonei [Letter]. *Lancet* 1959;2:846.
96. Jones CM, Homesley HD. Successful treatment of pseudomyxoma peritonei of ovarian origin with cisplatin, doxorubicin, and cyclophosphamide. *Gynecol Oncol* 1985;22:257.
97. Sugarbaker PH, Kern K, Lack E. Malignant pseudomyxoma peritonei of colonic origin: natural history and presentation of a curative approach to treatment. *Dis Colon Rectum* 1987;30:772.

23
Quality of Life Issues in Ovarian Cancer

George J. Olt and Joanna Cain

The phrase "quality of life" is frequently encountered in medical literature. At first glance the concept seems simple and intuitive. If one attempts to define quality of life, however, it becomes a complex and personal mixture of social, mental, and physical health issues. Indeed, no one definition of quality of life is agreed upon, and the concept means different things to different people at different times. Jonsen and associates (1) thought that it "expresses a value judgment. The experience of living, as a whole or in some aspect, is judged to be 'good' or 'bad,' 'better' or 'worse.'" Cella and Cherin (2), preferring to compare to an ideal state, defined it as "patients' appraisal of and satisfaction with their current level of functioning as compared to what they perceive to be possible or ideal." In a more psychological orientation, Shumaker and associates (3) defined quality of life as "individuals' overall satisfaction with life and their general sense of personal well-being." Schipper (4) defined quality of life in terms of functionality: "a pragmatic, day-to-day, functional representation of a patient's physical, psychological, and social response to a disease and its treatment." Regardless of differing approaches, quality of life is an individual patient's perception of her particular circumstances.

Although an exact definition of quality of life cannot be agreed on, all accept the importance of its evaluation and use. It has been suggested that the emotional suffering cancer causes may exceed that of the physical suffering (5). The impact that ovarian cancer and its therapies have on quality of life begins with diagnosis, extends through treatment, and continues beyond cure in those fortunate enough to achieve that state. A patient's perception of her quality of life changes dramatically from the time of diagnosis, throughout her therapy, and during remission. Understanding and acknowledging each patient's perception of quality of life, especially as it changes throughout the course of her disease, is necessary to provide the most compassionate and complete care possible.

The scope of the physician's responsibility for patient well-being has traditionally been defined by each physician. Historically, physicians directed the care of their patients. Although most physicians took into consideration the patient's general preferences and points of view, actual patient input in decision making was minimal. Physicians are increasingly being held responsible for quality-of-life and health issues that they may believe are more properly the concerns of the individual or society. Many physicians waver between the borders of too much involvement and not enough, in an attempt to restore the elusive composite called "health" and to maximize quality of life.

To address quality of life as health, we must examine both the quantity of time a patient survives after diagnosis, with or without treatment, and the quality of that time. Health providers have always had to consider the impact of specific treatments. This assessment has often been made through the "voice" of the caregiver rather than that of the patient. We are now attempting to include the patient's voice during experimental protocols by including the aggregate voices of quality-of-life assessments. However, a choir does not sing with the same voice as an individual, and we must be vigilant about orienting quality of life to the individual patient's perspective.

Presently, our knowledge about the quality of life of women with ovarian cancer is rudimentary. Only during the last decade has assessment of quality of life been incorporated into large clinical trials. Cella and Tulsky (6) succinctly presented the desired research goals directed toward the measurement of quality of life: (a) to identify the full range of side effects and impacts of the treatments in order to assess rehabilitation needs; (b) to compare treatments in a trial; and (c) to use quality-of-life ratings as a predictor of response to future treatment. Certainly, the enlarging role of managed health care will increase the importance of fulfilling these goals.

This chapter examines particular time points in the course of therapy for ovarian cancer when the perspectives of the patient, the physician, and society can be in conflict. It also highlights aspects of quality of life that should properly be the responsibility of caregivers, or at least considerations during the planning of care.

INITIATION OF THERAPY

Case. Patient A, with stage IIIC grade 3 serous ovarian adenocarcinoma, presents for a discussion of chemotherapy. She had suboptimal cytoreduction with a difficult recovery, and she is experiencing continued problems with bowel function and early satiety. After presentation of the risks and benefits of carboplatin and paclitaxel chemotherapy, she states, "No, I've read all about it and I don't want any chemotherapy. Besides, the government doesn't allow any of the effective treatments into this country; all the books say so. You've told me my chance for cure is low, so why bother anyway? I just want to go to sleep and die."

The initial education that a patient receives about ovarian cancer had a sustained effect on the quality of her relationship with her physician and, therefore, on her quality of life. Truthful information, given with sensitivity for the educational level and emotional status of the patient, requires attention to her perceptions rather than the perspective of the physician. For example, Patient A may be giving provocative statements regarding a need for recognition of her fear and distress. An acknowledgement of these feelings may allow her to consider chemotherapy. On the other hand, she may have a fixed, if false, view that the government does not allow effective treatment, a view that would render further discussion of chemotherapy futile. From this patient's perspective, treatment is useless, and it would be a greater burden than benefit. Her "experience of living," which physicians would expect to improve with chemotherapy, would seem to her to be worsened by the side effects of therapy that has "no chance" of helping her. This discrepancy between the facts that the physician perceives and the patient's perspective can be frustrating. However, even the irrational choices made by patients must be respected if they cannot be persuaded to change them.

Patients differ in their individual perceptions of the burdens and benefits of care. One patient may accept aggressive, highly toxic, initial protocol treatment because her contribution to medical knowledge is important to her sense of self. For such a patient, her sense of value as a person is intrinsic to her perception of quality of life. For another patient, a single day of mild nausea with treatment may be too great a burden. The experience of a symptom does not comprise quality of life; rather, quality of life is dependent on the filter through which symptoms are viewed. An individual patient's perceptions cause her to judge her existence as good or poor.

The planning of any therapy includes an examination of what quality of life is for a particular patient. This subject needs reassessment during the entire course of therapy, in light of current problems and overall health status. Our knowledge of how perceptions about quality of life change over the course of a disease is still emerging. However, we know that readjustment to new physical circumstances can lead to alterations in perceptions of quality of life. In fact, physical discomfort and anatomic changes that would previously have been totally unacceptable may be perceived as minor after refocusing occurs.

The initiation of a treatment plan is the first time during therapy when physicians may encounter the gap between their own perceptions of quality of life and those of the patient. Newcomb and Carbone (7) suggested that many clinicians assume that older patients do not want to be treated as aggressively as younger patients do. For example, a physician might expend more effort trying to convince Patient A of the need for initial therapy if she were 40 years old, a banker, and the mother of two small children than if she were 75 years old, diabetic, morbidly obese, partially blind, and living alone. However, a patient in either situation might have exactly the same response to therapy in terms of symptom control (diminution of ascites and increased food tolerance) and increased survival. Each might view her present circumstances as equally satisfactory. The responses of physicians to patients in various circumstances are based on their own views of what constitutes quality of life. The fact that physicians do not always perceive quality of life in the same way their patients do is a reality that we would be wise to reflect on before initiating therapy (8).

Another area of concern to the patient with ovarian cancer is the constancy of the relationship that she can expect from her physician. Will the physician continue to see her if she finds the course to be too great a burden, or if her disease does not respond to treatment? The constancy of the patient-physician relationship has a major impact on quality of life. It is not adequate to assume that a patient understands that an individual physician is willing to care for her during the course of her illness, whether she accepts the prescribed therapy or not. Physicians must acknowledge their willingness to care for patients who refuse to follow standard treatment patterns and those who are in the terminal phase of their disease. If a physician is not willing to provide terminal care, patients should be told that the physician's involvement is only with a particular treatment and that others will handle subsequent aspects of disease management.

A strong patient-physician relationship can be encouraged by a discussion, as Katz (9) stated, "in which both, appreciative of their respective inequalities, make a genuine effort to voice and clarify their uncertainties and then arrive at a mutually satisfactory course of action." The patient can then make a choice about care that includes the burden and sense of loss that a change of physician or a number of physicians involved in her care might cause. Patient autonomy is respected, and a maximal experience of living is supported.

ISSUES RAISED BY RESEARCH PROTOCOLS: CONFLICT OF INTEREST OVER QUALITY-OF-LIFE ISSUES

Clinical trials can present ethical problems for the physician because the roles of physician and researcher may contain inherent conflicts. For example, Hellman and Hellman (10) differentiated between the physician as "a practicing empathetic professional who is primarily concerned with each patient as an individual" and the scientist who is "determining the validity of a formally constructed hypothesis." Accrual to protocols must come through physicians who desire to increase knowledge about treatment options but want to protect the patients' best interests as well. Therefore, physicians must believe that both arms of a study are equal in benefit and in quality of life. The idea of clinical equipoise (11) has been promoted to deal with the conflict of an "honest, professional disagreement among expert clinicians" about the outcomes of two alternative therapies. The balance of effectiveness between two therapies, based on assessments of groups of expert clinicians, is intended to be unbalanced, or solved, by the outcome of the randomized trial.

Errors, particularly about quality-of-life issues, can affect accrual to clinical trials. The proposed morbidity, survival advantage, and scientific basis of two treatments may seem to be the same on the surface, but a patient or an individual physician may notice major quality-of-life issues that have not been considered. Preservation of body structures (e.g., mastectomy versus radiation only) may be enough of an issue to prevent accrual to the surgery arm of a study. The intuition of scientists about quality-of-life issues may be wrong in seemingly clear cases. For example, in studies of limb sparing for sarcoma (12), the issue of unanticipated sexual dysfunction outweighed that of limb sparing. Other issues may be more subtle. Clinical experts may agree that there is no proof that adjuvant therapy after a negative second-look laparotomy for ovarian cancer improves survival. However, the patient and her physician, both well informed about the disease, may decide that the lack of treatment is psychologically unacceptable to both, which would lead to poor accrual to a protocol with a no treatment arm. Although such a protocol may be the most scientifically satisfying option, the knowledge that treatment has stopped may create a problem for the patient, even if treatment has not been shown to have an advantage. In this case, the concerns of the physician as an "empathetic professional" looking at a quality-of-life issue in the psychological domain outweigh the concerns of the same physician as a "scientist."

Quality-of-life assessments have been encouraged in clinical research to better establish the way treatment outcomes affect patients' social, psychological, physical, and spiritual existence. Potential benefits for cancer patients are recognized to have two components: length of survival and the quality of that time. Short- and long-term diminution of quality of life clearly weighs against the quantity. Ideally, we want to provide our patients with information about the quality-of-life aspects of the various treatments. Because such data are often unavailable, we have had to discuss these issues from our perspective as caregivers and not from the perspective of the person receiving therapy.

A society with the responsibility to allocate health care dollars should attempt to choose therapies that maximize both survival time and quality of life. The Oregon prioritization project approached allocation of their health care dollars for Medicaid programs with exactly this focus. They attempted to address ethical concerns about using quality-of-life assessments for allocation of resources. To minimize the bias inherent in quality-of-life assessments, they viewed quality of life as a change in health status over time, rather than as an evaluation of status at one point in time. Quality of life was considered to be the "net benefit, realized from a treatment that matters, not the point-in-time quality of life of a patient" (13). The project looked at the "quality-adjusted life year" (QALY) to estimate the outcome of intervention in terms of percentages of normal quality of life. Information about quality of life may be used to decide whether society (e.g., insurance companies, the government) sees the benefits of various new therapies as worthwhile in view of the changes in quality of life or survival time that result from them.

QUALITY-OF-LIFE SCALES

The general issues in the objective evaluation of quality of life are as follows: (a) attention to the needs of individual patients cannot be replaced by objective quality-of-life measurements, nor can the considerable subjectivity of quality of life ever be objectified; (b) potential errors of timing may miss important changes; and (c) failure to assess adequately all the components of quality of life that are pertinent to therapy will lead to erroneous conclusions.

Quality-of-life scales should give physicians a reasonable measure of the relative levels of suffering that result from various therapies. For example, the finding that the loss of sexual function is perceived by most patients as greater suffering than the loss of a limb is not necessarily predictable, but it is clearly valuable information if the survival benefit for each treatment is the same. However, limb loss may seem to some patients to be a far greater threat than loss of sexual function (14,15), and limb loss would therefore cause greater suffering for those particular patients. Quality-of-life scales can give us overall measures, but they can never replace the complex understanding that an individual physician can have of an individual patient's quality of life. The elements of the complex understanding between physician and patient are important if accurate data about quality of life are to be obtained.

Multiple assessments over time rather than at one point in time are more likely to reflect the real impact of therapies. Graphically, this idea can be seen in Figure 23.1, adapted from Bush (16). With ovarian cancer, we most frequently deal with what Bush would consider "complicated failure" as an outcome. In terms of quality of life, measurements at A and B in Figure 23.1 would suggest that treatment 1 is superior to treatment 2 because quality of life is better at point A (initial measure) and equal at point B (second measure). However, if only survival is measured, treatment 2 has the advantage at point C. Individual patients might prefer the treatment that results in a shorter, higher quality of life to the one that results in a longer, lower quality of life. However, to make such discrete data available to patients, measures between A and B and

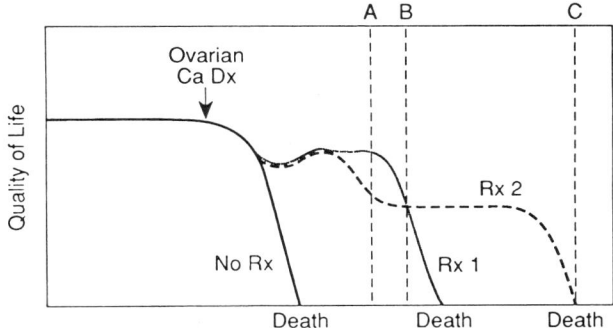

FIG. 23.1. Quality of life variant over time in patients given two alternate therapies. (From Bush R. Endpoints for evaluating treatment. In: Bush R, ed. *Malignancies of the ovary, uterus and cervix.* Chicago: Edward Arnold 1979, with permission.)

after B would have to occur. The evaluation becomes cumbersome and costly, even when it is done entirely by patient self-evaluation. Expert clinical judgment about time points in the disease process that are most frequently reported by patients as times of improved or diminished quality of life will help in scheduling testing so that it most accurately reflects the true curve.

Many scales have been used to measure quality of life in cancer patients (Table 23.1). Most early scales, such as the one developed by Karnofsky and Burchenal (17) are unidimensional and focus primarily on physical parameters. This may be helpful in delineating tolerance to therapy, but it fails to assess spiritual elements which can significantly affect a patient's perception of her existence. This is of greater importance late in the disease process, because spiritual elements of quality of life tend to dominate as physical elements decline. Other scales were developed for cancers other than ovarian or for other diseases and may overlook important concerns of women with ovarian cancer, such as loss of sexuality or reproduction. Cella and associates (18) developed a general cancer quality of life measure, called the Functional Assessment of Cancer Therapy (FACT) scale, to evaluate patients receiving cancer treatment. Subsequently, this scale was modified for individual cancer sites including ovary (FACT-O) (Table 23.2).

TABLE 23.1. *Dimensions*

Scale ref. no.	Population studied	Patient-designed	Patient-weighted	Physical	Psychological	Social	Global	Deficits in psychometric validity	Comments
Karnofsky and Burchenal (17)	General cancer patients			X					Only physical domain
Coates et al. (LASA) (41)	Melanoma, lung, ovary			X		X			Global assessment only
Schipper et al. (FLIC) (42)	Unselected cancer patients	X	X	X	X	X		Lacks reliability measures, visual analog score	Weighted toward physical and psychological; can get item scores
Spitzer et al. (43)	General cancer patients		X	X	X	X		Test/retest reliability and concurrent validity	Weighted toward physical domain; no dimension scores; index better for long-term disease
Cella et al. (18) (FACT-G)	Breast, lung, colon	X	X	X	X	X			Items developed by patients and specialists
(FACT-O)	Ovary	X	X	X	X	X	X		Useful to modify individual treatment

TABLE 23.2. FACT-O

Patient's name _____
Institution _____
Patient ID no. _____
Date of assessment _____

Below is a list of statements that other people with your illness have said are important. By circling one number per line, please indicate how true each statement has been for you during the past 7 days.

Physical Well-Being

During the past 7 days:	not at all	a little bit	somewhat	quite a bit	very much
1. I have a lack of energy..	0	1	2	3	4
2. I have nausea..	0	1	2	3	4
3. Because of my physical condition, I have trouble meeting the needs of my family....................	0	1	2	3	4
4. I have pain...	0	1	2	3	4
5. I am bothered by side effects of treatment.............	0	1	2	3	4
6. I feel sick...	0	1	2	3	4
7. I am forced to spend time in bed............................	0	1	2	3	4

8. Looking at the above seven questions, how much would you say your PHYSICAL WELL-BEING affects your quality of life? (circle one number)

```
    0       1       2       3       4       5       6       7       8       9       10
not at all                                                                      very much so
```

Social/Family Well-Being

During the past 7 days:	not at all	a little bit	somewhat	quite a bit	very much
9. I feel distant from my friends................................	0	1	2	3	4
10. I get emotional support from my family..................	0	1	2	3	4
11. I get support from my friends and neighbors..........	0	1	2	3	4
12. My family has accepted my illness.........................	0	1	2	3	4
13. Family communication about my illness is poor.......	0	1	2	3	4
14. I feel close to my partner (or the person who is my main support)...	0	1	2	3	4
15. Have you been sexually active during the past year? No__ Yes__ If yes: I am satisfied with my sex life...	0	1	2	3	4

16. Looking at the above seven questions how much would you say your SOCIAL/FAMILY WELL-BEING affects your quality of life? (circle one number)

```
    0       1       2       3       4       5       6       7       8       9       10
not at all                                                                      very much so
```

Relationship with the Doctor

During the past 7 days:	not at all	a little bit	somewhat	quite a bit	very much
17. I have confidence in my doctor(s)...........................	0	1	2	3	4
18. My doctor is available to answer my questions........	0	1	2	3	4

19. Looking at the above two questions how much would you say your RELATIONSHIP WITH THE DOCTOR affects your quality of life? (circle one number)

```
    0       1       2       3       4       5       6       7       8       9       10
not at all                                                                      very much so
```

Emotional Well-Being

During the past 7 days:	not at all	a little bit	somewhat	quite a bit	very much
20. I feel sad...	0	1	2	3	4
21. I am proud of how I am coping with my illness.........	0	1	2	3	4
22. I am losing hope in the fight against my illness.......	0	1	2	3	4
23. I feel nervous..	0	1	2	3	4
24. I worry about dying..	0	1	2	3	4
25. I worry that my condition will get worse..................	0	1	2	3	4

26. Looking at the above six questions how much would you say your EMOTIONAL WELL-BEING affects your quality of life? (circle one number)

```
    0       1       2       3       4       5       6       7       8       9       10
not at all                                                                      very much so
```

(continued)

TABLE 23.2. *(continued)*

Functional Well-Being

During the past 7 days:	not at all	a little bit	somewhat	quite a bit	very much
27. I am able to work (include the work in home)..	0	1	2	3	4
28. My work (include work in home) is fulfilling..........	0	1	2	3	4
29. I am able to enjoy life..	0	1	2	3	4
30. I have accepted my illness...................................	0	1	2	3	4
31. I am sleeping well...	0	1	2	3	4
32. I am enjoying the things I usually do for fun	0	1	2	3	4
33. I am content with the quality of my life right now..	0	1	2	3	4

34. Looking at the above seven questions how much would you say your FUNCTIONAL WELL-BEING affects your quality of life? (circle one number)

```
0     1     2     3     4     5     6     7     8     9     10
not at all                                              very much so
```

Additional Concerns

During the past 7 days:	not at all	a little bit	somewhat	quite a bit	very much
35. I have swelling in my stomach area..................	0	1	2	3	4
36. I am losing weight...	0	1	2	3	4
37. I have control of my bowels..............................	0	1	2	3	4
38. I have been vomiting..	0	1	2	3	4
39. I have been bothered by hair loss	0	1	2	3	4
40. I have a good appetite......................................	0	1	2	3	4
41. I like the appearance of my body.....................	0	1	2	3	4
42. I am able to get around my home by myself	0	1	2	3	4
43. I am able to feel like a woman..........................	0	1	2	3	4
44. I have cramps in my stomach area..................	0	1	2	3	4
45. I am interested in having sex............................	0	1	2	3	4
46. I have concerns about my ability to have children...	0	1	2	3	4

47. Looking at the above 12 questions how much would you say your ADDITIONAL CONCERNS affect your quality of life? (circle one number)

```
0     1     2     3     4     5     6     7     8     9     10
not at all                                              very much so
```

Items used in this questionnaire were generated through interview input from cancer patients as well as cancer specialists. They are grouped into six logical categories which are weighted by importance to the individual patient, allowing institution of therapeutic modifications based on individual patient preferences. When the results from multiple patients are combined, the data can be used to define treatment regimens and develop managed health care policy. This measurement scale has been extensively validated and has been shown to be brief, reliable, and responsive to change. The Gynecologic Oncology Group currently utilizes FACT-O in ovarian cancer trials having a quality-of-life component.

QUALITY OF LIFE AT THE END OF LIFE

Case. Patient B, 57 years old, presents with an enterocutaneous fistula after previous chemotherapy, whole-abdomen irradiation, and a phase II drug trial 4 months before her presentation. She was placed on total parental nutrition (TPN) last week when the status of her disease was unknown. Now, biopsies of the fistula tract demonstrate persistent disease. She has had persistent neutropenia and thrombocytopenia since her last treatment cycle 4 months ago, and no further therapy can be initiated because of this. One year ago, she had surgery for a small bowel obstruction that required removal of half of her small bowel and required dietary supplementation to maintain her weight. The attending surgeon plans an exploratory laparotomy to resect the fistula and debulk the disease.

Despite persistent efforts to treat patients with epithelial ovarian cancer, many eventually die from their disease. Among the admonitions of Hippocrates to physicians is a piece of advice that is easily forgotten in this era of high-technology medicine: Do not treat those who are overmastered by their disease. It is difficult to halt treatment when we have access to artificial means of support such as TPN and mechanical ventilation.

Often, the best method for exposing the lack of benefit of proposed interventions is to ask the simple question, "What is the best quality of life for the patient that can result from this intervention?" This question must be asked from the point of view of the patient and the onlooker.

In the case of Patient B, we could reasonably describe the best outcome in quality-of-life terms as resection of the fistula and decreased skin irritation. However, the likelihood of dependence on TPN and continued progressive disease are the best we can hope for. We will not be able to treat the underlying disease because of the status of the patient's bone marrow. Therefore, the temporary decrease in quality of life produced by surgery will not improve quality of life in the long run. The worst outcome would be multiple fistulae, infection, TPN dependence, and progressive disease. Framed in this overall view, the medical indication or benefit of the proposed surgery is very limited. For patient B, it is best termed futile. It fails to reach the ultimate goal of medicine that "any treatment should [lead to] improvement of the patient's prognosis, comfort, well-being or general state of health. A treatment that fails to provide such a benefit, even though it produces a measurable effect, should be considered futile" (19).

Should Patient B be offered the proposed surgery? Does our strong cultural bias for patient autonomy demand that patients be given all the options or treatments they request, even if the ultimate goal of medicine is not met? Tomlinson and Brody (20) argued that "patients do not have an unqualified right to demand 'treatment' that has no benefit." Furthermore, they argued that "if physicians are still to be permitted the judgment that an intervention would do more harm than good, therefore, it must be assumed that they have some authority to make comparative judgments of good and evil." Physicians continue to carry the duty of making judgments based on relative values without absolute certainty, and they should not be seduced into pushing all the decisions onto patient's shoulders. Hackler and Hiller (21) summarized the issue as follows: "Respect for patient autonomy does not require that the physician initiate discussion of medically pointless procedures. If there is no case to be made for a procedure, there should be no need to make one against it." Forcing issues of futile therapy as "decisions" for the patient can lead to psychological and social harm and to physically prolonged pain and suffering. Patients and families view choices as recommendations or as statements of potential improvements in quality of life. Often, such discussions fail to present honestly the fact that the patient is dying and the only appropriate interventions are palliative. In order to bring the best quality of life to the dying patient, sensitive but honest discussions must occur.

The need to treat and to offer assistance affects all physicians. As Jonsen and colleagues (1) pointed out, "the initiation of treatment expresses some measure of hope and assuages the uncertainty that besets medicine." Discomfort can arise during the change from an aggressive, curative goal to a palliative goal and when a decision is made to forego therapeutic options because of new medical problems. For example, in the case of patient B, if her renal function falters from obstruction, should ureteral stents be placed or antibiotics started? These troubling decisions must be faced as physicians continually clarify the goals of intervention and reassure themselves that it is appropriate to provide comfort to the dying patient and to respect her clear directives about the dying process. Time-limited trials of interventions such as antibiotic administration, in which no harm is done to the patient and unsuccessful therapies can be withdrawn, are successful means of dealing with some of these decisions.

TERMINAL CARE: THE QUALITY OF DYING

When the health care team recognizes that further care is futile, or the patient or surrogate requests that aggressive interventions be stopped, the patient-physician relationship has reached a critical point. Honest, well-timed, open-ended discussions of the terminal course can turn a fearful experience into a positive, supportive time of communication for the patient and her family. It is important to recognize pitfalls that can occur in this process (22). Particularly important is the continued awareness that patients and families can interpret palliative therapy as curative and can confuse simple healing (after surgery, perhaps) as a sign of improvement. In situations that involve multiple physicians, such as an intensive care setting (neurology, cardiology, pulmonary, and renal consultants), the potential for confusion about outcomes increases substantially. For example, a simple statement that "the PO is improved" or "now she has some urine output" may imply an improvement in the overall prognosis that is not warranted by the overall picture. The oncologist, as a central figure, should be responsible for communicating the overall prognosis. The oncologist must convey the fact that despite improvement in some aspects of the patient's condition, the expected terminal outcome is still inevitable. An understanding of the goals that the patient can and wants to achieve before death is essential to respect for her autonomous decisions about quality of life.

Advance directives and discussions about palliative care during the dying process are important issues for patients, physicians, and staff to discuss even before the terminal care setting. The Patient Self-Determination Act (part of the Omnibus Reconciliation Act of 1990) requires that all patients entering a hospital that accepts Medicaid and Medicare reimbursement have the opportunity to receive information about advance directives. The presentation of this information is recorded, but it does not require completion of documents that indicate patient or surrogate acceptance. Information about advance directives and discussions about them early in care can lead to an education process that may, for many dying patients, lessen fears of the unknown and increase their control over the dying process. Discussions can elicit values and goals that may facilitate decisions about terminal care (23). Discussions on issues such as nutrition and TPN in the context of dying might be easier if the patient has previously given thought to the issues. The limits of the supportive care offered to patients can be framed by the patients themselves or by their surrogates. Limitation of suffering and the provision of measures to help patients realize their goals (e.g., time at home, a visit with one's sister) become the goals of therapy.

Palliation often requires a greater intensity of care than curative therapy. Unfortunately, insurance carriers continue to reimburse preferentially for high-technology interventions in preference to the "hands-on" care that may be more acutely needed in a terminal setting (22). Therefore, although hospice-centered home care may be the best choice for maximizing quality of life, its availability may be limited by insurance coverage and lack of local programs. Palliative care may have to be given in a hospital setting where "helping patients cope with the technologically complicated medical environment that often surrounds them at the end of life... requires the act of deliberately creating a medical environment that allows a peaceful death" (24). The physician has the obligation to continue to provide the best care, now palliative, for the patient. That care will determine the quality of life of the patient's existence until death.

ENHANCING QUALITY OF LIFE IN PALLIATIVE/TERMINAL CARE

Health professionals must address an inherent conflict in the care of cancer patients before adequate palliative care can be delivered. The ultimate goals of cancer care and of the physician are oriented toward cure; if cure cannot be achieved for a particular patient, the possibility still exists that her experience might be useful for the benefit of others. The reinvestment of emotional and intellectual interest in intensive palliative care, in which cure cannot be effected under any circumstances, is challenging at best. The failure to clearly, openly, and aggressively focus on palliative care for dying patients produces odd concerns for some health practitioners, such as concerns about addiction to narcotics and concern for respiratory depression, that can interfere with administration of adequate pain control. Concern may even focus on the possibility that the center or hospital might become known for "good deaths" and that the accrual of potentially curable patients might somehow change. However, palliation, rather than representing the ultimate failure of the physician to defend health and provide cure, is the ultimate expression of another goal of medicine: "relief of symptoms including psychological suffering and physical distress" (1). It is as compelling a goal as cure of disease, and when cure cannot be achieved, it is the only goal. "Extreme responsibility, extraordinary sensitivity, and heroic compassion" (24) are the measures required for palliative care.

The first area to treat, and the area of greatest anxiety for many patients (25), is pain. The reality of pain is individual. It involves areas such as the psychological and cultural meaning of pain, the psychological status of the patient, the duration of the pain, and the general physical status of the patient. Failure to recognize and treat significant depression (26–28) may doom any attempt at pain control. Disregard of a cultural or individual concern about the development of tolerance or addiction to narcotics may hamper the administration of an adequate dose of pain medicine (28). The experience of pain as suffering, which directly diminishes the quality of life of the patient, should not be understood as the experience of pain as nociception. The multiple facets of suffering must be explored in order to palliate all of the patient's symptoms of discomfort or distress.

Effective pain management requires flexibility and often involves combined approaches (29). A frequent misconception is that an intravenous route will be adequate. Although absorption by the oral route is likely to be an issue for terminal ovarian cancer patients, the use of short-acting and long-acting analgesics by transdermal, sublingual, rectal, oral, or even subcutaneous administration is still valid (30–32). In one study, 64% of advanced cancer patients used oral routes up to 4 weeks before death, although only 21% were able to use this route effectively during the last 24 hours of life (33). The oral or transdermal routes allow a far greater freedom of action for the patient. Indwelling epidurals can be particularly effective for pelvic sources of pain and can reduce the need for large oral doses (34). Corticosteroids can be helpful, particularly when bony areas are sources of pain (35). The use of a base method of pain control, including the possibility of multiple modalities, should always have a "rescue" analgesic as a backup. This relieves the patient's anxiety about the control of pain and allows identification of failing control when use of the backup becomes more frequent.

The greatest errors made in the control of pain are inadequate dosage and lack of an aggressive yet flexible approach to management. The dying process is irreversible, and the physician's duties are to comfort the patient and treat her symptoms. In this regard, "the proper dose of pain medication is the dose that is sufficient to relieve pain and suffering, even to the point of unconsciousness" (24). Philosophers may argue over the fine points of intent or the principle of "double effect" (36), but physicians have always had to weigh the benefits of adequate pain dosage against the foreseen and often unavoidable side effects of respiratory depression and even unconsciousness. As when weighing other medical interventions in terminal care, the intent or benefit—adequate pain control to relieve suffering—must be clear. The pain technology that is available for terminal patients should never be denied to them.

In keeping with an aggressive approach to palliative care for the terminal patient, the provision of oxygen for relief of dyspnea is appropriate (37). Narcotics can also diminish the distress caused by dyspnea. Adequate control of nausea, muscle cramps (38), and sleep disturbances (39) is a reasonable expectation for aggressive palliative care. The changes in symptoms during terminal care can be acute, and reassessment of the clinical picture with adjustment of therapy should take place on a regular basis.

EUTHANASIA/SUICIDE

Euthanasia, a good death, has become part of the public consciousness. Whether it is called "assisted suicide" or "death with dignity," the idea of suicide is inextricably linked to lack of quality of life and fear of suffering at the end of life. Suicide itself and suicide plans in cancer patients can result from lack of information about dying, untreated underlying depression, or fear that the medical community and the physician will either abandon aggressive care for symptoms not leading to cure or will not respect the patient's desires for withholding or withdrawing medical technology. In these aspects, the physician is responsible and obligated to the patient. However, most patients fear loss of autonomy due to illness or loss of control of bodily functions. These are clearly patient-initiated issues that should be respected by their physicians. In 1997, the state of Oregon legalized physician-assisted suicide. Chin and associates (40) have published the experience of the first year of physician-assisted suicide. Fifteen patients who died after taking prescriptions for lethal medications were compared with controls made up of a cohort of patients who died from similar diseases but were not given lethal medication prescriptions. The case patients (lethal prescriptions) were more likely than the controls to have never married ($p = .04$) and were more likely to be concerned about loss of autonomy due to illness ($p = .01$) and loss of control of bodily functions ($p = .02$). Interestingly, only 1 of the 15 patients who died after using lethal medications expressed concern about inadequate control of pain, perhaps reflecting the overall adequacy of thoughtful terminal care.

Should we embrace the idea that the same technology that often uselessly prolongs life (as well as preserves it) can be used to intentionally terminate life at the hands of physicians? Is providing death at a patient's request a reasonable part of relieving suffering? Advocates of euthanasia state that it is the ultimate respect for patient autonomy. Others question whether the intent of causing death can be reconciled with the physician's obligation to preserve life and ensure its quality. Even with meticulous, aggressive terminal care, some patients with ovarian cancer will be unable to experience relief of pain or other sources of distress related to the disease. However, if physicians maintain a clear view of the benefits of medical interventions and attempt to improve quality of life for their patients—defined by the patient's perspective—this should be a rare dilemma.

REFERENCES

1. Jonsen A, Siegler M, Winslade W, eds. *Clinical ethics*, 2nd ed. New York: Macmillan, 1986.
2. Cella DF, Cherin EA. Quality of life during and after cancer treatment. *Compr Ther* 1988;14:69–75.
3. Shumaker SA, Anderson RT, Czajkowski SM. Psychological tests and scales. In: Spilker B, ed. *Quality of life assessments in clinical trials*. New York: Raven Press, 1990:95–113.
4. Schipper H. Guidelines and caveats for quality of life measurement in clinical practice and research. *Oncology* 1990;4:51–57.
5. Silberfarb PM. Psychiatric problems in breast cancer. *Cancer* 1984;53:820–824.
6. Cella DF, Tulsky DS. Quality of life in cancer: definition, purpose, and method of measurement. *Cancer Invest* 1993;11:327–336.
7. Newcomb PA, Carbone PP. Cancer treatment and age: patient perspectives. *J Natl Cancer Inst* 1993;85:1580–1584.
8. Presout CA. Quality of life in cancer patients. *Am J Clin Oncol* 1984;7:571–578.
9. Katz J. The physician-patient interaction. In: Milbursky GT, ed. *Genetics and the law*, vol 2. New York: Plenum, 1980.
10. Hellman D, Hellman S. Of mice but not men: problems of the randomized clinical trial. *N Engl J Med* 1991;324:1585–1589.
11. Freedman B. Equipoise and the ethics of clinical research. *N Engl J Med* 1991;3:141–145.
12. Osoba D. Measuring the effect of cancer on quality of life. In: Osoba D, ed. *Effect of cancer on quality of life*. Boca Raton: CRC Press, 1991:25–40.
13. Hadorn D. The Oregon priority-setting exercise: quality of life and public policy. *Hastings Cent Rep* 1991;21:11–16.
14. Cassell E. Recognizing suffering. *Hastings Cent Rep* 1991;21:24–31.
15. Cassell E. The nature of suffering and the goals of medicine. *N Engl J Med* 1982;306:639–645.
16. Bush R. Endpoints for evaluating treatment. In: Bush R, ed. *Malignancies of the ovary, uterus, and cervix*. Chicago: Edward Arnold, 1979:1–22.
17. Karnofsky DA, Burchenal HH. The clinical evaluation of chemotherapeutic agents in cancer. In: McLeod CM, ed. *Evaluation of chemotherapeutic agents*. New York: Columbia University Press, 1949:191–205.
18. Cella DF, Tulsky DS, Gray G, et al. The functional assessment of cancer therapy scale: development and validation of the general measure. *J Clin Oncol* 1993;11:570–579.
19. Schneiderman L, Jecker N, Jonsen A. Medical futility: its meanings and ethical implications. *Ann Intern Med* 1990;112:949–954.
20. Tomlinson T, Brody H. Futility and the ethics of resuscitation. *JAMA* 1990;264:1276–1280.
21. Hackler CJ, Hiller FC. Family consent to orders not to resuscitate: reconsidering hospital policy. *JAMA* 1990;10:264.
22. Cain J, et al. The quality of dying: financial, psychological and ethical dilemmas. *Obstet Gynecol* 1990;76:1.
23. Emanuel L. PSDA in the clinic. *Hastings Cent Rep* 1991;1:S7–S8.
24. Wanzer S, et al. The physician's responsibility toward hopelessly ill patients: a second look. *N Engl J Med* 1989;320:844–849.
25. Chapman C. Psychologic and behavioral aspects of cancer pain. In: Bonica J, Venta G, eds. *Advances in pain research and therapy*, vol 2. New York: Raven Press, 1989:44–56.

26. Doan B, Wadden N. Relationships between depressive symptoms and descriptions of chronic pain. *Pain* 1989;36:75–84.
27. Holland J, et al. A randomized clinical trial of alprazolam versus progressive muscle relaxation in cancer patients with anxiety and depressive symptoms. *J Clin Oncol* 1991;9:1004–1011.
28. Donepaal K, Aaronson N, Van Daam F. Pain experience and pain management among hospitalized cancer patients. *Cancer* 1989;63:593–598.
29. Levy M. Effective integration of pain management into comprehensive cancer care. *Postgrad Med J* 1991;67:S35–S43.
30. Walsh T, Saunders C. Oral morphine for relief of chronic pain from cancer. *N Engl J Med* 1981;305:1417–1420.
31. Adams J, Diebel L, Wilson J. Ambulatory use of high dose intravenous morphine for severe pain. *J Intel Clin Pharm* 1984;18:138–140.
32. Ferrell B, et al. Effects of controlled release morphine on quality of life for cancer pain. *Nurs Oncol Forum* 1989;16:521–526.
33. Coyle N, et al. Character of terminal illness in the advanced cancer: pain and other symptoms during the last few weeks of life. *J Pain Symptom Manage* 1990;5:83–93.
34. Coombes D, et al. Outcomes and complications of continuous intraspinal narcotic analgesia for cancer pain control. *J Clin Oncol* 1984;2:1414–1420.
35. Ettinger A, Portenoy R. The use of corticosteroids in the treatment of symptoms associated with cancer. *J Pain Symptom Manage* 1988;3:99–103.
36. Gillon R. The principle of double effect and medical ethics. In: Gillon R. *Philosophical medical ethics*. Chichester, England: Wiley, 1986:133–139.
37. Swinburn C, et al. Symptomatic benefit of supplemental oxygen in hypoxemic patients with chronic lung disease. *Am Rev Respir Dis* 1991;143:913–915.
38. Steiner I, Siegal T. Muscle cramps in cancer patients. *Cancer* 1989;63:574–577.
39. Hu D, Silberfarb P. Mangement of sleep problems in cancer patients. *Oncology* 1991;5:23–27.
40. Chin AE, et al. Legalized physician-assisted suicide in Oregon: the first year's experience. *N Engl J Med* 1999;340:577–583.
41. Coates A, et al. On the receiving end: II. Linear analogue self assessment (LASA) in evaluation of aspects of the quality of life of cancer patients receiving therapy. *Eur J Cancer Clin Oncol* 1983;19:1633–1637.
42. Schipper H, et al. Measuring the quality of life of cancer patients: the functional living index-cancer. Development and validation. *J Clin Oncol* 1984;2:472–483.
43. Spitzer W, et al. Measuring the quality of life of cancer patients: a concise quality of life index for use by physicians. *J Chronic Dis* 1981;34:585–597.

Subject Index

Note: Page numbers followed by f indicate figures; those followed by t indicate tables.

A

Actinomycin D. *See also* Chemotherapy
   for germ cell tumors, 373, 375
   for stromal tumors, 387, 388
Acute cerebellar degeneration, 103
Adenoacanthoma, 114
Adeno-associated viral vectors, 58t, 60–61
Adenocarcinoma
   endometrioid, 114, 114f
   metastatic to ovary, vs. endometrioid carcinoma, 115
Adenosarcoma, 115
Adenosquamous carcinoma, 114
Adenoviral E1A, in gene therapy, 70
Adenoviral vectors, 58t, 58–60, 59f, 60f
Adoptive T-cell immunotherapy, 79–83
   clonal expansion techniques in, 81–82
   cross-presentation in, 80
   limitations of, 81–83
   monoclonal antibodies in, 79
   principles of, 79
   T-cell costimulation in, 79, 80–81
Advanced cancer
   chemotherapy for, 262–269. *See also* Chemotherapy
   diagnosis of, 241–242
   first-line treatment for, 301
   laparoscopic management of, 232
   staging of, 241–242, 242t. *See also* Staging
   surgery for, 241–255. *See also* Cytoreductive surgery; Palliative care
   treatment guidelines for, 352
Advance directives, 427
Age
   incidence and, 167, 168t, 182
   mortality and, 167
AKT2, 29t, 31, 33
Alkylating agents. *See also* Chemotherapy *and specific agents*
   intraperitoneal, 321
   resistance to, 47–51. *See also* Chemoresistance
Allele-specific oligonucleotide analysis, 192–193
Allergic reaction, to paclitaxel, 267–268
α-fetoprotein
   in clear cell carcinoma, 119
   in germ cell tumors, 371, 372t
   in yolk sac tumors, 138
Americans with Disabilities Act, 194

Amplicon vectors, 61
Amsterdam criteria, 190, 190t
Analgesia, 428
Anaphylaxis, paclitaxel-induced, 267–268
Androblastomas. *See* Sertoli-Leydig cell tumors
Anthracyclines. *See also* Chemotherapy
   for advanced disease, 263
Antibodies
   antitumor, 85
   monoclonal. *See* Monoclonal antibodies
Antigen(s)
   T-cell, 73
   tumor-associated, 76t
   tumor-specific, 77
Antigen-based tumor vaccines, 76t, 77–79, 79t, 87t
Antigenicity, tumor, cytokines and, 83
Anti-HER-2 antibody, 70, 85–86
Antimüllerian hormone, in granulosa cell tumors, 385
Antisense oligonucleotides, in gene therapy, 69
Antitumor immune response. *See* Immune response, antitumor
Aortic lymph nodes, biopsy of, 211–212, 212f
Apoptosis
   Fas/FasL system and, 82
   inhibition of, chemoresistance and, 51–52
   in malignant transformation, 26–27
Appendix
   mucinous cystadenoma in, 112
   mucocele of, in pseudomyxoma peritonei, 414
Asbestos, 169–170
Ascites, 205, 336–338
   fibromas and, 389
   mucinous, in pseudomyxoma peritonei, 412, 412f, 413
   tumors of low malignant potential and, 406
Ashkenazi Jews, BRCA mutations in, 12, 12t, 186t, 186–188
   tests for, 191–192
Aspiration, laparoscopic, 221–222

B

Bacille Calmette-Guérin, 74–75
Basic fibroblast growth factor, 26t, 29
bax
   in apoptosis, 27
   in corrective gene therapy, 69

bcl-2
  in apoptosis, 27
  in chemoresistance, 51–52
bcl-X_L, in apoptosis, 27
bcl-X_S, in apoptosis, 27
Bethesda criteria, 190, 190t
Bimanual examination
  intraoperative, 208
  in screening, 174, 195
  in surveillance, 195
Biologic agents. *See also* Immunotherapy
  intraperitoneal, 323
  intrapleural, 340
Biopsy. *See also* Staging
  lymph node, 211–212, 212f
  in second-look laparotomy, 277
Birth control pills. *See* Oral contraceptives
Bleomycin. *See also* Chemotherapy
  for dysgerminomas, 373–374, 374t
  intrapleural, 340
  for nondysgerminomatous tumors, 376
  for stromal tumors, 387, 388
Blood, ovarian vein, sampling of, 100, 103
Bone marrow transplantation, for high-dose chemotherapy, 269
Borderline tumors. *See* Tumors of low malignant potential
Bowel obstruction, 329–336
  intraperitoneal chemotherapy and, 318
Brain metastasis, radiotherapy for, 360
BRCA1/2, 10, 11, 12–13, 171–173, 172t, 184–188
  in breast and ovarian cancer syndrome, 9, 10, 10t, 11–13, 12t, 171–173
  as caretaker gene, 186
  in corrective gene therapy, 68–69
  functions of, 13f, 13–15, 185–186
  isolation of, 184–185
  mutations in, 11–12, 12t, 35, 172–173
    founder, 186–187
    inheritance of, 183, 183f
    prevalence of, 186t, 186–187
    tests for, 191–192
  penetrance of, 172, 183, 186, 187–188, 193f
  structure of, 11, 12, 185
  as tumor suppressor gene, 35–36, 185
Breast and ovarian cancer syndrome, 8–10, 9f, 10t, 11–13, 12t, 172, 183–184. *See also* Hereditary ovarian cancer
  BRCA1 in, 9, 10t, 10–11, 12t
  BRCA2 in, 9
  breast cancer screening in, 197
  founder mutations in, 186–187
  genetic susceptibility testing for, 189–194. *See also* Genetic susceptibility testing
  prophylactic mastectomy for, 197
  prophylactic oophorectomy for, 173
Breast cancer
  estrogen replacement therapy and, 196–197
  HER-2/*neu* in, 30

  hereditary. *See* Breast and ovarian cancer syndrome
  metastatic to ovary, 123–124
  prevention of, in BRCA mutation carriers, 197
  screening for, in BRCA mutation carriers, 197
Brenner tumors, 109, 119t, 119–120, 120f
  of broad ligament, 126
Broad ligament
  carcinoma of, 126
  cystic lesions of, 125–126

C

CA 125
  in borderline tumors, 407
  in malignancy risk assessment, 220, 221
  normal, in persistent disease, 275t, 275–276
  in screening, 174–175, 195
  in surveillance, 195
CAG repeat-length polymorphism, 188
Call-Exner bodies, 151
Canalicular multispecific organic anion transporter, cisplatin resistance and, 50
Cancer. *See also specific sites and types*
  hereditary, 3–8, 171. *See also* Molecular genetics
  vs. sporadic cancer, 4, 4f
  two-hit model of, 5, 32, 185
Cancer family syndrome. *See* Hereditary nonpolyposis colorectal cancer syndrome
Cancer growth kinetics, 243f, 243–245, 244f
Carbon dioxide pneumoperitoneum, tumor spread and, 226
Carboplatin. *See also* Chemotherapy
  for advanced disease, 263–264
  vs. cisplatin, 265
    with paclitaxel, 268–269
  for germ cell tumors, 373–374, 375, 378
  high-dose, 269
  for intestinal obstruction, 330–331
  intraperitoneal, 320
    as first-line therapy, 323–324, 324t
  leukemia induction by, 379–380
  with paclitaxel, in salvage therapy, 304t, 304–306, 305t
  in salvage therapy, 282, 303–306, 304t, 305t
    with radiotherapy, 353–356
  toxicity of, 265, 268–269
Carcinogenesis
  molecular genetics and, 7f, 7–8, 23, 24t
  two-hit model of, 5, 32, 185
Carcinoid tumors. *See also* Germ cell tumors
  histopathology of, 143–145, 144f
  metastatic to ovary, 125, 125f
  vs. Sertoli-Leydig cell tumors, 158–159
Carcinoma of low malignant potential, 399. *See also* Tumors of low malignant potential
Caretaker genes, BRCA1/2 genes as, 186
Caspases, in cytotoxic gene therapy, 63
CDKs, 36f, 36–37
Cell cycle, 243f, 243–244

Cell growth kinetics, 243f, 243–245, 244f
Cell proliferation
　in malignant transformation, 26
　measurement of, 26
Cellular fibromas, 156. See also Fibromas
　vs. adult granulosa cell tumor, 153
Cellular senescence, in malignant transformation, 27
c-erbB2. See HER-2/neu
Cerebral metastasis, radiotherapy for, 360
Chemoresistance, 43–53
　to alkylating agents, 47–51
　apoptosis inhibition and, 51–52
　to cisplatin, 47f, 47–51, 48f, 49t
　cross-resistance in, 43–44, 45f
　definition of, 303t
　dose intensity and, 269
　MDR1 and, 45
　mechanisms of, 44t
　molecular basis for, 51–52
　multidrug phenotype in, 45–46
　to natural products, 44–47
　p53 and, 35
　to platinum analogs, 303t
　radioresistance and, 282
　salvage chemotherapy and, 303t, 303–304, 304t, 306, 306t
　tumor size and, 245
Chemosensitivity
　definition of, 303t
　salvage therapy and, 303–305, 304t, 305t
Chemotherapy, 259–270. See also generic names of specific drugs
　adjuvant, survival after, 249–250, 250t
　for advanced disease, 262–269
　　agents for, 263–264
　　future directions in, 269–270
　　with optimal vs. suboptimal cytoreduction, 263
　　single-agent vs. combination, 264–265
　for ascites, 338
　for borderline tumors, 409–411
　cell cycle-specific, 243f, 243–244
　for early-stage disease, 259–262
　　in 1970s, 259–260
　　in 1980s, 260–261
　　cisplatin-based, 261–262
　future directions for, 269–270
　for germ cell tumors, 373–374, 374t
　　late effects of, 378–379
　　salvage, 378
　high-dose, 269
　in salvage therapy, 312
　in interval cytoreduction, 251–252, 252f, 273, 289–290, 295–297, 296f, 296t, 297f
　for intestinal obstruction, 330–331
　intraperitoneal, 315–324
　　for ascites, 338
　　drug delivery in, 67, 316–317
　　drug distribution in, 316

　　drugs used in, 318–323
　　in early-stage disease, 261
　　as first-line therapy, 323–324
　　historical perspective on, 315
　　indications for, 324t
　　pharmacokinetic advantages of, 315–316, 316t
　　principles of, 315–317
　　for pseudomyxoma peritonei, 414–415
　　in salvage therapy, 312, 318–323
　　toxicity of, 317–318, 321
　intrapleural, for malignant effusion, 340
　for nondysgerminomatous germ cell tumors, 373–374, 374t, 375–376
　for pseudomyxoma peritonei, 414
　with radiotherapy, 353t, 353–356, 354t
　　future directions in, 366
　　toxicity of, 366
　resistance to. See Chemoresistance
　response rates for, 44t
　response to, residual disease and, 246t, 246–247, 247t
　results of, 204
　salvage, 281–282
　　high-dose, 312
　　immediate vs. delayed, 303–304
　　with immunotherapy, 281–282
　　intraperitoneal, 312
　　in platinum-resistant disease, 303t, 304t, 306t, 306–307, 311, 311t
　　in platinum-sensitive disease, 303–305, 304t, 305t, 310
　　with radiotherapy, 353t, 353–356, 354t
　　regimen for, 310–312, 312t
　　single-agent vs. combination, 305–306
　second malignancy and, 379
　as sole vs. adjuvant therapy, 204
　for stromal tumors, 387t, 387–388
　T cell dysfunction and, 82–83
Chest tube, for pleural effusion, 340
Choriocarcinoma, 374–375. See also Germ cell tumors
　histopathology of, 139–140, 140f
　serum markers in, 372t
Cisplatin. See also Chemotherapy
　for advanced disease, 263–264
　for borderline tumors, 410
　for early-stage disease, 261–262, 269
　for germ cell tumors, 373–374, 374t, 375, 378
　high-dose, 269
　for intestinal obstruction, 330–331
　intraperitoneal, 313–319, 319t
　　vs. carboplatin, 320
　　with etoposide, 320, 322
　　as first-line therapy, 323–324, 324t
　with intraperitoneal ^{32}P-chromic phosphate, 358–359
　leukemia induction by, 379–380
　in monotherapy vs. combination therapy, 264–265
　with paclitaxel, 265–269
　　vs. carboplatin, 265, 268–269
　　in salvage therapy, 304t, 304–306, 305t

Cisplatin (continued)
  sequential vs. concurrent administration of, 266–267
  as standard of care, 267
  for pseudomyxoma peritonei, 415
  with radiotherapy, 353–356, 366
    toxicity of, 366
  resistance to, 45–46, 47f, 47–51, 48f, 49t. See also Chemoresistance
    cell line studies of, 48, 48f, 49t
    decreased drug accumulation and, 48–50
    DNA damage tolerance and, 50–51
    increased efflux and, 49
    melphalan resistance and, 48–49
  response rates for, 44t
  in salvage therapy, 266, 282, 303–306, 304t, 305t
    with radiotherapy, 353–356
  for stromal tumors, 387, 388
Clear cell tumors, 116–119, 117t
  carcinoma, 117f, 117–119
    vs. juvenile granulosa cell tumor, 155
    vs. steroid cell tumors, 162
  of low malignant potential, 117
Clinical trials. See also Chemotherapy and specific drugs
  ethical aspects of, 421–422
Clonal evolution/expansion, 7f, 7–8
  in adoptive T-cell immunotherapy, 81
cMOAT, cisplatin resistance and, 50
c-myc, 29t, 32
Coffee, 169
Colorectal cancer
  clonal evolution in, 7f, 7–8
  hereditary. See Hereditary nonpolyposis colorectal cancer syndrome
  metastatic to ovary, 123–124
  tumorigenesis in, 7f, 7–8
Computed tomography
  in malignancy risk assessment, 221
  for persistent disease, 276
Conflicts of interest, clinical trials and, 421–422
Corrective gene therapy, 67–70, 68t
  genes delivered in, 68t
  gene targets in, 68t
  neutralization, 69–70
  replacement, 67–69
Corynebacterium parvum, intraperitoneal, 323
Cross-presentation, in T-cell activation, 80
Cross-resistance, to chemotherapy, 43–44, 44f
Culdocentesis cytology
  in persistent disease, 276
  in screening, 174
Cushing's syndrome, steroid cell tumors and, 160–161
Cutaneous paraneoplastic syndromes, 103
Cyclin-dependent kinase inhibitors, 36f, 36–37
Cyclin-dependent kinases, 36f, 36–37
Cyclins, 36f, 36–37

Cyclophosphamide. See also Chemotherapy
  for borderline tumors, 410
  for early-stage disease, 261
  for germ cell tumors, 373, 375, 378
  intraperitoneal, 321
  for pseudomyxoma peritonei, 415
  response rates for, 44t
  in salvage therapy, 304, 304t
    with radiotherapy, 353, 355, 356
  for stromal tumors, 387, 388
Cyst(s)
  of broad ligament, 125–126
  inclusion, 101
  intraoperative rupture of, 208–209
    during laparoscopy, 224–225, 226
  laparoscopic aspiration of, 221–222
Cystadenofibroma, serous nodules in, 100f
Cystadenoma
  mucinous, in appendix, 112
  serous, 104, 105f
Cystectomy, for borderline tumors, 408
Cystic epithelial tumors, 125
Cytokines
  in immunotherapy, 83–85
  intraperitoneal administration of, 84
  therapeutic use of, 75t
  toxicity of, 84
Cytologic washings, 208
Cytoreductive surgery, 203, 242–255
  benefits of
    clinical, 245–251
    theoretical, 243–245, 245t
  for germ cell tumors, 373
  interval, 251–252, 252f, 273, 289–290
    results of, 295–297, 296f, 296t, 297f
  vs. laparoscopic management, 232
  optimal
    procedures in, 251, 251t
    rate of, 251
    vs. suboptimal, 248–249, 263, 289
  residual disease after, 248–249, 263, 289
    chemotherapy response and, 246t, 246–247, 247t
    survival and, 247–251, 248f, 249f, 250t, 251t
  roles of, 242t
  scope of, 251, 251t, 255
  secondary, 273, 289–298
    clinical settings for, 289–290, 291t
    complications of, 290–292, 291t
    failure of, 298
    feasibility of, 290, 291t
    indications for, 289–290
    interval, 251–252, 252f, 273, 289–290, 295–297
    optimal, 290, 291t
    results of, 290, 291t, 292–295, 293t, 294f, 295f
    survival after, 292–295, 293t, 294f, 295f
  technique of, 252–255, 253f, 254f
  for ureteral obstruction, 341–342

Cytosine deaminase/5-fluorocytosine, in cytotoxic gene therapy, 64t, 64–65
Cytotoxic gene therapy, 63–67, 64t, 65f, 65t, 66f, 67t
 antitumor immune mechanisms in, 65, 65t, 66
 bystander effect in, 64, 65f
 efficacy of, 66f, 66–67, 67t
 transgene/prodrug systems for, 63–64, 64t
Cytotrophoblasts, in choriocarcinoma, 140, 140f

D

Dactinomycin. See also Chemotherapy
 for germ cell tumors, 373, 375
 for stromal tumors, 387, 388
Debulking. See Cytoreductive surgery
Demographic factors, 167, 168f, 168t, 182
Dendritic cells
 antitumor action of, 72, 72f, 73, 74, 78
 cytokine effects on, 83
Denver shunt
 for ascitic fluid, 338
 for pleural effusion, 340
Dermatomyositis, 103
Diagnosis. See also Screening and specific modalities
 histologic, problems in, 99–100
 intraoperative, accuracy of, 209t, 209–210
Diet, 169
Discrimination, genetic susceptibility testing and, 194
Disseminated intravascular coagulation, 103
DNA damage tolerance, in cisplatin resistance, 50–51, 52f
DNA mismatch repair genes, 6
 in cisplatin resistance, 51, 52f
 in hereditary nonpolyposis colorectal cancer syndrome, 15–16, 16f, 173, 184, 188–189
 in hereditary ovarian cancer, 173, 188–189
 mutations in, 188–189
  tests for, 192
 in sporadic ovarian cancer, 25
DNA ploidy, of borderline tumors, 402
DNA repair
 BRCA proteins in, 13–15, 185–186
 cisplatin resistance and, 50–51, 52f
 DNA mismatch repair system in, 51, 52f. See also DNA mismatch repair genes
 epithelial mutations and, 25
 nucleotide excision repair system and, 50–51
DNA vaccines, 79
DOC2, 37
Docetaxel, in salvage therapy, 306–307
Doppler ultrasonography, in risk of malignancy assessment, 220–221
Dose intensity, chemoresistance and, 269
Doxorubicin. See also Chemotherapy
 for advanced disease, 263
 for borderline tumors, 410
 intraperitoneal, 320–321
 for pseudomyxoma peritonei, 415

 response rates for, 44t
 in salvage therapy, 304, 304t, 306t, 307–308, 311
  with radiotherapy, 353
Drainage
 of ascitic fluid, 338
 of pleural effusion, 340
Dysgerminomas, 374 See also Germ cell tumors
 chemotherapy for
  late effects of, 378–379
  salvage, 378
 clinicopathology of, 372
 gonadoblastomas and, 146
 histopathology of, 135–136, 136f
 salvage therapy for, 378
 second-look laparotomy for, 376–377
 staging of, 372, 377–378
 surgery for, 372, 377–378
 treatment of, 372–374, 374t, 377–378
 tumor markers for, 221

E

E1A, in gene therapy, 70
Early-stage cancer
 chemotherapy for, 259–262. See also Chemotherapy
 definition of, 201
 first-line treatment for, 301
 incidence and frequency of, 202–203, 203t
 metastasis in, 211–212
  distant, 206
  retroperitoneal, 205–206
 patterns of spread of, 204–206
 prognostic factors in, 260
 second-look laparotomy in, 275
 surgery for, 201–214. See also Surgery
  abdominal exploration in, 211
  with chemotherapy, 259–262
  complications of, 213
  cytologic washings in, 208
  fertility preservation in, 210
  historical perspective on, 201–202
  incision in, 208
  vs. laparoscopy, 213–214, 215f
  organ removal in, 208–210
  pelvic examination for, 208
  preoperative considerations for, 206–208
  results of, 204, 210
  surgical approach in, 206
  tumor rupture in, 208–209
  with/without adjuvant therapy, 204
 survival in, 204
 treatment guidelines for, 352
Embryonal carcinoma, 374–375. See also Germ cell tumors
 histopathology of, 138–139
 serum markers in, 372t
Endodermal sinus tumors. See Yolk sac tumors
End-of-life issues, 425–429

Endometrial cancer
  in hereditary nonpolyposis colorectal cancer
      syndrome, 10, 10t
    screening for, 197–198
  with ovarian cancer, 115
Endometrial clear cell carcinoma, metastatic, 118
Endometrioid tumors, 112t, 112–115
  carcinoma, 113f, 113–114
    vs. adult granulosa cell tumor, 153
    vs. Sertoli-Leydig cell tumors, 158
  etiology of, 112
  histogenesis of, 112
  of low malignant potential, 112–113, 401
  proliferative, 112, 112f
  stromal, 116
Endosalpingosis, 107
  atypical, 126
Enzymes, in cytotoxic gene therapy, 63–67, 64t, 65f, 65t, 66f, 67t
Epidemiology, 167–168
Epidermal growth factor, 28–29, 30
  receptor for, 26t, 29–31, 30
Epirubicin. *See also* Chemotherapy
  for advanced disease, 263
Epithelial ovarian tumors
  Brenner, 119t, 119–120, 120f
    of broad ligament, 126
  classification of, 99, 100t
  clear cell, 116–119
  endocrine effects of, 102–103
  endometrioid, 112t, 112–115
  epithelial-stromal, 115–116
  etiology of, 101–102
  grading of, 100
  histogenesis of, 101–102
  histopathology of, 99–122
  metastasis in, 102
  mixed epithelial borderline, 121
  mixed epithelial carcinoma, 121
  mortality in, 102
  mucinous, 108–112
  paraneoplastic syndromes and, 103–104
  primary squamous carcinoma, 119t, 121
  serous, 104–108
  specimens from, 100–101
  transitional cell carcinoma, 119t, 120–121
  unclassified, 122
  undifferentiated carcinoma, 121–122
    vs. small cell carcinoma, 121–122
Epithelial paraovarian tumors, 125–126
Epithelial-stromal tumors, 115f, 115–116
*erb*B family, 30. *See also* HER-2/*neu*
Estrogen replacement therapy
  breast cancer risk and, 196–197
  after prophylactic oophorectomy, 196–197
  as risk factor, 171
Ethical issues
  in clinical trials, 421–422
  in genetic susceptibility testing, 194

Etiology, 168–173, 169t
Etoposide
  for germ cell tumors, 373–374, 374t, 378
  intraperitoneal, 322
    with cisplatin, 320, 322
  oral, in salvage therapy, 306t, 307, 311
  for stromal tumors, 387, 388
Euthanasia, 428–429

F

FACT-O scale, 423t, 423–425, 424t–425t
Familial cancer. *See* Hereditary cancer; Hereditary ovarian cancer
Family history, 190–191
Fasciitis, 103
Fas/FasL system, T cell apoptosis and, 82
Fat, dietary, 169
Fertility
  impaired, as risk factor, 170, 173–174
  preservation of, 210
    in germ cell tumors, 379
α-Fetoprotein
  in clear cell carcinoma, 119
  in germ cell tumors, 371, 372t
  in yolk sac tumors, 138
Fibromas, 389–390
  vs. adult granulosa cell tumor, 153
  cellular, 156
    vs. adult granulosa cell tumor, 153
  malignant, 156
Fibrosarcoma, 156
FIGO staging system, 202, 203t, 241, 242t
5-Floxuridine. *See also* Chemotherapy
  intraperitoneal, 322
5-Fluorouracil. *See also* Chemotherapy
  for borderline tumors, 410
  intraperitoneal, 322
  with leucovorin, in salvage therapy, 306t, 309–310
  for pseudomyxoma peritonei, 415
Follow-up. *See* Persistent/residual disease; Surveillance
Founder effect, 186
Frozen section analysis, accuracy of, 209t, 209–210
Functional Assessment of Cancer Therapy (FACT) scale, 423t, 423–425, 424t–425t

G

Ganciclovir-monophosphate, in cytotoxic gene therapy, 63–67, 64t
Gastric carcinoma, metastatic to ovary, 123–124, 124f
Gastrin-secreting cells, 103
Gastrostomy tube, in intestinal obstruction, 335
Gatekeeper genes, 186
Gemcitabine, in salvage therapy, 306t, 308–309, 311
Gene therapy, 57–70
  bystander effect in, 64, 65f, 69
  corrective, 57, 67–70, 68t

cytokines in, 84
cytotoxic (suicide), 57, 63–67, 64t, 65f, 65t, 66f, 67t
definition of, 57
immunopotentiating, 57
intraperitoneal, 67
neutralization, 69–70
replacement, 67–69
tumor suppressor genes in, 69
tumor vaccines and, 77
types of, 57
vectors in, 58t, 58–63
    adeno-associated viral, 58t, 60–61
    adenovirus, 58t, 58–60, 59f, 60f
    construction of, 58, 58t
    herpes simplex virus, 58t, 61f, 61–62
    liposomal, 62–63
    retroviral, 58t, 62
Genetic factors. *See* Molecular genetics
Genetic susceptibility testing, 189–194
    allele-specific oligonucleotide analysis in, 192–193
    for BRCA mutations, 191–192
    counseling for, 193
    discrimination and, 194
    ethical aspects of, 193, 194
    false-negative results in, 192, 193–194
    family history for, 190–191
    heteroduplex analysis in, 192
    indeterminate results in, 192–193, 194
    indications for, 189t, 189–190
    informed consent for, 193, 193t
    interpretation of results in, 192–193
    limitations of, 193–194
    for mismatch repair gene mutations, 192
    protein truncation assay in, 193
    psychologic aspects of, 193, 194
    risk assessment models for, 190
    risks and benefits of, 193–194
    single-strand conformation polymorphism analysis in, 192
    survivor guilt and, 193
Geographic distribution, 167, 168f, 168t, 182
Germ cell tumors, 371–380. *See also specific types*
    chemotherapy for, 373–374, 374t, 378
        late effects of, 378–379
        salvage, 378
    classification of, 135, 371
    clinicopathology of, 371–376
    histopathology of, 135–147
    mixed malignant, 145–147
    nondysgerminomatous, 374–376
    in pregnancy, 371
    presentation of, 371–376
    salvage therapy for, 378
    second-look laparotomy for, 376–377
    serum markers for, 221, 371–372, 372t
    staging of, 377–378
    surgery for, 372, 377–378
    treatment of, 372–374, 374t, 377–378

Gompertzian phenomenon, 244
Gonadoblastoma, 146, 146f
G proteins, 29t, 31
Grade/grading
    of epithelial tumors, 100
    prognosis and, 260, 278
    of serous carcinoma 107–108
Granulocyte-macrophage colony-stimulating factor, in immunotherapy, 84–85
Granulosa cell tumors, 151–155, 383–388
    adult, 151–154
        differential diagnosis of, 153–154
        histopathology of, 151–152, 152f, 153f
        prognosis of, 153–154
        vs. Sertoli-Leydig cell tumors, 158
    chemotherapy for, 387t, 387–388
    clinical features of, 383–384
    follow-up for, 387–388, 388t
    juvenile, 154–155, 388
        differential diagnosis of, 155
        histopathology of, 154f, 154–155
        vs. small cell carcinoma, 123
        vs. thecoma, 155
    luteinized, 152
    management of, 384–388
    prognostic factors for, 384–385
    recurrent, 388
    ruptured, 385–386, 386f
    serum markers for, 385
    staging of, 385
    vs. steroid cell tumors, 162
    surgery for, 385–386
Growth factors, 26t, 23–29
    receptors for, 26t, 29–31
Growth kinetics, 243f, 243–245, 244f
Gynandroblastoma, 392

H

Hammerhead ribozymes, in gene therapy, 69
Hand-foot syndrome, doxil and, 307, 311
Hematologic complications, 103
Hematologic toxicity
    of doxorubicin, 307
    of etoposide, 307
    of gemcitabine, 309
    of ifosfamide, 309
    of paclitaxel, 265, 266, 268
    of topotecan, 308
HER-2/*neu*, 29t, 30–31
    monoclonal antibody against, 70, 85–86
    overexpression of, gene therapy for, 70
    as tumor-specific antigen, 78
    in vaccine therapy, 78
Hereditary breast and ovarian cancer syndrome. *See* Breast and ovarian cancer syndrome
Hereditary cancer, 3–8, 171. *See also* Molecular genetics
    vs. sporadic cancer, 4, 4f
    two-hit model of, 5, 32, 185

Hereditary nonpolyposis colorectal cancer syndrome, 10, 10t, 183, 184
 Amsterdam criteria for, 190, 190t
 Bethesda criteria for, 190, 190t
 endometrial cancer in, 10, 10t
  screening for, 197–198
 founder mutations in, 189
 genetic susceptibility testing for, 189–194. See also Genetic susceptibility testing
 management options for, 197–198
 mismatch repair gene mutations in, 15–16, 16f, 173, 184, 188–189
  tests for, 192
 prophylactic surgery for, 198
 screening for, 197–198
Hereditary ovarian cancer, 8–16, 171–173, 181–199
 BRCA genes in, 9, 10t, 10–13, 12t, 171–173, 184–188. See also BRCA1/2
 in breast and ovarian cancer syndrome, 8–10, 9f, 10t, 11–13, 12t, 172, 181, 183–184
 clinicopathology of, 172–173
 definition of, 8
 epidemiology of, 181–182
 family history for, 190–191
 founder mutations in, 186–187
 genetic susceptibility testing for, 189–194. See also Genetic susceptibility testing
 in hereditary nonpolyposis colorectal cancer syndrome, 10, 10t, 15–16, 16f, 183, 184
 histopathology of, 184
 incidence and prevalence of, 8, 9f
 management options for, 194–198
 mismatch repair gene mutations in, 173, 188–189
 molecular genetics of, 3–16. See also Molecular genetics
 odds ratio for, 171, 172, 181
 pedigree analysis for, 183f
 prevention of
  oophorectomy for, 173, 195–196
  oral contraceptives for, 195
 relative risk of, 171, 172, 181
 risk assessment for, 189–194
 screening for, 177. See also Screening
 site-specific, 184
 surveillance for, 194–195
 syndromes of, 182–184
 two-hit model of, 5, 32, 185
Herpes simplex virus
 as oncolytic agent, 70–71, 71t
 thymidine kinase of, in cytotoxic gene therapy, 63–67, 64t, 67t, 77
Heteroduplex analysis, 192
Hexamethylmelamine, in salvage therapy, 310, 311
Histopathology. See also specific tumors
 diagnostic problems and, 99–100
 of epithelial tumors, 99–103, 100t
 methodology of, 100–101
 of mucinous tumors, 108–112, 109t
 of serous tumors, 104t, 104–108, 105f, 106f
 specimens for, 100–101
 tumor classification and, 99, 100t
History, family, 190–191
Hormonal factors, etiologic, 170–171
Hormone replacement therapy
 breast cancer risk and, 196–197
 after prophylactic oophorectomy, 196–197
 as risk factor, 171
Hormone secretion, from luteinized cells, 103, 103f
HRAS1, 9–10
HRAS1 variable number of tandem repeats, 188
Human chorionic gonadotropin, in germ cell tumors, 371, 372t
Hyperalimentation, in intestinal obstruction, 333–335
Hypercalcemia, 103
 in small cell carcinoma, 122–123, 153
Hypercortisolism, steroid cell tumors and, 160–161
Hysterectomy. See also Surgery
 for borderline tumors, 408, 410
 prophylactic, 198
 protective effect of, 171, 182

I
Ifosfamide, in salvage therapy, 306t, 309, 311
 for germ cell tumors, 378
Iliac lymph nodes, biopsy of, 211–212, 212f
Imaging techniques. See also specific techniques
 in malignancy risk assessment, 221
Immature teratoma, 140–141, 141f, 374
 management of, 375–376
Immune response
 antitumor, 72f, 72–74, 73t
  in cytotoxic gene therapy, 65, 65t, 66
  deficiencies in, 80
  mechanisms of, 72f
  viral potentiation of, 75
 cytokines in, 83
 in cytotoxic gene therapy, 65, 65t, 66
 suppression of, in cancer, 82
Immunotherapy, 72f, 72–87, 73t
 active, 72
 adoptive T-cell, 79–83
 clinical trials of, 72–73
 cytokines in, 83–85
 development of, 72–73
 intraperitoneal, 323
 intrapleural, 340
 monoclonal antibodies in, 85–87
 passive (adoptive), 72
 principles of, 72f, 72–74
 radioimmunoconjugates in, 87
 salvage, 281–282
 tumor vaccines in, 74–79. See also Tumor vaccines
 viral oncolysates in, 75–77, 77t
Immunotoxins, monoclonal antibodies and, 86

Incessant ovulation theory, 25, 35, 173–174, 182
Incidence, 167, 168t, 202–203
Incision, lower transverse abdominal, 208
Inclusion cysts, 101
Industrial exposures, 169–170
Infertility
 prevention of, 210
 in germ cell tumors, 379
 as risk factor, 170, 173–174
Informed consent, for genetic susceptibility testing, 193, 193t
Inhibin, in granulosa cell tumors, 385
Insulin-like growth factor-1, 29
Interferon(s), in immunotherapy, intraperitoneal administration of, 323
Interferons(s), in immunotherapy, 83–84
Interleukin-10, therapeutic use of, 75t
Interleukins, in immunotherapy, 83–84
Interval cytoreduction, 251–252, 252f, 273, 289–290. *See also* Cytoreductive surgery
 results of, 295–297, 296f, 296t, 297f
Intestinal obstruction
 etiology of, 330
 incidence of, 329–330
 intraperitoneal chemotherapy and, 318
 medical management of, 330–331, 337f
 palliative therapy for, 331–336, 337f
 radiation-induced, 363
 surgery for, 331–336
  algorithm for, 337f
  complications of, 335–336
  nutritional support and, 333–335
  patient selection for, 331, 333–335
  preoperative planning for, 335–336
  procedures in, 336
  results of, 331–333, 332t, 333t
  technique of, 336
  tumor status and, 333
Intracavitary chemotherapy. *See* Chemotherapy, intraperitoneal
Intracranial metastasis, radiotherapy for, 360
Intraperitoneal administration
 of biologic agents, 323
 of cytotoxic agents. *See* Chemotherapy, intraperitoneal
 of radiocolloids. *See* ^{32}P-chromic phosphate
Intraperitoneal dissemination, 205, 205f
Intravenous pyelography, for ureteral obstruction, 341
Iproplatin, in salvage therapy, 304

J
Jews, Ashkenazi, *BRCA* mutations in, 12, 12t, 186t, 186–188
 tests for, 191–192
Juvenile granulosa cell tumor, 388
 vs. small cell carcinoma, 123
 vs. thecoma, 155

K
Karnofsky scale, 423, 423t
Kinases, 29t, 31
 cyclin-dependent, 36f, 36–37
K-*ras*, 29t, 31
Krukenberg tumors, vs. Sertoli-Leydig cell tumors, 158

L
Lactate dehydrogenase, in germ cell tumors, 371–372
Lactic acid dehydrogenase, in ascitic fluid, 337
Laparoscopy, 219–236
 for advanced cancer, 232
 for borderline tumors, 221–222, 231–232
 in cyst aspiration, 221–222
 diagnostic, 219–221, 222t, 222–223
  guidelines for, 227–229, 228f
 for early-stage cancer, vs. surgery, 213–214, 215f
 guidelines for, 227–229, 228f
 immediate vs. delayed surgical staging after, 225–226
 for moderate-risk tumors, 222–229
 port site metastasis and, 215f, 233–235, 234f
 results of, 226t, 226–227
 second-look, 232–233, 282–284
 staging, 213–214, 215f, 229–231, 230t
 in tumor resection, 223–224, 227
 tumor spillage during, 224–225, 226
 tumor spread via, 226
Laparotomy. *See* Surgery
Lentiviral vectors, 62
Leucovorin, with 5-fluorouracil, in salvage therapy, 306t, 309–310
Leukemia
 ovarian presentation of, 125
 platinum-induced, 379–380
Leveen shunt, for ascitic fluid, 338
Leydig cells, 157f, 157–158
Leydig cell tumors, 394
Liposome vectors, 62–63
Living wills, 427
Loss of heterozygosity
 in tumors of low malignant potential, 402
 in tumor suppressor genes, 5, 6f, 23–24, 32
LOTI, 37
Lower transverse abdominal incision, 208
Low malignant potential tumors. *See* Tumors of low malignant potential
Lung cancer, p53 gene therapy for, 69
Luteinized granulosa cell tumor, 152
Lymphadenectomy. *See also* Staging
 laparoscopic, 213–214, 229–231
Lymph node biopsy, 211t, 211–212
 in second-look laparotomy, 277
Lymph node metastasis. *See also* Metastasis
 retroperitoneal, 205–206
Lymphocyst, postoperative, 213
Lymphocytes, T. *See* T cells
Lymphoma, ovarian presentation of, 125

Lynch syndrome II. *See* Hereditary nonpolyposis colorectal cancer syndrome

M

Macrophage colony-stimulating factor, 29
   in germ cell tumors, 372
Magnetic resonance imaging
   in malignancy risk assessment, 221
   for persistent disease, 276
Malignant melanoma
   antigen-based vaccines for, 77–78
   metastatic to ovary, vs. juvenile granulosa cell tumor, 155
Malignant mesodermal mixed tumors, 115f, 115–116
Malignant mixed germ cell tumors, 145–147
Malignant pleural effusions, 338–340
Malignant transformation. *See also* Tumorigenesis
   mechanisms of, 25–27
   oncogenes in, 26t, 27–32, 28f, 29t. *See also* Oncogenes
   tumor suppressor genes in, 32–37. *See also* Tumor suppressor genes
Mastectomy, prophylactic, 197
MDR1, in chemoresistance, 45
Meigs syndrome, 389
Melanoma
   antigen-based vaccines for, 77–78
   metastatic to ovary, vs. juvenile granulosa cell tumor, 155
Melphalan. *See also* Chemotherapy
   for borderline tumors, 409, 411
   for early-stage disease, 261
   intraperitoneal, 321
   for pseudomyxoma peritonei, 414
Metastasis
   in early-stage cancer, 205–206, 211t, 211–212, 212f
   histopathology of, 102
   from ovary
      to brain, 360
      distant, 206
      peritoneal carcinoma and, 196
      retroperitoneal, 205–206
   to ovary, 123–125
      from breast, 123–124
      from carcinoid tumors, 145
      from colorectal cancer, 123–124
      vs. endometrioid carcinoma, 115
      from melanoma, vs. juvenile granulosa cell tumor, 155
      from nonovarian clear cell carcinoma, 118
      from renal carcinoma, 118, 119f
   port site, 215f, 233–235, 234f
   umbilical, 102, 215f
Micrometastasis, peritoneal carcinoma and, 196
Microsatellite instability
   in hereditary nonpolyposis colorectal cancer, 15–16
   in tumors of low malignant potential, 402
Mismatch repair genes. *See* DNA mismatch repair genes
Mitomycin C, for pseudomyxoma peritonei, 415

Mitoxantrone
   intraperitoneal, 321
   in salvage therapy, 310
Mixed epithelial borderline tumors, 121
Mixed epithelial carcinoma, 121
Mixed germ cell-sex cord-stromal tumors, 145–146
Mixed germ cell tumors, 374
   serum markers in, 372t
MLH1, in hereditary nonpolyposis colorectal cancer, 15, 16f
Molecular genetics. *See also under* Genetics
   of hereditary ovarian cancer, 3–16
   historical perspective on, 3
   principles of, 4–8
   of sporadic ovarian cancer, 23–37
   tumorigenesis and, 7f, 7–8, 23, 24t
Monoclonal antibodies, 85–87
   in adoptive T-cell immunotherapy, 79
   anti-HER-2, 70, 85–86
   bispecific, 86
   production of, 85
   in radioimmunotherapy, 87
   specificity of, 86–87
   toxicity of, 86–87
Monodermal teratomas, 143–145, 144f
Mortality, mechanisms of, 102
Mortality rates, 167, 168f
MSH2, in hereditary nonpolyposis colorectal cancer, 15, 16f
MSH6, in hereditary nonpolyposis colorectal cancer, 15, 16f
Mucinous tumors, 108–112
   benign, 109
   carcinoid, 145
   carcinoma, 111, 111f
   classification of, 108–109, 109f
   cystadenoma, in appendix, 112
   etiology of, 109
   histogenesis of, 109
   histopathology of, 108–112, 109–112
   of low malignant potential, 109f, 109–110, 400
   mural nodules in, 110–111
   pseudomyxoma ovarii and peritonei, 111–112, 112f
Mucocele, appendiceal, in pseudomyxoma peritonei, 414
Müllerian mucinous papillary borderline tumors, 401
Mumps virus, 170
Mutations. *See also* Molecular genetics *and specific genes*
   founder, 186–187
   in proto-oncogenes, 5
   in tumor suppressor genes, 5, 6f
myc genes, 29t, 32
Myelosuppression. *See* Hematologic toxicity

N

Narcotic analgesics, 428
Natural killer cells, 73
NDV vaccine, 75–77, 76t, 76t

Nephrostomy, percutaneous, for ureteral obstruction, 341–342
neu, 29t, 30–31
Neuregulins, 30
Neuroectodermal tumors, 145. See also Germ cell tumors
Neurologic complications, 103
Neurotoxicity
  of ifosfamide, 309
  of paclitaxel, 265, 266, 267
Neutralization gene therapy, 69–70
Neutropenia. See Hematologic toxicity
Newcastle disease virus vaccine, 75–77, 76t
Nodal metastasis. See also Metastasis
  retroperitoneal, 205–206
Nodules
  mucinous, 110
  serosal, 100f
NOEY2, 37
Nondysgerminomatous germ cell tumors. See Germ cell tumors and specific types
Nongestational choriocarcinoma, 139–140
Non-Hodgkin's lymphoma, ovarian presentation of, 125
Normal-sized ovarian carcinoma syndrome, 126–127
Nuclear factors, 29t, 31–32
Nucleotide excision repair system, in cisplatin resistance, 50–51
Nulliparity, as risk factor, 170, 173–174, 182
Nutritional support, in intestinal obstruction, 333–335

O

Oligonucleotides, in gene therapy, 69
Ollier disease, 391
Oncogenes, 4, 5, 27–32
  activation of, 28
  classification of, 26t, 28f, 29t
  overexpression of, corrective gene therapy for, 67–70, 68t
  peptide growth factors as, 26t, 28–29
  translocation of, 28
Oncogenesis, genetic factors in, 4f, 4–8, 6f, 7f. See also Molecular genetics; Tumorigenesis
Oncolysate vaccines, 75–77, 77t
Oncolytic agents, 70–72, 71t
Oncoretroviral vectors, 62
ONYX-015, 71–72
Oophorectomy. See also Surgery
  for borderline tumors, 407–408, 410, 410t
  for early-stage cancer, incision in, 208
  historical perspective on, 201–202
  pelvic examination for, 208
  preoperative considerations in, 206
  prophylactic, 173, 195–197
    peritoneal involvement after, 205
  surgical approach in, 206–208
Opioid analgesics, 428
Oral contraceptives
  for fertility preservation, 379
  protective effect of, 25, 171, 173, 182, 195

Ovarian cancer. See also specific types
  advanced. See Advanced cancer
  direct extension of, 204
  early-stage. See Early-stage cancer
  epidemiology of, 167–168
  etiology of, 168–173, 169t
  hereditary. See Hereditary ovarian cancer
  histopathology of. See Histopathology
  incidence of, 167, 168t, 202–203
  intraperitoneal dissemination of, 205, 205f
  persistent. See Persistent/residual disease
  recurrent. See Recurrence
  retroperitoneal dissemination of, 205–206
  screening for. See Screening
  site-specific, 184
  sporadic. See Sporadic ovarian cancer
  spread of, 204–206. See also Metastasis
Ovarian cystectomy, for borderline tumors, 408
Ovarian suppression, for chemoprotection, 379
Ovarian vein blood, sampling of, 100, 103
Ovariotomy. See also Surgery
  historical perspective on, 201–202
Ovary, metastasis to. See Metastasis, to ovary
OVCA1/2, 37
Ovulation, cancer risk and, 25, 35, 173–174, 182

P

p16, 36–37
  in corrective gene therapy, 69
p21$^{Waf1/Cip1}$, in chemoresistance, 51
p27, 37
p53
  chemoresistance and, 35
  in corrective gene therapy, 68, 68t, 69
  functions of, 33–34, 36f
  loss of, 68, 72
  mutations in, 33–35, 34f, 35f, 68, 72
  oncolytic therapy and, 71–72
p170, in chemoresistance, 45–46, 46t
Paclitaxel, 265–269. See also Chemotherapy
  allergic reaction to, 267–268
  with cisplatin, 265–269
    vs. Carboplatin, 268–269
    concurrent vs. sequential administration of, 266–267
    in salvage therapy, 304t, 304–306, 305t
    as standard of care, 267
  clinical trials of, 265–269
  vs. cyclophosphamide, 265–266
  development of, 265
  dosage of, 267
  for early-stage disease, 269
  infusion of, duration of, 267–268
  intraperitoneal, 322–323. See also Chemotherapy, intraperitoneal
    as first-line therapy, 324
  mechanism of action of, 46–47
  with radiotherapy, 366–367

Paclitaxel (*continued*)
   resistance to, 45t, 45–47. *See also* Chemoresistance
   response rates for, 44t
   in salvage therapy, 266, 282, 304t, 304–307
      for platinum-resistant disease, 306–307
      for platinum-sensitive disease, 304t, 304–306, 305t
   in single-agent vs. combination therapy, 266–267
   toxicity of, 265, 266, 267, 268
Pain management, 428
Palliative care, 273, 329–342
   for ascites, 336–338
   for intestinal obstruction, 330–336, 337f. *See also* Intestinal obstruction
   pain management in, 428
   for pleural effusions, 338–340
   quality of life and, 427–428
   radiotherapy in, 359–360
Papillary tumors, peritoneal, 126–127
Papillomas, surface, of low malignant potential, 106, 106t
Paracentesis, for ascites, 338
Paraneoplastic syndromes, 103
Paraovarian epithelial tumors, 125–127
Parathyroid hormone-related peptide, 103
Parenteral nutrition, in intestinal obstruction, 333–335
Parity
   incidence and, 167, 170, 173–174, 182
   mortality and, 168, 168f
Pathogenesis, 173–174
Pathologic specimens, collection and preparation of, 100
Pathology. *See* Histopathology
Patient autonomy
   suicide and, 428–429
   treatment decisions and, 426, 427
Patient-physician relationship, 421
^{32}P-chromic phosphate, intraperitoneal
   administration of, 346t, 346–349
   vs. cisplatin, 261–262
   in consolidation/salvage therapy, 358–359
   for early-stage disease, 261, 346–349
   vs. melphalan, 261
   after negative second-look laparotomy, 280
   vs. phenylalanine mustard, 261
   randomized trials of, 347t, 347–349
Pedigree analysis, 183f
Pelvic examination
   intraoperative, 208
   in screening, 174, 195
   in surveillance, 174, 195
Penetrance, of *BRCA* genes, 187–188
Peptide growth factors, 26t, 28–29
Percutaneous nephrostomy, for ureteral obstruction, 341–342
Peritoneal carcinoma
   after prophylactic oophorectomy, 196
   serous papillary, 126–127

Peritoneal implants, of borderline serous tumors, 106–107
Peritoneal papillary tumors, 126
Peritoneovenous shunt, for ascitic fluid, 338
Persistent/residual disease, 248–249, 263, 289
   CA 125 normalization in, 275
   chemotherapy for, 281–282
      response to, 246t, 246–247, 247t
   chemotherapy response and, 246t, 246–247, 247t
   computed tomography for, 276
   culdocentesis cytology for, 276
   cytoreduction for, 274, 280–281, 289–298. *See also* Cytoreductive surgery, secondary
   cytoreductive surgery for, 273, 289–298. *See also* Cytoreductive surgery, secondary
   evaluation for, 275–276
   magnetic resonance imaging, 276
   predictors of, 278
   salvage therapy for. *See* Salvage therapy
   second-look laparotomy for, 273–284. *See also* Second-look laparotomy
   survival and, 247–251, 248f, 249f, 250t, 251t
Peutz-Jeghers syndrome, 171
   sex cord tumors with annular tubules in, 159–160, 160f, 393
P-glycoprotein, in chemoresistance, 45–46, 46t
Phenylalanine mustard. *See also* Chemotherapy
   for early-stage disease, 259, 260–261
Phosphatases
   as tumor suppressor proteins, 32–33
   tyrosine kinases and, 31
Phosphate, radioactive. *See* ^{32}P-chromic phosphate
Physician-assisted suicide, 428–429
Physician-patient relationship, 421
PIK3CA, 31, 33
Plantar-palmar erythrodysesthesia, doxorubicin and, 307, 311
Platelet-derived growth factor, 29
Platinum-based therapy. *See also* Carboplatin; Chemotherapy; Cisplatin
   for advanced cancer, 264
   for dysgerminomas, 375
   high-dose, 269
   for intestinal obstruction, 330–331
   intraperitoneal, 318–320, 319t
      as first-line therapy, 323–324, 324t
   leukemia induction by, 379–380
   with paclitaxel, 265–269
   resistance to, 303t. *See also* Chemoresistance
      salvage therapy and, 303–306, 304t, 305t, 311, 311t
   salvage, 303–306, 304t, 305t, 311, 311t
      with radiotherapy, 353–356
   sensitivity to, 303t
      salvage therapy and, 303–306, 304t, 305t, 310
   in single-agent vs. combination therapy, 264–265
Pleural effusions, 338–340
Ploidy, of borderline tumors, 402
Pneumoperitoneum, CO_2, tumor spread and, 226

Polyembryomas, 375. *See also* Germ cell tumors
  histopathology of, 139
  serum markers in, 372t
Polymer microspheres, for intraperitoneal drug delivery, 67
Port site metastasis, 215f, 233–235, 234f
Pregnancy
  borderline tumors in, 404
  protective effect of, 167, 170, 173–174, 182
Premalignant lesions, 101–102
Prodrugs, in cytotoxic gene therapy, 63–67, 64t, 65f, 65t, 66f, 67t
Prognostic factors, 278
  in early-stage disease, 260
Programmed cell death
  Fas/FasL system and, 82
  inhibition of, chemoresistance and, 51–52
  in malignant transformation, 26–27
Prophylactic colectomy, 198
Prophylactic hysterectomy, 198
Prophylactic mastectomy, 197
Prophylactic oophorectomy, 173, 195–197
  peritoneal involvement after, 205
Prostate cancer, in BRCA mutation carriers, 184, 188
Protein truncation assay
  for BRCA mutations, 192
  for mismatch repair gene mutations, 192
Proto-oncogenes, 5
Psammocarcinoma, 108
Pseudomyxoma ovarii, 111–112, 112f
Pseudomyxoma peritonei, 112, 112f, 412t, 412–415
Psychosocial concerns. *See also* Quality of life
  in genetic susceptibility testing, 193, 194
PTEN, 32–33

Q

Quality-adjusted life year, 422
Quality of life, 419–429
  assessment tools for, 422–425, 423t–425t
  clinical trials and, 421–422
  definition of, 419
  at end of life, 425–428
  initiation of therapy and, 420–421
  palliative care and, 427–428
  patient-physician relationship and, 421
  survival time and, 422
  treatment planning and, 420–421

R

Race, mortality and, 168
Radiation, as etiologic agent, 170
Radiation therapy, 345–367
  in advanced disease, 352–359
  advantages and disadvantages of, 282
  for borderline tumors, 408–409, 409t
  with chemotherapy, 353t, 353–356, 354t
  future directions in, 366
  toxicity of, 366
  in early-stage disease, 345–352
    patient selection for, 345–346
  future directions in, 366–367
  for granulosa cell tumor, 388
  with intraperitoneal ^{32}P, 346–349. *See also* ^{32}P-chromic phosphate
  palliative, 359–360
  patient selection for, 345–346
  for pseudomyxoma peritonei, 414
  results of, 204
  in salvage therapy, 282
  as sole vs. adjuvant therapy, 204
  whole-abdomen
    in advanced disease, 352–358, 353t
    in consolidation/salvage therapy, 353t, 353–358
    dosage for, 361–362
    in early-stage disease, 349–352
    pelvic boost in, 361, 365
    shielding in, 360f, 360–361, 361f
    technique of, 360–362
    toxicity of, 362–366
Radioimmunoconjugates, intrapleural, 340
Radioimmunotherapy, 87
ras, 29t, 31
RB1, as gatekeeper gene, 186
Rb gene, 36
RCAS1, 73
Reassessment laparotomy, 273
Recurrence
  after conservative surgery, 210
  after negative second-look laparotomy, 279–280
  palliative surgery for, 329–342. *See also* Palliative care
  residual disease and, 247–251, 248f, 249f, 250t, 251t
  risk factors for, 210
  second-look laparotomy for, 273–284. *See also* Second-look laparotomy
  treatment of, 301–312. *See also* Salvage therapy
Renal cell carcinoma, metastasis from, 118, 119f
Renal ultrasonography, for ureteral obstruction, 341
Reproductive factors, etiologic, 170–171, 182
Residual disease. *See* Persistent/residual disease
Restaging laparoscopy, 232–233, 282–284
  complications of, 233
  vs. laparotomy, 232–233, 283
Retinoblastoma tumor suppressor gene, 36, 186
Retroperitoneal metastasis, 205–206, 212, 213. *See also under* Lymph node
Retroviral vectors, 58t, 62
Risk assessment
  family history for, 190–191
  genetic testing in, 189–194. *See also* Genetic susceptibility testing
Risk factors, 168–171, 169t, 182, 182t
Risk of malignancy index, 220
Rokitansky's protuberance, 142, 142f
Rupture, tumor, intraoperative, 208–209, 224–225, 226

S

Salpingo-oophorectomy. *See also* Surgery
   for borderline tumors, 407–408, 410, 410t
Salvage therapy
   chemotherapy in, 281–282, 303–312. *See also*
      Chemotherapy, salvage
   cytoreductive surgery in, 273, 289–298. *See also*
      Cytoreductive surgery, secondary
   immunotherapy in, 281–282
   patient populations for, 302t, 302–303
   radiation therapy in, 282
Sarcoma, 123
   metastasis of, 102
Schiller-Duval bodies, in yolk sac tumor, 137, 137f, 374
Sclerosants, for pleural effusion, 340
Sclerosing stromal tumor, 390
Screening, 174–177
   algorithm for, 177f
   bimanual examination in, 174
   for BRCA mutation carriers, 194–195
   CA 125 in, 174–175
   clinical trial of, 177
   for colorectal cancer, in mutation carriers, 197–198
   cost-effectiveness of, 176
   for endometrial cancer, in mutation carriers, 197–198
   recommendations for, 176–177
   ultrasonography in, 175–176, 194–195
Second-line therapy. *See* Salvage therapy
Second-look laparoscopy, 232–233, 282–284
   complications of, 233
   vs. laparotomy, 232–233, 283
Second-look laparotomy, 204, 273–284
   benefits of, 273, 282
   for borderline tumors, 410–412
   complications of, 278
   cytoreductive. *See* Cytoreductive surgery, secondary
   definition of, 273
   disease evaluation prior to, 275–276
   in early-stage disease, 275
   for germ cell tumors, 376–377
   history of, 274–275
   indications for, 275–276, 284
   vs. laparoscopy, 232–233
   limitations of, 273, 274–275, 282
   negative findings at, 279–280
      chemotherapy after, 279–280
      intraperitoneal ^{32}P chromic phosphate after, 280
      recurrence after, 279–280
   patient selection for, 275–276, 284
   positive findings at, 278t, 278–279, 280–282
   predictive value of, 278–279
   results of, 274–275
   as standard of care, 273
   technique of, 276–277
   timing of, 277
Senescence, in malignant transformation, 27
Serosal nodules, 100f
Serous micropapillomatosis, 126

Serous ovarian tumors
   carcinoma, 107–108
   classification of, 104, 104t
   cystadenocarcinoma, 107, 108f
   cystadenoma, 104, 105f
   histopathology of, 104–108
   of low malignant potential, 104–107, 105f, 106f,
      400, 400f
   nodules in, 100f
   papillary projections of, 101f
Serous peritoneal tumors, 126–127
Sertoli cells, 157, 157f, 158, 158f
Sertoli cell tumors, 156
Sertoli-Leydig cell tumors, 156–159, 390–392
   classification of, 156
   clinical features of, 390–391
   differential diagnosis of, 158–159
   histopathology of, 156–158, 157f, 158f
   management of, 391–392
   presentation of, 156
   prognosis of, 159
Sertoli-stromal cell tumors, 156–159, 390–392
Sex cord-stromal tumors, 151–156, 383–388
   classification of, 152t
   clinical features of, 383–384
   granulosa cell, 151–155, 383–388. *See also* Granulosa
      cell tumors
   histopathology of, 151–160
   management of, 384–388
   Sertoli-stromal cell, 156–159, 390–392
   sex cord tumor with annular tubules, 159–160, 160f,
      392–393
   thecoma-fibroma type, 156, 389–390
   unclassified, 160, 393
Sex cord tumors with annular tubules, 159–160, 160f,
   392–393
Shunts
   for ascitic fluid, 338
   for pleural effusion, 340
Single-strand conformation polymorphism analysis,
   192
Site-specific ovarian cancer, 184
Skin lesions, 103
Small bowel obstruction, 329–336. *See also* Intestinal
   obstruction
   intraperitoneal chemotherapy and, 318
Small cell carcinoma, 122–123
   vs. adult granulosa cell tumor, 153
   vs. juvenile granulosa cell tumor, 155
SPARC, 37
Specimens, collection and preparation of, 100
Sporadic ovarian cancer
   apoptosis in, 26–27
   cell proliferation in, 26
   genetic alterations in, 23–37
      chromosomal gain and loss, 23
      clonality and, 24–25
      etiology of, 24t, 24–25

loss of heterozygosity, 23–24
mechanisms of, 25–27
tumor grade and, 24
tumor histology and, 23
senescence in, 27
Squamous carcinoma, 119t, 121
Staging
FIGO system for, 202, 203t, 241, 242t
laparoscopic, 213–214, 215f, 229–231, 230t
vs. surgical staging, 226–227, 229–231
surgical, 202. *See also* Surgery
abdominal exploration in, 211
accuracy of, 203–204, 207–208
of advanced cancer, 241–242
of borderline tumors, 213, 404–405, 405t
complications of, 213
criteria for, 202, 203t
cytologic washings in, 208
of dysgerminomas, 372, 377–378
of early-stage cancer, 202–214
frozen section analysis in, 209t, 209–210, 210f
of germ cell tumors, 372, 377–378
of granulosa cell tumors, 385
immediate vs. delayed, 225–226
vs. laparoscopic staging, 226–227, 229–231
lymph node sampling in, 211t, 211–212, 212f
procedures in, 207t
secondary, 273
of serous carcinoma, 108
visualization/palpation vs. pathologic findings in, 212–213
Stem cell transplantation, for high-dose chemotherapy, 269
Stents, ureteral, 341–342
Sterilization, surgical, protective effect of, 171, 182
Steroid cell tumors, 160–162, 393–395
classification of, 152t
differential diagnosis of, 162
histopathology of, 161f, 161–162
sTN-KLH vaccine, 78–79
Stomach cancer, metastatic to ovary, 123–124, 124f
Stromal luteinization, 103, 103f
Stromal luteoma, 393–394
Stromal tumors. *See also* Sex cord-stromal tumors
endometrioid, 116
management of, 383
sclerosing, 390
Struma ovarii, 143. *See also* Germ cell tumors
Suicide, 428–429
Suicide gene therapy, 63–67, 64t, 65f, 65t, 66f, 67t
Surface papillomas, of low malignant potential, 106, 106t
Surgery
for advanced cancer, 241–255. *See also* Cytoreductive surgery; Palliative care
diagnosis during, accuracy of, 209t, 209–210
for early-stage cancer, 201–214. *See also* Early-stage cancer, surgery for; Staging, surgical
laparoscopic, 219–236. *See also* Laparoscopy

prophylactic. *See under* Prophylactic
reassessment, 273
secondary, types of, 273
for staging. *See* Staging, surgical
Surveillance
for hereditary ovarian cancer, 194–195
for tumors of low malignant potential, 411–412
Survivor guilt, 193
Syncytiotrophoblastic giant cells
in choriocarcinoma, 139, 140f
in dysgerminoma, 135–136, 136f
in embryonal carcinoma, 139
in polyembryoma, 139

T
Talc
as etiologic agent, 169–170
for pleural effusion, 340
Tamoxifen, in salvage therapy, 306t, 310
Taxanes. *See also* Docetaxel; Paclitaxel
resistance to, 45–47. *See also* Chemoresistance
in salvage therapy, for platinum-resistant disease, 306t, 306–307
Taxol. *See* Paclitaxel
T cells
abnormalities of, in cancer, 82
activation of, 80–81
in adoptive immunotherapy, 79–83
antitumor action of, 72, 72f, 73–74
chemotherapy effects on, 82–83
costimulation of, 80–81, 86, 86t
cytokine effects on, 83
deficiency of, in ovarian cancer, 79t
Fas-mediated apoptosis of, 82
monoclonal antibodies and, 86
Telomerase, 27
Teratomas, 374. *See also* Germ cell tumors
classification of, 141
histopathology of, 140–143, 141f, 142f
immature, 140–141, 141f, 374
management of, 375–376
mature, 141–143, 142f
monodermal, 143–145, 144f
serum markers in, 372t
treatment of, 375
Tetracycline, intrapleural, 340
Thecomas, 389, 390
vs. adult granulosa cell tumors, 153, 389
vs. juvenile granulosa cell tumors, 155
malignant, 156
vs. steroid cell tumors, 162
Therapy. *See* Treatment
Thiotepa, intraperitoneal, 321
Thoracentesis, for pleural effusion, 340
Thoracostomy tube, for pleural effusion, 340
Thymidine kinase, of herpes simplex virus, in cytotoxic gene therapy, 63–67, 64t, 67t, 77

Topotecan. *See also* Chemotherapy
  response rates for, 44t
  in salvage therapy, 306t, 308, 311
Total parenteral nutrition, in intestinal obstruction, 333–335
TP53, in chemoresistance, 51
Transabdominal ultrasonography, in screening, 175. *See also* Ultrasonography
Transcription, *BRCA* proteins in, 13f, 13–14
Transforming growth factor-α, 28–29, 30
Transforming growth factor-β, 33
  therapeutic use of, 75t
Transgene/prodrug systems, in cytotoxic gene therapy, 63–67, 64t
Transitional cell carcinoma, 119t, 120–121
Transplantation, stem cell, for high-dose chemotherapy, 269
Transvaginal ultrasonography. *See also* Ultrasonography
  in screening, 175–177, 177f, 194–195
  in surveillance, 194–195
Trastuzumab, 70, 86
Treatment. *See also* Chemotherapy; Immunotherapy; Radiation therapy; Surgery
  withholding/withdrawal of, 426–429
Treatment planning, quality of life and, 420–421
Triplex-forming oligonucleotides, in gene therapy, 69
Tubal ligation, protective effect of, 171, 182
Tube feeding, in intestinal obstruction, 333–335
Tubulin, in paclitaxel resistance, 46–47
Tumor(s). *See also specific types*
  antigenicity of, 73
    cytokines and, 83
  immune response to, 72–74, 73t, 75, 80
  intraoperative rupture of, 208–209, 224–225, 226
  size of
    chemoresistance and, 245
    optimal vs. suboptimal, 248–249, 263, 289
Tumor-associated antigens, 76t
Tumor debulking. *See* Cytoreductive surgery
Tumor growth, kinetics of, 243f, 243–245, 244f
Tumorigenesis. *See also* Malignant transformation
  molecular genetics and, 7f, 7–8, 23, 24t
  two-hit model of, 5, 32, 185
Tumor markers. *See also specific types*
  for germ cell tumors, 221, 371–372, 372t
  in malignancy risk assessment, 221
Tumor necrosis factor, intraperitoneal, 323
Tumors of low malignant potential, 399–415
  Brenner, 120
  clear cell, 117
  diagnosis of, 401–402
  early-stage
    proportion of, 404–405, 405t
    treatment of, 407–409, 408t–410t
  endometrioid, 112–113, 401
  epidemiology of, 402–404
  historical perspective on, 399
  incidence of, 402–403
  laparoscopic management of, 221–222, 231–232
  loss of heterozygosity in, 402
  metastatic, 406–407
  microcystic, 400
  microinvasive, 400, 401
  microsatellite instability in, 402
  mixed epithelial, 121
  mucinous, 109f, 109–110, 400
  oncogene expression in, 402
  pathology of, 399–402, 400f
  patterns of spread of, 404–407
  peritoneal serous papillary, 126
  ploidy of, 402
  in pregnancy, 404
  pseudomyxoma peritonei and, 414
  recurrence of, 411–412, 412t
  second-look laparotomy for, 410–412
  serous, 400, 400f
    histopathology of, 104–107, 105f, 106f
  serum markers in, 407
  size of, 405
  staging of, 213, 404–405, 405t
  surveillance of, 411–412
  symptoms of, 404–405
  terminology for, 399
  treatment of, 407–412
    in advanced disease, 409–412
    in early-stage disease, 407–409
  tumor suppressor genes in, 402
Tumor-specific antigens, 77
Tumor spillage, 208–209
  during laparoscopy, 224–225, 226
Tumor suppressor genes, 4, 5–7, 6f, 32–37
  BRCA genes as, 35–36, 185
  classification of, 26
  in corrective gene therapy, 69
  extranuclear, 32–33
  inactivation of, 5, 6f, 23–24, 32
  loss of heterozygosity in, 5, 6f, 23–24, 32
  mutations in, 32
  p53 as, 33f, 33–35, 34f
  retinoblastoma, 36
  transforming growth factor-β as, 33
  two-hit model and, 5, 32, 185
Tumor vaccines, 74–83
  in adoptive T-cell immunotherapy, 80
  antigen-based, 77–79, 76t, 79t
  cytokine, 84
  design and application of, 74
  oncolysate, 75–77, 77t
  preparation of, 76t
  preventive, 74
  T-cell costimulation and, 80
  therapeutic, 74
  whole-cell, 74–77, 75t–77t
Two-hit model, 5, 32, 185
Tyrosine kinases, 29t, 31

U

Ultrasonography
　in malignancy risk assessment, 219–221
　in screening, 175–176, 194–195
　in surveillance, 194–195
　in ureteral obstruction, 341
Umbilical metastasis, 102
　port site, 215f, 233–235, 234t
Undifferentiated carcinoma, 121–122
　vs. juvenile granulosa cell tumor, 155
　vs. small cell carcinoma, 123
Ureteral obstruction, 340–342
Uterine cancer. See Endometrial cancer

V

Vaccines, tumor, 74–83. See also Tumor vaccines
Vectors
　liposome, 62–63
　viral, 58t, 58–62
　　adeno-associated, 58t, 60–61
　　adenoviral, 58t, 58–60, 59f, 60f
　　construction of, 58, 58t
　　herpes simplex, 58t, 61f, 61–62
　　retroviral, 58t, 62
Vinblastine, for germ cell tumors, 373, 375
　in salvage therapy, 378
Vincristine, for stromal tumors, 387, 388
Vinorelbine, in salvage therapy, 306t, 309, 311
Viral oncolysates, tumor vaccines and, 75–77

Viral vectors. See Vectors, viral
Virilization
　differential diagnosis of, 391
　Sertoli-Leydig cell tumors and, 156, 390–391
Viruses
　oncogenic, 170
　as oncolytic agents, 70–72, 71t
　for tumor vaccines, 75–76, 75–77, 75t, 78t. See also Tumor vaccines
　as vectors. See Vectors, viral
Vision loss, 103
Vitamin A, protective effect of, 169
VP-16. See Etoposide

W

Whole-cell tumor vaccines, 74–77, 75t–77t

Y

Yolk sac tumors, 136, 374. See also Germ cell tumors
　histopathology of, 136–138, 137f
　vs. juvenile granulosa cell tumors, 155
　vs. Sertoli-Leydig cell tumors, 159
　serum markers in, 372t
　treatment of, 375

Z

Zollinger-Ellison syndrome, 103